WITHDRAWN

SCSU
H.C. BULEY LIBRARY
MAR 1 2 1991
New Haven, CT 06515

Biological Effects and Health Implications of Radiofrequency Radiation

Biological Effects and Health Implications of Radiofrequency Radiation

Sol M. Michaelson
University of Rochester School of Medicine and Dentistry
Rochester, New York

and

James C. Lin
University of Illinois
Chicago, Illinois

Plenum Press • New York and London

Library of Congress Cataloging in Publication Data

Michaelson, Sol M.
Biological effects and health implications of radiofrequency radiation.

Includes bibliographies and index.
1. Radio waves—Physiological effect. I. Lin, James C. II. Title. [DNLM: 1. Radio Waves—adverse effects. WD 605 M621b]
QP82.2.R33M53   1987   612′.014481   86-30589
ISBN 0-306-41580-1

QP
82.2
.R33
M53
1987

© 1987 Plenum Press, New York
A Division of Plenum Publishing Corporation
233 Spring Street, New York, N.Y. 10013

All rights reserved

No part of this book may be reproduced, stored in a retrieval system, or transmitted in any form or by any means, electronic, mechanical, photocopying, microfilming, recording, or otherwise, without written permission from the Publisher

Printed in the United States of America

Preface

The study of electromagnetic bioeffects is multidisciplinary; it draws heavily from the disciplines of physics, engineering, mathematics, biology, chemistry, medicine, and environmental health. This book is about these disciplines and how they mutually integrate in the study of electromagnetic pathophysiology.

Over a period of years, the authors have become increasingly aware of the difficulty in locating information concerning interaction of electromagnetic energy and biological tissues. There are numerous reports and publications, but no single comprehensive source in the American literature where such information is readily accessible. Regrettably, much of the important information is contained in government documents and reports, some of which are inaccessible, or spread through many diverse journals, making retrieval and analysis of the material difficult.

Although this book is primarily clinically oriented, it also focuses on those biophysical, biochemical, and fundamental molecular studies and findings that provide the basis for understanding the presence or absence of pathophysiological manifestations of exposure to radiofrequency, including microwave, energies. Detailed discussion and analysis of the relevant comprehensive physics, engineering, and biophysics are contained in Chapters 2-5.

Because the treatment is multidisciplinary, wherever possible analysis is begun with basic background information that may appear elementary to some readers but is essential to understanding for those from a different discipline. Most confusion and controversies that exist in the field today arise from individuals of one discipline not appreciating basic facts or theories from another.

One purpose of this book, therefore, is to review the literature on radiofrequency bioeffects and to list pertinent references. The authors do not wish to inflict personal views on the reader. The extensive reference lists are presented to overcome potential misunderstanding. They are provided as a stimulus for further literature research by the reader to permit the formation of individual opinions from a knowledgeable base. Direct quotations from the appropriate literature are used to provide greater accuracy and to put the material in proper perspective. This also obviates the possibility of misinterpretation or bias, which has become so prevalent in this field.

Although the authors have endeavored to maintain scientific objectivity, they are acutely aware that their own judgments will dominate the presentation. In this controversial field, it could be no other way; nor should it be. The authors make no apologies for their own opinions or judgments, for it is felt that the latter are the result of careful evaluation of the problem.

It is with gratitude and love that the authors thank their families for their patience and forbearance during the many years it took to write this book. The many graduate students who read and critiqued many of the chapters as they were being prepared are also acknowledged with gratitude.

Sol M. Michaelson
James C. Lin

Contents

1. HISTORICAL PERSPECTIVE 1
2. PHYSICAL DESCRIPTION OF RADIO AND
   MICROWAVE RADIATION 11
   2.1. Fundamentals of Wave Propagation 11
        2.1.1. Maxwell's Equations 12
        2.1.2. Boundary Conditions 14
        2.1.3. Wave Equations 16
        2.1.4. Energy Storage and Power Flow 16
        2.1.5. Plane Waves 17
        2.1.6. Polarization of Plane Waves 18
   2.2. Propagation of Plane Waves 19
        2.2.1. Plane Waves in Free Space 19
        2.2.2. Plane Waves in Lossy Media 20
        2.2.3. Reflection and Transmission at Interfaces 23
        2.2.4. Refraction of Electromagnetic Waves 26
   2.3. Waves in Enclosed Space 28
        2.3.1. Waveguides 28
        2.3.2. Cavities 32
        2.3.3. Waveguide and Cavity Excitation 35
   2.4. Radiation of Electromagnetic Energy 36
        2.4.1. The Short Dipole 37
        2.4.2. Near Fields 39
        2.4.3. Receiving Characteristics 43
   References 45

3. RADIO AND MICROWAVE DOSIMETRY AND
   MEASUREMENT 47
   3.1. Quantities and Units 47
   3.2. Irradiation of Biological Systems 48
        3.2.1. Applicators for Partial-Body Irradiation 48
        3.2.2. TEM Chambers 52
        3.2.3. Microstrip Exposure Systems 55

	3.2.4.	Waveguide Chambers	56
	3.2.5.	Multimode Cavity	62
	3.2.6.	Anechoic Chambers	63
3.3.	Field Measuring Methods		66
	3.3.1.	Isotropic Instruments	66
	3.3.2.	Other Instruments	73
3.4.	Absorption Measuring Methods		74
	3.4.1.	Whole-Body Absorption	75
	3.4.2.	Distribution of Absorbed Energy—Probe Measurements	79
	3.4.3.	Distribution of Absorbed Energy—Thermographic Measurements	84
References			88

4. RADIO AND MICROWAVE DIELECTRIC PROPERTIES OF BIOLOGICAL MATERIALS ... 93

4.1.	Introduction		93
4.2.	Relaxation Mechanism		95
	4.2.1.	Low-Loss Dielectric Materials	97
	4.2.2.	Lossy Dielectrics at Low Frequencies	98
	4.2.3.	Biological Materials	102
4.3.	Temperature Dependence of Dielectric Properties		102
4.4.	Methods of Permittivity Measurement		103
	4.4.1.	Radiofrequency Techniques	104
	4.4.2.	Microwave Techniques	111
4.5.	Permittivity of Water		117
4.6.	Dielectric Properties of Biological Materials		120
4.7.	Dielectric Properties of Tumor Tissue		132
References			134

5. PROPAGATION AND ABSORPTION IN TISSUE MEDIA ... 137

5.1.	Planar Tissue Geometries		138
	5.1.1.	Reflection and Transmission	138
	5.1.2.	Multiple Layers of Tissue	141
5.2.	Bodies of Revolution		146
	5.2.1.	Spherical Tissue Models	146
	5.2.2.	Prolate Spheroidal Tissue Models	160
5.3.	Complex Tissue Models		171
	5.3.1.	Computational Schemes	171
	5.3.2.	Models of the Human Body	177
5.4.	Scaled Dielectric Bodies		195
	5.4.1.	Thermographic Measurements	196
	5.4.2.	Probe Measurements	202

CONTENTS

    5.5. Laboratory Animal Models 204
        5.5.1. Whole-Body Absorption 204
        5.5.2. Distribution of Absorbed Energy 211
    References 218

6. CRITERIA FOR EVALUATION OF BIOLOGICAL LITERATURE 223
    6.1. Principles of Animal Experimentation 223
    6.2. Analysis of Scientific Literature 225
    6.3. The Nature of Causality 228
    6.4. Scaling 230
    References 238

7. MOLECULAR, CELLULAR, INVERTEBRATE BIOLOGY 241
    7.1. Macromolecules 241
    7.2. Cell Membranes 244
    7.3. Mitochondria 244
    7.4. Effects on Microogranisms 245
        7.4.1. Bacteria, Viruses, and Fungi 245
        7.4.2. Mechanisms of Microbial Action 250
    7.5. Effects on Protozoa and Other Unicellular Organisms ... 256
    7.6. Chromosome–Genetic Effects 258
    7.7. Hyperthermia and Cell Kinetics 269
    7.8. Effects on Invertebrates 272
        7.8.1. Genetic Effects 273
        7.8.2. Specific Effects: Insect Control 275
    References 277

8. REPRODUCTION, DEVELOPMENT, AND GROWTH ... 287
    8.1. Reproduction 287
    8.2. Embryonic Development 294
    References 310

9. THERMOREGULATION 317
    9.1. Physiologic Regulation 319
    9.2. Thermoregulation 321
    9.3. The Physiology of Thermoregulation 327
    9.4. Adaptation 339
    9.5. Thermal Stress 339
    9.6. Response to Absorbed RF Energy 342
    9.7. Acute Lethality 344
    9.8. Response to Local Exposure to MW/RF Energies 348
    9.9. Comparison of Exposure to Microwaves and Infrared ... 349

9.10. Therapeutic Application of RF/MW Energies
(Diathermy) 349
9.11. Summary 352
References 354

10. NEURAL EFFECTS OF MICROWAVE/RADIOFREQUENCY ENERGIES 361
10.1. Anatomy and Physiology of the Nervous System 361
10.2. Fundamentals of Electromagnetic Energy–Neural Tissue Interaction 366
10.3. *In Vitro* Studies 370
10.4. Effects in Experimental Animals 376
    10.4.1. Electroencephalographic Changes 377
    10.4.2. Biochemical Changes 379
    10.4.3. Histopathology 384
    10.4.4. Influence of Drugs 387
10.5. Effects on the Blood–Brain Barrier 389
10.6. Observations in the Human 395
10.7. The Soviet Approach to Biology and Medicine 399
References 402

11. BEHAVIORAL EFFECTS 413

12. NEUROENDOCRINE EFFECTS 425
12.1. Introduction to Neuroendocrine Physiology 425
12.2. Neuroendocrine and Endocrine Effects 430
12.3. Hypothalamic–Hypophysial–Adrenal Response 430
12.4. Hypothalamic–Hypophysial–Thyroidal Response 434
12.5. Growth Hormone 437
12.6. Neuroendocrine/Metabolic Correlations 438
12.7. Neuroendocrine Activity and Cardiovascular Function . 439
12.8. Localized Exposures 439
12.9. Conclusion 441
References 445

13. CARDIOVASCULAR EFFECTS 451
13.1. Animal Experiments 451
    13.1.1. *In Vitro* Preparations 451
    13.1.2. Whole-Body or Regional Exposure 452
    13.1.3. Atherosclerosis 459
    13.1.4. Pharmacodynamics 459
    13.1.5. Conclusion 459
13.2. Reported Observations in the Human 460

	13.3.	Implanted Electronic Cardiac Pacemaker Interference .	472
		13.3.1. Normal Cardiac Function	472
		13.3.2. The Electronic Cardiac Pacemaker	473
		13.3.3. Pacemaker Interference	473
		13.3.4. Clinical Reports	475
		13.3.5. Laboratory Tests	478
		13.3.6. Control of Potential Hazards	481
	References	484

14. EFFECTS ON HEMATOPOIESIS AND HEMATOLOGY . 489
14.1. *In Vitro* Studies 489
14.2. Animal Experiments 492
14.3. Reported Observations in the Human 505
References 508

15. EFFECTS ON IMMUNE RESPONSES 513

16. BIOCHEMICAL EFFECTS 523
16.1. Enzyme Activity 525
16.2. Metabolism 527
    16.2.1. Carbohydrate and Lipid Metabolism 527
    16.2.2. Protein Metabolism 529
16.3. Histamine Release 530
16.4. Clinical Chemistry, Serum Proteins, Electrolytes 531
References 534

17. THE COMMON INTEGUMENT (SKIN) 539
17.1. Anatomy and Physiology 539
17.2. Thermal Perception 542
17.3. Pain Perception 546
17.4. Biochemistry 549
17.5. Pathology (Burns) 550
References 555

18. CATARACTS AND OTHER OCULAR EFFECTS 559
18.1. Introduction 559
18.2. Anatomy and Physiology of the Eye 559
    18.2.1. Definition of Cataract 563
    18.2.2. Classification and Appearance 565
    18.2.3. Age Factors 566
    18.2.4. Mechanisms of Opacification 568
    18.2.5. Incidence of Cataract 568
    18.2.6. Etiology of Cataract 570

	18.3.	Spectral Transmission of the Ocular Media	574
	18.4.	Radiation Cataracts	575
	18.5.	Effects of Microwaves on the Ocular Lens	579
		18.5.1. Animal Experiments	579
		18.5.2. Biochemical Changes	585
		18.5.3. Frequency Specificity	586
		18.5.4. Modulation Effects	587
		18.5.5. Far-Field Exposures	587
	18.6.	Thermal Aspects of Microwave Cataractogenesis	589
	18.7.	Concept of Threshold and Cumulative Effect	592
	18.8.	Problems in Simulation Studies and Extrapolation to the Human	595
	References		597

19. EPIDEMIOLOGICAL AND OTHER INVESTIGATIONS IN THE HUMAN ... 603

- 19.1. Nervous System and Cardiovascular Effects ... 609
- 19.2. Ocular Effects ... 611
- 19.3. Fertility and Sterility ... 623
- 19.4. Growth and Development ... 624
- 19.5. Cancer ... 626
- 19.6. Critique of Epidemiological Studies ... 626
- References ... 631

20. PERSONNEL PROTECTION, PROTECTION GUIDES, AND STANDARDS ... 637

- 20.1. Protective Clothing and Eye Shields ... 637
- 20.2. Personal Monitors ... 637
- 20.3. Ancillary Hazards Associated with Electromagnetic Interference ... 637
- 20.4. Exposure Standards ... 638
  - 20.4.1. Occupational Standard (USA) ... 640
  - 20.4.2. Product Emission Standard ... 640
  - 20.4.3. American National Standards Institute (ANSI) ... 642
  - 20.4.4. Standards in Various Countries ... 644
  - 20.4.5. Criteria for Setting Tolerance Levels and Exposure Standards ... 647
- References ... 656

21. PROBLEMS AND RECOMMENDATIONS ... 659

INDEX ... 663

1

Historical Perspective

Life on earth has developed in a natural radiation environment. Man is continually exposed to electromagnetic radiation from the sun, to radioactivity inside and outside the body, and to cosmic rays. Within our planetary system the sun is the largest source of natural radiant energy.

Ordinarily, man exists in equilibrium within very narrow ranges of physical influences of the earth such as temperature, pressure, electromagnetic radiant energies, and geomagnetic fields. Harmful as well as beneficial effects of these physical forces on man, animals, and vegetation have been known for thousands of years.

Beginning in the 1940s, man's hopes and aspirations for better or for worse came under the direct influence of the nuclear age. This challenge to man's potential has been rightfully dramatized so that today people in all walks of life are fairly cognizant of the benefits and dangers attending the exploration and development of nuclear energy. During this same period, there has been a parallel but less sensational development in the generation and utilization of nonionizing electromagnetic energy. Especially in recent years, there has been increased utilization of equipment and devices that emit various nonionizing electromagnetic energies for communications, military, industrial, entertainment, consumer use, and medical applications. Thus, all sectors of society, including a large portion of our economy, are in one way or another affected by various segments of the nonionizing electromagnetic spectrum.

Strictly speaking, the electromagnetic spectrum comprises all energy that may be propagated electromagnetically in space, and hence includes low-frequency 50- and 60-Hz electric and magnetic energies used for power line transmission, radiofrequencies (including microwaves), infrared through visible light to ultraviolet, X rays, and gamma rays. For theoretical and practical convenience, the spectrum is subdivided into two spectra according to whether or not the radiation involved is of a wavelength shorter than or longer than that required to produce ionization. Radiation at wavelengths shorter than this ionization wavelength are in the ionizing spectrum; those longer are in the nonionizing radiation spectrum, as shown in Fig. 1-1. For practical purposes, the

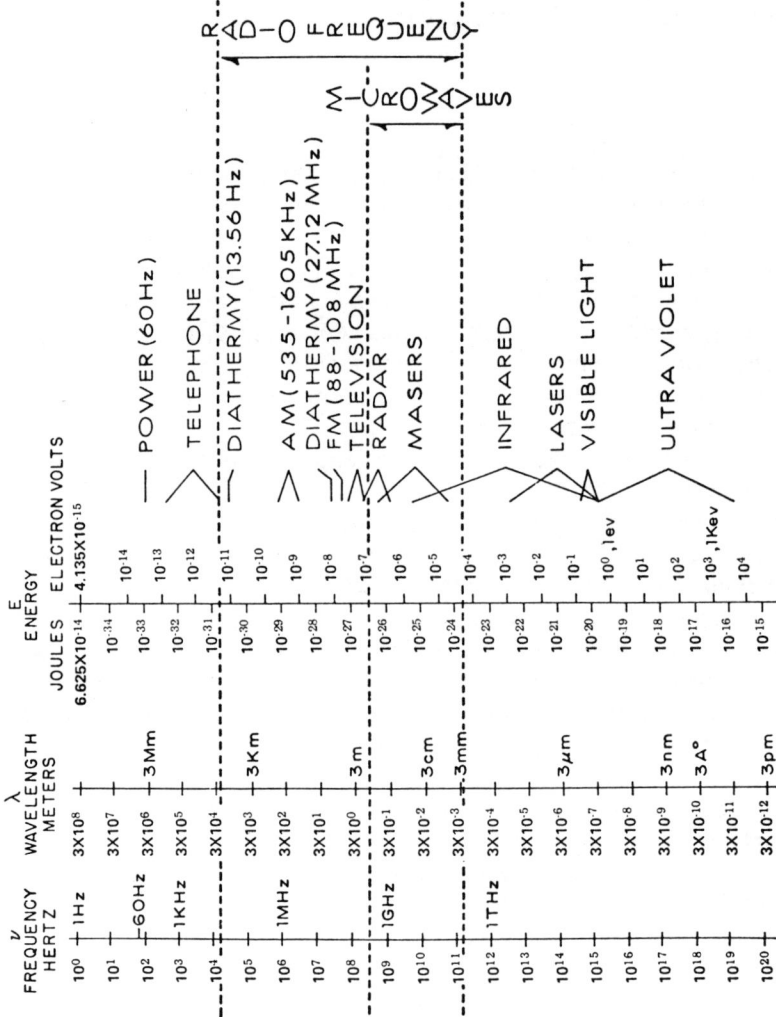

FIGURE 1-1. Nonionizing electromagnetic radiation. Adapted from Air Force Manual AFM 161-8, 1969.

nonionizing spectrum is further subdivided into three spectra, historically termed optical, radiofrequency, and electrical, because they were once thought to be separate entities. Although they coalesce as shown in Fig. 1-1, these spectra are technologically different.

The electrical spectrum is that in which energy is usually transmitted along wires or cables. By far the greatest part of the man-made electromagnetic energy is in this spectrum, as 25-, 50-, and 60-Hz electric power generation, transmission, and utilization. The electrical spectrum also covers the bulk of electronic devices, from control mechanisms to audio amplifiers. Its upper limit is traditionally a bit above the upper limit of human hearing, or about 20 kHz. Frequencies in this spectrum may, of course, radiate and hence propagate in space as do higher-frequency electromagnetic waves.

The radiofrequency spectrum includes frequencies both below and above those of traditional radio, in which energy usually is caused to travel in space and is generated, directed, contained, detected, or utilized by electric or electronic means. It is considered to extend from 10 kHz [very low frequency (VLF)] to 300,000 MHz [extremely high frequency (EHF)]. On an operational basis, frequencies in the range from 100 to 300,000 MHz (300 GHz) are designated as microwaves.

The optical spectrum is that in which energy traditionally is associated with light or its neighboring radiations in the spectrum and is generated, focused, contained, detected, and utilized by optical means. Radiofrequency techniques have invaded the optical spectrum as light-emitting diodes and as lasers (acronym for light amplification by stimulated emission of radiation). But as even these devices rely mostly on optical techniques for their effective utilization, they still belong in the optical spectrum.

This book is concerned with the biological effects of electromagnetic radiation in the radiofrequency part of the nonionizing spectrum. By their very nature, the biological effects of ionizing radiation are a completely different subject. The biological effects of optical radiation are also a separate subject, although some workers in bioeffects have erroneously discussed lasers along with radiofrequency devices and have thus contributed to the confusion of the biological effects involved.

Interest in the biological effects of "high-frequency" currents goes back to the work of D'Arsonval (1893) who, at the end of the 19th century, reported physiological effects from a device capable of delivering a frequency of several hundred thousand oscillations per second. This was followed by the introduction of "ultrashortwave" therapy in the early part of the 20th century (Schereschewsky, 1926). Through the 1930s and 1940s, the development and therapeutic applications of radiofrequency energy were further stimulated by the work and writing of Schliephake

(1935), Liebesny (1935, 1938), Rajewsky (1938), Schaefer and Schwan (1943, 1947), and Pätzold and Schaefer (1948).

Some of the early investigators of the electrical properties of biological tissues made numerous contributions that are essential for understanding the interaction of microwave and radiofrequency fields with biological tissues. For original reviews of the electrical properties of tissues, the publications by Schwan (1957a,b, 1958a,b, 1975) should be consulted. It is of interest, nevertheless, to mention some of the highlights during this period. By the early 1910s, Höber (1912, 1913) had determined the resistivity inside erythrocytes using high-frequency current and proposed the membrane theory. During primarily the 1930s and 1940s, the principles of biological impedance were formulated in classic papers by Cole (1928), Cole and Cole (1941, 1942), Cole and Curtis (1936, 1941, 1960), Curtis and Cole (1938), Fricke (1933), Fricke and Curtis (1934), Fricke et al. (1956), Hodgkin (1947), and Schwan and Cole (1960). These principles led to the formulation of the Hodgkin–Huxley equations (1952) and modern membrane biophysics and electrophysiology came into being.

During this period, extensive work on tissue properties was also carried out in the laboratories of Rajewsky (1938), and by Osswald (1937), Schaefer and Schwan (1943), and Pätzold and Schaefer (1948). Schwan (1948, 1953) continued this work immediately after World War II by measuring blood properties and used these data to calculate depth-of-penetration values in anticipation of increasing interest in the use of microwaves (Schwan and Piersol, 1954, 1955). Another important contribution during the late 1930s and early 1940s was the classic work of Oncley (1942, 1943) on proteins, which provided a major step in our understanding of the effects of electrical fields on biopolymers. This work was continued to the early 1960s through many other investigators, including Takashima (1962) with his work on nucleic acids.

During World War II, the magnetron, an efficient high-power source of microwave energy, was developed for and extensively used in military radar transmitters. During the latter part of the war, the U.S. military services became aware of and interested in the possible hazards to personnel associated with the employment of electronic equipment emitting microwaves. The average power output generated by early military electronic equipment was low and was not considered a serious hazard. However, later development of radars with peak powers in the megawatt region, and communications equipment with effective radiated power of several megawatts, necessitated reevaluation of the exposure hazard problem. Thus, World War II can be considered as the time at which the study of the bioeffects of unintentional exposure to man-made nonionizing electromagnetic radiation started. As the wartime radars operated at microwave frequencies, the initial and still dominant bioeffects work is concerned with the microwave spectrum. The wartime investigations of the bioeffects of radiating sources were hampered by the lack of sophisticated testing equipment, which only recently has become available and is continually being improved.

Shortly after the war, the Mayo Clinic became a major center of microwave bioeffects studies primarily for diathermy applications under Krusen *et al.* (1947), Krusen (1950, 1951), Herrick and Krusen (1953), Herrick (1958) as well as Wakim *et al.* (1948a,b) and Worden *et al.* (1948). This activity culminated in a symposium organized by Herrick in 1955, the proceedings of which provided the background for future studies in the United States (Herrick and Krusen, 1956).

In 1948 the U.S. Office of Naval Research (ONR) initiated research on the biological effects of microwaves (Anne, 1963; Ely and Goldman, 1959; Imig *et al.*, 1948; McAfee, 1959; Richardson, 1958; Richardson *et al.*, 1948; Schwan, 1955, 1957a,b, 1958a,b, 1964, 1970; Schwan and Li, 1956; Schwan and Sher, 1967).

In 1953, ONR organized a conference to discuss tolerance levels for exposure to microwaves. H. P. Schwan submitted a memo to ONR suggesting 10 mW/cm^2 as an appropriate guide number or standard for microwave exposure of humans. The acceptability and implications of this guide number will be discussed in subsequent chapters.

Another milestone was reached in 1956 when the U.S. Department of Defense assigned to the Air Force the responsibility of Tri-Service coordination to assess the biological effects and potential hazards of microwave exposure and to initiate research in this area of interest. Thus, the "Tri-Service Program" was initiated (Michaelson, 1971).

At the time the Tri-Service Program was organized, a review of existing information on microwave bioeffects indicated:

1. Microwave radiation injury had been qualitatively demonstrated in animals but had not been observed clinically in radar personnel.
2. Experimentally induced injury appeared to be thermal in nature.
3. Reliable information on power densities for radar beams in use was not readily available, and the parameters of potentially injurious exposure were unknown.

Based on the evidence that injury could be produced in experimental animals and could possibly occur in personnel, all available information was reviewed in an effort to establish a safe exposure level to microwaves. Many variables were considered, such as the frequency of the energy to which an individual might be exposed, the nature of the exposure including duration, field strength, and other aspects.

Research was undertaken to investigate whether there were effects other than thermal, and whether biological effects were frequency dependent. There was also interest in whether there were "biological windows" in the frequency spectrum, i.e., regions of the spectrum that give a more pronounced effect than others or regions of no effect. There was also the desire to determine whether the pulse repetition frequency for pulsed radars was of any importance from the biological point of view.

The findings of these studies were reported in several publications, including the Tri-Service reports (Pattishall, 1957; Pattishall and Banghart, 1958; Susskind, 1959; Peyton, 1961; Michaelson *et al.*, 1967), which are now considered to be classic contributions to the early understanding of the biological effects of microwaves.

Numerous summaries and commentaries, reviews, chapters in books and compendiums, conference and Congressional Hearing proceedings, and translations of foreign books, discuss these as well as other studies. This material will be referenced in the following chapters. It is worth noting here, however, the extensive bibliography by Glaser (1971, *et seq.*).

In 1965, $10\,\text{mW}/\text{cm}^2$ was accepted as the personnel exposure standard by the U.S. Department of Defense (DOD, 1965). In 1966, after reviewing all the available information, the American National Standards Institute (ANSI), formerly USASI, also recommended $10\,\text{mW}/\text{cm}^2$ as the standard (ANSI, 1966); it was reaffirmed in 1973.

With passage in the United States of the "Radiation Control for Health and Safety Act of 1968" (PL 90-602) and the "Occupational Safety and Health Act of 1970" (PL 91-596), there has been an increase in interest in the biological effects of exposure to nonionizing electromagnetic energies. The Radiation Control for Health and Safety Act provides for the protection of the public from unnecessary exposure to radiation from electronic products. The Secretary of Health, Education and Welfare is authorized by the act to promulgate performance standards for electronic products and regulations pertaining to record keeping, reporting, certification, and notification. The Bureau of Radiological Health is responsible for administering the act. The Occupational Safety and Health Act of 1970, designed to assure safe and healthful working conditions for workers, provides broad authority to the Departments of Labor and Health, Education and Welfare to promulgate, modify, and improve mandatory occupational safety and health standards as they relate to employee exposure to potentially toxic substances including physical agents.

REFERENCES

American National Standards Institute (1966) Safety Level of Electromagnetic Radiation with Respect to Personnel. United States of America Standards Institute (USASI), New York, USASI-C 95.1.

Anne, A. (1963) Scattering and Absorption of Microwaves by Dissipative Dielectric Objects: The Biological Significance and Hazard to Mankind. Ph.D. thesis, University of Pennsylvania, Philadelphia.

Cole, K. S. (1928) Electric impedance of suspensions of Arbacia eggs. *J. Gen. Physiol.* **12**:37.

Cole, K. S., and R. H. Cole (1941) Dispersion and absorption in dielectrics. I. Alternating current characteristics. *J. Chem. Phys.* **9**:341.

Cole, K.S., and R. H. Cole (1942) Dispersion and absorption in dielectrics. II. Direct current characteristics. *J. Chem. Phys.* **10**:98.

Cole, K.S., and H. J. Curtis (1936) Electric impedance of nerve and muscle. *Cold Spring Harbor Symp. Quant. Biol.* **4**:73.

Cole, K. S., and H. J. Curtis (1941) Membrane potential of squid axon during current flow. *J. Gen. Physiol.* **24**:551.

Cole, K. S., and H. J. Curtis (1960) Bioelectricity: Electric physiology. In: *Medical Physics*, Vol. II, O. Glasser (ed.). Year Book Medical, Chicago, p. 82.

Curtis, H. J., and K. S. Cole (1938) Electric impedance of single marine eggs. *J. Gen. Physiol.* **21**:583.

D'Arsonval, M. A. (1893) The generation of high-frequency and high-intensity currents and their physiological effects. *C. R. Soc. Biol.* **45**:122.

Department of Defense (1965) Control of Hazards to Health from Microwave Radiation. TB MED 270/AFM 161-7, Departments of the Army and Air Force.

Ely, T. S., and D. E. Goldman (1957) Heating characteristics of laboratory animals exposed to ten centimeter microwaves—Summary. In: *Proceedings of the Tri-Service Conference on Biological Hazards of Microwave Radiation*, E. G. Pattishall (ed.). George Washington University, Washington, D.C., p. 64.

Fricke, H. (1933) Electric impedance of suspensions of biological cells. *Cold Spring Harbor Symp. Quant. Biol.* **1**:117.

Fricke, H., and H. J. Curtis (1934) Specific resistance of interior of red blood corpuscle. *Nature (London)* **133**:651.

Fricke, H., H. P. Schwan, K. Li, and V. Bryson (1956) Dielectric study of the low-conductance surface membrane in *E. coli. Nature (London)* **177**:134.

Glaser, Z. R. (1971, *et seq.*) Bibliography of Reported Biological Phenomena ("Effects") and Clinical Manifestations Attributed to Microwave and Radio-Frequency Radiation. U.S. Nav. Med. Res. Inst., Bethesda.

Herrick, J. F. (1958) Pearl-chain formation. In: *Proceedings of the Second Annual Tri-Service Conference on Biological Effects of Microwave Energy*, E. G. Pattishall and F. W. Banghart (eds.). University of Virginia, Charlottesville, p. 88.

Herrick, J. F., and F. H. Krusen (1953) Certain physiologic and pathological effects of microwaves. *Electrical Eng.* **72**:239.

Herrick, J., and F. Krusen (1956) Problems which are challenging investigators in medicine. *IRE Trans. Med. Electron.* **PGME-4**: 10.

Höber, R. (1912) Ein zweites Verfahren, die Leitfahigkeit im Innern von Zellen zu messen. I. *Arch. Ges. Physiol.* **148**:189.

Höber, R. (1913) Ein zweites Verfahren, die Leitfahigkeit im Innern von Zellen zu messen. II. *Arch. Ges. Physiol.* **150**:15.

Hodgkin, A. L. (1947) Membrane resistance of non-medullated nerve fibre. *J. Physiol. (London)* **106:**305.
Hodgkin, A. L., and A. F. Huxley (1952) Quantitative description of membrane current and its application to conduction and excitation in nerve. *J. Physiol. (London)* **117:**500.
Imig, C. J., J. D. Thomson, and H. M. Hines (1948) Testicular degeneration as a result of microwave irradiation. *Proc. Soc. Exp. Biol. Med.* **69:**382.
Krusen, F. H. (1950) Medical applications of microwave diathermy: Laboratory and clinical studies. *Proc. R. Soc. Med.* **43:**641.
Krusen, F. H. (1951) New microwave diathermy director for heating large regions of the human body. *Arch. Phys. Med.* **32:**695.
Krusen, F.H., J. F. Herrick, U. Leden, and K. G. Wakim (1947) Microkymatotherapy: Preliminary report of experimental studies of the heating effect of microwaves (radar) in living tissues. *Proc. Mayo Clin.* **22:**209.
Liebesny, P. (1935) *Short and Ultrashort Waves in Biology.* Urban & Schwarzenberg, Munich.
Liebesny, P. (1938) Athermic short wave therapy. *Arch. Phys. Ther. (Chicago)* **19:**736.
McAfee, R. D. (1959) Neurophysiological effects of microwave irradiation. In: *Proceedings of the Third Annual Tri-Service Conference on Biological Effects of Microwave Radiating Equipments,* C. Susskind (ed.). University of California, Berkeley, p. 314.
Michaelson, S. M. (1971) The tri-service program—A tribute to George M. Knauf, USAF (MC). *IEEE Trans. Microwave Theory Tech.* **MTT-19:**131.
Michaelson, S. M., R. A. E. Thomson, and J. W. Howland (1967) Biologic Effects of Microwave Exposure. Tech. Rep. RADC-TR-67-461, Griffiss AFB, Rome Air Development Center, Rome, N.Y. Also: U.S. Senate, 90th Congress, Second Session on S2067, S3211, and HR 10790, 1968; Radiation Control for Health and Safety Act of 1967, pp. 1443–1570.
Oncley, J. L. (1942) Investigation of proteins by dielectric measurements. *Chem. Rev.* **30:**433.
Oncley, J. L. (1943) The electric moments and relaxation times of proteins as measured from their influence upon the dielectric constants of solutions. In: *Proteins, Amino Acids, and Peptides as Ions and Dipolar Ions,* E. J. Cohn and J. T. Edsall (eds.). Reinhold, New York, pp. 543–568.
Osswald, K. (1937) High frequency conductivity and dielectric constants of biological tissues and fluids. *Hochfrequenztech. Elektroakust.* **49:**40.
Pattishall, E. G. (ed.) (1957) *Proceedings of the Tri-Service Conference on Biological Hazards of Microwave Radiation.* George Washington University, Washington, D.C.
Pattishall, E. G., and F. W. Banghart (eds.) (1958) *Proceedings of the Second Annual Tri-Service Conference on Biological Effects of Microwave Energy.* University of Virginia, Charlottesville.
Pätzold, J., and H. Schaefer (1948) Biophysical foundations of the therapeutic aspects of high frequency electrical fields. In: *Natural Sciences and Medicine in Germany, 1934–1946,* Vol. 22, B. Rajewsky (ed.). Biophysics II, Wiesbaden, pp. 17–19.
Peyton, M. F. (ed.) (1961) *Biological Effects of Microwave Radiation: Proceedings of the Fourth Annual Tri-Service Conference.* Plenum Press, New York.
Rajewsky, B. (ed.) (1938) *Ergebnisse der Biophysikalischen Forschung in Einzeldarstellungen,* Vol. I. Thieme, Stuttgart.
Richardson, A. W. (1958) Review of the work conducted at the University of St. Louis (USN sponsored). In: *Proceedings of the Second Annual Tri-Service Conference on Biological Effects of Microwave Energy,* E. G. Pattishall and F. W. Banghart (eds.). University of Virginia, Charlottesville, p. 169.

Richardson, A. W., T. D. Duane, and H. M. Hines (1948) Experimental lenticular opacities produced by microwave irradiation. *Arch. Phys. Med.* **29:**765.

Schaefer, H., and H. Schwan (1943) Concerning the question of selective heating of small particles in the ultrashort wave condenser field. *Ann. Phys. (Leipzig)* **43:**99.

Schaefer, H., and H. Schwan (1947) Concerning the question of selective overheating of single cells in biological tissue by means of ultrashort wave currents. *Strahlentherapie* **77:** 123.

Schereschewsky, J. W. (1926) The physiological effects of currents of very high frequency (135,000,000 to 8,300,000 cps). *Public Health Rep.* **41:**1939.

Schliephake, E. (1935) *Short Wave Therapy—The Medical Use of Electrical High Frequencies.* Actinic Press, London.

Schwan, H. P. (1948) Temperature dependence of the dielectric constant of blood at low frequencies. *Z. Naturforsch.* **3b:**361.

Schwan, H. P. (1953) Electrical properties of blood at ultrahigh frequencies. *Am. J. Phys. Med.* **32:**144.

Schwan, H. P. (1955) Applications of UHF impedance measuring techniques in biophysics. *IRE Trans. Med. Electron.* **PGME-4:**75.

Schwan, H. P. (1957a) Influence of Electromagnetic Radiation on Biological Material. Final report from the University of Pennsylvania on ONR Contract (1 July 1954 to 30 June 1957), AD 149535.

Schwan, H. P. (1957b) Electrical properties of tissues and cell suspensions. *Adv. Biol. Med. Phys.* **5:**147.

Schwan, H. P. (1958a) Biophysics of diathermy. In: *Therapeutic Heat,* S. H. Licht (ed.). E. Licht, New Haven, Conn., p. 55.

Schwan, H. P. (1958b) Molecular response characteristics to ultra-high frequency fields. In: *Proceedings of the Second Annual Tri-Service Conference on Biological Effects of Microwave Energy,* E. G. Pattishall and F. W. Banghart (eds.). University of Virginia, Charlottesville, p. 33.

Schwan, H. P. (1964) Non-Thermal Effects of Alternating Electrical Fields on Biological Structures. Final report from the University of Pennsylvania on ONR Contract, AD 600263.

Schwan, H. P. (1970) Non-Thermal Effects of Alternating Electrical Fields on Biological Structures. Final report from the University of Pennsylvania on ONR Contract (March 1964 to December 1969).

Schwan, H. P. (1975) Dielectric properties of biological materials and interaction of microwave fields at the cellular and molecular level. In: *Fundamental and Applied Aspects of Nonionizing Radiation,* S. M. Michaelson, M. W. Miller, R. Magin, and E. L. Carstensen (eds.). Plenum Press, New York, p. 3.

Schwan, H. P., and K. S. Cole (1960) Bioelectricity: Alternating current admittance of cells and tissues. In: *Medical Physics,* Vol. III, 0. Glasser (ed.). Year book Medical, Chicago, p. 52.

Schwan, H. P., and K. Li (1956) Hazards due to total body irradiation by radar. *Proc. IRE* **44:**1572.

Schwan, H. P., and G. M. Piersol (1954) The absorption of electromagnetic energy in body tissues, a review and critical analysis. Part I. Biophysical aspects. *Am. J. Phys. Med.* **33:**371.

Schwan, H. P., and G. M. Piersol (1955) The absorption of electromagnetic energy in body tissues, a review and critical analysis. Part II. Physiological and clinical aspects. *Am. J. Phys. Med.* **34:**425.

Schwan, H. P., and L. D. Sher (1967) Non-Thermal Effects of Alternating Electric Fields on Biological Structures. University of Pennsylvania Progress Report to ONR (AD 656736).

Susskind, C. (ed.) (1959) *Proceedings of the Third Annual Tri-Service Conference on Biological Effects of Microwave Radiating Equipments*. University of California, Berkeley.

Takashima, S. (1962) Dielectric properties of water of absorption on protein crystals. *J. Polym. Sci.* **62**:233.

Wakim, K. G., J. W. Gersten, J. F. Herrick, E. C. Elkins, and F. H. Krusen (1948a) The effects of diathermy on the flow of blood in the extremities. *Arch. Phys. Med.* **29**:583.

Wakim, K., J. Herrick, E. Parkhill, and W. Benedict (1948b) Effects of microwave diathermy on the eye. *Am. J. Physiol.* **155**:432.

Worden, R. E., J. F. Herrick, K. G. Wakim, and F. H. Krusen (1948) The heating effects of microwaves with and without ischemia. *Arch. Phys. Med.* **29**:751.

2

Physical Description of Radio and Microwave Radiation

An understanding of the interaction of radio and microwave radiation with biological systems requires a knowledge of some of the laws describing the characteristics of radio and microwave radiation. The physical processes of radio and microwave radiation are governed by four principles now known as Maxwell's equations. These equations represent mathematical expressions of experimental observations. From these four principles or laws of electromagnetics, one may deduce with mathematical vigor and exactness, all macroscopic electromagnetic phenomena.

The fundamentals of radio and microwave radiation are presented in this chapter to promote a basic understanding. Those properties of radio and microwave radiation that are of the greatest interest in biological interactions are stressed, rather than trying to give a short summary of all that radio and microwave radiation entails. The reader interested in a detailed physical account of radio and microwave radiation is referred to some readily available texts devoted entirely to these topics (Adams, 1969; Gandhi, 1981; Kraus and Carver, 1973; Jordan and Balmain, 1968; Collin, 1966; Collin and Zucker, 1969; Ramo *et al.*, 1965; Harvey, 1963).

2.1. FUNDAMENTALS OF WAVE PROPAGATION

Radio and microwave radiation consists of electric and magnetic fields that vary with position and time, and is propagated through free space at the speed of light, 2.998×10^8 m/sec. The variation in this speed in material medium through which the wave propagates is dependent on the permittivity and permeability of the medium. The propagation, scattering, and transmission of radio and microwave radiation are governed by Maxwell's equations. These equations, in fact, describe all electromagnetic phenomena in continuous media that are stationary with respect to the coordinate system employed. They are valid for linear or nonlinear, isotropic or anisotropic, homogeneous or nonhomogeneous medium in the frequency range from zero to the highest microwave frequencies, including many phenomena at optical frequencies. Maxwell's equations are macroscopic laws that define the relationship between space and time-averaged electric and magnetic fields. They apply to regions or volumes whose dimensions are larger than atomic dimensions. Time intervals of observation are assumed to be long enough to allow for an averaging of atomic fluctuations.

2.1.1. Maxwell's Equations

The integral forms of Maxwell's equations are

$$\oint \mathbf{E} \cdot \mathbf{dl} = -\int_s \frac{\partial \mathbf{B}}{\partial t} \cdot \mathbf{ds} \qquad \text{(Faraday's law)} \qquad (2.1)$$

$$\oint \mathbf{H} \cdot \mathbf{dl} = \int_s \left(\mathbf{J} + \frac{\partial \mathbf{D}}{\partial t} \right) \cdot \mathbf{ds} \qquad \text{(Ampere–Maxwell's law)} \qquad (2.2)$$

$$\oint \mathbf{D} \cdot \mathbf{ds} = \int_v \rho \, dv \qquad \text{(Gauss's electric law)} \qquad (2.3)$$

$$\oint \mathbf{B} \cdot \mathbf{ds} = 0 \qquad \text{(Gauss's magnetic law)} \qquad (2.4)$$

where

$\mathbf{E}$ = electric field strength (volt/meter)
$\mathbf{H}$ = magnetic field strength (ampere/meter)
$\mathbf{D}$ = electric flux density (coulomb/square meter)
$\mathbf{B}$ = magnetic flux density (weber/square meter)
$\mathbf{J}$ = conduction current density (ampere/square meter)
ρ = charge density (coulomb/cubic meter)

According to Faraday's law (2.1) the total voltage induced in an arbitrary closed path is equal to the time rate of change of magnetic flux through the area bounded by the closed path. Therefore, a time-varying magnetic field generates an electric field. There is no restriction on the nature of the medium.

Ampere's law (2.2) states that the line integral of the magnetic field strength around a closed path is equal to the total current enclosed by the path. The total current may consist of two parts: a conduction current with density $\mathbf{J}$ and a displacement current with density $\partial \mathbf{D}/\partial t$. Thus, Ampere's law implies that a magnetic field can only be produced by movement of charges. The displacement current was first introduced by

PHYSICAL DESCRIPTION OF RF RADIATION

Maxwell and allowed him to unify the separate laws governing electricity and magnetism into an electromagnetic theory. It also led to the postulate of electromagnetic waves that can transport energy and the concept that light is an electromagnetic wave.

Equation (2.3) is Gauss's electric law, which states that the net outward flow of electric flux through a closed surface is equal to the charge contained in the volume enclosed by the surface. Gauss's law for the magnetic field (2.4) states that the net outward flow of magnetic flux through a closed surface is zero. Therefore, magnetic flux lines are always continuous and formed closed loops.

Although (2.1) through (2.4) lend to ready physical interpretation, they are not in forms most suitable for the analysis of physical problems. It is often expedient to solve differential equations to obtain field quantities. The desired differential equations may be derived by using Stokes's and divergence theorems from vector analysis. As a result, Maxwell's equations in differential form are

$$\nabla \times \mathbf{E} = -\frac{\partial \mathbf{B}}{\partial t} \tag{2.5}$$

$$\nabla \times \mathbf{H} = \mathbf{J} + \frac{\partial \mathbf{D}}{\partial t} \tag{2.6}$$

$$\nabla \cdot \mathbf{D} = \rho \tag{2.7}$$

$$\nabla \cdot \mathbf{B} = 0 \tag{2.8}$$

It is seen from the right-hand sides of (2.6) and (2.7) that the sources of electromagnetic fields and waves are charges and currents. When the electromagnetic fields are harmonically oscillating functions with a single frequency, f, all field quantities may be assumed to have a time variation represented by $\exp(j\omega t)$, where $\omega = 2\pi f$ in radians, is the angular frequency. Under this assumption, the time derivatives in Maxwell's equations may be replaced by a multiplier $j\omega$, and the common factor $\exp(j\omega t)$ may be omitted from these equations. Maxwell's equations can be written as

$$\nabla \times \mathbf{E} = -j\omega \mathbf{B} \tag{2.9}$$

$$\nabla \times \mathbf{H} = \mathbf{J} + j\omega \mathbf{D} \tag{2.10}$$

$$\nabla \cdot \mathbf{D} = \rho \tag{2.11}$$

$$\nabla \cdot \mathbf{B} = 0 \tag{2.12}$$

Note the use of boldface letters for the vectors that are complex functions of space coordinates.

A set of auxiliary equations relating the fields and flux densities are required to determine the electric and magnetic fields produced by a given current and charge distributions. For a linear, isotropic, and homogeneous medium, the field quantities are related as follows:

$$\mathbf{D} = \varepsilon \mathbf{E} \tag{2.13}$$

$$\mathbf{B} = \mu \mathbf{H} \tag{2.14}$$

$$\mathbf{J} = \sigma \mathbf{E} \tag{2.15}$$

The free space or vacuum is such a medium in which the permittivity is given by

$$\varepsilon = \varepsilon_0 = 8.854 \times 10^{-12} \, \text{farad/m} \tag{2.16}$$

permeability is given by

$$\mu = \mu_0 = 4\pi \times 10^{-7} \, \text{henry/m} \tag{2.17}$$

and conductivity, $\sigma = 0$. For other simple media, it is conventional to introduce the dimensionless ratios

$$\varepsilon_r = \varepsilon/\varepsilon_0 \tag{2.18}$$

$$\mu_r = \mu/\mu_0 \tag{2.19}$$

which are usually labeled the relative dielectric constant and relative permeability, respectively. Living things generally have relative permeabilities close to that of free space and relative dielectric constants that show characteristic dependence on frequency.

2.1.2. Boundary Conditions

The behaviour of electric and magnetic fields in situations where the physical properties of the medium change abruptly across one or several interfaces is governed by certain boundary conditions to be satisfied at the interfaces. These conditions may be derived by applying Maxwell's equations (2.1–2.4) to infinitesimal regions containing these interfaces. If medium 1 and medium 2 are separated by a common boundary (see Fig. 2-1), the boundary conditions at the interface may be summarized as

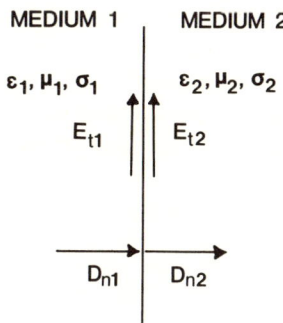

FIGURE 2-1. Boundary between two different media.

follows:

1. The tangential components of the electric field strengths are continuous across the boundary, i.e.,

$$E_{t1} = E_{t2} \tag{2.20}$$

2. The normal components of the electric flux densities differ by an amount equal to the surface charge density, i.e.,

$$D_{n1} - D_{n2} = \rho_s \tag{2.21}$$

If there is no surface charge on the boundary, $\rho_s = 0$, which is the usual case for dielectric materials, then

$$D_{n1} = D_{n2} \tag{2.22}$$

3. The tangential components of magnetic field strength differ by an amount equal to the surface current density, i.e.,

$$H_{t1} - H_{t2} = J_s \tag{2.23}$$

In all cases except that of a perfect conductor, the surface current density is vanishingly small, then

$$H_{t1} = H_{t2} \tag{2.24}$$

4. The normal components of magnetic flux density are continuous across a boundary, i.e.,

$$B_{n1} = B_{n2} \tag{2.25}$$

When dealing with fields in an infinite region of space, the radiation condition requires that the field at infinity must be an outward propagating wave with finite amount of energy. Alternatively, electric and magnetic fields must vanish rapidly so that the energy stored in the fields and the energy flow at infinity are zero.

2.1.3. Wave Equations

Equations (2.9) and (2.10) are a set of coupled equations both containing electric and magnetic field quantities. If we assume for the moment that the conduction current density is zero in the region of interest, these two equations may be combined to give two second-order differential equations, one containing the electric field strength and the other containing the magnetic field strength:

$$\nabla^2 \mathbf{E} + \omega^2 \mu \varepsilon \mathbf{E} = 0 \quad (2.26)$$

$$\nabla^2 \mathbf{H} + \omega^2 \mu \varepsilon \mathbf{H} = 0 \quad (2.27)$$

where we have taken the charge density as zero. It is customary to let $k^2 = \omega^2 \mu \varepsilon$, where k is the wave number and has the following relations:

$$k = \omega(\mu\varepsilon)^{1/2} = \omega/v = 2\pi/\lambda \quad (2.28)$$

Equations (2.26) and (2.27) are wave equations. The solutions represent electromagnetic waves propagating with velocity v equal to $(\mu\varepsilon)^{-1/2}$. The wavelength λ is equal to v/f, where f is the frequency. In free space, v is equal to the speed of light, $c = 2.998 \times 10^8$ m/sec.

In a medium with finite electrical conductivity σ, a conduction current density $\mathbf{J} = \sigma \mathbf{E}$ will exist and this will give rise to energy loss to Joule heating. The wave equations in media of this type have a loss term,

$$(\nabla^2 + \omega^2 \mu \varepsilon - j\omega\mu\sigma)\mathbf{E} = 0 \quad (2.29)$$

$$(\nabla^2 + \omega^2 \mu \varepsilon - j\omega\mu\sigma)\mathbf{H} = 0 \quad (2.30)$$

It should be mentioned that a finite conductivity is equivalent to an imaginary component in the permittivity ε. Comparing (2.26) with (2.29), it is seen that the equivalent permittivity is $\varepsilon - j\sigma/\omega$.

2.1.4. Energy Storage and Power Flow

Electromagnetic energy is either stored in the electric and magnetic fields or radiated away in the form of electromagnetic waves. For a region in which permittivity and permeability are functions of position but not time, the energy density at a point is given by

$$W = (1/2)(\varepsilon E^2 + \mu H^2) \qquad (2.31)$$

where $(1/2)\varepsilon E^2$ is the energy stored per unit volume in the electric field and $(1/2)\mu H^2$ is the energy stored per unit volume in the magnetic field. The stored energy is partitioned between electric and magnetic fields and is transferred from electric to magnetic fields and back again as a function of time.

In regions with finite conductivity, part of the electromagnetic energy is dissipated as heat. The term

$$P_a = (1/2)\sigma E^2 \qquad (2.32)$$

represents the density of power converted to heat energy and is called dissipated power or *absorbed power density*. It also equals the rate of energy absorption or *specific rate of absorption* (SAR).

The instantaneous density of power that flows across a surface bounding a given region is given by the Poynting vector **P**,

$$\mathbf{P} = \mathbf{E} \times \mathbf{H} \qquad (2.33)$$

Thus, the direction of power flow is perpendicular to **E** and **H**, and is in the direction of the Poynting vector **P**. It can be shown by an application of the Poynting theorem that the total power flowing into a region is equal to the total power dissipated within the region plus the time rate of increase of energy stored within the region. For electric and magnetic fields that vary sinusoidally with time, the time-average power flow or rate of energy flow per unit area is

$$P_d = (1/2)\,\mathrm{Re}(\mathbf{E} \times \mathbf{H}^*) \qquad (2.34)$$

where $\mathbf{H}^*$ is the complex conjugate of **H** and P_d is given by the real part of the product of sinusoidal quantities.

2.1.5. Plane Waves

The radiated energy of a small antenna (a point source) in free space is in the form of a spherical wave in which the wavefronts are concentric spherical shells. The spherical wavefronts expand as the wave propagates outward from the source. At points far from the source, the wavefront would essentially appear as a plane. This is analogous to the situation of an observer on earth who sees the earth's surface as a plane, since he is able to view only a small portion of the total surface of the earth. Both electric and magnetic fields of the wave lie in the plane of the wavefront. They vary only in the direction of propagation and are uniform in planes normal to the direction of propagation. Such a wave is called a *plane wave*. It is a very important practical case since fields radiated by any transmitting antenna appear as plane waves at distances far from the source. Moreover, through Fourier analysis a suitable combination of plane waves may be made to represent a wave of any desired form in space and time.

2.1.6. Polarization of Plane Waves

To specify the orientation of radio and microwave radiation in space, it is necessary to specify the orientation of one of the field vectors. Since the magnetic field vector is always perpendicular to the electric field vector, a knowledge of the orientation of the latter is sufficient to describe the orientation of the wave. The *polarization* of a plane wave refers to the time-varying character of the electric field at a given location in space. If the electric field of the wave always lies in a specific direction, the wave is said to be *linearly polarized*. An example would be a linearly polarized plane wave in the x direction of a rectangular coordinate system. If both E_x and E_y are present and are in time phase, the resultant electric field has a direction dependent on the relative magnitude of E_x and E_y. The angle that this direction makes with the x axis, however, is constant with time. The wave is therefore also linearly polarized (see Fig. 2-2a).

If E_x and E_y are equal in magnitude and E_y leads E_x

$$\mathbf{E} = E_x \mathbf{x} + jE_y \mathbf{y} \tag{2.35}$$

E_x and E_y reach their maximum values at different instants of time, the direction of the resultant electric field will vary with time. It can be shown that the locus of the endpoint of the resultant electric field will be a circle. The wave is said to be *circularly polarized*. Moreover, it may be seen that looking in the direction of propagation, the rotation of the electric field vector is that of a left-handed screw advancing in the direction of propagation. The wave is therefore also said to be left *circularly polarized* (see Fig. 2-2b). If the x component of the electric field leads the y component instead, a reversal of the direction of rotation is obtained.

The most general form of polarization is *elliptical polarization*. This happens when E_x and E_y differ in magnitude as well as time phase.

PHYSICAL DESCRIPTION OF RF RADIATION

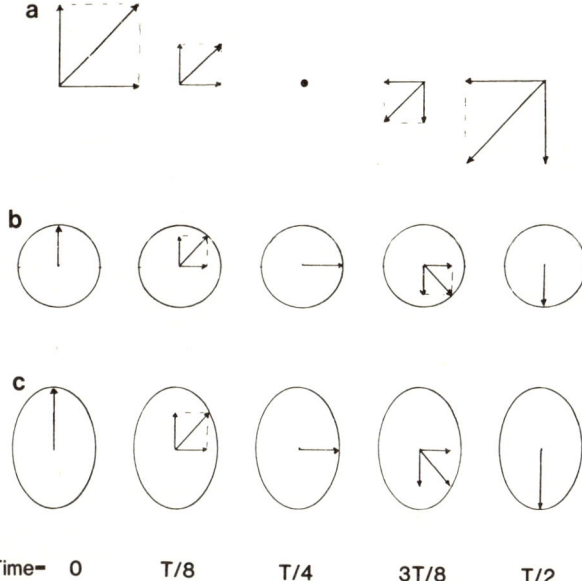

FIGURE 2-2. Polarization of plane waves: (a) linear polarization; (b) circular polarization; (c) elliptical polarization. Arrows indicate directions of electric field and its components.

Assuming again E_y leads E_x by 90°, since E_x and E_y are not equal in magnitude the endpoint of the resultant field traces out an ellipse in the plane normal to the direction of propagation (see Fig. 2-2c). The circular polarization is in fact a special case of elliptical polarization.

2.2. PROPAGATION OF PLANE WAVES

A wave propagating in a given direction has no field variations in planes normal to the direction of propagation and is a linearly polarized plane wave. In this section we shall describe the properties of plane wave propagation in free space, lossy media, and media involving plane boundaries.

2.2.1. Plane Waves in Free Space

Assume that the electric field is polarized in the x direction and the wave propagating in the z direction, the wave equation (2.26) reduces to

$$(d^2 E_x / dz^2) + k_0^2 E_x = 0 \qquad (2.36)$$

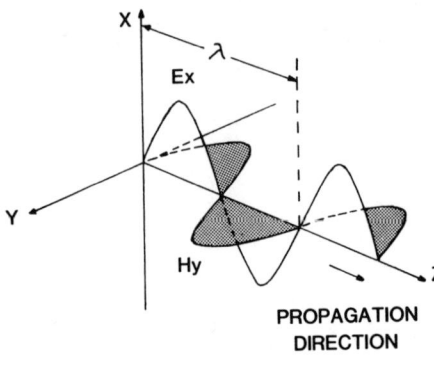

FIGURE 2-3. A plane wave propagating in the positive z direction. The directions of electric and magnetic fields are everywhere perpendicular and both are perpendicular to the direction of propagation.

where $k_0 = \omega(\mu_0\varepsilon_0)^{1/2}$ is the *free space wave number*. The solution to this equation is

$$E_x = E_0 e^{-jk_0 z} \tag{2.37}$$

The associated magnetic field is related to the electric field through Maxwell's equation (2.9), thus

$$H_y = (\varepsilon_0/\mu_0)^{1/2} E_x \tag{2.38}$$

The ratio of E_x to H_y has the dimension of impedance and is called the *intrinsic impedance*. The intrinsic impedance of free space is

$$\eta_0 = (\mu_0/\varepsilon_0)^{1/2} = 120\pi \simeq 377 \text{ ohms} \tag{2.39}$$

Figure 2-3 shows the electric and magnetic fields as a function of distance at some instant of time. The wavelength λ_0 is defined as the distance over which the sinusoidal waveform passes through a full cycle of 2π radians. Note that the electric and magnetic fields are in time phase but in space quadrature.

The time-average power flow or average power density associated with this wave is

$$P_d = (1/2)(E_0^2/\eta_0) \tag{2.40}$$

The direction of power flow is normal to both electric and magnetic field vectors and is in the direction of wave propagation.

2.2.2. Plane Waves in Lossy Media

In the case of a plane wave propagating through a homogeneous isotropic medium with dielectric loss or finite conductivity, the governing equation (2.29) becomes

$$(d^2E_x/dz^2) - \gamma^2 E_x = 0 \tag{2.41}$$

γ is the *propagation factor* given by

$$\gamma = [j\omega\mu(\sigma + j\omega\varepsilon)]^{1/2} \tag{2.42}$$

The solution of (2.41) for a wave propagating along the positive z direction is

$$E_x = Ee^{-\gamma z} \tag{2.43}$$

The corresponding solution for the magnetic field is

$$H_y = (\gamma/j\omega\mu)Ee^{-\gamma z} \tag{2.44}$$

The intrinsic impedance of a medium was previously defined as the ratio of electric field to magnetic field. Thus,

$$\eta = E_x/H_y = j\omega\mu/\gamma = [j\omega\mu/(\sigma + j\omega\varepsilon)]^{1/2} \tag{2.45}$$

For a lossless dielectric medium, $\sigma = 0$, the intrinsic impedance reduces to

$$\eta = (\mu/\varepsilon)^{1/2} \tag{2.46}$$

As shown earlier, η has a value of 377 ohms for free space. Since dielectric media have approximately the same permeability of free space and have permittivities greater than free space, it follows that the intrinsic impedance of free space is the upper limit of attainable value for dielectric materials.

The real and imaginary parts of complex propagation factor γ may be represented by α and β such that

$$\gamma = \alpha + j\beta \tag{2.47}$$

and

$$\alpha = \omega\{(\mu\varepsilon/2)[(1 + \sigma^2/\omega^2\varepsilon^2)^{1/2} - 1]\}^{1/2} \tag{2.48}$$

$$\beta = \omega\{(\mu\varepsilon/2)[(1 + \sigma^2/\omega^2\varepsilon^2)^{1/2} + 1]\}^{1/2} \tag{2.49}$$

where α and β are referred to as *attenuation coefficient* and *propagation*

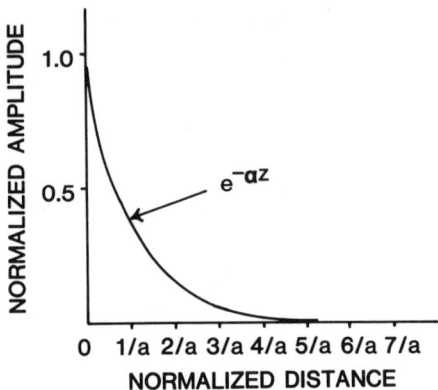

FIGURE 2-4. Attenuation of plane waves in a lossy medium.

coefficient, respectively. It is clear from (2.43), (2.44), and (2.47) that the amplitude of the wave decreases as it advances in the lossy medium and the reduction is exponential in nature (see Fig. 2-4). Furthermore, since α is related to ω and σ, the rate of attenuation is proportional to frequency and conductivity. When $\sigma \gg \omega\varepsilon$, such as for a good conductor, α and β may be simplified to yield

$$\alpha = \beta = (\omega\mu\sigma/2)^{1/2} \qquad (2.50)$$

The time-average power density associated with a plane wave propagating through a lossy media is

$$P_d = (1/2)\text{Re}[(E^2 e^{-2\alpha z})/\eta] \qquad (2.51)$$

It is easily seen from (2.51) that the average power density decreases according to $e^{-2\alpha z}$ as the wave propagates in the lossy medium. This is as expected since the field decreases exponentially $(e^{-\alpha z})$ as it travels in the medium. At $z = \delta$, both electric and magnetic field strengths decrease to $1/e$, 36.8% of their value at the surface or the point of entry into the lossy medium (the term *conducting medium* is also used to mean *lossy medium*).

The quantity δ is known as the *depth of penetration* or *skin depth* and is given by

$$\delta = 1/\alpha \qquad (2.52)$$

Therefore, the depth of penetration is inversely proportional to the conductivity and the frequency. It should be mentioned that the fields do not fail to penetrate beyond the depth of δ; this is merely the point at

PHYSICAL DESCRIPTION OF RF RADIATION

which they have decreased to 37% of their initial value. The power density will decrease to 14%, accordingly.

The concept as presented here applies strictly to planar media. It may be extended, however, to bodies of other geometry so long as the depth of penetration is much smaller than the radius of curvature of the body surfaces.

2.2.3. Reflection and Transmission at Interfaces

When radio and microwave radiation propagating in one medium impinges on a second medium having different electromagnetic properties, partial reflection occurs at the boundary between the two media. A portion of the incident radiation may also be transmitted into the second medium. If intrinsic impedances of the two media are approximately equal, most of the energy is transmitted into the second medium and the reflected radiation is relatively small. Conversely, if intrinsic impedances differ greatly, the transmitted radiation is small and the reflected radiation is relatively large. If the wave impinges normally on the boundary surface, the resulting reflected wave propagating back toward the source combines with the incident wave to form a *standing wave* in the first medium. An example of the standing wave created by a perfect conductor is shown in Fig. 2-5. The term *standing wave ratio* (SWR) is defined as the ratio of maximum to minimum electric field strength in a standing wave. It is used as a measure of the degree of impedance mismatch or of differences between the electromagnetic properties of the two media.

The essential features of the behavior of radio and microwaves at the surface between two media may be deduced from an analysis of the

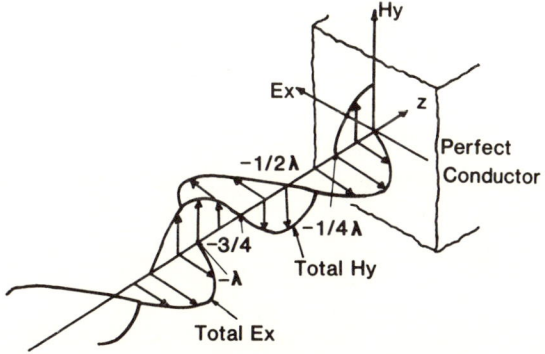

FIGURE 2-5. A standing wave created when a plane wave impinges normally on a perfect conductor. The fields are shown at time $t = T/8$.

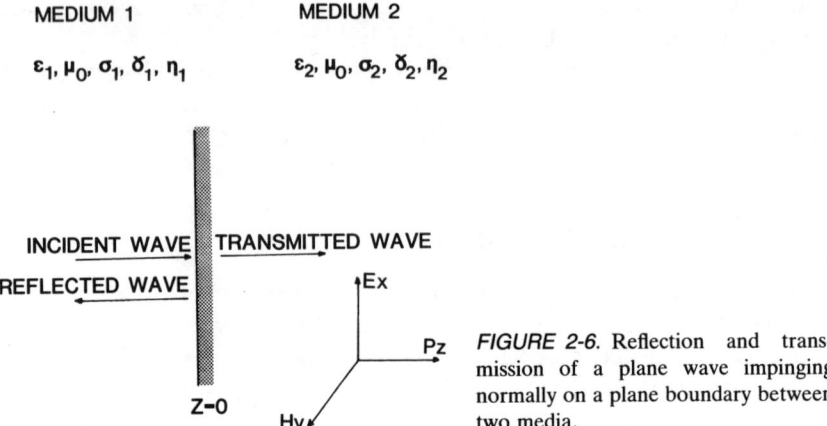

FIGURE 2-6. Reflection and transmission of a plane wave impinging normally on a plane boundary between two media.

simple situation of a plane wave incident normally upon a plane surface between two media (see Fig. 2-6). Both media are assumed to be infinite in extent in all directions except at the boundary ($z = 0$). At any plane z we may define a wave impedance as the ratio of total electric to total magnetic fields at that plane:

$$Z(z) = E_x(z)/H_y(z) \tag{2.53}$$

For the wave propagating along the positive z direction in medium 2, $Z = \eta_2$ is the intrinsic impedance. Similarly, for the incident plane wave traveling positively in medium 1, $Z = \eta_1$; however, there is also a negatively traveling wave having a $Z = -\eta_1$. The combination of the incident and reflected components gives rise to a wave impedance that varies with z in medium 1, such that

$$Z(z) = \eta_1 \left(\frac{\eta_2 + \eta_1 \tanh \gamma_1 z}{\eta_1 + \eta_2 \tanh \gamma_1 z} \right) \tag{2.54}$$

where γ_1 is the propagation factor in medium 1.

The reflected radiation is characterized by the *reflection coefficient R*, which is defined as the ratio of the reflected electric field strength to the incident field strength at the boundary and is given by

$$R = (\eta_2 - \eta_1)/(\eta_2 + \eta_1) \tag{2.55}$$

In a similar manner, the *transmission coefficient T* is defined as the ratio of the transmitted electric field strength to that of the incident field at the boundary,

$$T = 2\eta_2/(\eta_2 + \eta_1) \tag{2.56}$$

It is seen from (2.55) and (2.56) that when $\eta_2 = \eta_1$, i.e., the electrical properties of the media are approximately equal, there is no reflection and transmission is maximal. On the other hand, there is complete reflection when η_2 is zero. As shall be seen later, for biological materials, microwave reflection and transmission behaviors fall between the two extremes. The latter of the two extremes may be encountered when metallic components are involved in research on biomedical aspects of radio and microwave radiation.

The SWR may be expressed in terms of the magnitude of the reflection coefficient as

$$\text{SWR} = (1 + |R|)/(1 - |R|) \tag{2.57}$$

It may be shown using the results of the last paragraph that the SWR = 1 when there is equality of media. Any mismatch of the two media will result in an SWR greater than unity.

For the situation illustrated in Fig. 2-6, the electric and magnetic fields may be expressed as

$$E_{1x} = E_i(e^{-\gamma_1 z} + Re^{\gamma_1 z}) \tag{2.58}$$

$$H_{1y} = (E_i/\eta_1)(e^{-\gamma_1 z} - Re^{\gamma_1 z}) \tag{2.59}$$

$$E_{2x} = E_i T e^{-\gamma_2 z} \tag{2.60}$$

$$H_{2y} = (E_i/\eta_2) T e^{-\gamma_2 z} \tag{2.61}$$

where the reflection coefficient R and transmission coefficient T are as defined previously. E_i is the incident electric field strength.

The time-average density of power transmitted across the interface is

$$P_t = \frac{1}{2}\frac{E^2}{\eta_1}(1 - |R|^2) \tag{2.62}$$

The difference between the incident and transmitted power must be that reflected, or

$$P_r = \frac{1}{2}\frac{E^2}{\eta_1}|R|^2$$

Let us consider for example the case of a metal conductor ($\eta_2 = 0$); according to (2.55) the reflection coefficient $R = -1$. There will not be any transmitted energy. The incident and reflected components of the electric and magnetic fields will combine as indicated in (2.58) and (2.59). If we further assume the medium is lossless, then

$$E_x = -2jE_i \sin \beta z \tag{2.63}$$

$$H_y = (2E_i/\eta) \cos \beta z \tag{2.64}$$

These equations represent a wave that is stationary in space. The values of E and H are sine and cosine functions of z, respectively. The maxima and minima do not move in the z direction but remain at a fixed position as time passes (Fig. 2-5). Note also that E_x is 90° apart in time phase from H_y and the peak values of E do not occur at the same point in space as H field. In other words, the electric and magnetic energies of a standing wave are in space and time quadrature. The energy is not transferred but oscillates back and forth from the electric form to the magnetic form over a distance $\lambda/4$.

The situation involving a plane wave incident upon several parallel layers of dielectric materials is also of practical interest. The problem may be treated by considering quantities in each medium and use of an impedance formulation similar to (2.54). Examples of wave propagation in layers of biological material are given in Chapter 5.

2.2.4. Refraction of Electromagnetic Waves

The refraction or transmission of a plane wave at a plane interface depends on the frequency, polarization, and angle of incidence of the wave, and on the dielectric constant and conductivity of the tissue. A wave of general polarization usually is decomposed into its orthogonal linearly polarized components whose electric or magnetic field is parallel to the interface. These components are called E and H polarizations, respectively, and can be treated separately and combined afterward. The reflection coefficients for H and E polarizations are (Kraus and Carver, 1973)

$$R_h = \frac{-(\varepsilon_2/\varepsilon_1)\cos\theta + [(\varepsilon_2/\varepsilon_1) - \sin^2\theta]^{1/2}}{(\varepsilon_2/\varepsilon_1)\cos\theta + [(\varepsilon_2/\varepsilon_1) - \sin^2\theta]^{1/2}} \tag{2.65}$$

$$R_e = \frac{\cos\theta - [(\varepsilon_2/\varepsilon_1) - \sin^2\theta]^{1/2}}{\cos\theta + [(\varepsilon_2/\varepsilon_1) - \sin^2\theta]^{1/2}} \tag{2.66}$$

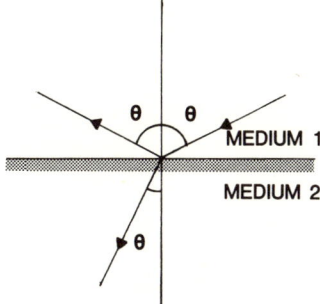

FIGURE 2-7. Plane wave incident upon a boundary surface at an angle.

and the transmission coefficients are given by

$$T_h = (1 + R_h) \frac{\cos \theta}{[1 - (\varepsilon_1/\varepsilon_2) \sin^2 \theta]^{1/2}} \qquad (2.67)$$

$$T_e = 1 + R_e \qquad (2.68)$$

where θ is the angle of incidence (Fig. 2-7) and ε_1 and ε_2 are the complex permittivity of the medium in front of and behind the interface, respectively. In particular, $\varepsilon = \varepsilon_0[\varepsilon_r - j(\sigma/\omega\varepsilon_0)]$ with free-space permittivity ε_0 and radian frequency $\omega = 2\pi f$. It is noted that the angle of reflection is equal to the angle of incidence, while the angle of transmission is given by Snell's law of refraction,

$$\sin \theta_t = (\varepsilon_1/\varepsilon_2)^{1/2} \sin \theta \qquad (2.69)$$

An examination of (2.65) shows that, for H polarization, it is possible to find an angle so that $R_h = 0$ and the wave is totally transmitted. This angle, referred to as the *Brewster angle* θ_B, can be obtained by setting the numerator of (2.65) equal to zero such that

$$\theta_B = \tan^{-1}(\varepsilon_1/\varepsilon_2)^{1/2} \qquad (2.70)$$

Note that a Brewster angle exists for either $\varepsilon_1 > \varepsilon_2$ or $\varepsilon_1 < \varepsilon_2$. Thus, a circularly polarized wave incident at θ_B becomes linearly polarized upon reflection since there will be no reflection for the H-polarized component.

There is a second phenomenon that applies to both polarizations. For a wave that is incident from a medium with a larger permittivity onto a medium with a smaller permittivity, total reflection can take place at the interface between the two dielectric media. This incident angle is called the *critical angle*

$$\theta_c = \sin^{-1}(\varepsilon_2/\varepsilon_1)^{1/2} \tag{2.71}$$

Under these conditions, the incident wave is totally internally reflected back into the medium with larger permittivity. The wave in the medium with smaller permittivity will decay exponentially away from the interface.

2.3. WAVES IN ENCLOSED SPACE

Waveguides and cavities are used to transport and to store energy in electromagnetic systems. They differ from conventional transmission lines and resonators in that they are either partially or completely enclosed metallic structures. Apart from their intended use in communication systems, they are widely used in microwave power application as applicators of microwave energy for treating biological material.

2.3.1. Waveguides

The common forms of waveguides are the rectangular and circular ones. They consist of enclosed cylindrical metallic tubes of rectangular and circular cross sections, respectively; each offers some distinct advantages for certain applications. Because the theory and operation are not sufficiently different, only the rectangular waveguide will be described in detail in this section.

For the rectangular waveguide illustrated in Fig. 2-8, the wave equations (2.26) and (2.27) may be solved in rectangular coordinates for the electric and magnetic fields that correspond to waves propagating along the z axis. There are two wave types that can propagate in a hollow

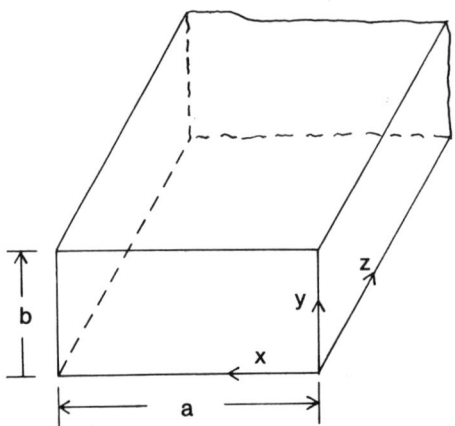

FIGURE 2-8. Schematics of a rectangular waveguide.

rectangular waveguide. A wave having no electric field component in the direction of propagation is called a transverse electric (TE) wave or mode. One having no magnetic field component in the direction of propagation is called a transverse magnetic (TM) wave or mode. However, the waves are characterized by zero tangential components of electric field at the conducting walls. This leads to a characteristic set of values that determine the possible fields or modes in a given waveguide. The cutoff frequency and wavelength may be written as

$$(f_c)_{mn} = [1/2(\mu\varepsilon)^{1/2}][(m/a)^2 + (n/b)^2]^{1/2} \quad (2.72)$$

$$(\lambda_c)_{mn} = 2ab/(m^2b^2 + a^2n^2)^{1/2} \quad (2.73)$$

The cutoff frequency is the lowest source frequency below which no wave can propagate in the waveguide and the cutoff wavelength is the longest source wavelength above which wave propagation is not allowed in the waveguide for a given mode. There are therefore a doubly infinite number of possible modes for each wave type corresponding to all the combinations of the integers m and n. A transverse electric wave with m half-sine variations in the x direction and n half-sine variations in the y direction is denoted as a TE$_{mn}$ mode. A transverse magnetic wave with m half-sine in x, n in y, is denoted as a TM$_{mn}$ mode.

The mode with the lowest cutoff frequency in a particular waveguide is called the *dominant mode*. The dominant mode in a rectangular waveguide is the TE$_{10}$ mode. Higher values of m and n give higher-order modes, i.e., modes with higher cutoff frequencies. It is seen from (2.73) that the cutoff wavelength of the TE$_{10}$ mode is $\lambda_c = 2a$. That is, wave propagation can take place in a rectangular waveguide only when its widest side is greater than one-half the intrinsic wavelength of the dielectric material filling the waveguide.

The rectangular waveguide is usually operated so that only the dominant mode propagates. The important quantities for the TE$_{10}$ mode are summarized here. There are three components of the electric and magnetic fields:

$$E_y = E \sin\left(\frac{\pi x}{a}\right) e^{-\gamma z} \quad (2.74)$$

$$H_x = -\left(\frac{E}{Z_{TE}}\right) \sin\left(\frac{\pi x}{a}\right) e^{-\gamma z} \quad (2.75)$$

$$H_z = \frac{jE}{\eta}\left(\frac{f_c}{f}\right) \cos\left(\frac{\pi}{a}\right) e^{-\gamma z} \quad (2.76)$$

where η is the intrinsic impedance of the dielectric material filling the waveguide and f is the operating frequency. The cutoff frequency is given by

$$f_c = 1/2a(\mu\varepsilon)^{1/2} \tag{2.77}$$

and the characteristic impedance is given by

$$Z_{TE} = \eta/[1 - (f_c/f)^2]^{1/2} \tag{2.78}$$

The propagating factor $\gamma = \alpha + j\beta$ above cutoff reduces to $\gamma = j\beta$ when the medium is loss-free, and is given by

$$\gamma = j\beta = j\omega\{\mu\varepsilon[1 - (f_c/f)^2]\}^{1/2} \tag{2.79}$$

Attenuation due to lossy material filling the waveguide is characterized by

$$\alpha = \sigma\eta/2[1 - (f_c/f)^2]^{1/2} \tag{2.80}$$

Thus, the wave is attenuated in the direction of propagation when a lossy material fills the waveguide.

It is interesting to note that the forms of the attenuation produced by a lossy material are the same for all modes and in fact all shapes of waveguides. However, the amount of attenuation is a function of the cutoff frequency, which does depend on the waveguide and the mode.

The average power transfer along the waveguide can be obtained by integrating the axial component of the Poynting vector over the cross-sectional area. Thus,

$$P_d = \int_0^a \int_0^b \frac{1}{2}(E_y H_x^*) \, dx \, dy = \frac{ab |E|^2}{2Z_{TE}} e^{-2\alpha z} \tag{2.81}$$

The average power dissipation is given by the rate of decrease in P_a versus z,

$$P_a = -\frac{dP_d}{dz} = 2\alpha P_d = \frac{\alpha ab |E|^2}{Z_{TE}} e^{-2\alpha z} \tag{2.82}$$

This is the time-average rate of energy absorption due to a lossy material in the waveguide. When both lossy material and imperfectly conducting waveguide walls need to be considered, the total attenuation is given merely by the sum of the two losses.

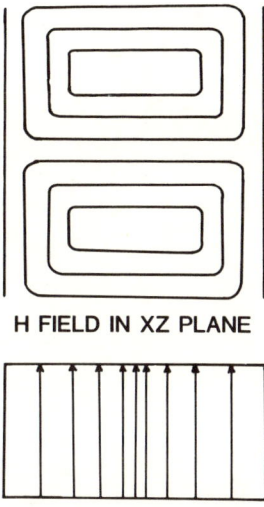

FIGURE 2-9. Electric and magnetic field distributions inside a rectangular waveguide (TE_{10} mode).

The field configuration or mode pattern for the TE_{10} mode is shown in Fig. 2-9. Note that the electric field component that passes between top and bottom of the guide does not vary in the y conducting walls, while varying as a half-sine curve in the x direction. The magnetic field forms closed paths surrounding the vertical electric field.

Many of the above concepts and expression apply very closely to the corresponding situation for the circular waveguide, but there are noticeable differences in field functions and structures. The modes that may exist in the circular waveguide are the higher-order TE and TM modes. The TE_{11} mode will propagate at a lower frequency than any other mode; it is therefore the dominant mode. As shown in Fig. 2-10a, the electric field for the TE_{11} mode in the circular waveguide is maximum in the center of the guide and the direction of the electric field is curved. The TE_{01} mode is of particular interest because of its low attenuation characteristics in practical waveguides having finite wall conductivity and circularly symmetric electric field distribution. It can be seen from Fig. 2-10 that the electric field forms concentric circles around the axis of the guide and has nulls at the center and the wall of the guide.

However, the use of the TE_{01} mode presents several problems that stem from the fact that it is not the mode with the lowest cutoff frequency. The guide must always be operated at a frequency where many modes can propagate. Any irregularity in the guide causes some of the power carried in the TE_{01} mode to be converted into power in other undesired modes (at least four if the operating frequency is just above

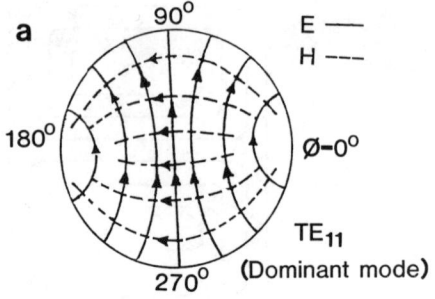

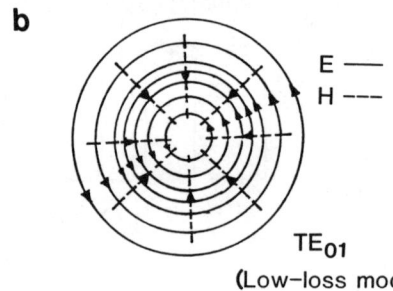

FIGURE 2-10. Electric field (———) and magnetic field (– – –) in hollow cylindrical waveguides for (a) TE_{11} (dominant mode) and (b) TE_{01} (low-loss mode).

cutoff: otherwise many more modes are in the propagating range). This in combination with different phase velocities of the several modes leads to distortion of the field. Fortunately, mode filters that discriminate against the undesired modes but cause negligible attenuation to the desired one can be devised to eliminate field distortion arising from this mode conversion (Collin, 1966).

2.3.2. Cavities

A radio or microwave cavity is a volume completely enclosed by conducting walls, with the electromagnetic energy confined to the inside. The cavities are used as the resonant elements in microwave circuits, as wavemeters to measure frequency, for converging microwave energy into foodstuff, as well as for many other applications. Since the principal difference between cavities of various shapes is the detailed field distribution, an understanding of the behavior of waves in rectangular cavities provides a clue to the operation of cavities of other shapes. In this section the basic properties of the simple rectangular cavity shown in Fig. 2-11 will be discussed in some detail.

An exact mathematical analysis based on the solution of Maxwell's equations subject to the boundary conditions may be obtained for the electric and magnetic fields. However, the electric and magnetic fields

PHYSICAL DESCRIPTION OF RF RADIATION

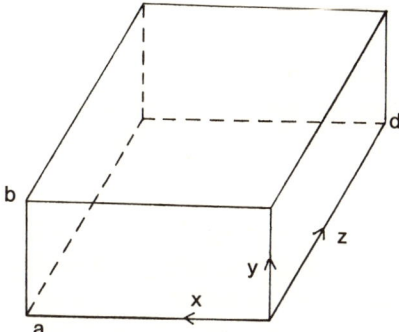

FIGURE 2-11. A rectangular cavity.

inside the rectangular cavity are readily constructed from physical arguments and from the corresponding solutions for the rectangular waveguide. For example, the cavity in Fig. 2-12 may be considered as a part of the rectangular waveguide. The desired field solutions are expressions having zero tangential components of the electric field over the entire metallic boundary. The TE_{10} mode already satisfies this

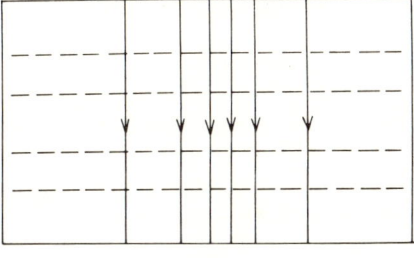

SIDE

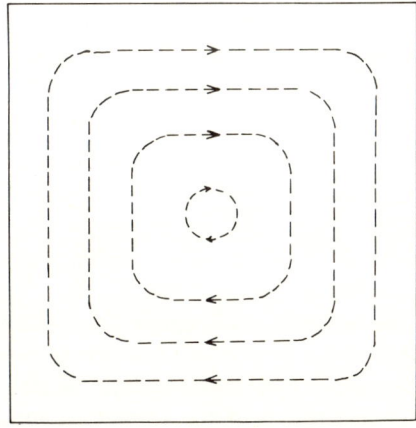

FIGURE 2-12. Electric field (———) and magnetic field (- - -) in an empty cavity for TE_{101} mode.

TOP

condition over four of the walls. Let a TE_{10} mode propagate in the positive z direction, and let a conducting plate be placed at $z = d$, complete reflection will take place. The electric field in a loss-free medium according to (2.67) will be

$$E_y = -2jE \sin(\pi x/a)\sin \beta z \qquad (2.83)$$

At any plane where $\sin \beta z$ vanishes, another conducting plate can be placed to obtain a rectangular cavity. On the other hand, if the ends of the cavity are chosen at $z = 0$ and $z = d$, then

$$\sin \beta d = 0$$

or

$$\beta = p\pi/d, \quad p = 1, 2, 3, \ldots \qquad (2.84)$$

For the TE_{10} mode with a single half-sine variation along z, $p = 1$ and $\beta = \pi/d$, therefore according to (2.72), we have

$$2\pi fd\{\mu\varepsilon[1 - (f_c/f)^2]\}^{1/2} = 2\pi fd[\mu\varepsilon - (1/2af)^2]^{1/2} = \pi \qquad (2.85)$$

The resonant frequency $f = f_s$ is obtained from solving (2.78), i.e.,

$$f_s = (1/2ad)[(a^2 + d^2)/\mu\varepsilon]^{1/2} \qquad (2.86)$$

The mode of oscillation is designated as the TE_{101} mode, since there is only a single standing wave variation in the x and z directions and none in the y direction. The solutions for the magnetic field components associated with the TE_{101} mode are

$$H_x = \frac{2aE}{\eta(a^2 + d^2)^{1/2}} \sin\left(\frac{\pi x}{a}\right)\cos\left(\frac{\pi z}{d}\right) \qquad (2.87)$$

$$H_z = -\frac{2dE}{\eta(a^2 + d^2)^{1/2}} \cos\left(\frac{\pi x}{a}\right)\sin\left(\frac{\pi z}{d}\right) \qquad (2.88)$$

The electric and magnetic fields in a cavity are 90° out of phase; therefore, E is maximum when H is minimum and vice versa. The field distributions at some instant of time are shown in Fig. 2-12. It is seen that the electric field for the TE_{101} mode is greatest near the center of the cavity.

PHYSICAL DESCRIPTION OF RF RADIATION

In addition to the TE_{101} mode, there are an infinite number of possible modes of oscillation in a rectangular cavity corresponding to the TE and TM waveguide modes. The resonant frequencies for the higher-order modes are given by the expression

$$f_r = \frac{1}{2(\mu\varepsilon)^{1/2}} \left[\left(\frac{m}{a}\right)^2 + \left(\frac{n}{b}\right)^2 + \left(\frac{p}{d}\right)^2 \right]^{1/2} \qquad (2.89)$$

The time-averaged electric and magnetic energies stored in the cavity are equal. Since the total energy stored in the cavity is independent of time, therefore,

$$W = 2(\varepsilon/4) \iiint_{\text{cavity}} E^2 \, dv \qquad (2.90)$$

where ε is the dielectric constant for the material filling the cavity and **E** is the magnitude of the electric field strength. Thus, from (2.83) and (2.90) the total time-averaged energy stored in a rectangular cavity supporting a TE_{101} mode is

$$W = (1/8) abd\varepsilon E^2 \qquad (2.91)$$

In the absence of dielectric loss, the cavity oscillations may build up the field strengths to very large values. A relatively small amount of energy is needed to compensate for the energy lost to the finite conductivity of the walls. The relatively large amount of stored energy is essentially constant and passing back and forth between electric and magnetic fields. If there are imperfections in the construction and losses in the dielectric material filling the cavity, either partially or completely, extra energy must then be supplied to sustain the electromagnetic field oscillations inside the cavity.

2.3.3. Waveguide and Cavity Excitation

Electromagnetic waves in cavities and waveguides may be excited or coupled to coaxial transmission lines by means of small loops or probes. Loops are used to couple to the magnetic field of the wave and are therefore located at a point where the magnetic field is large and its direction normal to the plane of the loop. Probes must be introduced in the direction of the electric field and located at a point where the electric field is maximum.

Moreover, the cavity may be coupled to a waveguide by means of a small hole in a common wall between the cavity and a driving waveguide. The hole must be located so that some field component in the cavity has a

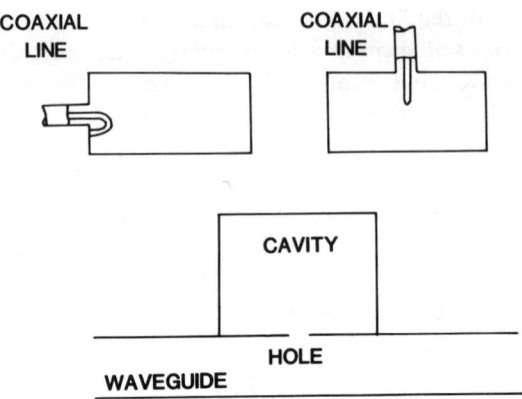

FIGURE 2-13. Methods for exciting electromagnetic waves in waveguides and cavities.

direction common to that in the waveguide. These coupling methods are illustrated in Fig. 2-13.

2.4. RADIATION OF ELECTROMAGNETIC ENERGY

Radio and microwaves are radiated into space or material media through antennas or radiators that serve as transitions between the transmission system and space or material medium. Thus, an antenna can also be used as a device to receive radio and microwave radiation. The distribution of electromagnetic energy from an antenna as a function of direction is given by the *antenna pattern.* The pattern usually consists of several lobes. The lobe with the largest maximum is referred to as the main lobe, while the smaller lobes are called minor or side lobes. If the pattern is measured sufficiently far from the antenna so that there is no change in pattern with distance, the pattern is called the far-field or radiation pattern. Measurement at lesser distances gives near-field patterns, which are functions of both angle and distance.

Generally speaking, antennas involved in biomedical applications are of the order of one wavelength in size, and include such diverse types as dipoles, slots, horns, and apertures. Their far-field radiated energy is distributed broadly in space. Therefore, these antennas are referred to as broad-beam antennas. Another class of antennas, called narrow-beam antennas, radiate energy into small volumes and are mostly used in communication and target acquisition situations.

Another important parameter of an antenna is the *power gain,* or simply the gain, G, of an antenna; this may be defined as the ratio of the maximum radiation intensity to the radiation intensity from a lossless isotropic antenna radiating the same total power. In this case the radiation intensity is the average power radiated per unit solid angle and an isotropic antenna is one that radiates uniformly in all directions. It should be noted that the gains of an antenna may also be defined with respect to any reference antenna. Furthermore, the gain of an antenna is applicable to all antennas regardless of its particular function. That is, the gain of an antenna where used for transmitting is the same as its gain where used for receiving.

The near- and far-field characteristics of radio and microwave antennas will be briefly discussed using the example of a short dipole. The short dipole is an elementary antenna but a very important one theoretically. For example, any linear antenna may be regarded as a series of short dipoles, and large antennas of other shapes may be regarded as being composed of many short dipoles. Thus, a knowledge of the properties of the short dipole is useful in determining the properties of larger antennas of complex shape.

2.4.1. The Short Dipole

For the short dipole illustrated in Fig. 2-14, the length l is short compared with a wavelength ($l \ll \lambda$) and the diameter is small compared with its length. It is energized by a transmission line that does not radiate. Hence, for purposes of analysis the short dipole may be considered simply as a thin conductor of length l carrying a uniform current I. It can be shown (Jordan and Balmain, 1968) that the electric and magnetic fields from the dipole have only three components E_θ, E_ϕ, and H_ϕ in the spherical coordinate system (Fig. 2-15) and are given by

$$E_r = \frac{\eta I l e^{j(\omega t - \beta r)} \cos \theta}{2\pi} \left(\frac{1}{r^2} + \frac{1}{j\beta r^3} \right) \quad (2.92)$$

$$E_\theta = \frac{\eta I l e^{j(\omega t - \beta r)} \sin \theta}{4\pi} \left(\frac{j\beta}{r} + \frac{1}{r^2} + \frac{1}{j\beta r^3} \right) \quad (2.93)$$

$$H_\phi = \frac{I l e^{j(\omega t - \beta r)} \sin \theta}{4\pi} \left(\frac{j\beta}{r} + \frac{1}{r^2} \right) \quad (2.94)$$

The components E_ϕ, H_r, and H_θ are zero at all points.

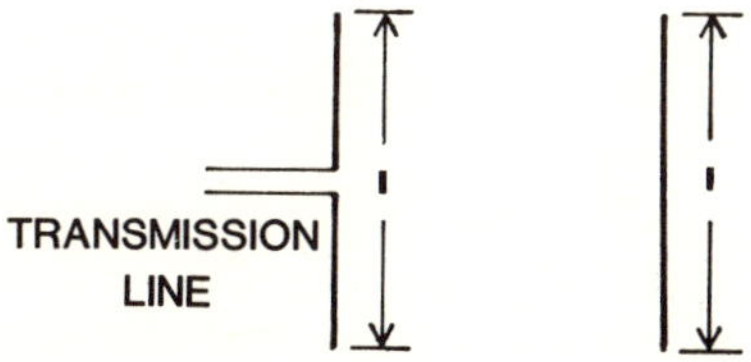

FIGURE 2-14. The short dipole antenna fed by a 2-conductor transmission line and its mathematical equivalent.

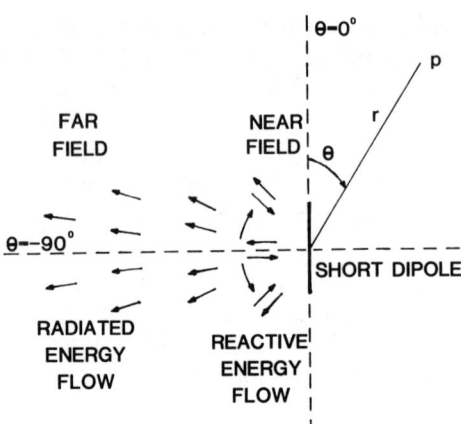

FIGURE 2-15. Energy flow in the near and far fields of a short dipole. (From Kraus and Carver, 1973.)

At points far from the dipole, r is large, the terms involving $1/r^2$ and $1/r^3$ in (2.92)–(2.94) can be neglected in comparison with terms involving $1/r$. Thus, in the *far field*, there are only two field components given by

$$E_\theta = j(\eta I \beta l / 4\pi r) e^{j(\omega t - \beta r)} \sin \theta \qquad (2.95)$$

$$H_\phi = j(I \beta l / 4\pi r) e^{j(\omega t - \beta r)} \sin \theta \qquad (2.96)$$

It is seen that the wave impedance in the far field, i.e., the ratio of E_θ to H_ϕ as given by (2.95) and (2.96), is the same as the intrinsic impedance of the medium. Also, E_θ and H_ϕ in the far field are in time phase and at right angles to each other. Thus, the electric and magnetic fields in the far field of a short dipole are related in the same fashion as in a plane wave. Further, the direction and time-average flow of energy per unit area are given by the Poynting vector (2.33 and 2.34),

$$\mathbf{P} = \eta (I \beta l / 4\pi r)^2 \sin^2 \theta \hat{r} \qquad (2.97)$$

Clearly, energy flow in the far field is real and is entirely in the radial direction. The energy is hence radiated, and the term *radiation field* is synonymous with *far field*. In the far field, the intensity of radiated energy decreases as $1/r^2$ with increasing distance.

It is instructive to separate the far-field expression of (2.95) and (2.96) into seven basic physical quantities. For example, E_θ may be written as

$$E_\theta = \tfrac{1}{2} I (l/\lambda)(1/r) \eta j e^{j(\omega t - \beta r)} \sin \theta \qquad (2.98)$$

where 1/2 is a constant (magnitude) factor, I is the dipole current, l/λ is the dipole length expressed in wavelengths, $1/r$ is the distance factor, η is the intrinsic impedance of the medium, $je^{j(\omega t - \beta r)}$ is the phase factor, and $\sin \theta$ is the pattern factor specifying the field variation with angle. In general, the far-field description of any antenna will involve these seven factors.

2.4.2. Near Fields

Examination of the expressions for E_r, and E_θ and H_ϕ shows that, at points close to the short dipole where r is small, the $1/r^2$ and $1/r^3$ terms become predominant and equations (2.92)–(2.94) reduced to

$$E_r = -j(\eta Il/2\pi\beta r^3)e^{j(\omega t - \beta r)} \cos \theta \tag{2.99}$$

$$E_\theta = -j(\eta Il/4\pi\beta r^3)e^{j(\omega t - \beta r)} \sin \theta \tag{2.100}$$

$$H_\phi = (Il/4\pi r^2)e^{j(\omega t - \beta r)} \sin \theta \tag{2.101}$$

Consequently, both components of the electric field are in time quadrature with the magnetic field. Thus, the electric and magnetic fields in the near field are related as in a standing wave. The maxima and minima of electric and magnetic field do not occur at the same point in space. The ratio of electric to magnetic field strength varies from point to point, giving rise to widely divergent field impedances.

Furthermore, the terms that vary as $1/r^3$ in the expression for E_r and E_θ correspond exactly to the field of an oscillatory electrostatic dipole; these $1/r^3$ terms are referred to as *electrostatic fields*. The terms that vary inversely as r^2 are just the fields that would be obtained by a direct application of Ampere's law. Thus, the field represented by the $1/r^2$ term is called the *induction field* and becomes predominant at points close to the dipole.

If the Poynting vector is invoked, it will be clear that the electrostatic and induction terms contribute to energy that is stored in the field during one-quarter of a cycle and returned to the dipole during the next without any net or average outward flow. In the near field the energy flow is largely reactive; only the $1/r$ terms contribute to an average outward flow of energy. The energy transfer characteristics are illustrated in Fig. 2-15 where the arrows represent the direction of energy flow at successive instants of time (Kraus and Carver, 1973).

The criterion of distance most commonly used to demarcate near and far fields is that the phase variation of the field from the antenna not exceed $\lambda/16$ (Silver, 1949). This boundary occurs at a conservative distance of

$$R = 2D^2/\lambda \tag{2.102}$$

where D represents the largest dimension of the antenna aperture. In the far field, the field strengths decrease as $1/r$, and only transverse field components appear. The near field can be divided into two subregions: the radiative near-field region and the reactive near-field region. In the *radiative near-field region*, the region closer than $2D^2/\lambda$, the radiation pattern varies with the distance from the antenna. The region of space surrounding the antenna in which the reactive components predominate is known as the *reactive near-field region*. The extent of this region varies for different antennas. For most antennas, however, the outer limit is of the order of a few wavelengths or less. For the special case of a short dipole, the reactive component predominates to a distance of approximately $\lambda/2\pi$, where the radiating and reactive components are equal.

The three field regions are illustrated in Fig. 2-16. In this case, the boundary between the radiative and reactive near-field regions has been conservatively assumed to be 1λ away from the antenna (Hansen, 1964). It should be noted that at low frequencies, the wavelengths are long, and the induction field may extend to very large distances from the source. The corresponding wavelengths at high frequencies are quite short, and the induction field may not exist at all.

In the far-field region, the electric and magnetic fields are outgoing waves with plane wavefronts and the power density along the axis of the antenna in free space is given by

$$P_c = PG/4\pi r^2 \tag{2.103}$$

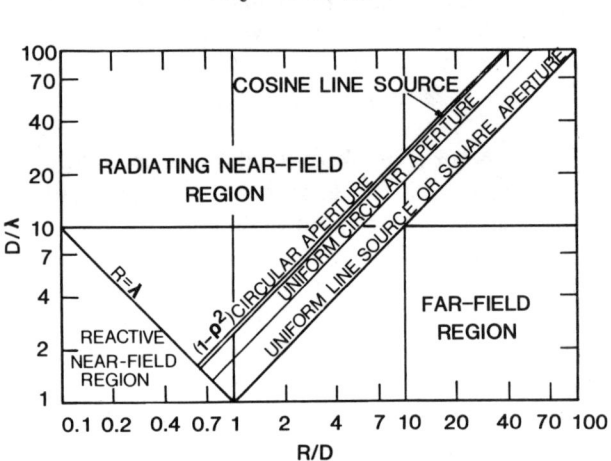

FIGURE 2-16. The three field regions surrounding an antenna. (From Hansen, 1964.)

where P is the total radiated power, G is the gain of the antenna, and r is the distance from the antenna. Clearly, in the far field, the power density along the beam axis falls off inversely with the square of the distance.

Power density in the near field is not as uniquely defined as in the far field, since the electric and magnetic fields and their ratio vary from point to point. Further, the angular distribution is actually dependent on the distance from the antenna. It is therefore necessary to individually arrive at a quantitative estimate of the power density even along the axis. In general, the near-field power density depends on the antenna shape and aperture field distribution. Analyses have been reported for several types of antennas (Hansen, 1964). Figure 2-17 illustrates the calculated on-axis power density for a uniform line source such as a narrow slot on a rectangular waveguide. The values are normalized to unity at $R = 2D^2/\lambda$. Observe the $1/R$ dependence in the reactive near-field region and the merging of oscillations with the $1/R^2$ line as the distance gets closer to $2D^2/\lambda$ (actually starts at D^2/λ).

The square antenna on-axis power density is shown in Fig. 2-18, where the dashed line indicates the envelope of maximum power density obtained. It is seen that at points close to the antenna ($2D^2/\lambda < 0.1$), the power density oscillates about a normalized value of 4.5. It reaches a peak normalized value of 13.3 at $0.18D^2/\lambda$ in the radiative near-field region. But the power density falls below the $1/R^2$ value for distances less than D^2/λ. The on-axis power density for a circular aperture is given in Fig. 2-19. The normalized value at a point close to the antenna is about 26. The peak power density occurs at about $0.2D^2/\lambda$ and is nearly 42 times the value at $2D^2/\lambda$.

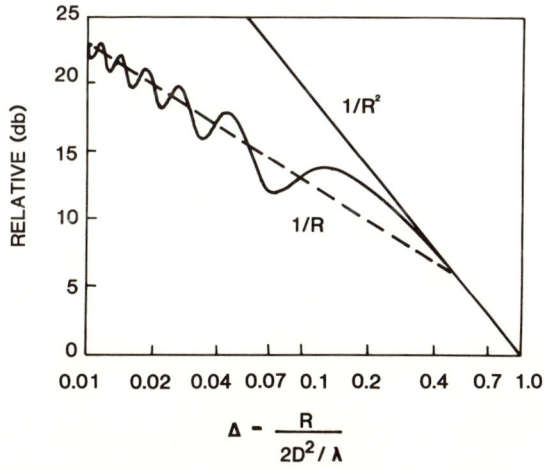

FIGURE 2-17. The on-axis power density of a uniform line source. (From Hansen, 1964.)

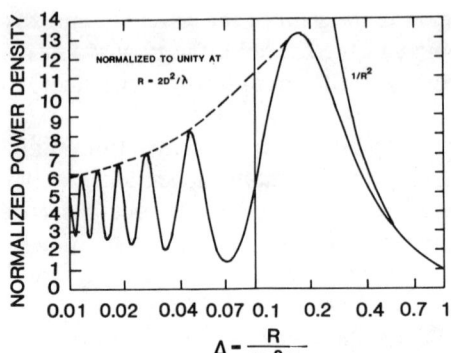

FIGURE 2-18. The on-axis power density of a uniform square antenna. (From Hansen, 1964.)

These graphical data indicate that the transition point between reactive and radiative near-field regions occurs from 0.2 to 0.4 D^2/λ. Moreover, they give average and maximum near-field power densities such that for

1. Square antenna with uniform field distribution:

$$P_d = 0.88 P/A \text{ average} \tag{2.104}$$

$$P_d = 2.61 P/A \text{ maximum} \tag{2.105}$$

2. Circular antenna with uniform field distribution:

$$P_d = 3.01 P/A \text{ average} \tag{2.106}$$

$$P_d = 4.86 P/A \text{ maximum} \tag{2.107}$$

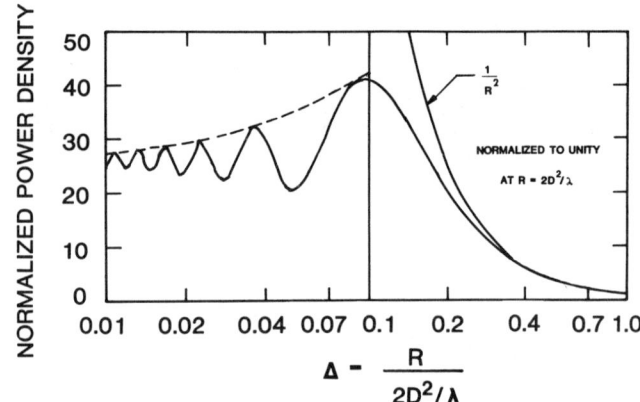

FIGURE 2-19. The on-axis power density of a tapered circular aperture. (From Hansen, 1964.)

where P is the total radiated power and A is the area of the antenna. Thus, the maximum near-field power density that can exist on the axis of a practical aperture antenna is about $5P/A$. It should be noted that these formulas do not include the effect of ground reflections, which could cause a value of power density that is four times the free-space volume (Mumford, 1961). Thus, the electromagnetic radiation in the far field is quite different from that in the near field although there is a smooth transition from one to the other. It is important to note that radiation is largely confined to within a cylinder whose cross section is the antenna aperture until the distance from the antenna approaches the transition range. This characteristic is also indicated by the on-axis power density, which at large distances varies inversely as the square of the distance but in the near field oscillates about a constant value.

2.4.3. Receiving Characteristics

Thus far, we have been mainly concerned with transmitting antennas that radiate energy. As mentioned earlier, an antenna can also be used to receive radio and microwave radiation. This is because the performance of an antenna when used for transmitting is the same as its performance when used for receiving according to the *reciprocity theorem*. However, a more direct characterization of receiving antenna performance is effective cross section or effective area. The *effective cross section* is defined as the area of an ideal antenna that absorbs the same amount of energy from an incident plane wave as the actual antenna. The effective cross section has particular significance when applied to horns and reflector antennas that have well-defined physical apertures. For these antennas the ratio of the effective cross section to the actual aperture is a direct measure of the antennas' effectiveness in radiating or receiving the energy to or from the desired direction. Normal values of this ratio for reflector antennas vary from 45% to 75%, depending on antenna type and design, with 65% considered rather good for the commonly used parabolic reflector antenna (Jordan and Balmain, 1968).

The total power or rate of energy extracted by a receiving antenna with the effective cross section S from an incident plane wave is therefore given by

$$P = P_d S \qquad (2.108)$$

Since the effective cross section is related to the gain of an antenna through

$$S = (\lambda^2/4\pi)G \qquad (2.109)$$

the total power received in the field of impinging plane wave for any antenna is

$$P = (\lambda^2/4\pi)P_d G \tag{2.110}$$

In particular, it can be shown that the rate of energy extraction for the short dipole antenna illustrated in Fig. 2-14 is

$$P = 1.5(\lambda^2/4\pi)P_d \tag{2.111}$$

A special case of interest is that of a thin dipole antenna of finite length, l. For this case, the maximum gain is (Harrington, 1961)

$$G = (\eta/\pi R_r)(1 - \cos \beta l/2)^2 \tag{2.112}$$

where η is the intrinsic impedance of the medium and R_r is the radiation resistance of an antenna defined by analogy to Ohm's law as

$$R_r = P/|I|^2 \tag{2.113}$$

where I is the antenna current. A graph of R_r versus l is shown in Fig. 2-20. The total received power is found using (2.110) as

$$P = (\eta \lambda^2 P_d / 4\pi^2 R_r)(1 - \cos \beta l/2)^2 \tag{2.114}$$

Because of the cosine term and the R_r term in the denominator of (2.114), the total power received or rate of energy extracted by a thin dipole antenna reaches a peak as a function of the antenna length expressed in terms of wavelength. That is, the antenna exhibits resonant

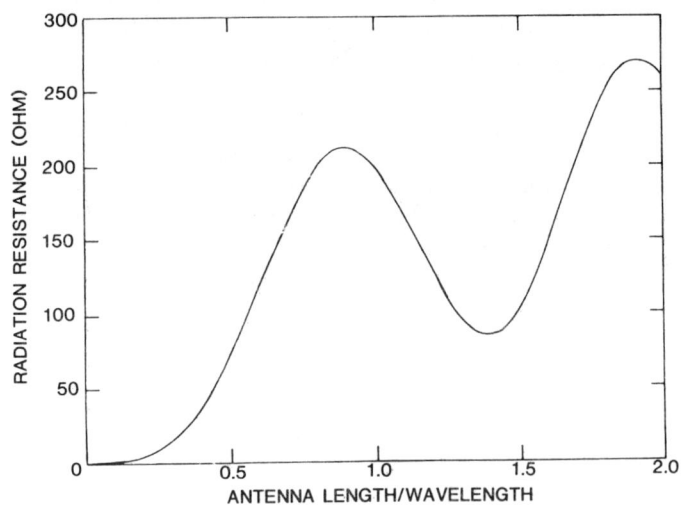

FIGURE 2-20. The radiation resistance of a dipole antenna.

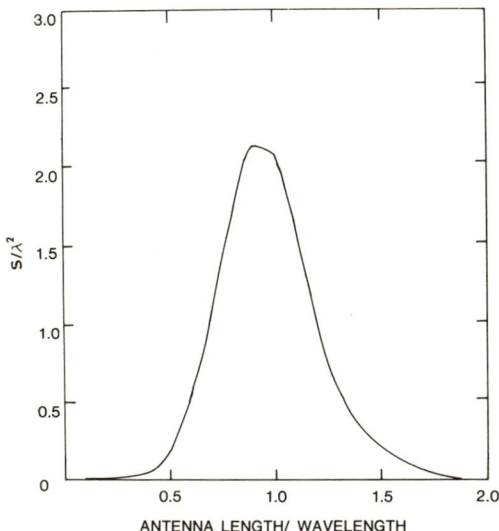

FIGURE 2-21. Resonant absorption characteristics of dipoles.

receiving characteristics. The total energy extracted from an impinging plane wave peaks for selected antenna lengths. The first of the resonant lengths occurs at a length l and equals 0.9λ (Fig. 2-21). These results are useful in both qualitative and quantitative descriptions of the coupling of radio and microwaves into biological bodies.

REFERENCES

Adams, S. F. (1969) *Microwave Theory and Applications*. Prentice-Hall, Englewood Cliffs, N.J.
Collin, R. E. (1966) *Foundations for Microwave Engineering*. McGraw-Hill, New York.
Collin, R. E., and F. Zucker (1969) *Microwave Antenna Theory and Design*. McGraw-Hill, New York.
Gandhi, O. P. (1981) *Microwave Engineering and Application*. Pergamon Press, New York.
Hansen, R. C. (ed.) (1964) *Microwave Scanning Antennas*, Vol. 1. Academic Press, New York.
Harrington, R. F. (1961) *Time Harmonic Electromagnetic Fields*. McGraw-Hill, New York.
Harvey, A. F. (1963) *Microwave Engineering*. Academic Press, New York.
Jordan, E. C., and K. G. Balmain (1968) *Electromagnetic Waves and Radiating Systems*. Prentice-Hall, Englewood Cliffs, N.J.
Kraus, J. F., and K. R. Carver (1973) *Electromagnetics*. McGraw-Hill, New York.
Mumford, W. W. (1961) Some technical aspects of microwave radiation hazards. *Proc. IRE* **49:**427.
Ramo, S., J. R. Whinnery, and T. Van Duzer (1965) *Fields and Waves in Communication Electronics*. Wiley, New York.
Silver, S. (ed.) (1949) *Microwave Antenna Theory and Design*. McGraw-Hill, New York.

3

Radio and Microwave Dosimetry and Measurement

Progress in understanding electromagnetic interaction with biological systems is closely linked to the advances in measurement capability. Measurement provides the means to describe physical phenomena in quantitative terms. As our ability to describe these phenomena with precision and reliability increases, the opportunity of advancing our understanding of the laws of nature increases and the capability of making use of this understanding also increases. Furthermore, the growing significance of international cooperation to arrive at a meaningful safety standard has made valid measurement a necessary means for the international exchange of scientific and engineering results.

This chapter begins with a description of the physical quantities relevant to radio and microwave interaction with biological systems and mentions the generally accepted units of measure for these quantities. In order to make constructive use of this quantitative information, there must be a means of measuring and controlling the relevant quantities. The remainder of the chapter describes techniques for irradiation of biological specimens in the laboratory and methods for measuring relevant electromagnetic quantities.

3.1. QUANTITIES AND UNITS

Many different concepts and quantities have been proposed and used to characterize propagation and absorption of electromagnetic energy in biological systems (Justesen, 1975). Some of the quantities and units that are now in use will be briefly described in this section.

Power density is the time rate of energy flow per unit area across a surface and is given by the value of the Poynting vector (equation 2.33) in watts per square meter, milliwatts per square centimeter, or microwatts per square centimeter. It expresses exposure in terms of incident power per unit area.

Specific absorption rate (SAR) is the time rate of energy absorption per gram of tissue from nonionizing electromagnetic radiation. It is expressed in watts per kilogram or milliwatts per gram and is the same as the absorbed-power density defined in the previous chapter. It is important that the term *whole-body SAR* is used to specify whole-body absorbed-power density to recognize the fact that the same SAR (in W/Kg) for whole-body and local absorption does not necessarily produce the same degree of biological response.

The term *SAR distribution* is used to indicate the SAR pattern inside the body. Incident radiation, body geometry, and orientation as well as dielectric property affect the SAR distribution. A highly nonuniform SAR distribution may result from a plane wave impinging on a biological object.

At lower frequencies, and under near-field irradiation conditions, the electric field strength and the magnetic field strength are used instead of power density to express the exposure. The field strengths may either be calculated or measured in the absence of the experimental object.

Furthermore, field strengths are useful measures for quantifying biological interactions that are field specific. In this case, the terms *internal electric* and *internal magnetic field strengths* may be used. They are expressed in volts per meter and amperes per meter, respectively. They are appropriate units for specifying incident as well as internal fields.

3.2. IRRADIATION OF BIOLOGICAL SYSTEMS

There are many different methods for irradiation of biological objects. The choice depends on the frequency, the power density required, the duration of exposure, the desired SAR and its distribution, the biological system involved, and the intent of the radiation. The various irradiation methods can be classified into two general categories: partial-body and whole-body or whole-organism irradiation. Each of these categories allows an abundant array of experimental arrangements.

3.2.1. Applicators for Partial-Body Irradiation

Partial-body irradiation procedures presently in use utilize two basic schemes for coupling microwave energy into tissue media: noncontact and direct-contact methods. In the noncontact case, antennas or applicators are normally spaced at a distance of 1.0 to 5.0 cm from the subject and may scatter microwave energy, which can result in unnecessary exposure to the subject and the experimenter. Since therapeutic applications require substantial power, direct-contact methods that minimize scattered radiation are preferred over noncontact ones. On the other hand, scattered radiation is employed in many diagnostic applications. Hence, both noncontact and direct-contact methods are useful. In this section, we describe several direct-contact applicators.

The direct-contact applicator is a good approach to localize electromagnetic energy to a particular area of the specimen. It is designed to operate in intimate contact with the surface of the body to be irradiated (Guy and Lehmann, 1966). The applicator is often filled with a low-loss dielectric material whose dielectric constant matches either that of the skin or that of the fat layer. In this way, the size of the applicator may be considerably reduced and energy coupling takes place entirely within the dielectric medium. Furthermore, this approach increases the coupling efficiency between the antenna and deep-lying tissues and reduces the power required for a given quantity of absorbed energy.

Among the many direct-contact applicators that have been developed, applicators operating at 915 and 2450 MHz are most widely used. Three such applicators are illustrated in Fig. 3-1. They all yield a relatively uniform SAR distribution and produce the highest temperature rise in muscles.

The 13-cm square applicator (Fig. 3-1a) is designed for 915-MHz operation with surface cooling capability (Guy *et al.*, 1978). It consists of a transition from a coaxial connector to a stripline power splitter that feeds power to the two side-by-side rectangular waveguides filled with a porous, lightweight, low-loss dielectric material. The applicator is equipped with an air inlet (on the back of the applicator) so that cooled air can be forced through the porous dielectric and a radome onto the surface to cool the skin and underlying subcutaneous tissue.

The 15.2-cm-diameter circular applicator (Fig. 3-1b) is designed for 2450-MHz operation (Kantor *et al.*, 1978). It consists of a circular waveguide and conically-flared horn output section that is surrounded by an annular choke to control radiation leakage. The waveguide is fed by a probe through a coaxial connector. Two sets of posts are placed in the

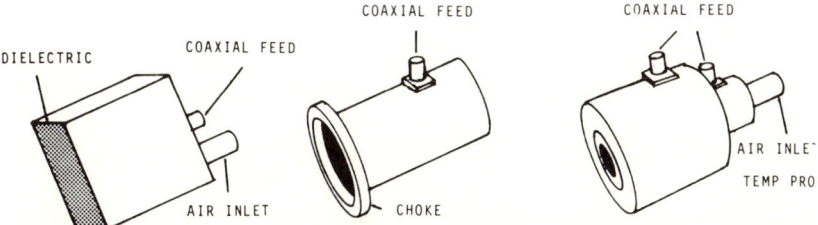

FIGURE 3-1. Three direct-contact microwave applicators: (a) 915-MHz square applicator; (b) 2450-MHz circular applicator; (c) 2450-MHz coaxial applicator.

forward portion of the waveguide to generate a circularly polarized wave. A resistive card is mounted at the center of the back-plate to minimize any mismatch that may result from tissue loading. This applicator does not have any provision for surface cooling.

The 10.2-cm-diameter coaxial applicator (Fig. 3-1c) is designed for dual-beam 2450-MHz operation (Lin *et al.*, 1978). It consists of three concentric, cylindrical tubes. Microwave energy is introduced into the outer and middle coaxial waveguide via coax-to-waveguide transitions that give rise to TE_{21} and TE_{11} modes of propagation, respectively. The TE_{21} mode has a null along the axis, while the TE_{11} mode is maximum along this direction. This produces a broad, combined heating pattern without a sharp temperature gradient. The applicator has several advantages over others in that the inner cylinder is inactive and serves as an inlet for circulating coolant to reduce surface temperature and as a port for inserting temperature-monitoring devices. It may also be used as a port for introducing ionizing radiation in combination therapy for cancer.

A comparison of some of the performance characteristics of these direct-contact applicators is given in Table 3-1. The maximum SARs were determined using planar fat–muscle models and thermographic procedures, and the power density measurements were made in the vicinity of the applicators in contact with the tissue-substitute models by using Narda 8300 meters. It can be seen that the input power required to produce an SAR of 150 W/kg in muscle was the highest for the square applicator, and leakage radiation at a distance of 5 cm from the applicator housing was either below or at 5 mW/cm^2.

Recent development in stripline design has yielded a number of stripline applicators whose characteristics are comparable to those described above. The stripline radiators are especially suited for direct-contact applications. They are lightweight, small, and capable of conforming to the body's contour. When properly designed, they may allow the subject to move about with only minimal restriction (Bahl *et al.*, 1980).

The strip applicator shown in Fig. 3-2a consists of a surface strip

TABLE 3-1
A Comparison of Direct-Contact Applicators

Type	Frequency (MHz)	Input power (W)	SAR (W/kg)	Leakage at 5 cm (mW/cm^2)
Square	915	50	150	5
Circular	2450	12.5	150	0.1
Coaxial	2450	17	150	0.3

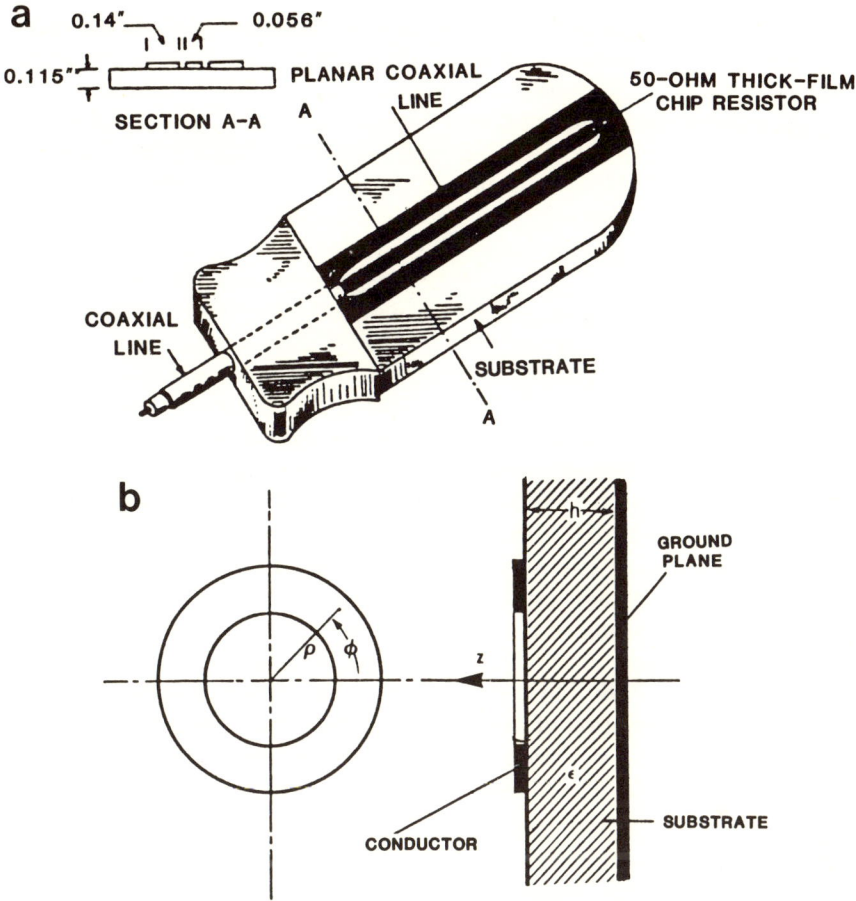

FIGURE 3-2. Stripline applicators: (a) coaxial transmission line applicator; (b) ring-type stripline applicator.

transmission line on a dielectric substrate that is terminated in a 50-ohm thick-film chip resistor. Microwave energy fed into the applicator via a flexible coaxial cable is confined to the regions around the transmission line and between the center conductor and ground planes on both sides of the center strip. When the applicator is placed in contact with the body surface, energy is efficiently transferred from the transmission line to the body through the discontinuity created at the contact area with minimal external leakage radiation. The energy coupling is maximal at the contact region and rapidly decreases with distance away from the contact region.

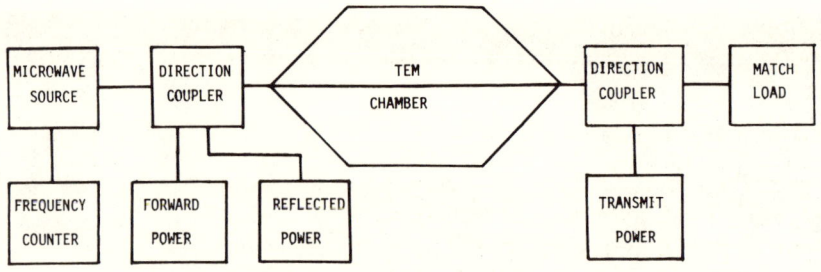

FIGURE 3-4. Instrumentation system for irradiation with TEM chamber.

The field or power density in the plane midway between the center conducting strip and the chamber wall is fairly uniform (Baird, 1974; Lin *et al.,* 1979b). The introduction of a biological specimen into the chamber alters the field distribution slightly, if the maximum dimensions of the specimen are less than a third of the transverse chamber dimension.

TEM chambers can be used to mimic free-space, near-field, and grounded conditions. The free-space or plane wave irradiation condition is obtained when the chamber is terminated in its characteristic impedance (50 ohms) and is the usual mode of operation. In the near-field case, field impedances vary from well below to values that are considerably above the free-space impedance of 377 ohms. This wide range of field impedances can be obtained by changing the termination from short circuit configuration through configurations with an endless combination of inductive and capacitive load and open circuit configuration. The differing load configurations give rise to reflections inside the chamber and result in standing waves with field impedances that range from zero to infinity. Finally, the grounded condition can be simulated by bringing the specimen in contact with the chamber and can be applied to near-field situations with variable impedances as well.

The TEM chambers can be made in various sizes to suit the experimental requirements. The width of the chamber must, however, be less than one-half the wavelength at the highest operating frequency to prevent higher-order-mode or multimoding effects, which result in complicated field distributions. The TEM chambers presently in use have upper frequency limits of 50, 150, 300, 500, and 1000 MHz. They provide electric field strengths from very low to extremely high values depending on the input power available. It is important to note that at higher frequencies the chambers are compact, portable, simple to build, and can be used for broadband operation up to the upper frequency limit. They also furnish fairly uniform and calculable fields. The major disadvantage of the TEM chamber is the restriction on specimen size imposed by the chamber dimensions, which is inversely proportional to the upper frequency limit (Donaldson *et al.*, 1978).

3.2.3. Microstrip Exposure Systems

Several methods have been developed for acute irradiation of small specimens, cell suspensions, and subcellular organelles under precisely controlled field and temperature conditions. They include coaxial transmission lines (Elder *et al.*, 1976; Guy, 1977), fluid-filled rectangular waveguide chambers (Courtney *et al.*, 1975; Lin, 1976), and compact microstrips (Friend and Howe, 1980). Figure 3-5 shows the configuration of a microstrip irradiator that was developed for 2450-MHz operation. The $8 \times 8 \times 3$-mm cavity provides a volume of about 200 mm^3, which is adequate for many biochemical and biophysical investigations. The electric field lines are straight and parallel, except in regions close to the edges, where fringing effects cause field distortions. It is estimated that the field is uniform over 90% of the chamber volume. Fluid channels are provided at two opposite corners of the chamber to facilitate fluid circulation and are perpendicular to the microstrip line to minimize field interference.

The system is matched to a 50-ohm transmission line when the cavity is empty and about 15% of the incident energy is absorbed when the chamber is filled with physiological saline solution. The system is unique in that it is self-contained and simple to operate. The external connections required are a microwave source and a power meter. Built-in directional couplers and a three-way switch allow determinations of rates

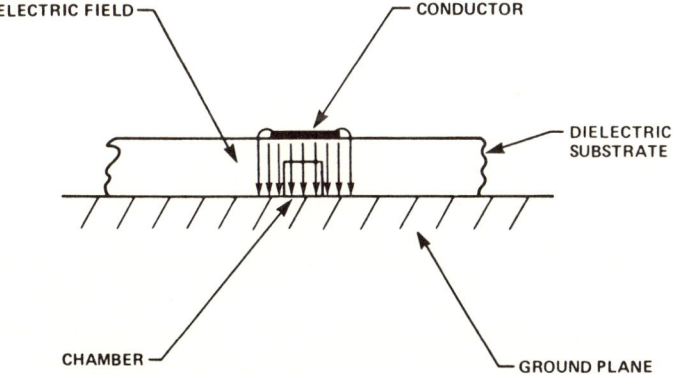

FIGURE 3-5. Configuration for microstrip irradiation chamber.

of absorbed energy by simple subtraction of the reflected and transmitted powers from the incident power. These measured parameters may then be used to calculate the field strength or power density by considering the boundary conditions and allowable solutions to the wave equation.

3.2.4. Waveguide Chambers

Hollow waveguide irradiation systems may be used to achieve a substantial exposure level with considerable less source power. Their small sizes make them most useful over frequencies in the gigahertz range. The fields inside a waveguide can be accurately calculated (Section 2.3) and, in some cases, are sufficiently uniform to justify it as the exposure method of choice.

A typical rectangular waveguide exposure system is illustrated in Fig. 3-6, which also shows some of the computerized data acquisition equipment that can be used with this exposure system. A matched resistive load is connected to the output end to prevent standing waves from occurring in the waveguide chamber. The whole-body SAR is determined through measurement of forward S_f, reflected S_r, and transmitted S_t powers using

$$\text{Whole-body SAR} = (S_f - S_r - S_t)/M \tag{3.3}$$

where M is the body mass and the loss due to imperfectly conducting

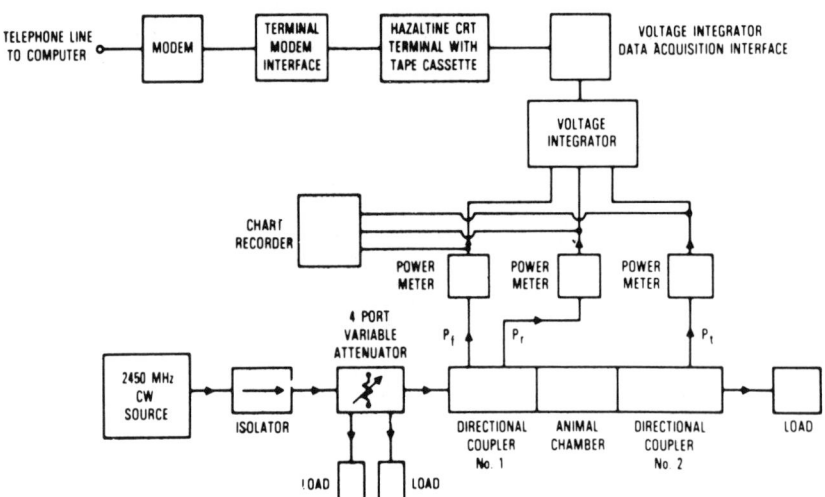

FIGURE 3-6. Schematic diagram of a waveguide irradiation system.

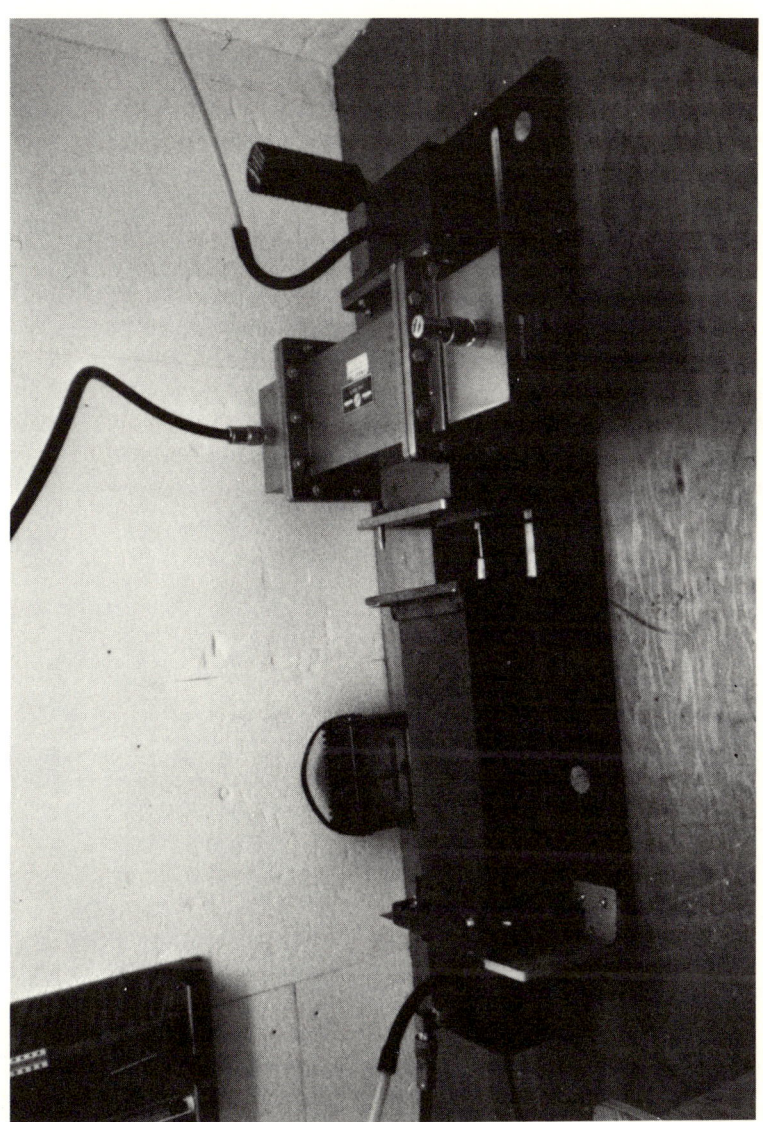

FIGURE 3-7. An S-band rectangular waveguide chamber for whole-body irradiation of small animals. (Courtesy of H. S. Ho, FDA, Washington, D.C.)

waveguide walls has been neglected. At microwave frequencies, energy absorbed by biological specimens is usually large compared to wall losses.

One disadvantage is that the maximum cross-sectional dimensions of the waveguide must be less than one-half the wavelength for the highest operating frequency in order to avoid higher-order modes, which result in complicated field distributions. Another is that field strength in waveguides is extremely sensitive to the size, shape, and location of the biological specimen being irradiated. It has been shown, however, that field strengths within a properly designed hollow waveguide exposure system can be established with an uncertainty of ±6% (Aslan, 1975).

Figure 3-7 shows an S-band rectangular waveguide chamber that is used for whole-body irradiation of small animals, such as mice and hamsters. The chamber is designed to operate between 1.7 and 2.6 GHz. It has been used with 2450-MHz sources that provide up to 100 W of power (Ho *et al.*, 1973, 1976).

The waveguide chambers also can be used for irradiating isolated tissue preparations such as cells and nerves (Courtney *et al.*, 1975; Chou and Guy, 1978; Lin and Peterson, 1977). The waveguide chamber shown in Fig. 3-8 is filled with a fluid whose dielectric constant and conductivity are similar to those of the specimen. Microwave energy is fed through a one-quarter-wavelength impedance transformer that matches the fluid medium to air on the incident side. The specimen to be irradiated is inserted into the chamber through small holes in the broader side walls

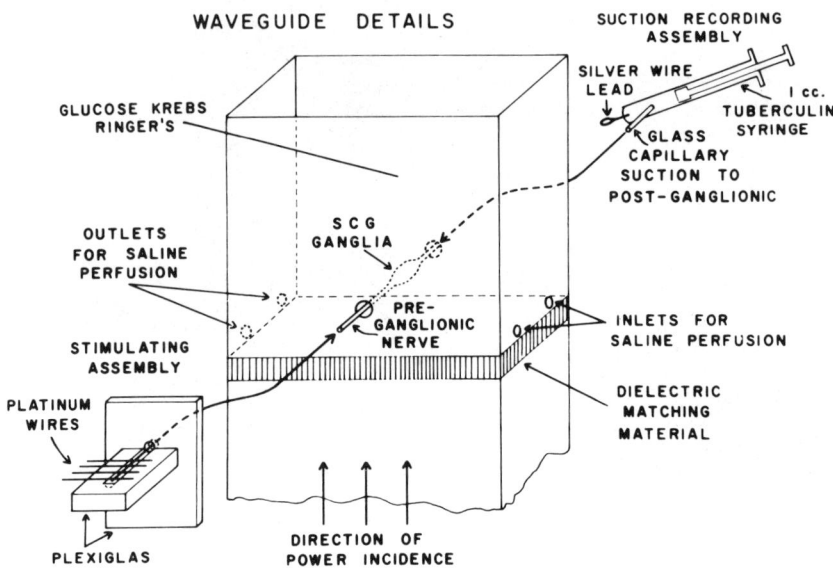

FIGURE 3-8. A fluid-filled waveguide irradiation chamber.

and positioned in the center of the waveguide where the field is uniform. The calculated power density at the center of the waveguide for 100-W input power at 2450 MHz is about 2000 mW/cm^2, which corresponds to an SAR of 2200 mW/g (see Section 2.3). A constant-temperature circulator is used to control the fluid temperature inside the chamber.

Waveguide chambers also have been designed for selective *in vivo* irradiation of an animal's head. An access hole in the wall of the waveguide allows insertion of only the head of the animal, thereby permitting selective irradiation. In order to facilitate microwave energy coupling efficiency to the head, rectangular waveguide chambers have been designed by incorporating holes in the broad wall and the short-circuiting endplates and by installing metallic shims (Lenox *et al.*, 1976) and shunting elements. Furthermore, waveguide tuners (stub and E-H tuners) are used to eliminate mismatches resulting from a large variety of loads (head sizes and geometries).

One design, as shown in Fig. 3-9, consists of an access hole in the broad rectangular waveguide (WR 430) wall where the electric field strength (TE$_{10}$ mode) is high and fairly uniform over an extended region. The waveguide is terminated in a short-circuiting metallic endplate. A pair of symmetric thin metallic, inductive shunting diaphragms extend

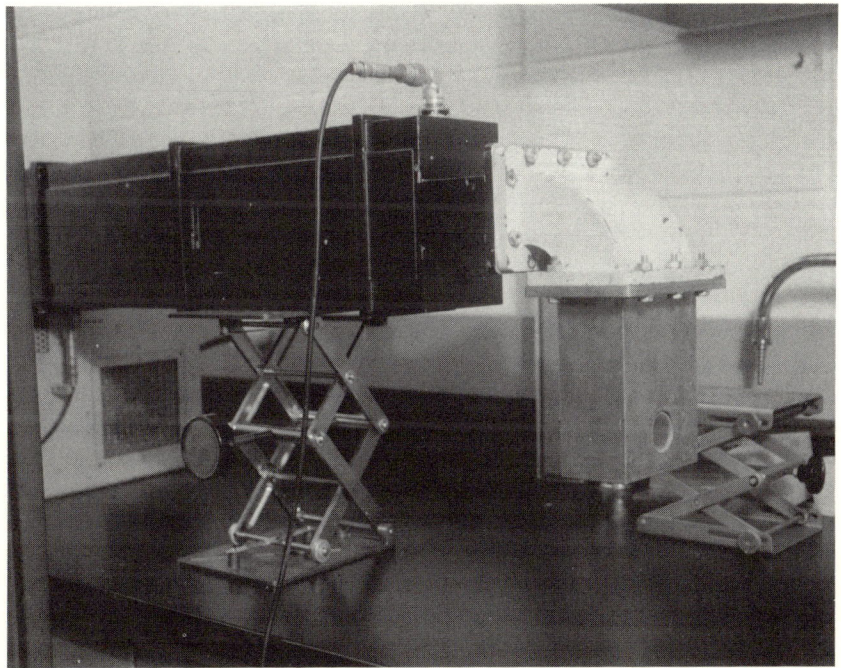

FIGURE 3-9. A rectangular waveguide chamber for irradiation of animal heads.

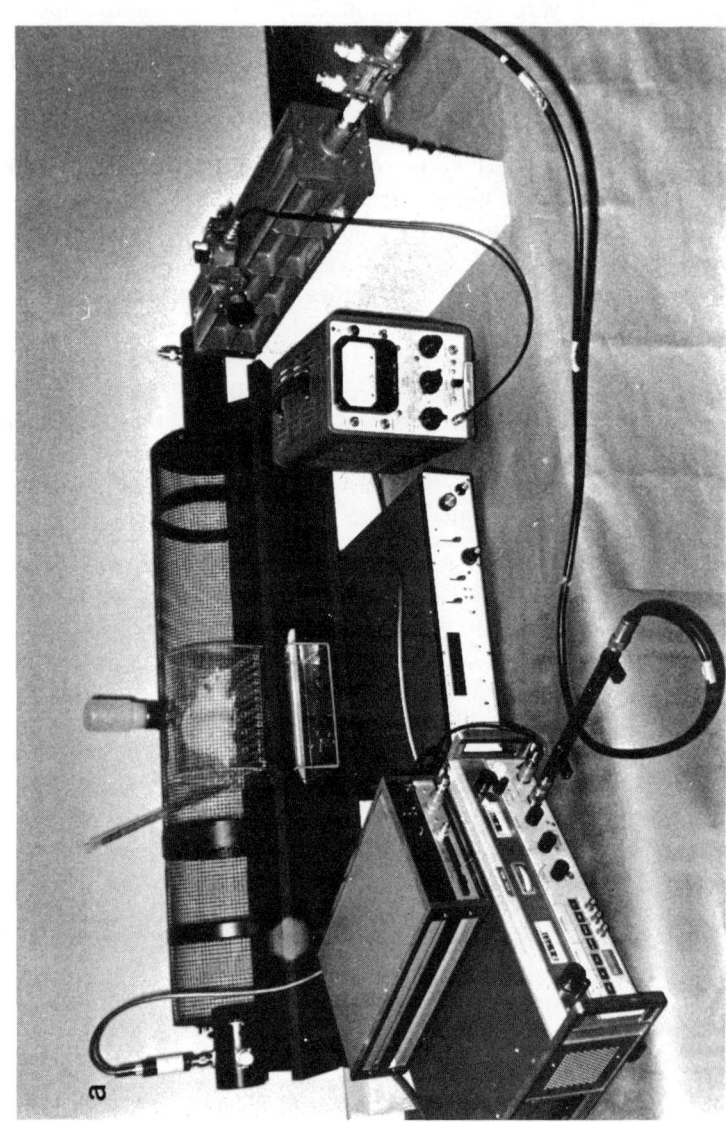

FIGURE 3-10. A hollow circular waveguide irradiation chamber. (a) Chamber with associated test instrumentation; (b) plastic cage containing a rat; the cage fits in the midsection of the chamber. (Courtesy of A. W. Guy, University of Washington, Seattle.)

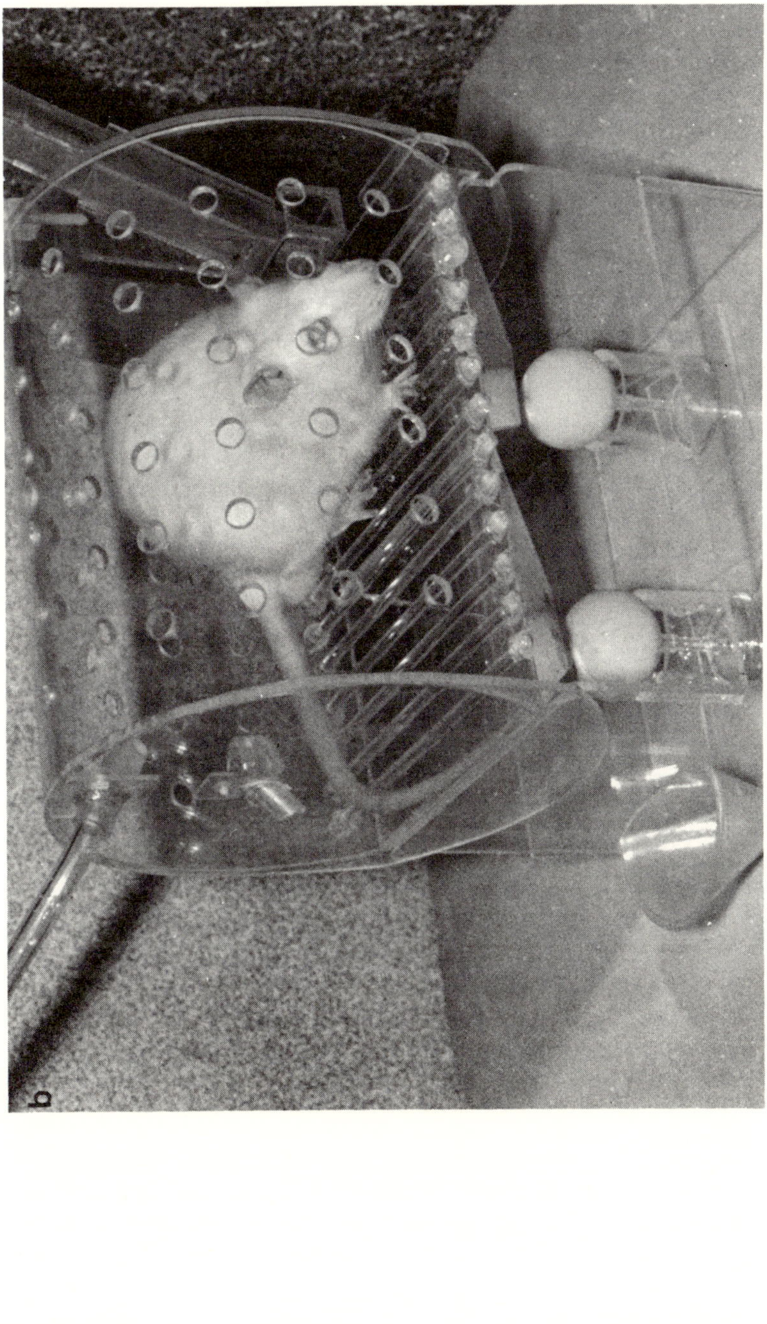

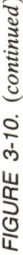

FIGURE 3-10. (continued)

across the narrow dimension of the waveguide to form a waveguide cavity chamber. When a TE_{10} mode impinges on these symmetric diaphragms, the shunt inductive elements match the chamber to the waveguide and permit maximum energy transfer to the load (a small animal's head). This chamber, when connected to a 2.5-kW, 2450-MHz source, can deposit sufficient microwave energy within 15 msec into the head of a mouse to allow rapid *in vivo* inactivation of brain enzymes (unpublished results).

An example of a different type of waveguide chamber that has been used for whole-body irradiation is shown in Fig. 3-10. The basic unit is a section of hollow circular waveguide operating in the dominant TE_{11} mode (see Section 2.3). Each end of the chamber contains two orthogonal excitation probes connected to standard four-terminal hybrid rings that adapt the probes to 50-ohm coaxial transmission lines. Microwave energy (915 or 2450 MHz) is fed through a 90° phase shifter to the two orthogonal probes at one end of the chamber, while the probes at the other end are terminated in matched resistive loads. The superposition of the two TE_{11} modes excited by the orthogonal probes produces a circularly polarized guided wave in the chamber (Guy and Chou, 1976; Guy *et al.*, 1979).

The field distribution is relatively uniform in the transverse dimension and the absorbed energy is nearly independent of animal movement, position, and posture. Moreover, the field distribution and whole-body SAR can be easily calculated from net power delivered to the chamber using equations found in many books containing circular waveguide theory (e.g., Collin, 1966; Ramo *et al.*, 1965). Guy and Chou (1976) described a 0.2-m-diameter waveguide chamber operating at 915 MHz to produce an average power density of 3 mW/cm² for a 1-W net input power. The corresponding whole-body SAR in a 330-g prolate spheroidal model of the rat is about 0.8 mW/g.

The system also contains a plastic cage of appropriate size to house rodents up to the size of guinea pigs under near-normal laboratory living conditions. Furthermore, the reflection coefficient for the chamber is sufficiently low that a number of these chambers may be connected through a power divider network to a single microwave source. Thus, the system is suitable for chronic exposure of a population of rodents to microwave radiation. One disadvantage of such a system is that it is only useful for frequencies below 2 or 3 GHz, hence the animal being irradiated must be small compared to the waveguide chamber.

3.2.5. Multimode Cavity

A multimode cavity is a small shielded enclosure, usually a rectangular metal box excited at frequencies well above the first resonant frequency of the cavity (Section 2.3). A commonly used multimode cavity in biological research on small animals and isolated tissue specimens is the microwave oven (Justesen et al., 1971; Chernovetz et al., 1975). It is generally designed for operation at 915 or 2450 MHz, two of the many frequencies assigned by the Federal Communications Commission for industrial, scientific, and medical uses.

To provide a degree of field uniformity, the available power is distributed in as many modes as possible within the enclosed volume. The field distribution inside the cavity without a biological specimen can be calculated as outlined in Section 2.3. In order to maintain stability of power coupling to the cavity and uniformity of field distribution under all load conditions, metal impeller mode-stirrers are often used. The mode-stirrer increases the number of resonant modes and changes the cavity mode structure. An elaborate mathematical analysis would then be required to describe the field distribution. A reasonable approximation to the average value of electric field strength can be obtained from equation (2.91) by neglecting wall losses and by using the relation

$$E = (8Pt/abd\varepsilon)^{1/2} \tag{3.4}$$

where P is the net power delivered to the cavity, t is the duration of irradiation, ε is the dielectric constant of material filling the cavity, and a, b, and d are the width, height, and depth of the rectangular cavity, respectively. The net power is given by the difference between forward and reflected powers measured with a directional coupler. Wall losses can be calculated or empirically determined for individual cavities, which would permit more precise determination of electric field strength values using equation (3.4).

A single biological specimen can be located at any point within the cavity except in close proximity of the walls. Several specimens can be simultaneously irradiated in the cavity with relatively constant energy absorption. The specimens must have similar geometry and dielectric property and be symmetrically positioned within the cavity.

A number of factors related to multimode cavity irradiation chambers should be noted. The technique requires the assumption that the losses are the same for each specimen tested. The specimen being irradiated is subjected to a composite field pattern, both in strength and in polarization; many local maxima in field strength are possible. Nevertheless, the multimode cavity chamber does provide a technique for simple and repeatable exposure of biological specimens.

3.2.6. Anechoic Chambers

A shielded microwave anechoic chamber is one of the best and often most desirable approaches for irradiating biological specimens. This type of chamber provides a nearly free-space test volume isolated from the outside environment. There are two basic types, the rectangular and tapered chambers. The rectangular anechoic chamber is usually designed to minimize reflected energy by using high-quality absorbing material (Emerson, 1973). Although the ceiling, floor, and side walls are covered with absorbing material, significant reflections can occur from these surfaces, especially for large angles of incidence. To limit the reflected energy for angles of incidence smaller than 70° to within acceptable levels (-25 dB at design frequency), the overall width and height of the chamber must be restricted to values such that

$$w > R/2.75 \qquad (3.5)$$

where w is the width or height of the chamber and R is the source antenna to specimen distance (Kummer and Gillespie, 1978). Furthermore, the chamber height, width, and the size of the antenna must be such that no part of the main beam of the source antenna impinges on the ceiling, floor, or side walls. The source antenna is usually a standard-gain horn or parabolic dish with well-defined gain and field strength characteristics. The interior of a rectangular anechoic chamber with a horn antenna is shown in Fig. 3-11.

The tapered anechoic chamber is configured in the shape of a pyramidal horn that tapers from the small source end to a large

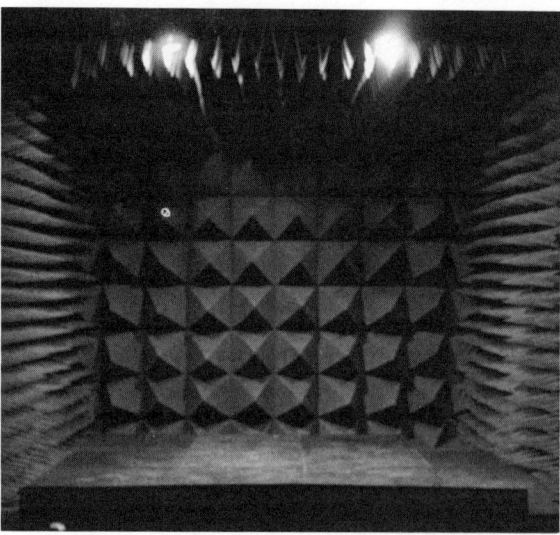

FIGURE 3-11. The interior of (or sectional view of) a microwave anechoic chamber.

rectangular test volume. A higher-gain source antenna is employed to suppress undesirable reflections.

Anechoic chambers are designed in such a manner that the region with field uniformity is maximized within the chamber. This region is usually referred to as the "quiet zone," and it is in this region that the specimen to be irradiated is placed. Animals, anesthetized or otherwise restrained in holders made of low-loss and low-dielectric-constant materials, are placed on Styrofoam blocks of appropriate height. Multiple exposure arrangements can be accomplished by three-dimensional placement of animals in the quiet zone. Placement is chosen to minimize scattering effect and to achieve a fairly equal level of exposure to each animal (Oliva and Catravas, 1977). Even though anechoic chambers are best utilized for whole-body irradiation, isolated tissue preparations, such as a cell suspension, can also be irradiated using an anechoic chamber. In this case, it will be necessary to continuously mix the suspension by rotating or shaking the specimen holder to ensure equal exposure to each cell.

The advantages of anechoic chambers include field uniformity over a large region to accommodate large variations of specimen size and broadband operation with predictable and stable levels of performance throughout the microwave frequencies of interest in this book. The power density P_d, in the quiet zone, at a point along the axis of the source antenna is given by

$$P_d = PG/4\pi r^2 \qquad (3.6)$$

where P is the net power delivered to the source antenna, G is the effective gain of the antenna, and r is the distance from the antenna aperture to the field point. The gain of the antenna is normally determined in advance. The most common procedure of measuring P is by means of a directional coupler, as shown in Fig. 3-12. The difference between forward and reflected powers gives the net power delivered to the source antenna. The disadvantages associated with anechoic chambers are the high cost of the chamber and difficulty in adapting it for chronic irradiation of a large number of animals and partial-body irradiation.

Finally, it should be emphasized that several of the arrangements discussed above are suitable for chronic or repeated exposure. It is obvious that all of these exposure techniques can be used to irradiate many types of biological materials. The examples discussed are chosen to illustrate a few of the experimental arrangements presently in use. Many other equally good exposure systems are in use in laboratories throughout the world.

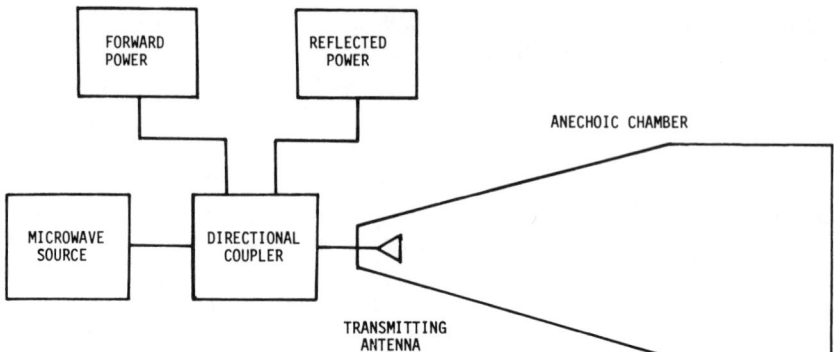

FIGURE 3-12. Simplified test arrangement for microwave power measurement associated with an anechoic chamber.

3.3. FIELD MEASURING METHODS

Although only the field induced or energy absorbed inside the body of an animal or human is relevant for judging the biological responses and potential health hazards of electromagnetic radiation, the ability to evaluate any effect or damage depends critically on knowledge of the field impinging on the subject. Accurate specification of the field or power incident on a subject therefore is important for safety reasons and to provide a basis for comparison of the experimental results of various laboratories. While measurements of both fields external to the subject and fields unperturbed by the presence of the subject are of interest, the latter approach is taken in a great number of experimental situations, and is the most practical for safety and survey purposes.

The field impinging on a biological subject can be determined through calculation, measurement, or both. In controlled laboratory experiments, there is the option to generate many known field configurations with the exposure systems described in Section 3.2. In each case the field strength or power density is calculated in terms of the measured power flow through, or the power delivered to the exposure system. A simpler approach is to measure the exposure field with a calibrated meter.

3.3.1. Isotropic Instruments

There are several meters that are widely used in measuring power densities in air. These instruments have been developed to respond to the magnitude of electric field strength over a wide frequency range in the presence of multipath contributions, reactive near-zone components, and arbitrary polarization.

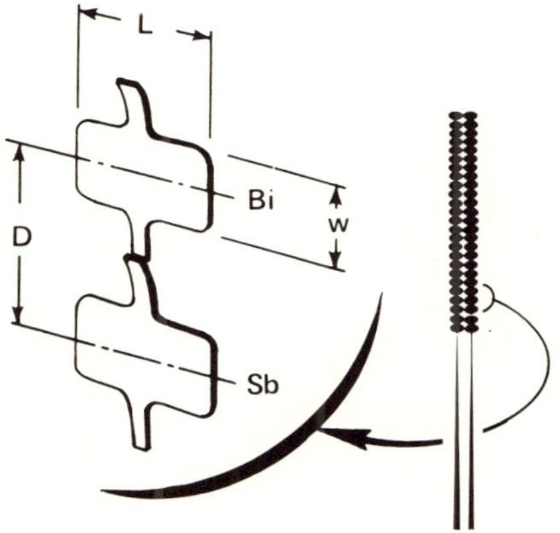

- Antenna Probe Element

- Sixty distributed resistive thermocouples that function as both antenna and detector.

- Resistive leads prevent perturbation of field.

- Hot and cold junction of thermocouple.

- Many squares for high resistance provides hot junction.

- Fraction of a square provides low resistance for cold junctions.

- Closeness of hot and cold junctions, independent of an ambient temperature drift.

- Three elements, series connected.

FIGURE 3-13. The electrothermia-sensing element of an isotropic radiation monitor. (Courtesy of Narda Microwave Corp., Plainview, N.Y.)

Aslan (1972) reported a radiation survey meter that is isotropic and has a wide-band response. The instrument is a sensor consisting of three orthogonal electrothermic elements that can be heated by the incident field (Fig. 3-13). Each element consists of a series of thin-film, antimony–bismuth thermocouple vacuum-deposited on a plastic substrate and secured to a low-density Polyfoam support (Fig. 3-14). The length of the thermocouple strip is small compared with the wavelength of the incident radiation; since the linear resistance of the strips is high, the sensor produces minimal perturbation to the incident field. The dc output of each strip is directly proportional to the square of incident electric field component parallel to the strip. The three outputs from the sensing elements are conducted via high-resistance wires and summed to provide a signal proportional to the square of the total electric field by a voltmeter. The meter is calibrated to read in milliwatts per square centimeter and has an adequate time constant to measure average equivalent plane-wave power density when used in modulated fields. A photograph of the instrument is shown in Fig. 3-15.

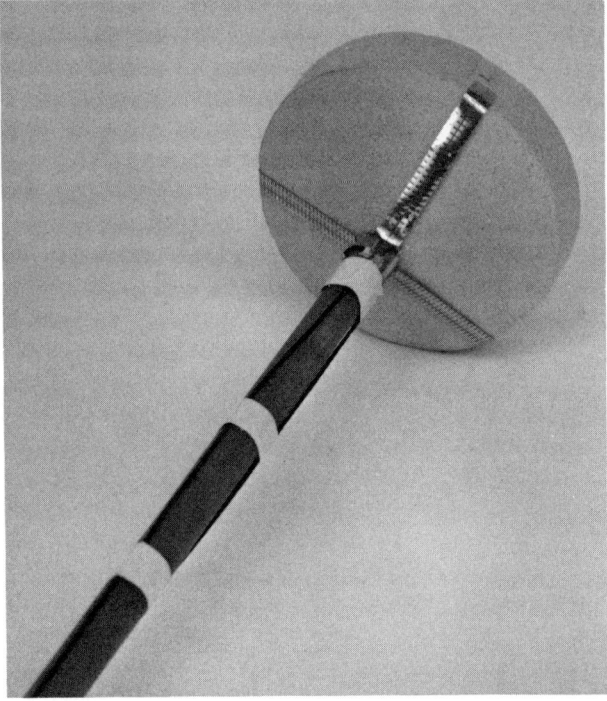

FIGURE 3-14. Antenna probe elements on a low-density Polyfoam support. (Courtesy of Narda Microwave Corp., Plainview, N.Y.)

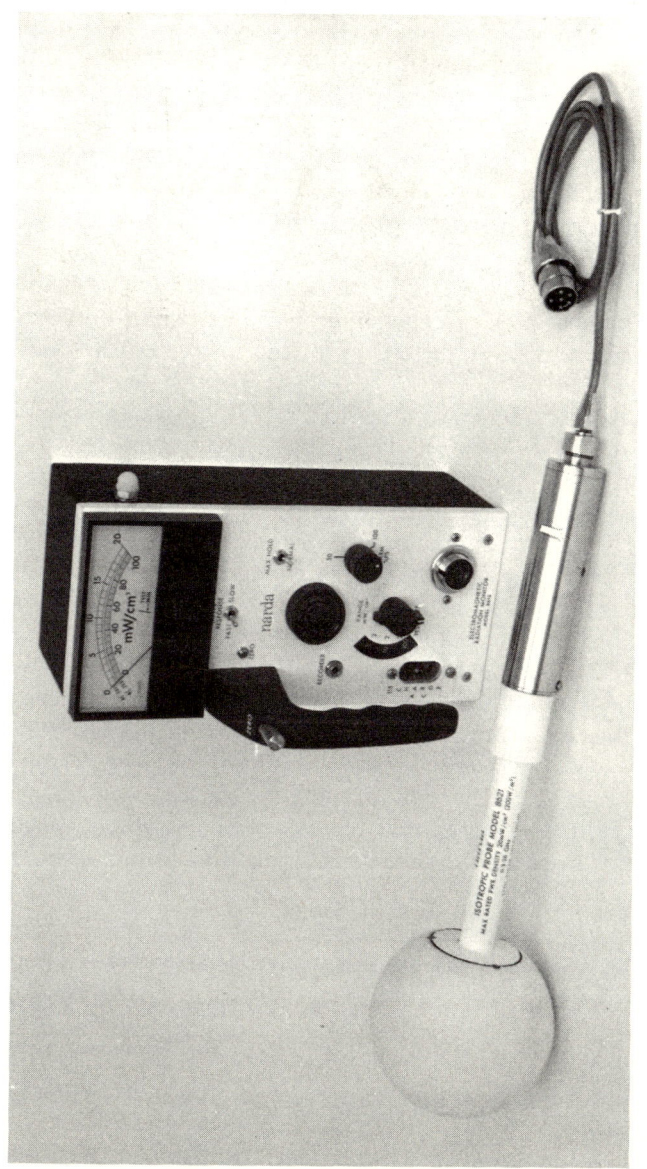

FIGURE 3-15. Model 8616 electromagnetic radiation monitor. (Courtesy of Narda Microwave Corp., Plainview, N.Y.)

Most of the heating occurs in the narrow portion of the resistive thermocouple (Fig. 3-13); the wide portion of the thermocouple serves as a heat sink. Also, since both hot and cold junctions of the thermocouple elements are at ambient temperature, the output of the instrument is reasonably independent of ambient conditions. In fact, the instrument has a low ambient temperature sensitivity of less than 0.05% per °C.

As shown in Fig. 3-14, the sensing element and the support are housed inside a 10-cm-diameter low-density Polyfoam sphere. It therefore cannot be used to measure fields closer than 5 cm from the surface of a radiating or scattering object. In general, the instrument can be used to accurately measure simple plane-wave as well as complicated fields. It has an overload capacity of 100–300 mW/cm^2 for continuous wave fields and 20–60 W/cm^2 for peak power, depending on the particular probe model and serial number. Other characteristics of the instrument are given in Table 3-2.

Actually, the instrument just described is an improved version of an earlier instrument (Aslan, 1970). This earlier instrument responds to either 2450- or 915-MHz radiation and consists of two orthogonal thin-film thermocouples of the same composition vacuum-deposited on a plastic substrate. As above, the thermocouples serve as both antenna and detector. The thermocouple elements are connected in series to give a total dc output independent of orientation and field polarization about the axis of the probe. The output is proportional to the square of the magnitude of the electric field and is calibrated to read in power density (mW/cm^2). If the relation between the electric and magnetic components of the field is constant or known, such as 377 ohms in the far field, the reading is equivalent to the actual power density of the field. In the near field, however, the meter indication is simply the square of the magnitude of the electric field divided by 377 ohms, which has sometimes been referred to as the "equivalent power density." It is important to bear this

TABLE 3-2
Comparison of Measuring Instrument Characteristics

	Narda 8606[a]	NBS/EDM[b]	RAHAM 3[c]
Frequency range for ±1-dB response to plane wave (GHz)	0.3–26	0.03–3	0.3–18
Dynamic range (mW/cm^2)	±0.5	±0.5	±0.5
Isotropic response (dB)	±0.5 dB	±1%	±0.5 dB
Continuous overload (mW/cm^2)	100–300	60,000	500
Peak overload (W/cm^2)	60–300	—	—

[a] The Narda Microwave Corporation, Plainview, New York.
[b] National Bureau of Standards, Boulder, Colorado.
[c] General Microwave Corporation, Farmingdale, New York.

in mind when using this type of instrument to measure external field conditions.

Another type of broadband, isotropic measuring instrument was discussed by Bowman (1971). This instrument makes use of three orthogonal dipoles with diodes connected between the arms of the dipoles. Each dipole is 8 mm in length. However, instead of connecting the diodes in series, as was done for the thermocouple sensors in the previously described instruments, each diode is connected individually to separate signal processing amplifiers using a pair of high-resistance wires. The instrument is shown in simplified block diagram form in Fig. 3-16. The high-resistance wires are made of carbon-impregnated Teflon and have a linear resistance of 3 to 30 kohm/cm depending on the instrument model. They therefore cause very little perturbation in the field being measured. For low-level fields whose wavelengths are long compared with the dipoles, the response of the sensing elements is proportional to the square of the electric field components along the axis of each dipole. The summing circuit shown in Fig. 3-16 equalizes the signals from the three orthogonal dipoles and provides an output proportional to the magnitude of the total electric field squared. For high field levels, the nonlinear behavior of the summing circuit provides the needed dynamic

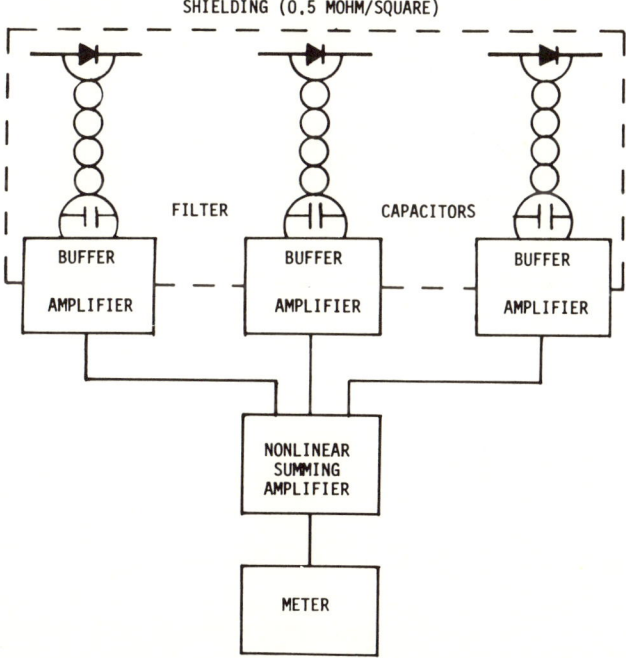

FIGURE 3-16. Simplified block diagram for the NBS energy density meter.

range. The instrument is calibrated to give electric-energy density in units of nanojoules per cubic centimeter. For a plane wave propagating in free space, the relation between power density P and energy density U is given by

$$P = cU \qquad (3.7)$$

where c is the speed of light. For example, if a plane wave has a power density of 1 mW/cm^2, the energy density is $3.33 \times 10^{-5} \text{ nJ/cm}^3$ and the electric field strength is 86.8 V/m.

Figure 3-17 is a diagram of one of the three identical dipole–diode sensing elements. The Nichrome thin-film resistance lines deposited on the substrate form a balanced twin-lead with resistances of approximately 50 kohm/cm and constitute the connection between the diode and the Teflon wires. The acute angle between each dipole and the Nichrome leads is 54.74°. In this way, when the three dipole–diode elements are arranged along the long edges to form an equilateral triangular tube, the three elements become orthogonal. The sensors along with the Polyfoam

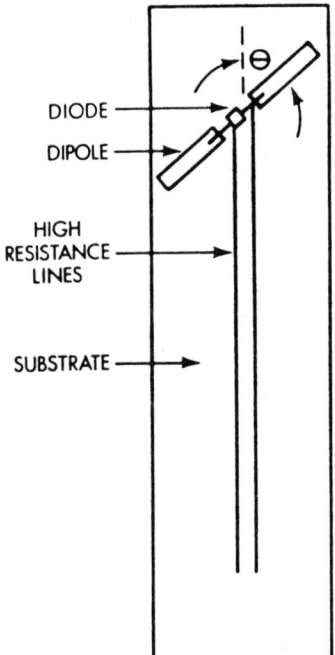

FIGURE 3-17. Diagram of dipole–diode detectors used in the NBS meter. (Courtesy of R. Bowman, NBS, Boulder, Colo.)

support are placed snugly inside a thin-walled plastic cylinder for protection. The protective cylinder is coated with a slightly conducting layer, which is continuously bonded to the metallic handle of the measuring probe with silver glue to reduce capacitive coupling in the high-resistance leads. The instrument cannot be used to measure multi-frequency fields with any certainty. It will, however, provide accurate measurements at a single frequency down to 0.0002 mW/cm^2. Some other characteristics of the instrument are given in Table 3-2.

RAHAM 3 is a portable battery-operated power density meter designed to measure microwave radiation in the range 0.3 to 18 GHz and power densities from 0.2 to 200 mW/cm^2. The isotropic probe employs three orthogonally oriented thin-film thermocouple arrays, which is equivalent to a resistance sheet whose surface resistivity is high relative to the intrinsic impedance of free space. This provides an almost constant effective aperture throughout the frequency range such that the frequency sensitivity over the operating band is within ± 1 dB.

It is seen from Table 3-2 that the accuracy, range, and sensitivity of Narda model 8606 and RAHAM model 3 are comparable, whereas the NBS electric-energy density meter is the only instrument that is sensitive enough to measure fields lower than 0.01 mW/cm^2. Although none of the instruments described are ideal from the standpoint of not perturbing the field being measured, the degree of perturbation is small in most cases. It must be borne in mind that in studies of microwave interaction with biological systems, the goal of ideal instrumentation is seldom realized. The accuracy, reliability, and reproducibility of the probe measurement must be established by calibration. This is usually done by careful comparison of probe measurement with standard field (Baird, 1974; Larson, 1979). The standard field is established with precisely known field variations through calculation, measurement, or both, in much the same manner as that described in Section 3.2. The instrument under test is then placed in the standard field and the meter reading is compared with the known field.

3.3.2. Other Instruments

There are a number of other power density meters currently in use. For example, the Holaday model H1 1500 (Holaday Industries, Hopkins, Minn.) survey meter has been developed for measuring microwave radiation at a fixed frequency of 2450 MHz. The instrument can accurately measure power densities from 0.1 up to 100 mW/cm^2 in three sequentially switched ranges to within ± 1 dB. It has a unique detection probe that makes the measurement independent of field polarization. The probe is connected to the indicating device by a shielded cable and the combination of probe and connecting cable design minimizes perturbation of the field due to its presence. It has a maximum power density measuring capacity of 1.5 W/cm^2 and a fast response time of 1 sec and a slow response time of 3 sec.

At lower frequencies under near-field conditions, both electric field strength and magnetic field strength should be measured. It has been shown (Lin *et al.*, 1973a) that in the lower-frequency region, magnetic field-induced energy absorption predominates in humans and animals. It is therefore necessary to measure both electric and magnetic fields.

The Narda model 8607 isotropic radiation monitor is designed to provide accurate near- and far-field power density measurement over the frequency range 10 to 300 MHz. Three mutually perpendicular sets of square low detectors that respond equally to magnetic fields with arbitrary orientation and polarization permit the addition of magnetic field sensed from all directions. The meter is calibrated to give "equivalent plane-wave power density," using the free-space impedance of 377 ohms. The range extends from 0.02 to 100 mW/cm^2, corresponding to mean square magnetic field strength of 0.02 to 1.6 A/m. The general characteristics of the instrument are comparable to the other Narda probe previously described.

It is important to emphasize that measurement accuracy involved with probe measurement, in general, depends critically on the placement of the probe. As slight a difference as a few millimeters can change the meter readings by 5 to 10%, especially in the near field.

3.4. ABSORPTION MEASURING METHODS

A clear understanding of the biological responses of radio and microwave radiation must be based on a quantitative understanding of the relationship between the field impinging on the subject, the energy absorbed in the tissues, and the observed effect. Internal fields and absorbed energy, in principle, can be directly measured *in vivo* by implanted probes transparent to electromagnetic radiation. However, accurate, reliable implanted probes still remain to be developed. Currently, there are two distinctive approaches toward quantification of induced field and absorbed energy. These are the whole-body absorption and the spatial distribution of absorbed energy. While each has its own merit, clarification of the biological responses and hazards of radio and microwave radiation demands knowledge of both in most situations. In the following paragraphs a description of some techniques used for determination of whole-body absorption is given first, followed by a discussion of methods used for measuring the spatial distribution of absorbed energy.

3.4.1. Whole-Body Absorption

Whole-body absorption is the simpler of the two problems. As mentioned in Section 3.2, the total electromagnetic energy absorbed by animals and humans in a TEM exposure system can be simply determined using precision directional couplers and power meters. The power incident on, reflected by, and transmitted through a chamber containing the subject are measured as a function of time and used to compute the total absorbed energy. Similarly, energy absorbed by small animals such as mice and rats in a waveguide-type irradiation chamber can be ascertained in the same manner. This technique is simple to use and does not require that a device or instrument be implanted in the subject. It is therefore nonperturbing so far as the electromagnetic field is concerned. Moreover, the subject may even be mobile. The limitation of the system is that it is only adaptable to situations where transmission lines and waveguides are used.

For closed-space irradiation, such as in a large TEM chamber or multimode cavity with appreciable internal surface area, the energy absorbed can be calculated from measures of forward and reflected powers. In addition, losses caused by the finite conductivity of the chamber walls must be evaluated. For a good conductor, the magnetic fields at the walls are essentially those associated with the loss-free field solutions (Section 2.3) and the power loss in the walls is given by

$$P_1 = \frac{1}{2\sigma\delta} \iint_{\text{walls}} |H_{\text{tan}}|^2 \, ds \tag{3.8}$$

where H_{tan} is the tangential component of the magnetic field at the surface of the chamber walls. Thus, the net power delivered to a cavity or chamber when a biological specimen is present is

$$P = P_{\text{f}} - (P_{\text{r}} + P_{\text{l}}) \tag{3.9}$$

This is the time rate of energy absorbed by the specimen, and the whole-body SAR is obtained by dividing body mass into equation (3.9). It is important to note that wall losses remain unchanged for specimen sizes that are small compared with the dimensions of the chamber or cavity. This only needs to be evaluated once for a given exposure system.

An important parameter associated with a multimode cavity is the quality factor Q (Collin, 1966). Changes in cavity Q when a biological specimen is present can also be used to calculate whole-body SAR.

To measure whole-body SAR directly, the technique of calorimetry involving models or animal carcasses may be employed (Justesen and King, 1970; Hunt and Phillips, 1972). This technique has also been

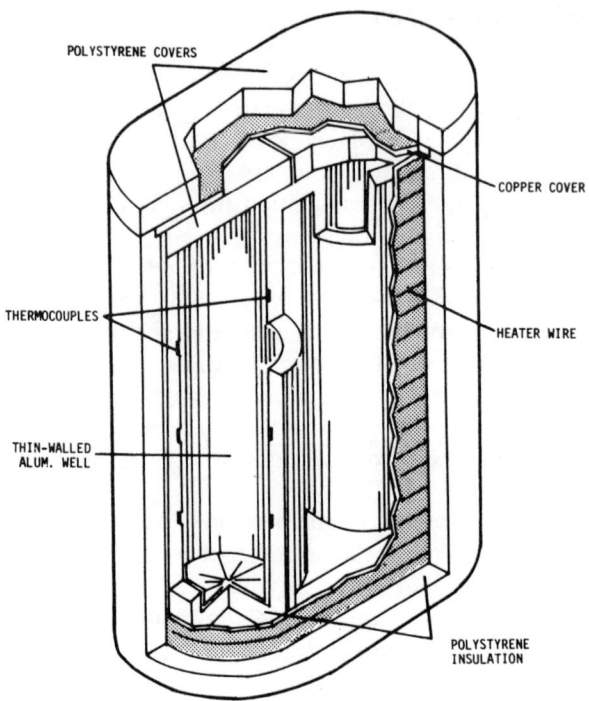

FIGURE 3-18. The construction of a twin-well calorimeter.

applied to determine absorbed energy in rats exposed in an anechoic chamber (Phillips *et al.*, 1975). It involves a twin-well calorimeter (Fig. 3-18) and is based on the amount of heat generated in a fresh animal carcass by microwave irradiation. The procedure consists of placing a pair of freshly killed animals of equivalent body mass into the calorimeter and measuring the differential body heat content of the animals. This technique provides a physical method of sufficient precision to be useful in investigations on the biological effects of microwave radition involving small animals.

The twin-well calorimeter, shown schematically in Fig. 3-18, is composed of two thin-walled, thermally insulated aluminum wells, which serve as isothermal reference planes for the thermopile. There are 24 iron–constantan thermocouples connected in series and positioned in alternating sequence on the outside surfaces of the wells. The voltage generated by differential well temperatures is amplified and recorded on a strip chart recorder. The ambient temperature level for the calorimeter is kept constant by a copper jacket surrounding the insulated wells. The jacket is maintained at $29.6 \pm 0.05°C$ by controlled heating of a

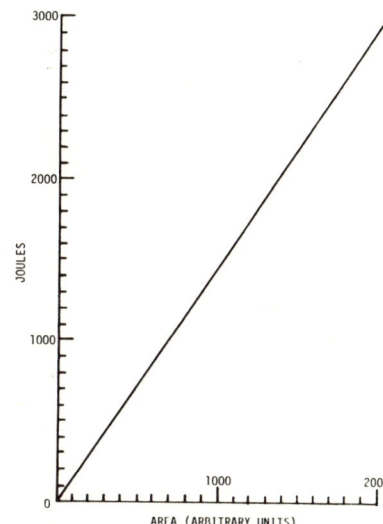

FIGURE 3-19. Typical calibration curve for energy deposition as a function of the area under a voltage–time curve.

constant-resistance, manganin alloy coil wrapped around the jacket. The heater is controlled by a thermistor (attached to the jacket) that is used to provide a signal to a null-seeking bridge circuit operating the voltage controller for the heater.

The calorimeter is calibrated by adding known quantities of heat to one of the wells and measuring the area of the resultant voltage–time curve. A typical calibration curve is shown in Fig. 3-19. In this case, a plastic rod to which heat could be added electrically was loaded into one well (Phillips et al., 1975). It is seen that the curve area depends linearly on the total energy.

To determine the total energy absorbed by animals exposed to microwave radiation, pairs of animals are selected that are matched closely in body mass. The animals are killed with an intraperitoneal injection of sodium pentobarbital, and the carcasses placed in the calorimeter. The resultant voltage–time curve between the two carcasses is recorded. The shape of the initial portion of the curve is highly variable among different pairs, depending on whether one of the animals is excited just before death, and other factors. In general, approximately $2\frac{1}{2}$ hrs later and at least 1 hr after the curve reaches the maximum, it exhibits an exponential decay toward thermal equilibrium (Fig. 3-20). The time constant of the exponential decay is directly proportional to the size of the carcass.

Approximately 1 hr after the exponential decay of the differential heat curve is clearly evident, both carcasses are removed from the calorimeter and loaded in polystyrene holders. As a rule, the warmer one

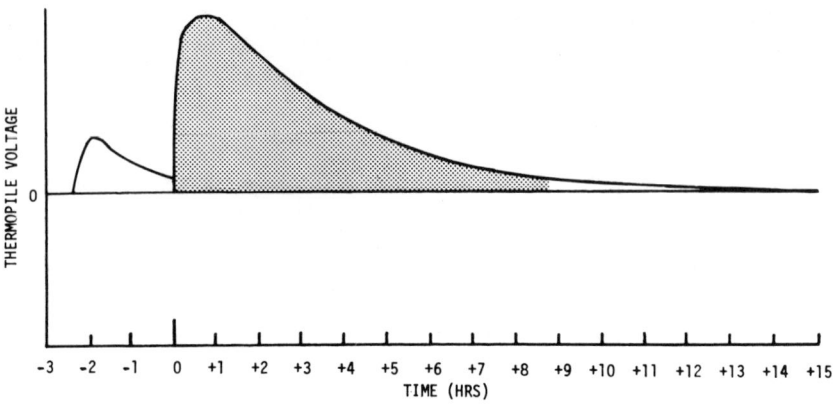

FIGURE 3-20. Typical voltage–time curves obtained in a twin-well calorimeter.

is exposed for a short duration at a moderate power level. (For example, exposure is 1 min with a net power of 100 W for animals irradiated in a 2450-MHz cavity.) During the exposure the other animal carcass is placed in an identical cavity. Immediately following the brief exposure, both carcasses are promptly returned to the calorimeter in the same sequence as they were removed. The total amount of energy absorbed by the whole animal is measured from the calibration curve shown in Fig. 3-20 using the area under the voltage–time curve or differential residual body heat curve. Since the curve area depends on the total energy and not on the rate of heating, the whole-body SAR is simply given by

$$\text{whole-body SAR} = \text{total energy}/tM \qquad (3.10)$$

where t is exposure duration and M is body mass.

This method of measuring total absorption or average absorption per unit body mass has several advantages. It is very accurate: the accuracy in determinations of whole-body absorption by animals has been shown to be within 0.8% (Phillips *et al.*, 1975). It makes no assumption regarding the geometry of the subject or the frequency of the impinging radiation. Moreover, the use of dead animals eliminates the problem of normal thermoregulation with its consequences on heat production and loss. It requires, however, the assumption that the electrical properties of the animal tissue remain unaltered within the first few hours of death. The total absorption is still a function of orientation of the subject with respect to the source. For larger animals, the time required to reach thermal equilibrium may be inordinately long and the associated complications tend to make this technique unreliable.

It is interesting to note that the twin-well calorimetry method also provides an empirical technique of sufficient precision to allow estimation of wall and other intrinsic losses associated with multimode cavity exposure chambers. The energy stored in the cavity can be calculated from the difference between forward and reflected powers measured with calibrated meters. The difference between energy stored in the cavity and the total energy absorbed by a specimen represents energy loss in the exposure system.

3.4.2. Distribution of Absorbed Energy—Probe Measurements

The most obvious technique for measuring the internal field distribution would be measurement of the electric field induced inside the subject. However, to date, electric field sensors that function in the tissue have not been commercially available. Since absorption of microwave energy produces heat inside the specimen, the temperature rise may be measured by a number of existing temperature sensors of small size. The temperature rise may then be converted to magnitude of the internal field as a function of position. There are some serious difficulties, however, involved in using internal temperature rise as a measure of the induced field and absorbed energy. Nevertheless, it has been shown that implanted thermocouple and thermistors can be used to measure field-related quantities in test animals or humans.

Osborne and Frederick (1948) used thermocouples, inserted in the eyes of dogs, to obtain temperature rises as a result of microwave heating. The thermocouple was inserted before and after microwave irradiation. Richardson *et al.* (1948) applied a thermocouple to the rabbit eye in their cataract studies to measure temperature increases as a result of microwave irradiation. Lehmann *et al.* (1968, 1970) used thermistors in the thighs of human volunteers and live swine under experimental shortwave and microwave diathermy treatment. The problems associated with the use of thermistors or thermocouples for measuring absorbed power include: (1) the device senses only tissue temperature, which is also subject to a number of other factors such as heat diffusion, blood circulation, and the general thermoregulatory activity of the specimen; (2) if the temperature sensors (conventional thermocouples and thermistors) are left in the tissue during irradiation, they can introduce significant perturbation to the field surrounding the sensor and selectively absorb incident radiation and therefore alter the tissue temperature and the meter reading; (3) current temperature sensors require appreciable temperature rise for detection, and thus are relatively insensitive to a low SAR.

Most of these problems can be minimized by using a small-diameter

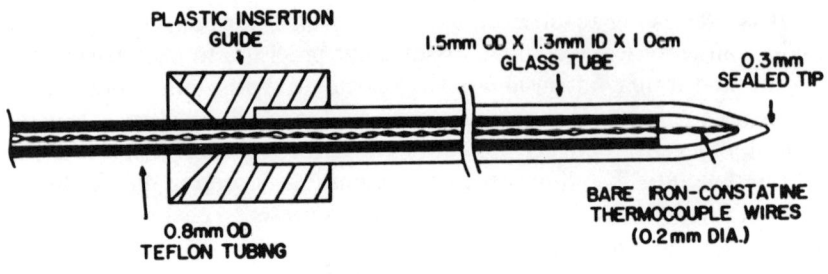

FIGURE 3-21. Metallic thermocouple in a glass pipette guide.

plastic or glass pipette sealed at one end and implanted at the location where the absorbed energy information is desired. The pipette shown in Fig. 3-21 must be long enough so that the open end, fitted with a plastic guide, protrudes from the tissue. A thin thermocouple is inserted into the pipette with the junction right at the probe tip and an initial temperature is recorded. The thermocouple is quickly withdrawn from the pipette and the specimen is irradiated under the same experimental configuration. Instead of using the power level normally chosen for the experiment, the specimen is subjected to a short but high-power irradiation sufficient to reproduce appreciable temperature rises. The thermocouple is then reintroduced into the pipette and advanced to its original position and the temperature is measured for several minutes. Since a short lapse of time is unavoidable, the temperature versus time curve must be extrapolated back in time to the instant the power was turned off and, based on the density and specific heat of the tissue, the SAR can be calculated from the difference in initial and final extrapolated temperature. The short irradiation period ensures that there is no loss of heat due to convection or diffusion, so that the expression

$$P_a = 4186 c \Delta T / t \qquad (3.11)$$

may be used to calculate the SAR, P_a in watts per kilogram. c is the specific heat of the tissue (kcal/kg per °C), ΔT is the temperature change (°C), and t is the duration of irradiation (sec). The measured SAR can then be used to relate the incident power to the absorbed energy in the tissue under normal exposure conditions.

It should be noted that this technique is slow and cumbersome to implement when SARs at a large number of points are desired. Furthermore, it is not always clear where to implant the probes since the region of maximum absorption in the specimen is generally unknown.

The last few years has seen a large increase in the number of specialized temperature probes developed for radio and microwave biology research (Larsen *et al.*, 1974; Rozzell *et al.*, 1974; Cetas, 1975; Bowman, 1976; Wickersheim and Alves, 1981). The probes not only allow temperature measurement without prior implantation of electrically nonconducting tubes, but also produce negligible direct heating due to induced currents on the probe such that they can be used during microwave irradiation.

The first significant development was the production of fiber-optic-liquid-crystal temperature probes in commercial quantities (Ramal, Sandy, Utah). The probe consists of two bundles of optic fibers inside a thin-walled polyvinyl chloride tube. The fiber bundles are used to transmit light to and receive light reflected from the liquid-crystal temperature sensor at the tip of the probe. A red light given off by a gallium arsenide phosphide light-emitting diode (LED) is used as a source and the light reflected by the liquid crystal is detected using a photo-transistor. The output of the photo-transistor is a voltage proportional to the reflected light intensity, which is a function of the temperature surrounding the liquid crystal. The output voltage may be calibrated to read either in temperature or in absorbed energy (Rozzell *et al.*, 1974). The probe causes little perturbation to microwave fields and contributes a negligible amount of heat to the surrounding tissue materials. It is potentially useful in determination of absorbed microwave energy. However, a number of difficulties, including stability, reproducibility, and hystereses, must be resolved before they can be used to give consistent and reproducible results.

A probe that has much greater sensitivity, stability, and dynamic range than the one described above is the Electro-thermia Monitor (Vitek, Boulder, Colo). The probe uses a small carbon thick-film thermistor for a temperature sensor and leads made from carbon-loaded plastic (PTFE) that are slightly conductive. The thermistor resistance is sensed by injecting a small current from a constant-current generator through one pair of leads and measuring the voltage developed across the thermistor with a high-input-impedance amplifier connected to the other pair of high-resistance leads. The probe is slightly more than 1 mm in diameter. The electronic package provides a digital readout in degrees Celsius and an analog signal for recording. The nonlinearity is less than 0.03°C from 25 to 45°C. The precision offset allows measurement of temperature differences as small as 0.01°C.

Since the probe interacts minimally with radio and microwave radiation, it may be used to continuously record temperature changes in animals undergoing irradiation (Lin and Lin, 1981). Figure 3-22 illustrates the use of an indwelling carbon thick-film thermistor probe for measuring the temperature changes in a rat undergoing selective micro-

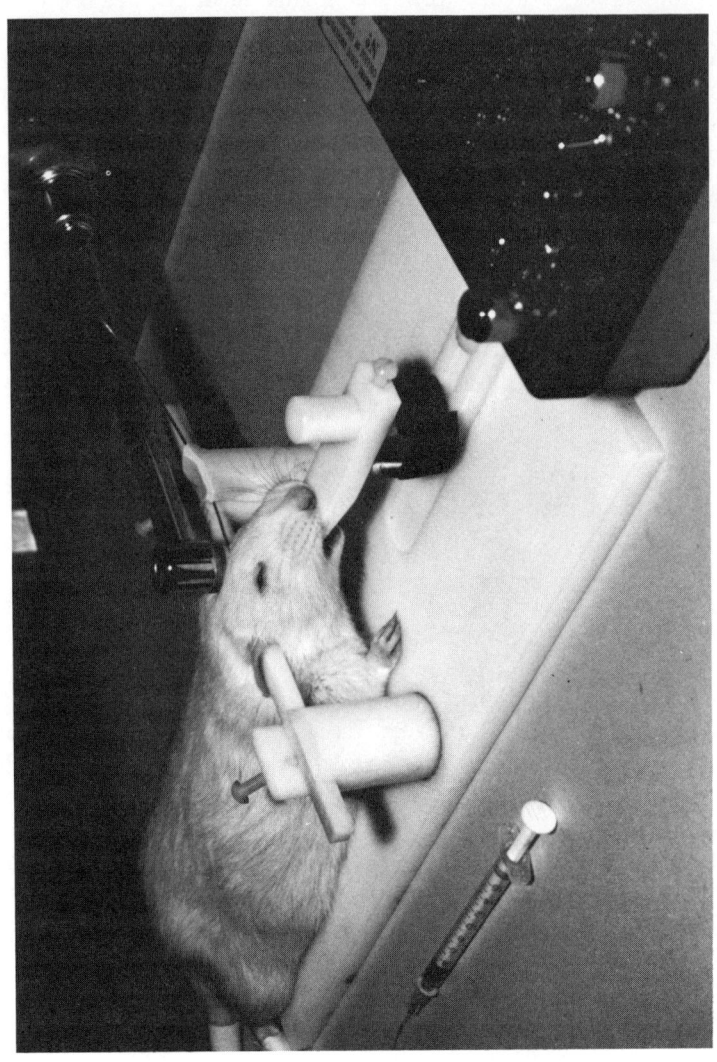

FIGURE 3-22. An indwelling carbon thermistor probe for temperature measurements in a rat brain undergoing selective head irradiation.

wave irradiation of the brain by a contact applicator at the animal's head. The tip of the probe was implanted in the cerebral cortex beneath the applicator.

More recently an optical instrument based on phosphor/fiber-optic technique has been developed by Wickersheim and Alves (1981). This unique Fluoroptic thermometer (Luxtron, Mountain View, Calif.) permits temperature measurements in the presence of radio and microwave radiation as well as other electromagnetic fields. It can be inserted into liquids, tissues, and other biological bodies to obtain direct temperature measurements with no perturbation of the irradiation process.

The temperature probe consists of a small quantity of rare earth phosphor bonded to the tip of an optical fiber about 0.7 mm in diameter and ranging from 2 to 15 m in length. This thin optical probe is coupled to an instrument package containing an optical head, microprocessor, and signal processing electronics (Fig. 3-23). A high-intensity tungsten–halogen lamp sends ultraviolet light along the fiber to the tip where it

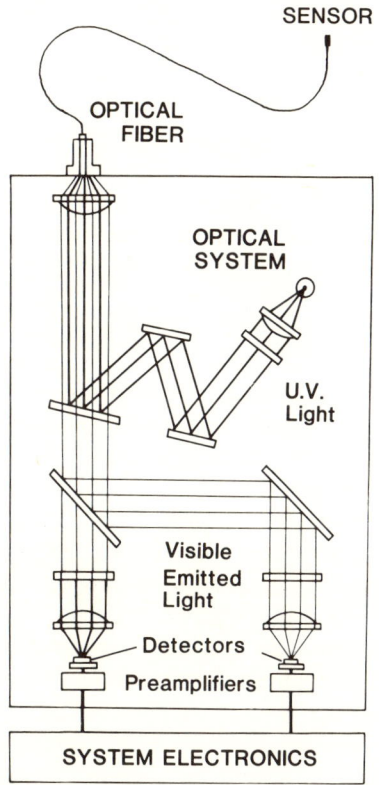

FIGURE 3-23. Schematic diagram of the Fluoroptic temperature sensor.

excites the phosphor. The visible fluorescence emitted by the phosphor, containing the desired temperature information, is transmitted to the instrument by the same fiber and analyzed by means of a two-channel spectrometer. The intensities of the two lines of interest are measured with silicon photodiodes. After suitable signal integration, the ratio of the two intensities is computed. A microprocessor then compares this ratio with a previously stored calibration table, determines the corresponding temperature, and sends the information to the instrument display and to analog and digital output ports.

The probe is constructed from plastic-clad silica fiber with an FPA Teflon jacket to prevent ambient light from being scattered into the system. Moreover, the instrument package is well shielded to minimize electromagnetic interference. With an integration time of 1 sec, a precision of 0.1°C is readily achieved over the full range from −50 to 250°C.

3.4.3. Distribution of Absorbed Energy—Thermographic Measurements

A method for rapid evaluation of the SAR distribution over a surface inside a specimen of arbitrary shape and dielectric properties when irradiated with radio and microwaves has been developed by Guy *et al.* (1968; Guy, 1971). The method, valid for both far and near-zone fields, involves the use of a thermograph camera for recording temperature patterns produced by energy absorption in models of tissue structures or animal carcasses. The absorbed energy or magnitude of the electric field may be obtained anywhere in the body as a function of the heating pattern.

The models consist of polyfoam cavities with geometric properties similar to those of the tissue structures they represent and are filled with synthetic dielectric materials having the same microwave and thermal properties as biological tissues (see Table 3-3). The models are designed to separate along particular planes where SAR distributions are desired. A thin 0.25-mm polyethylene film or silk screen is placed over the precut surfaces to prevent evaporation and to facilitate separation following irradiation. To obtain the SAR distribution, the model is first irradiated in the same exposure configuration as during the experiment for a short duration (15 sec or less) at high power density. The model then is quickly disassembled and the temperature pattern over the surface of separation is recorded with a thermograph camera. Since the duration of irradiation is very brief, the temperature pattern will not be altered by thermal conduction or convection. Under these conditions, the temperature increase due to radio and microwave irradiation is a linear function of irradiation time and is related to the SAR through equation (3.10).

TABLE 3-3
Composition and Properties of Tissue Modeling Materials

Tissue model	Frequency (MHz)	Temp. (°C)	Dielectric constant	Conductivity (mmho/cm)	Specific heat (cal/g-°C)	Density (g/cm)	Composition		Reference
Muscle	200	23	58	10.3	0.86	1.0	15.2	Polyethylene powder	Guy (1971)
	500	23	55	13.2	0.86	1.0	0.91	Sodium chloride	
	915	23	52	13.2	0.86	1.0	8.45	Super Stuff	
	2,450	23	50	22.5	0.86	1.0	75.44	Water	
	8,500	20	43.6	63.8	0.84	1.0	15.2	Polyethylene powder	Cheung and Koopman (1976)
	10,000	20	40.9	66.9	0.84	1.0	0.91	Sodium chloride	
							8.45	Super Stuff	
							75.44	Water	
Bone and fat	200	23	6.2	0.38	0.27	1.30	14.5	Aluminium powder	Guy (1971)
	500	23	5.7	0.44	0.27	1.30	0.24	Acetylene black	
	915	23	5.5	0.62	0.27	1.30	0.45	Catalyst	
	2,450	23	4.9	1.10	0.27	1.30	84.81	Laminac 4110	
	8,500	20	4.26	2.76	0.29	1.30	14.5	Aluminium powder	Cheung and Koopman (1976)
	10,000	20	4.07	3.16	0.29	1.30	0.5	Acetylene black	
							0.45	Catalyst	
							84.55	Laminac 4110	
Brain	200	23	37	6.7	0.83	0.96	29.8	Polyethylene powder	Guy (1971)
	500	23	35	6.8	0.83	0.96	0.76	Sodium chloride	
	915	23	35	7.8	0.83	0.96	7.0	Super Stuff	Lin et al. (1973)
	2,450	23	33.5	12.3	0.83	0.96	62.44	Water	

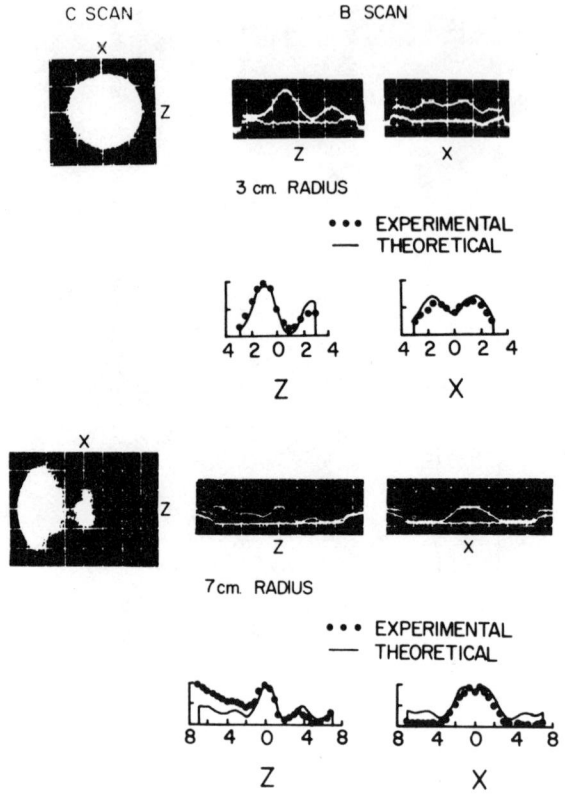

FIGURE 3-24. Comparison of theoretical and thermographically measured SAR distribution in spherical brain models.

A comparison of theoretical and experimental SAR distribution thus determined in spherical brain models is given in Fig. 3-24. The thermograms at the left of Fig. 3-24 are "C" scans taken over the surface of the separated hemispheres where brightness is proportional to absorbed power and each division is equivalent to 2 cm. The thermograms in the middle are "B" scans taken before and after exposure to the microwave sources where vertical deflection is proportional to absorbed power along the z axis of the sphere. The thermograms at the right are also "B" scans taken along the x axis of the sphere. The graphs below the "B" scans are comparisons of the theoretical and measured absorbed power. The results agree well with the exception of the deviation between the theoretical and experimental value for the large sphere exposed to 915-MHz energy. This is due to the diverging fields of the

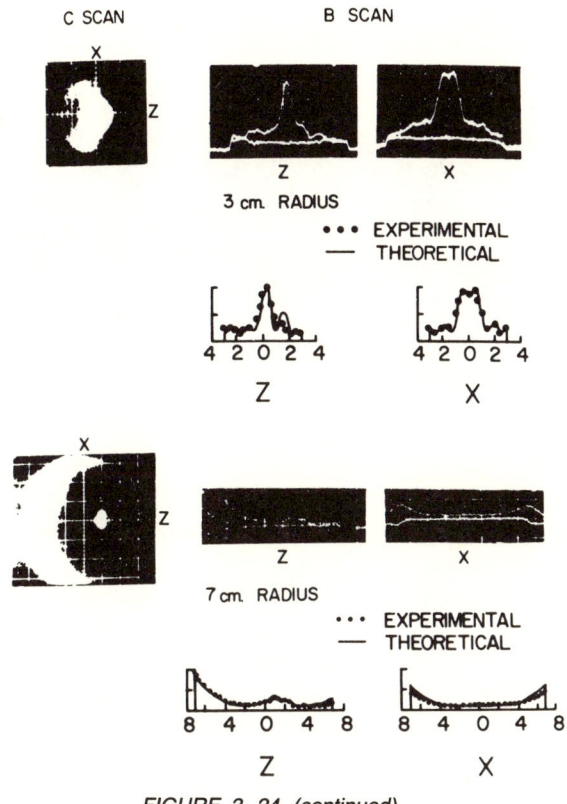

FIGURE 3–24. (continued)

finite aperture source that was used to irradiate the phantom model at this frequency.

In the case of animals, the experimental animal or a different animal of the same species, size, and other characteristics must be killed. The animal is frozen in the same position and orientation as during the experiment. It is then cast in a polyfoam block and bisected along a plane where the SAR distribution is desired. Each half of the animal is then covered with a plastic film or silk screen and the bisected body is returned to room temperature. The procedure just described for models is then used to obtain two-dimensional SAR distributions over the internal surface of the bisected animal.

A photograph illustrating the use of thermography over a parasagittal section of a rat is shown in Fig. 3-25. A thermogram is taken first of the bisected rat's body. The rat is then reassembled and exposed for a

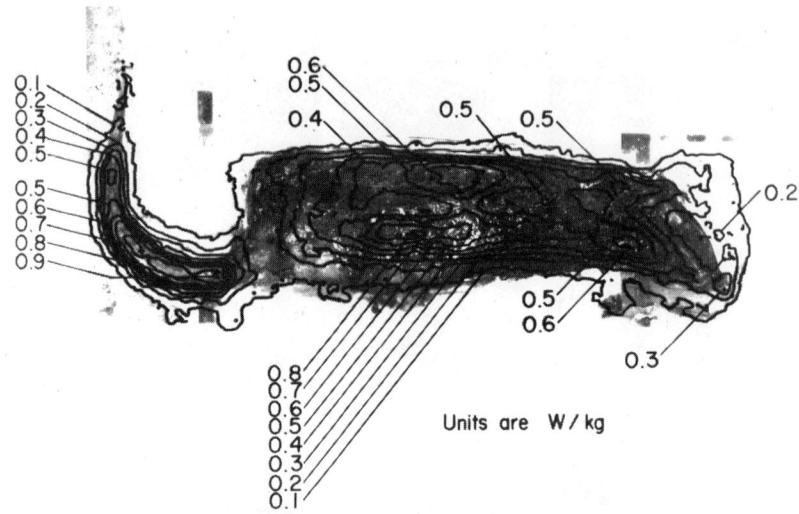

FIGURE 3-25. Thermogram of a parasagittal section of a rat body (Lin *et al.*, 1977).

short time to high-power radiation. Another thermogram of the rat's body over the surface of separation is taken immediately following irradiation. The difference in temperature distributions between the successive thermograms represents the absorbed energy.

An obvious disadvantage of the thermographic procedure is the requirement that the specimen be static. It is therefore restricted to cadavers or equivalent models of animal bodies. The infrared technique also is limited in that it is useful only for surface measures with known emissivities and it has poor sensitivity in the lower temperature ranges. Furthermore, the resolution of the technique is such that it is only applicable to specimens whose dimensions are greater than a few millimeters.

REFERENCES

Allen, S. J. (1975) Measurement of power absorption by human phantoms immersed in radio-frequency fields. *Ann. N.Y. Acad. Sci.* **247**:494.

Aslan, E. (1970) Electromagnetic radiation survey meter. *IEEE Trans. Instrum. Meas.* **IM-19**:368.

Aslan, E. (1972) Broad-band isotropic electromagnetic radiation monitor. *IEEE Trans. Instrum. Meas.* **IM-21**:421.

Aslan, E. (1975) Simplify leakage probe calibration. *Microwaves* **14**:52.

Bahl, I. J., S. S. Stuchly, and M. A. Stuchly (1980) A microstrip antenna for medical application. *IEEE MTT-S Int. Microwave Symp. Digest,* Washington, D.C., pp. 358–360.

Baird, R. C. (1974) Methods of calibrating microwave hazard meters. In: *Biological Effects and Health Hazards of Microwave Radiation*, P. Czerski, K. Ostrowski, M. L. Shore, C. Silverman, M. J. Suess, and B. Waldeskog (eds.). Polish Medical Publishers, Warsaw, pp. 228–236.

Bowman, R. R. (1971) An isotropic electric energy-density probe for high-level fields. Presented at *International Union Radio Science, USNC Meeting*, April, Washington, D.C.

Bowman, R. R. (1976) A probe for measuring temperature in radio-frequency heated material. *IEEE Trans. Microwave Theory Tech.* **MTT-24**:43.

Cetas, T. C. (1975) Temperature measurement in microwave diathermy fields: Principles and probes. In: *Proc. Int. Symp. Cancer Therapy by Hyperthermia and Radiation*, Washington, D.C., pp. 193–203.

Chernovetz, M. E., D. R. Justesen, N. W. King, and J. E. Wagner (1975) Teratology, survival and reversal learning after fetal irradiation of mice by 2430-MHz microwave energy. *J. Microwave Power* **10**:391.

Cheung, A. Y., and D. W. Koopman (1976) Experimental development of simulated biomaterials for dosimetry studies of hazardous microwave radiation. *IEEE Trans. Microwave Theory Tech.* **MTT-24**:669.

Chou, C. K., and A. W. Guy (1978) Effects of electromagnetic fields on isolated nerve and muscle preparations. *IEEE Trans. Microwave Theory Tech.* **MTT-26**:141.

Collin, R. E. (1966) *Foundations for Microwave Engineering*. McGraw-Hill, New York.

Courtney, K., J. C. Lin, A. W. Guy, and C. K. Chou (1975) Microwave effect on rabbit superior cervical ganglion. *IEEE Trans. Microwave Theory Tech.* **MTT-23**: 809.

Crawford, M. L. (1974) Generation of standard EM fields using TEM transmission cells. *IEEE Trans. Electromagn. Compat.* **16**:189.

Donaldson, E. E., W. R. Free, D. W. Robertson, and J. A. Woody (1978) Field measurement made in an enclosure. *Proc. IEEE* **66**:464.

Elder, J. A., J. S. Ali, M. D. Long, and G. E. Anderson (1976) A coaxial air-line microwave exposure system: Respiratory activity of mitochondria irradiated at 2–4 GHz. In: *Biological Effects of Electromagnetic Waves*, Vol. I, C. C. Johnson, and M. L. Shore (eds.). HEW Publ. (FDA) 77-8010, pp. 352–365.

Emerson, W. H. (1973) Electromagnetic wave absorbers and anechoic chambers through the years. *IEEE Trans. Antennas Propag.* **21**:484.

Friend, A. W., and H. Howe (1980) A microstrip microwave biological exposure system. *IEEE MTT-S Int. Microwave Symp. Digest*, Washington, D.C., pp. 345–346.

Guy, A. W. (1971) Analyses of electromagnetic fields induced in biological tissues by thermographic studies on equivalent phantom models. *IEEE Trans. Biomed. Eng.* **BME-19**:205.

Guy, A. W. (1977) A method for exposing cell cultures to electromagnetic fields under controlled conditions of temperature and field strength. *Radio Sci.* **12**:87S.

Guy, A. W., and C. K. Chou (1976) System for quantitative chronic exposure of a population of rodents to UHF fields. In: *Biological Effects of Electromagnetic Waves*, Vol. II, C. C. Johnson, and M. L. Shore (eds.) HEW Publ. (FDA) 77-8011, pp. 389–411.

Guy, A.W., and J. F. Lehmann (1966) On the determination of an optimum microwave diathermy frequency for a direct contact applicator. *IEEE Trans. Biomed. Eng.* **BME-13**:76.

Guy, A. W., J. F. Lehmann, J. A. McDougall, and C. C. Sorensen (1968) Studies on therapeutic heating by electromagnetic energy. In: *Thermal Problems in Biotechnology*. ASME, New York, pp. 26–45.

Guy, A. W., J. F. Lehmann, J. B. Stonebridge, and C. C. Sorensen (1978) Development of a 915-MHz direct-contact applicator for therapeutic heating tissues. *IEEE Trans. Microwave Theory Tech.* **MTT-26:**550.

Guy, A. W., C. K. Chou, J. F. Lehmann, W. Farnham, and J. A. McDougall (1979) Specific absorption rates in mice exposed to 918 and 2450 MHz circularly polarized guided EM fields. Presented at *Bioelectromagnetics Symp.*, Seattle.

Hill, D. A., (1982) Human whole-body radiofrequency absorption studies using a TEM-cell exposure system. *IEEE Trans. Microwave Theory Tech.* **MTT-30:** 1847.

Ho, H. S., E. E. Ginn, and C. L. Christman (1973) Environmentally controlled waveguide irradiation facility. *IEEE Trans. Microwave Theory Tech.* **MTT-21:**837.

Ho, H. S., M. R. Foster, and M. L. Swicord (1976) Microwave irradiation apparatus design and dosimetry. In: *Biological Effects of Electromagnetic Waves,* Vol. II, C. C. Johnson, and M. L. Shore (eds.). HEW Publ. (FDA) 77-8011, pp. 423–434.

Hunt, E. L., and R. D. Phillips (1972) Absolute dosimetry for whole animal experiments. In: *Joint Army/Georgia Inst. Tech. Microwave Dosimetry Workshop,* Walter Reed Army Institute of Research, Washington, D.C., pp. 74–77.

Iskander, M. F., and C. H. Durney (1980) Electromagnetic techniques for medical diagnosis: A review. *Proc. IEEE* **68:**126.

Justesen, D. R. (1975) Toward a prescriptive grammar for the radiobiology of non-ionizing radiation. *J. Microwave Power* **10:**343.

Justesen, D. R., and N. W. King (1970) Behavioral effects of low-level microwave irradiation in the closed space situation. In: *Biological Effects and Health Implications of Microwave Radiation,* S. F. Cleary (ed.). HEW Publ. BRH/DBE 70-2, pp. 154–179.

Justesen, D. R., D. M. Levinson, R. L. Clarke, and N. W. King (1971) A microwave oven for behavioral and biological research. *J. Microwave Power* **6:**237.

Kantor, G., D. M. Witters, and J. W. Greiser (1978) The performance of a new direct-contact applicator for microwave diathermy. *IEEE Trans. Microwave Theory Tech.* **MTT-26:**563.

Kummer, W. H., and E. S. Gillespie (1978) Antenna measurements—1978. *Proc. IEEE* **66:**483.

Larsen, L. E., R. A. Moore, and J. A. Acevedo (1974) A microwave decoupled brain-temperature transducer. *IEEE Trans. Microwave Theory Tech.* **MTT-22:**438.

Larson, E. B. (1979) Technique for producing standard EM fields from 10 kHz to 10 GHz for evaluating radiation monitors. In: *Electromagnetic Fields in Biological Systems,* S. S. Stuchly (ed.). IMPI, Edmonton, Canada, pp. 96–112.

Lehmann, J. F., A. W. Guy, B. J. Delateur, J. B. Stonebridge, and C. G. Warren (1968) Heating patterns produced by short-wave diathermy using helical induction coil applicators. *Arch. Phys. Med. Rehabil.* **44:**193.

Lehmann, J. F., A. W. Guy, C. G. Warren, B. J. Delateur, and J. B. Stonebridge (1970) Evaluation of a microwave contact applicator. *Arch. Phys. Med. Rehabil.* **51:**143.

Lenox, R. H., O. P. Gandhi, J. L. Meyerhoff, and H. M. Grove (1976) A microwave applicator for in vivo rapid inactivation of enzymes in the central nervous system. *IEEE Trans. Microwave Theory Tech.* **MTT-24:**58.

Lin, J. C. (1976) A new system for investigating nonthermal effects of microwaves on cells. In: *Biological Effects of Electromagnetic Waves,* Vol. II, C. C. Johnson, and M. L. Shore (eds.) HEW Publ. (FDA) 77-8011, pp. 350–355.

Lin, J. C., and M. F. Lin (1980) Studies on microwave and blood–brain barrier interaction. *Bioelectromagnetics* **1:**313.

Lin, J. C., and M. F. Lin (1981) Temperature–time profile in rats subjected to selective irradiation of the brain. *IEEE Trans. Biomed. Eng.* **BME-28:**29.

Lin, J. C., and W. D. Peterson (1977) Cytological effects of 2450 MHz CW microwave radiation. *J. Bioeng.* **1:**471.

Lin, J. C., A. W. Guy, and C. C. Johnson (1973a) Power deposition in spherical model of man exposed to 1–20 MHz electromagnetic fields. *IEEE Trans. Microwave Theory Tech.* **MTT-21:**791.

Lin, J. C., A. W. Guy, and G. H. Kraft (1973b) Microwave selective brain heating. *J. Microwave Power* **8:**275.

Lin, J. C., A. W. Guy, and L. R. Caldwell (1977) Thermographic and behavioral studies of rats in the near field of 918-MHz radiations. *IEEE Trans. Microwave Theory Tech.* **MTT-25:**833.

Lin, J. C., G. Kantor, and M. Grods (1978) A class of new microwave therapeutic applicators. Presented at *URSI Int. Symp. Biol. Effects of Electromagnetic Waves*, Helsinki; also in *Radio Sci.* (1982) **17:**119S.

Lin, J. C., R. J. Meltzer, and F. K. Redding (1979a) Microwave-evoked brainstem potentials in cats. *J. Microwave Power* **14:**211.

Lin, J. C., J. C. Nelson, and M. E. Ekstrom (1979b) Effects of repeated exposure to 148-MHz radio waves on growth and hematology of mice. *Radio Sci.* **14:**173S.

Magin, R. L., and G. Kantor (1977) Comparison of heating patterns of small microwave applicators. *J. Bioeng.* **1:**493.

Meyers, P. C., N. L. Sadewsky, and A. H. Barrett (1979) Microwave thermography: Principles, methods and clinical applications. *J. Microwave Power* **14:**105.

Oliva, S. A., and G. N. Catravas (1977) A multiple-animal array for equal power density microwave irradiation. *IEEE Trans. Microwave Theory Tech.* **MTT-25:**433.

Osborne, S. J., and J. N. Frederick (1948) Microwave radiation: Heating of human and animal tissues by means of high-frequency current with wavelength of 12-cm. *J. Am. Med. Assoc.* **137:**1030.

Phillips, R. D., E. L. Hunt, and N. W. King (1975) Field measurements, absorbed dose, and biologic dosimetry of microwaves. *Ann. N.Y. Acad. Sci.* **247:**499.

Ramo, S., J. R. Whinnery, and T. Van Duzer (1965) *Fields and Waves in Communication Electronics.* Wiley, New York.

Richardson, A. W., T. D. Duane, and H. M. Hines (1948) Experimental lenticular opacities produced by microwave irradiation. *Arch. Phys. Med.* **29:**765.

Rozzell, T. C., C. C. Johnson, C. H. Durney, J. L. Lords, and R. G. Olsen (1974) A non-perturbing temperature sensor for measurements in electromagnetic fields. *J. Microwave Power* **9:** 421.

Wickersheim, K. A., and R. V. Alves (1981) A new optical technique for measuring temperature precisely in the presence of RF and microwave fields. *Digest Microwave Power Symposium*, Toronto, Canada, pp. 173–175.

4

Radio and Microwave Dielectric Properties of Biological Materials

4.1. INTRODUCTION

Dielectric properties of tissue materials have been extensively studied (Schwan, 1957, 1963, 1965). A basic understanding has been achieved of the mechanisms and structures that determine the electromagnetic properties of tissue materials. It has been demonstrated that tissue materials are nearly nonmagnetic, and thus have permeabilities close to that of free space and are independent of frequency. On the other hand, the electrical properties of tissue materials have been shown to display a characteristic dependence on frequency. They possess very high dielectric constants compared with many other types of homogeneous liquids and solids. This is because biological tissues are nonhomogeneous, and are composed of cells, macromolecules, and other membrane-bound substances. An example of the frequency-dependent character of tissue materials is given in Fig. 4-1. There are three principal regions of dispersions described as α, β, and γ, respectively. Each dispersion is defined by either a single relaxation frequency or a small group of relaxation frequencies.

The α dispersion at extremely low frequencies (< 1 kHz) apparently results from variation with frequency of cell membrane capacitance. However, the precise mechanism responsible for the decrease in dielectric constant is at present unknown. The membrane capacitance undergoes a pronounced decrease from about 20 μf/cm^2 to near 1 μf/cm^2 as the frequency increases. It is possible that the frequency-dependent membrane capacitance stems from ionic gating currents through the "pores" in the membrane, counterion displacement surrounding the charged membrane, or connections between inner and outer membrane systems (Schwan, 1957, 1975, 1977).

The β dispersion has been shown to originate from the non-homogeneous nature of biological tissues. At frequencies of 1 kHz to 10 MHz, the applied electric field causes charges to accumulate at boundaries separating tissue regions of different dielectric property

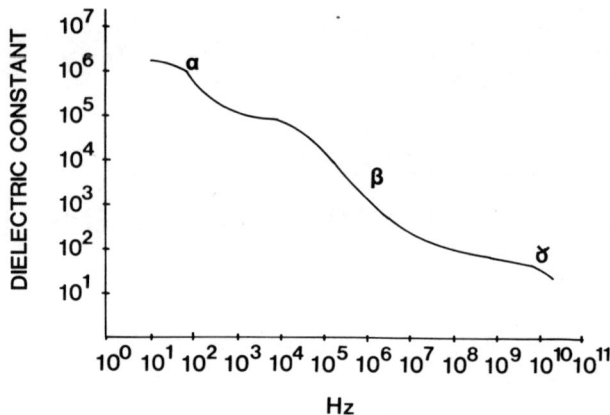

FIGURE 4-1. Dielectric constant of muscle tissue.

(membranes separating intra- and extracellular fluids, for example). Finite periods of time are required before the boundaries can reach charge neutrality, giving rise to the relaxation phenomenon.

As the frequency increases, insufficient time is provided during each cycle to allow complete charging of the cell membranes. The total charges per cycle must decrease, along with the membrane capacitance, as the frequency is increased. This is manifested as a decrease in the dielectric constant.

As the frequency increases still further, the membrane capacitance change stabilizes until the rotational properties of polar molecules in water become important and cause the γ dispersion. This dispersion is characterized by a single relaxation frequency slightly lower than that of pure water, which is due to macromolecule-bound water and to contributions from the macromolecule itself.

Although not shown in Fig. 4-1, there appears to be a minor relaxation termed the δ dispersion, occurring between the γ and β dispersions. This is thought to be partially caused by the relaxation of water molecules bound to the surface of macromolecules, and rotation of amino acids as well as charged side groups of proteins (Schwan, 1975, 1977; Grant et al., 1978).

The conductivities of biological materials change in a similar manner. Cell membranes have a relatively high capacitance (about $1\,\mu f/cm^2$) at frequencies near the β dispersion. They become progressively short-circuited for frequencies above the β dispersion, permitting the intracellular fluid to participate in current conduction. This causes the conductivity to increase as the frequency increases. In the γ dispersion region, the rotation of water molecules is accompanied by viscous loss which accounts for the principal mechanism of increased conductivity.

It is apparent from the dispersion behavior of muscle tissue summarized above that the dielectric and conductivity properties of biological materials in the radio and microwave frequency range are largely determined by the relaxation properties of biological membranes and tissue water. This chapter briefly describes the relaxation process. It also summarizes the measured tissue dielectric constants and conductivities as a function of frequency and temperature.

More detailed description may be found in Debye (1929), von Hippel (1954), Fröhlich (1958), and Daniel (1967). For additional information on the dielectric properties of biological materials, the reader is referred to Schwan (1957), Cole (1968), Hill et al. (1969), and Grant et al. (1978).

4.2. RELAXATION MECHANISM

The frequency-dependent nature of the electrical properties of biological materials may be described by relaxation processes associated with many physical materials displaying a time-dependent response to sudden excitation. Polar molecules and cellular components rotate in response to an applied electric field. This rotation is impeded by inertia and by viscous forces. Therefore, the orientation of polar molecules does not occur instantaneously, giving rise to the time-dependent behavior (relaxation). Moreover, cells and tissues composed of structural components of different properties, when subjected to a step function electrical stimulation, require a finite length of time for charges to accumulate at the interfaces. The accumulation of charges at the interfaces continues until a condition of current equilibrium is reestablished; thus, the relaxation. Many types of relaxation processes can occur in tissue material, owing to dipoles and charges existing in the material.

When the dipole distribution is uniform, the positive charges of one dipole cancel the effect of the negative charge from an adjacent dipole. But when the dipole distribution changes from point to point, this complete cancellation cannot occur. At an interface especially, the ends of the dipoles leave an uncancelled charge on the surface, which becomes an equivalent "bound" charge in the material. The relaxation behavior may therefore be examined by considering the response of bound charges in an applied electric field. For the model shown in Fig. 4-2, the dynamic force equation is

$$m\frac{d^2x}{dt^2} = qE - m\omega_s^2 x - mv\frac{dx}{dt} \qquad (4.1)$$

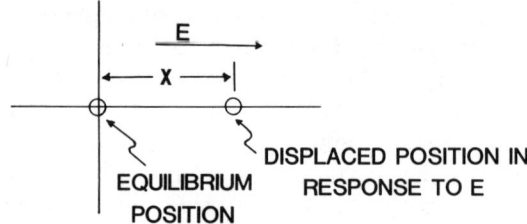

FIGURE 4-2. Behavior of bound, charged particle in an applied electric field.

where x is the particle displacement, E is the electric field, and q and m are the particle charge and mass, respectively. The force given by mass times particle acceleration, on the left-hand side of the equation, consists of the electric driving force qE, an elastic restoring force proportional to displacement x with spring constant conveniently denoted as $m\omega_s^2$, and a retarding damping force proportional to velocity dx/dt with damping constant $m\nu$. The spring and damping constants are chosen in this notation because ω_s is the characteristic frequency of the spring–mass system and ν is the particle collision frequency.

If the field varies harmonically in time ($e^{j\omega t}$), (4.1) may be rearranged to give

$$x(\omega) = \frac{(q/m)/E}{\omega_s^2 - \omega^2 + j\omega\nu} \tag{4.2}$$

Note that the equilibrium position for the charge ($x = 0$) represents local electrical neutrality in the medium. When the charge is displaced from its equilibrium position, a dipole field is established between the charge itself and the "hole" left behind bound in the molecular or membrane structure. A dipole moment p of charge q times the displacement x is formed. For a medium with volume-bound charge density ρ, the total dipole moment per unit volume or polarization P is

$$P = \rho p = \frac{\rho(q^2/m)E}{\omega_s^2 - \omega^2 + j\omega\nu} \tag{4.3}$$

The electric flux density D may be expressed in terms of the electric field E and polarization P as $D = \varepsilon_0 E + P$. For isotropic media the permittivity ε may be related to D by the expression $D = \varepsilon E$. These relations, together with (4.3), give an expression for the permittivity,

$$\varepsilon = \varepsilon_0\left(1 + \frac{\omega_p^2}{\omega_s^2 - \omega^2 + j\omega\nu}\right) \tag{4.4}$$

where

$$\omega_p^2 = \rho q^2/m\varepsilon_0$$

and ε_0 is the free-space permittivity. Clearly ε is a complex number and can be denoted by

$$\varepsilon = \varepsilon' - j\varepsilon'' \qquad (4.5)$$

where ε' and ε'' are the real and imaginary parts of the permittivity and can be obtained by equating the real and imaginary parts of (4.4) and (4.5).

The velocity of bound charge motion $v = dx/dt$ is obtained from (4.2):

$$v(\omega) = \frac{(q/m)E}{v - j[(\omega_s^2 - \omega^2)/\omega]} \qquad (4.6)$$

The finite velocity of charge motion in the material indicates that the particles cannot respond instantaneously to a suddenly applied electric field. This time-delay phenomenon gives rise to a frequency-dependent behavior of charge displacement leading to changes in permittivity with frequency or relaxation.

It was mentioned earlier that relaxation is exhibited by all biological tissues and many physical materials. In what follows, the general development will focus on two classes of dielectric materials of interest to the biophysical aspects of electromagnetic interaction with biological systems.

4.2.1. Low-Loss Dielectric Materials

For low-loss dielectric materials characterized by low collision frequency, v, ε', and ε'' can be easily derived from (4.4) with $\omega \neq \omega_s$:

$$\varepsilon'/\varepsilon_0 = 1 + [\omega_p^2/(\omega_s^2 - \omega^2)] \qquad (4.7a)$$

$$\varepsilon''/\varepsilon_0 = \omega v \omega_p^2/(\omega_s^2 - \omega^2)^2 \qquad (4.7b)$$

A graphical representation of this result is shown in Fig. 4-3. The real part of the permittivity is usually high at low frequencies, increasing to extremely high values at the characteristic frequency ω_s and then returning to ε_0 at higher frequencies. The imaginary part of the permittivity is small at all frequencies except near ω_s. It is high there because of the large particle displacement at the characteristic frequency,

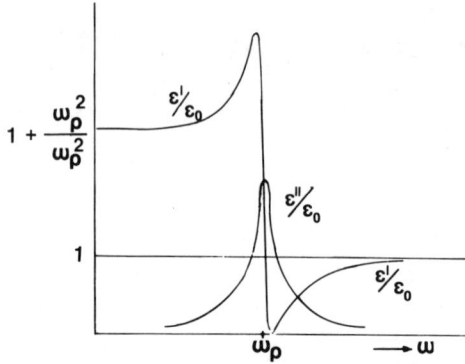

FIGURE 4-3. Frequency permittivity associated with low-loss dielectric materials.

giving rise to large collisional and thus absorption effects. For most solid dielectric materials of practical interest to microwave biophysics (e.g., Plexiglas), the frequency ω_s is in the optical spectrum or above. They are thus characterized by low loss and slowly increasing dielectric constant with frequency. Values of $\varepsilon'/\varepsilon_0$ and $\varepsilon''/\varepsilon'$ for some low-loss materials are given in Table 4-1, as a function of frequency.

4.2.2. Lossy Dielectrics at Low Frequencies

At frequencies low compared to the characteristic frequency ($\omega \ll \omega_s$), (4.4) reduces to

$$\frac{\varepsilon}{\varepsilon_0} = 1 + \frac{\omega_p^2/\omega_s^2}{1 + j\omega v/\omega_s^2} \qquad (4.8a)$$

This equation may be expressed in terms of the permittivity at zero frequency,

$$\varepsilon(0) = \varepsilon_0(1 + \omega_p^2/\omega_s^2)$$

and the permittivity at infinite frequency $\varepsilon(\infty) = \varepsilon_0$. Note that both these limiting values of complex permittivity are real numbers. Thus, (4.8a) written in the Debye form becomes

$$\varepsilon = \varepsilon(\infty) + \frac{\varepsilon(0) - \varepsilon(\infty)}{1 + j\omega\tau} \qquad (4.8b)$$

where $\tau = v/\omega_s^2$ is the relaxation time and is inversely related to the

TABLE 4-1
Electrical Properties of Low-Loss Dielectric Materials at 25°C[a]

	$\varepsilon'/\varepsilon_0$				$\varepsilon''/\varepsilon'$			
	\multicolumn{8}{c}{Frequency (Hz)}
	10^6	10^8	3×10^9	2.5×10^{10}	10^6	10^8	3×10^9	2.5×10^{10}
Fused quartz	3.78	3.78	3.78	3.78	1×10^{-4}	2×10^{-4}	6×10^{-5}	2.5×10^{-4}
Glass–soda borosilicate	4.84	4.84	4.82	4.65	3.6×10^{-3}	3×10^{-3}	5.4×10^{-3}	9×10^{-3}
Foamed polystyrene	1.03	1.03	1.03	1.03	2×10^{-4}	2×10^{-4}	1×10^{-4}	1×10^{-4}
Polystyrene	2.26	2.26	2.26	2.26	2×10^{-4}	2×10^{-4}	3.1×10^{-4}	6×10^{-4}
Teflon (polytetrafluoroethylene)	2.1	2.1	2.1	2.08	2×10^{-4}	2×10^{-4}	1.5×10^{-4}	6×10^{-4}
Beeswax	2.53	2.45	2.39		9.2×10^{-3}	9×10^{-3}	7.5×10^{-3}	

[a] Modified from Westman (1968).

relaxation frequency ω_r. Relaxation time τ, proportional to ν, is a measure of how fast the charges move in response to an applied field. A low value of ν means fewer collisions and a faster response, giving rise to a shorter relaxation time τ. From (4.8b), the real and imaginary parts of ε may be written as

$$\varepsilon' = \varepsilon(\infty) + \frac{\varepsilon(0) - \varepsilon(\infty)}{1 + (\omega\tau)^2} \tag{4.9}$$

$$\varepsilon'' = \frac{\omega\tau[\varepsilon(0) - \varepsilon(\infty)]}{1 + (\omega\tau)^2} \tag{4.10}$$

The loss mechanism described above applies to a model in which there are only bound charges. In biological materials and many other liquids and solids, there exists an appreciable number of free charges. The loss mechanisms in these materials are described by the conductivity relating current density to applied field [see (2.15)]. This may be visualized as free charges moving randomly because of their thermal velocities and frequently experiencing collisions with other particles making up the material. The applied electric field produces a general drift in the direction of the applied field with a nonzero average velocity. This component of the velocity and the resulting current are in phase with the applied field at frequencies low compared with the collision frequency and represent an ohmic loss. At any given frequency, this loss and that for the bound charge add directly. If one is interested only in the macroscopic behavior, it is customary to include the conduction loss in the imaginary part of the permittivity or vice versa. If one is to be concerned with microscopic properties, it would then be necessary to keep the two mechanisms separate.

Moreover, in living matter it is impossible to separate the two contributions from measurements made at a given frequency. Therefore, the presence of a finite ε'' has the effect of producing a total electrical conductivity σ, and a finite conductivity is equivalent to a total imaginary part of the permittivity as ε''. The relationship between σ and ε'' may be derived from two of Maxwell's equations, (2.9) and (2.10), or

$$\sigma = \omega\varepsilon''$$

where σ, an equivalent conductivity representing all losses, is given by

$$\sigma = \frac{\omega^2\tau[\varepsilon(0) - \varepsilon(\infty)]}{1 + (\omega\tau)^2} \tag{4.11}$$

This equation for conductivity can be expressed in an alternate fashion such as

$$\sigma = \sigma(0) + [\sigma(\infty) - \sigma(0)] \frac{(\omega\tau)^2}{1 + (\omega\tau)^2} \qquad (4.12)$$

where $\sigma(0)$ and $\sigma(\infty)$ are the conductivity values far below and above the relaxation frequency ω_s. The conductivity term $\sigma(0)$ has been added to account for the ionic and frequency-independent contribution to σ. Equations (4.8b) and (4.12) are special cases of the Kramers–Kronig relationship (Boettcher, 1952). They show that the frequency response of the permittivity determines that of the conductivity and vice versa.

It is also convenient to define a relative dielectric constant by dividing ε' by the free-space permittivity ε_0:

$$\varepsilon_r = \varepsilon'/\varepsilon_0 \qquad (4.13)$$

This notation will be used often in this volume, as it simplifies the mathematical manipulations. It should be mentioned that ε_r is usually referred to simply as the dielectric constant [see also (2.18)].

The ratio $\varepsilon''/\varepsilon'$ is also a commonly used parameter for dielectric materials and is referred to as the loss tangent. For low-loss materials such as those given in Table 4-1, the loss tangent is much less than unity. On the other hand, biological materials are characterized by considerable amounts of losses and therefore have loss tangents close to or greater than one.

The results summarized in (4.9), (4.10), and (4.11) have been used to describe the electrical properties of biological tissues throughout the radio and microwave region. For a particular frequency range, the values

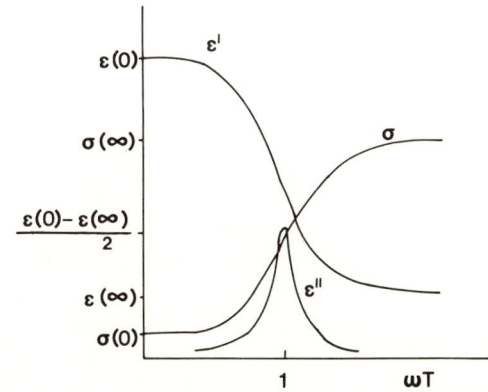

FIGURE 4-4. Frequency-dependent characteristics of permittivity and conductivity of a lossy dielectric material.

of $\varepsilon(\infty)$ and $\varepsilon(0)$ are taken to be the permittivity at frequencies far above and below the relaxation frequency ω_s.

The variation with frequency of the real and imaginary parts of the permittivity, and electrical conductivity is illustrated in Fig. 4-4. It is seen that the dielectric constant ε' falls from a high value $\varepsilon(0)$ to $\varepsilon(\infty)$ as the frequency increases through the dispersion region, while the conductivity rises from a small value $\sigma(0)$ to $\sigma(\infty)$. The imaginary part of the permittivity ε'' peaks at $\omega\tau = 1$ and falls off for both higher and lower frequencies.

4.2.3. Biological Materials

The dielectric properties of tissue materials are complex and require a distribution of relaxation processes for representation throughout the radio and microwave frequency region. In this case, the dielectric behavior may be modeled as a sum of relaxation processes, with each process being a non-instantaneous exponential relaxation from one state to another. The corresponding responses in the frequency domain are of the form

$$\varepsilon = \varepsilon_\infty + \sum_{n=1}^{N} \frac{\Delta\varepsilon_n}{1 + j\omega\tau_n} \qquad (4.14)$$

where $\Delta\varepsilon_n$ is the difference between the permittivity far below and far above the relaxation frequency, and τ_n is the relaxation time associated with each relaxation process.

As mentioned earlier, the dielectric properties of biological materials frequently are characterized by three distinct relaxation processes. Thus, the relaxation times are well separated such that $\tau_1 \gg \tau_2 \gg \tau_3$. The corresponding relaxation frequencies for each region are near 100 Hz, 50 kHz, and 25 GHz at body temperature.

4.3. TEMPERATURE DEPENDENCE OF DIELECTRIC PROPERTIES

In considering relaxation processes in Section 4.2, it was indicated that the electrical properties of biological tissues throughout the radio and microwave frequency range are governed by structural and rotational relaxation phenomena. There are in biological materials abundant layers of tissues and membranes with different dielectric constants and conductivities. When an electric field is applied, surface charges build up at the interface between two adjacent layers, thus generating a time-varying permittivity. Further, molecular dipoles tend to orient in an applied electric field. Since the reorientation of polar molecules does not occur instantaneously, it gives rise to a rotational relaxation effect.

The movement of charges, whether to accumulate at tissue interfaces or to realign through rotation, is hindered by collisions with other particles in the surrounding medium. The speed of movement depends, therefore, on temperature, among other factors. Thus, both dielectric constants and conductivities are temperature dependent.

A mathematical treatment of the temperature dependence of the dielectric constant and conductivity, however, is very difficult (Fröhlich, 1958). The few studies (Cook, 1952; Schwan and Li, 1953; Schwan and Foster, 1980) concerned with the temperature dependence of dielectric constants and conductivities have shown that the temperature dependence of the conductivity is much more pronounced than that of the dielectric constant. Near a relaxation frequency, the relationship

$$\frac{d\varepsilon}{\varepsilon} = \frac{d\sigma}{\sigma} \frac{\varepsilon(0) - \varepsilon(\infty)}{\varepsilon(0) + \varepsilon(\infty)} \tag{4.15}$$

may be derived for the relative change in dielectric constant to the relative change in conductivity (Schwan and Foster, 1980). Since $\varepsilon(0)$ and $\varepsilon(\infty)$ are fairly independent of temperature and $\varepsilon(0)$ is much larger than $\varepsilon(\infty)$, the change of the dielectric constant with temperature must be smaller than that of the conductivity.

As indicated earlier, the properties of biological materials are characterized by three distinct dispersion regions. For each dispersion, the temperature coefficient reflects those of $\varepsilon(0)$, $\varepsilon(\infty)$, and ω_s. The α dispersion may be due to frequency-dependent membrane capacitance arising from ionic gating currents through or counterions surrounding cell membranes. These ionic activities have temperature coefficients similar to that of the conductivity of electrolytes, i.e., about 2% per °C. The β dispersion is caused by polarization effects in which the cellular membranes are charged through the electrolytes. Hence, the temperature coefficient is equal to that of the conductivity of electrolytes. The γ dispersion originates from the rotational relaxation of water molecules. Hence, its temperature dependence is equal to that of water, which is again close to 2% per °C. Thus, the temperature coefficient of the conductivity for biological materials has a maximum value of about 2% per °C for tissues with higher water content.

4.4. METHODS OF PERMITTIVITY MEASUREMENT

A large number of techniques exist for measuring the complex permittivity of materials at radio and microwave frequencies. In this section, a few commonly used techniques will be described for the frequency ranges of interest. Most of these techniques require manual operation. Measurements of dielectric constants and conductivities have thus been extremely time-consuming, and consequently there has been a lack of comprehensive data on the dielectric properties of biological materials. Recent advances in instrumentation have made it possible to employ automated procedures for measuring the electrical properties of materials, including biological tissues. These techniques can rapidly and accurately measure the desired parameter over a wide frequency range under the control of a small laboratory computer. This development will undoubtedly help to resolve the multitudinous questions regarding the biological effects and potential hazards of electromagnetic radiation. It will also facilitate the medical and biological uses of these radiant energies. Therefore, a brief discussion of automated procedures is also presented.

4.4.1. Radiofrequency Techniques

At the lower edge of the radiofrequency region, common circuit elements may be used to measure the dielectric constant and conductivity of these materials. One such technique involves the use of a parallel plate capacitor serving also as a sample holder. The tissue sample is placed between the plates of the capacitor and the capacitance change due to the presence of the tissue sample may be measured using a sensitive impedance bridge. The dielectric constant and conductivity are related to the real and imaginary parts of the admittance Y_1 and Y_2, respectively, of the tissue-loaded capacitor through

$$\varepsilon_r = Y_2 d / \omega \varepsilon_0 A \tag{4.16}$$

$$\sigma = Y_1 d / A \tag{4.17}$$

where A is the cross-sectional area of the plate and d is the plate separation of the capacitor sample holder.

At higher frequencies, around 10 MHz, the above technique is no longer reliable. Transmission line techniques must then be utilized and a number of basic principles may be used to convert the measured parameters to dielectric constant and conductivity information. A very convenient and reliable technique for measuring dielectric properties of tissue materials over a wide frequency range is determination of the propagation constant of waves in a coaxial transmission line filled with tissue materials. This is a technique of controlled wave propagation. Since the wave in a coaxial transmission line has electric and magnetic fields strictly in the transverse plane, similar to a plane wave in a material medium, the dielectric constant and conductivity are related to the attenuation and propagation factors through (see Section 2.2)

$$\varepsilon_r = (\beta^2 - \alpha^2)/\omega^2 \mu_0 \varepsilon_0 \qquad (4,18)$$

$$\sigma = 2\alpha\beta/\omega\mu_0 \qquad (4.19)$$

Hence, a knowledge of the propagation characteristics of a tissue-filled coaxial transmission line will enable us to obtain the electrical properties of the tissue (Guy *et al.*, 1974; Toler and Seals, 1977).

Two related methods may be used to implement the technique outlined above. The first case involves a network analyzer (or vector voltmeter), a sweep frequency signal generator, a coaxial transmission line with a series of fixed probes, and a recording device. A typical experimental arrangement for the measurement is shown in Fig. 4-5. The attenuation and phase factor can be measured rapidly over a wide frequency range between a reference probe and several similar sensing probes inserted in the line at periodic intervals in the direction of propagation. The line should be sufficiently long to prevent any possible reflections due to the termination from reaching the measuring probes.

The second method is similar to the first except a slotted coaxial transmission line sample holder is used. A practical experimental

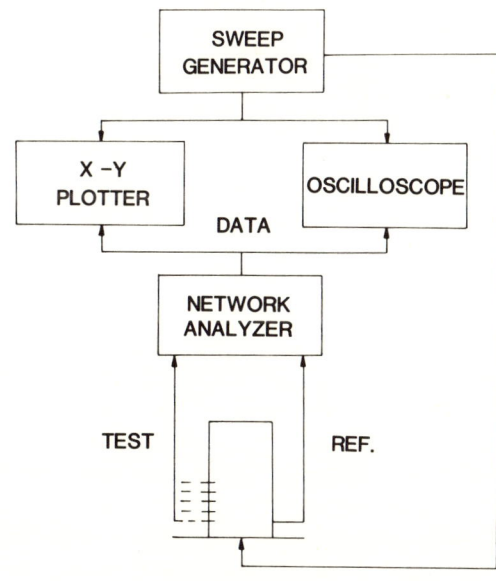

FIGURE 4-5. Equipment block diagram for fixed probe coaxial line measurements.

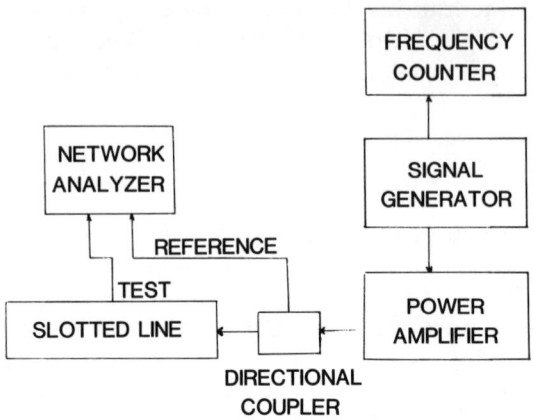

FIGURE 4-6. Equipment block diagram for slotted line measurements.

arrangement of the measuring system is shown in Fig. 4-6. In this case, the amplitude and phase are measured continuously as a function of distance along the loaded transmission line at a given frequency. Although this arrangement is useful for the entire radio and microwave range, and for any tissue material, it is most easily adapted to liquid media since the measuring probe may be moved freely along the slot on the transmission line filled with liquids. For solids or tissues of more condensed nature, it is necessary to provide a path for the probe and accurate measurements become difficult and highly dependent on the skill of the experimenter.

For frequencies below approximately 30 MHz, the real part of the complex permittivity becomes increasingly small compared with the imaginary part. Consequently, the conductivity is of primary interest in many practical situations. Under these conditions, $\alpha = \beta$ and the conductivity is simply given by

$$\sigma = \alpha/\eta_0 = \alpha(\varepsilon_0/\mu_0)^{1/2} \tag{4.20}$$

where $\eta_0 = (\mu_0/\varepsilon_0)^{1/2}$ is the intrinsic impedence of free space. Therefore, the conductivity is relatively constant and essentially independent of frequency in this range. The conductivity may be measured directly by filling a cylindrical plastic tube with tissue material, allowing a known current (applied via a pair of endplate electrodes) to pass through the material, and monitoring the voltage drop across a second pair of electrodes a known distance apart near the middle of the tube (see Fig. 4-7). The cross-sectional area of the tube and the distance between the

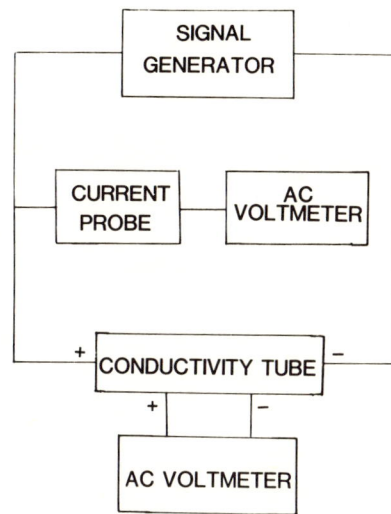

FIGURE 4-7. Equipment block diagram for conductivity measurements.

measuring electrodes may be adjusted so that the conductivity can be read directly from the voltmeter. Since

$$\sigma = l/RA = (l/A)(i/v) \qquad (4.21)$$

where l is the separation between the measuring electrodes, A is the cross-sectional area of the tube, R is the resistance, i is the current through, and v is the voltage drop across the measuring points. For l and A equal to unity and a known current, the conductivity is indeed given by the voltage measurement.

A major shortcoming of the method just described is that it requires a large tissue sample volume and it is practically useless under *in vivo* conditions. Recently, a four-electrode technique has been developed that can be used to measure the tissue conductivity in volumes as small as 1 cm³. The technique is suitable for both *in vitro* and *in vivo* measurements.

One of the problems in making conductivity measurements using implanted electrodes in tissues is the formation of an ionic sheath (electrode polarization) about the current-carrying electrodes. The four-electrode method minimizes this problem by using separate current-injecting and voltage-measuring electrodes. This method is a straightforward technique that has been used extensively in other conductivity or resistivity studies. The technique basically involves applying a current to a medium with one set of electrodes and measuring the resulting voltage between a second set of electrodes. The current flow established in the tissue can be determined by an external ammeter. The voltage may be measured using an extremely high-impedance voltmeter. In this way, the ionic sheath that can develop near the injection electrodes will have no disturbing effects on the voltage measurements as long as the voltage probes are at a reasonable distance away from the excitation point.

Another problem often encountered in measurements at these frequencies is stray capacitance. This may occur between tissues (especially *in vivo*), equipment leads, and metal structures in the proximity of the measuring system. Isolation transformers and electrical balancing can be used to minimize these problems.

Figure 4-8 shows the construction of a conductivity probe consisting of a set of outer electrodes (two rows of three hypodermic needles) acting as current-injecting electrodes, and two inner electrodes to sample the voltage drop across the medium under measurement. The spacing between needles is about 2 mm. Three needles are used for the outer electrodes to reduce field fringing effects. The nonparallel fringing fields are not eliminated, but a larger volume of material is within the electrode configuration and is exposed to a uniform field so that the magnitude of the fringe contributes less to the total measurement.

Two measuring circuits may be used. Figure 4-9 shows a simple system for use in the frequency range 3 to 300 Hz. The current injected into the sample medium is determined by measuring the voltage drop across the current-sampling resistor. The resulting electric field is calculated from the voltage measured between the two inner electrodes. A Tektronix P6046-type probe may be used as a voltage amplifier to obtain the high common mode rejection required and to provide the

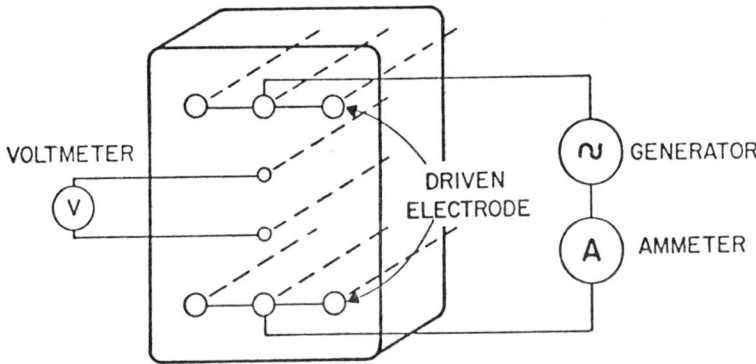

FIGURE 4-8. Probe construction using a guarded modification of the "four-electrode method."

DIELECTRIC PROPERTIES OF BIOLOGICAL MATERIALS

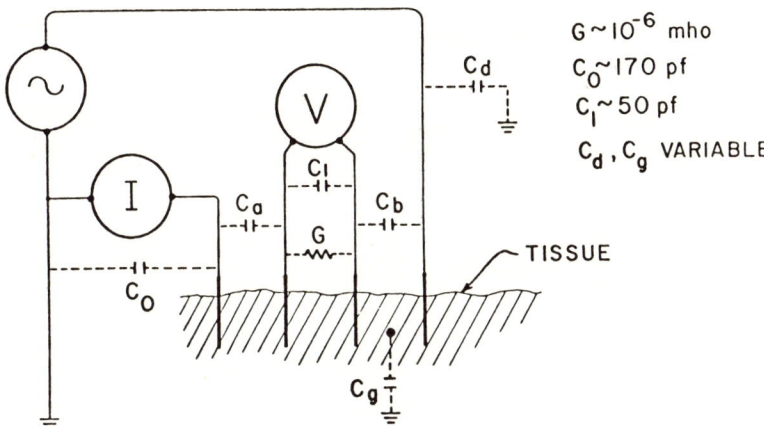

FIGURE 4-9. Low-frequency four-electrode technique. Parasitic capacitances are indicated.

necessary match between the high input impedance and the low impedance measuring devices.

At frequencies between 0.3 and 30 MHz, stray capacitances between the tissue specimen, various instrumentation, and movable items including the experimenter cause considerable difficulty. The system shown in Fig. 4-10 uses a doubly balanced isolation transformer to reduce the stray capacitance influences. The system employs two Tektronix P6046 probes; one measures via the sampling resistor, the current injected into the specimen, and the other measures the voltage drop across the inner

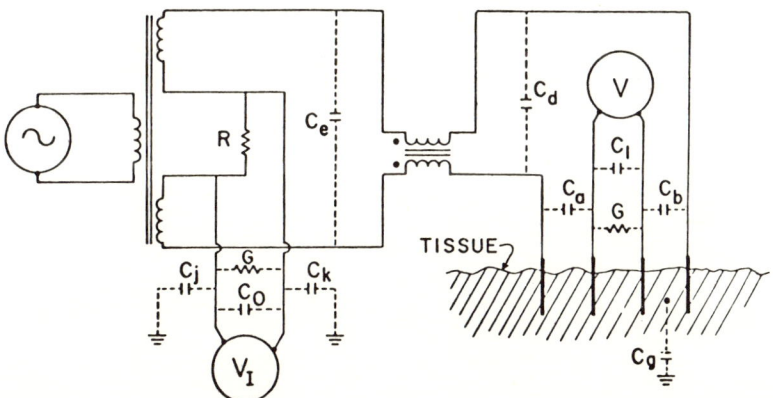

FIGURE 4-10. High and medium frequency circuit employing an isolation transformer and a current balancing transformer.

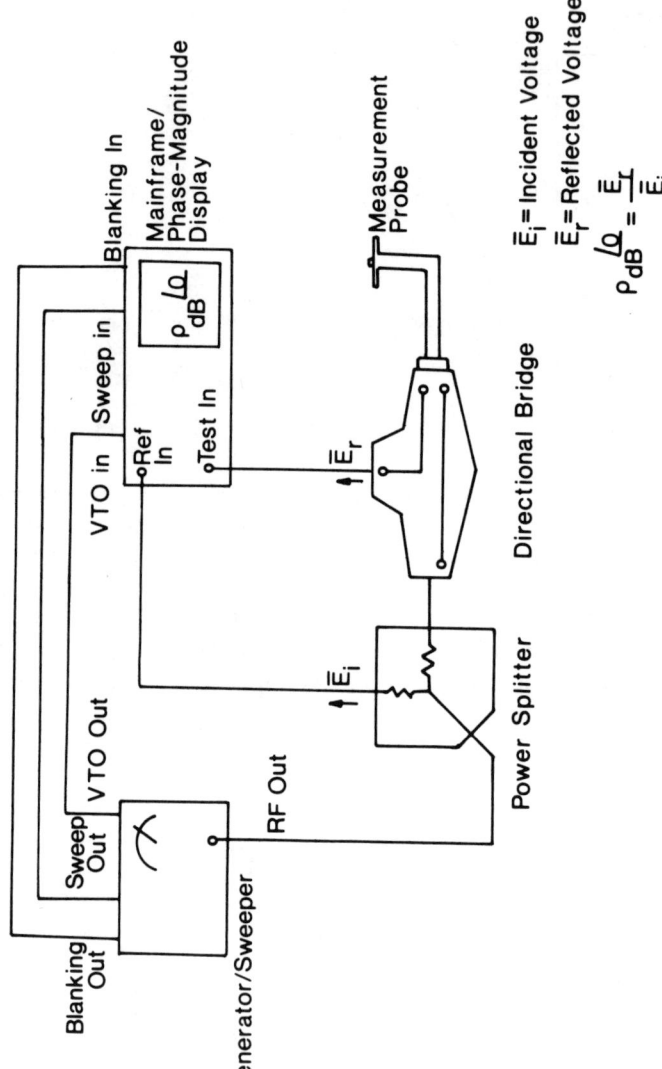

FIGURE 4-11. Block diagram of dielectric property measurement system consisting of probe, network analyzer, and associated instrumentation.

electrode pair. The outputs of these probes are fed into a network analyzer, which gives the ratio between the measured current and voltage. The conductivity of the specimen is found by using equation (4.21).

Another measurement technique that is suited for both *in vivo* and *in vitro* dielectric property determinations involves the use of a short monopole antenna probe and a network analyzer (Toler and Seals, 1977). A block diagram for the probe measurement system is shown in Fig. 4-11. The signal transmitted by the signal generator and the portion that is reflected from the monopole antenna in the specimen are sampled by the directional bridge and power splitter. These sampled signals are then routed to the network analyzer, which calculates the reflection coefficient, i.e., the ratio of signals reflected from the probe to those transmitted by the source. The input impedance is related to the reflection coefficient through [see (2.54) and (2.55)]

$$Z_i = Z_0[(1 + \rho)/(1 - \rho)] = R - jX \qquad (4.22)$$

It can be shown that the dielectric constant and conductivity are given, respectively, by

$$\varepsilon_r = \frac{\cos^2 \delta}{\omega X C} \qquad (4.23)$$

$$\sigma = \omega \varepsilon_r \varepsilon_0 \tan \delta \qquad (4.24)$$

where

$$\tan \delta = R/X \qquad (4.25)$$

and C is a constant associated with the probe configuration and is obtained by calibration against a medium of known dielectric properties.

4.4.2. Microwave Techniques

At microwave frequencies, a hollow waveguide is useful for electrical property determinations (Roberts and von Hippel, 1946; Wind and Rapaport, 1955). The measurement makes use of input impedance characteristics, referred to as the air–dielectric interface of a tissue sample in a waveguide. The tissue samples in the waveguide must be sufficiently deep so that reflections from the terminating endplate are minimized. The method requires manual standing wave pattern measurements in a slotted section. A block diagram for the experimental arrangement is shown in Fig. 4-12. The dielectric constant at a given frequency is related to the measured guide wavelength λ_g and cutoff

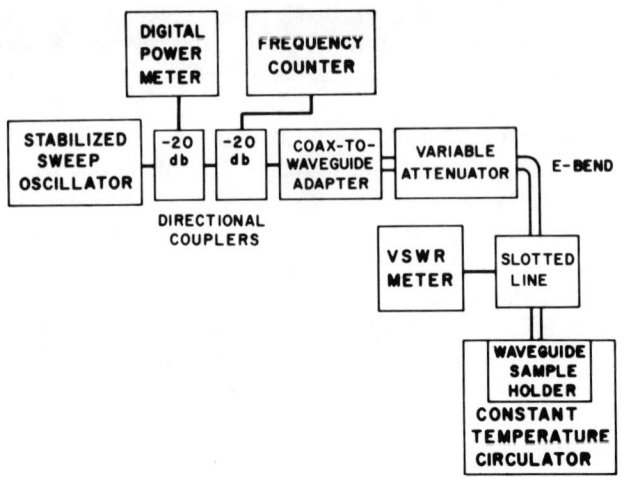

FIGURE 4-12. Block diagram for manual dielectric property measurement.

wavelength λ_c of the guide, voltage standing wave ratio S, and the null positions of the probe in the slotted section with and without the sample in the waveguide P_a and P_s through the following equation:

$$\varepsilon = [1 + (\lambda_c/\lambda_g)^2]^{-1} + [1 + (\lambda_g/\lambda_c)^2]^{-1} \\ \times [S - j \tan k(P_a - P_s)]^2/[1 - jS \tan k(P_a - P_s)]^2 \quad (4.26)$$

where $k = 2\pi/\lambda_g$. The values for ε_r and σ may be calculated with the aid of a small laboratory computer.

The accuracy of this technique depends critically on the sample conductivity. At higher conductivities, the reflection coefficient is relatively insensitive to the conductivity of the sample and, consequently, large potential errors may be encountered. An alternative approach is to use "tuned" samples that are nearly one-quarter of a wavelength long. In this case, the reflection coefficient is almost real and most sensitive to the dielectric constant and conductivity of the sample. The accuracy of this technique is largely determined by the accuracy of the sample thickness measurement. It has been shown, using a dial gauge, that measurement accuracy is better than 2% for tissues at microwave frequencies (Foster *et al.*, 1979). The disadvantage of the technique is that it requires the use of "tuned" samples. Thus, a different sample must be used at each frequency and the required sample thicknesses can be quite small, e.g., 1 mm for brain tissue at 10 GHz. These necessities cause a great increase in the scatter of data and make the technique labor intensive.

As mentioned previously, most of the techniques require manual determination of the standing wave characteristics in a dielectric loaded waveguide or transmission line. For this reason, measurements of complex permittivity have been extremely time-consuming, and consequently there has been a lack of comprehensive data on the dielectric properties of biological materials. Recent advances in the application of microwave energy in industry, science, biology, and medicine have created an urgent need for dielectric property information. Fortunately, new developments in electronic instrumentation have provided techniques capable of yielding dielectric properties rapidly and accurately over a wide range of microwave frequencies. This section describes a method for making dielectric constant measurements using a computer-controlled automatic network analyzer.

One such method is Fig. 4-13. The system is programmed to measure the scattering parameters of the dielectric sample in the holder at a set of predetermined discrete frequencies over a wide frequency range (Lin and Jacobi, 1975). The complex relative dielectric constants are computed from the measured scattering parameters in real time using the following equations in the data analysis:

$$\varepsilon_r = \frac{G + (\lambda_g/2a)^2}{1 + (\lambda_g/2a)^2} \quad (4.27)$$

$$\sigma = \frac{\omega B}{1 + (\lambda_g/2a)^2} \quad (4.28)$$

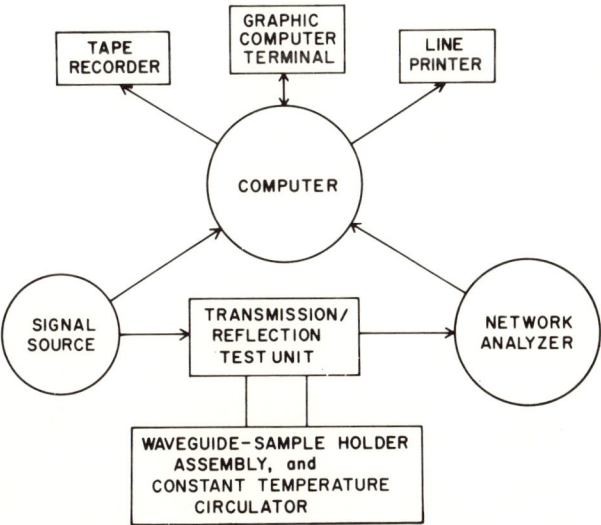

FIGURE 4-13. Automated dielectric property measurement system.

where λ_g is the guide wavelength in air, a is the broad dimension of the waveguide, G and B are the real and imaginary parts of

$$Y = \frac{(1 - S_{11})^2 - S_{12}^2}{(1 + S_{11})^2 - S_{12}^2} = G + jB \qquad (4.29)$$

where S_{11} and S_{12} are the scattering parameters, which are also the reflection coefficient at the air–dielectric interface and the transmission coefficient through the dielectric material, respectively. The validity of these equations can be verified by computing the reflection and transmission coefficients for a known slab of dielectric material and calculating the complex permittivities from these coefficients using (4.27)–(4.29).

The materials measured are either machined or shaped to fit perfectly in the sample holder (see Fig. 4-14). The holder consists of a washerlike waveguide or transmission line section having the same thickness as the dielectric sample. The sample holders are precision made to match the transmission and reflection ports (flanges). The system is therefore symmetric and consequently it is only necessary to consider S_{11} and S_{12}.

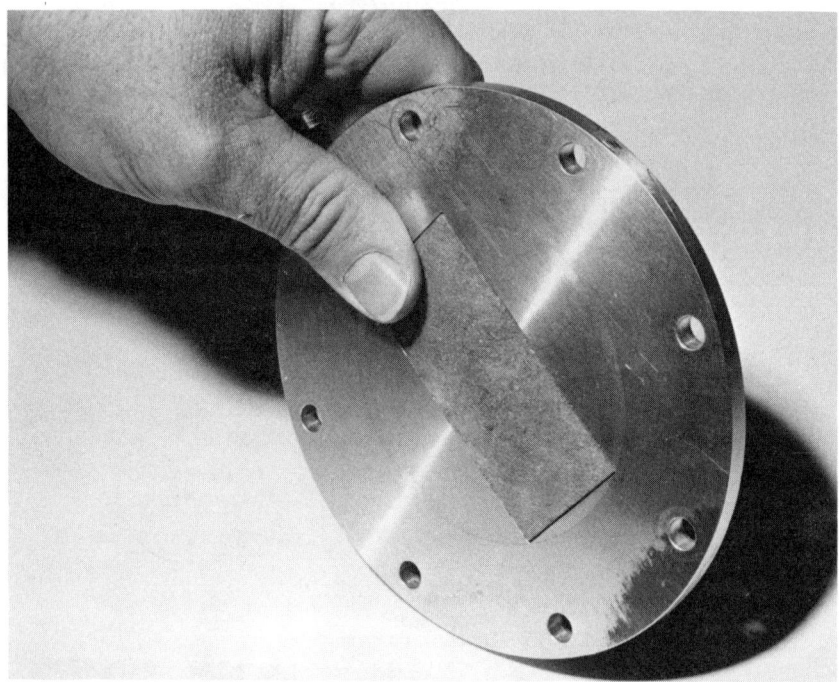

FIGURE 4-14. Precision waveguide tissue sample holder.

The use of a washerlike sample holder increases the accuracy of the measurements considerably, since the location of the sample is known to a much greater degree of precision and the sample holder eliminates the need to correct for the shift in reference planes.

The accuracy of the measurements is increased because the system applies a self-calibrating procedure that eliminates errors due to mismatch, cross talk, directivity, and frequency response. The accuracy is further enhanced by averaging the results of several successive measurements. It should be noted that while this technique was developed specifically for *in vitro* measurement, the concept of scattering parameter, in particular the reflection coefficient S_{11}, easily could be adopted for *in vivo* situations.

A probe technique for determination of the dielectric properties of living tissue *in situ* has in fact been developed by Burdette et al. (1980). The technique is based on the use of an infinitesimal monopole antenna and on the use of microprocessor-controlled microwave measurement instrumentation. It uses a network analyzer and a semiautomated data acquisition/processing system to accurately determine the electrical characteristics of the *in vivo* probe and tissue being measured.

The input impedance of an infinitesimal monopole antenna in free space is given by

$$Z(\omega, \varepsilon_0) = 1/j\omega C \qquad (4.30)$$

where C is a constant determined by the physical dimensions of the probe (Jordan and Balmain, 1968). It is seen that the probe impedance is totally reactive. The radiation resistance of the probe approaches zero and no power is radiated. According to the antenna modeling theorem (Tai, 1961), the input impedance of the antenna in a dielectric medium is related to the input impedance of the antenna in free space through

$$Z(\omega, \varepsilon)/\eta = Z(n\omega, \varepsilon_0)/\eta_0 \qquad (4.31)$$

where η_0 and η are the intrinsic impedance of free space and of the dielectric medium, respectively, and $n = (\varepsilon/\varepsilon_0)^{1/2}$. Using the antenna impedance given in (4.30), one obtains

$$Z(\omega, \varepsilon) = \varepsilon_0/j\omega\varepsilon C \qquad (4.32)$$

The equation may be expressed in terms of the dielectric constant and loss tangent, such that

$$Z(\omega, \varepsilon) = [j\omega\varepsilon_r C(1 - j\tan\delta)]^{-1} \qquad (4.33)$$

Since $Z = R + jX$, the real and imaginary parts of the impedance are given by

$$R = \tan \delta / \omega \varepsilon_r C (1 + \tan^2 \delta) \tag{4.34}$$

$$X = [\omega \varepsilon_r C (1 + \tan^2 \delta)]^{-1} \tag{4.35}$$

where R and X are measured using the network analyzer and C is the antenna constant. The solutions for ε_r and $\tan \delta$ are easily found by noting that $\tan \delta = R/X$.

The configuration of the *in vivo* probe that has been used most intensively is illustrated in Fig. 4-15. The probe is fabricated from 0.085-inch (0.22-cm)-diameter semirigid coaxial cable. An SMA-type connector is attached to one end of the probe to permit connection to the microwave instrumentation. The center conductor at the open end of the probe protrudes slightly to ensure good probe–tissue contact. Both center and outer conductors of the probe at the open end are gold-plated to minimize chemical reaction between the probe and the electrolyte in the tissue.

The impedance measurement and data acquisition/processing system is shown in Fig. 4-16. In addition to the probe, the system consists of a network analyzer, an interferface with A/D conversion, a microprocessor, a printer, an RF sweep oscillator, and a frequency counter. The network analyzer measures the impedance of the *in vivo* probe in terms of a complex reflection coefficient. The magnitude and phase angle of the reflection coefficient are fed to the computer, which corrects for systematic measurement errors and computes the dielectric constant and loss tangent using (4.34) and (4.35). This system (Burdette *et al.*, 1980) incorporates an error correction model that permits system calibration using known terminations (short-circuit, open-circuit, and matched load). Using the infinitesimal monopole probe, the system can accurately determine *in vivo* dielectric properties from below 0.1 GHz to above 10 GHz. Other advantages of this system include the ability to perform

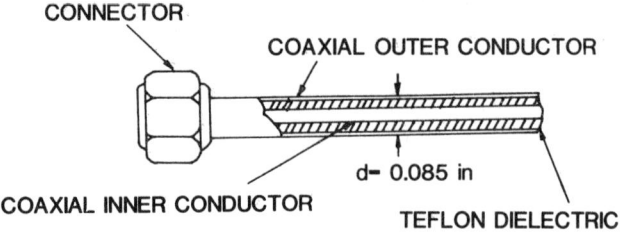

FIGURE 4-15. Configuration of the infinitesimal probe.

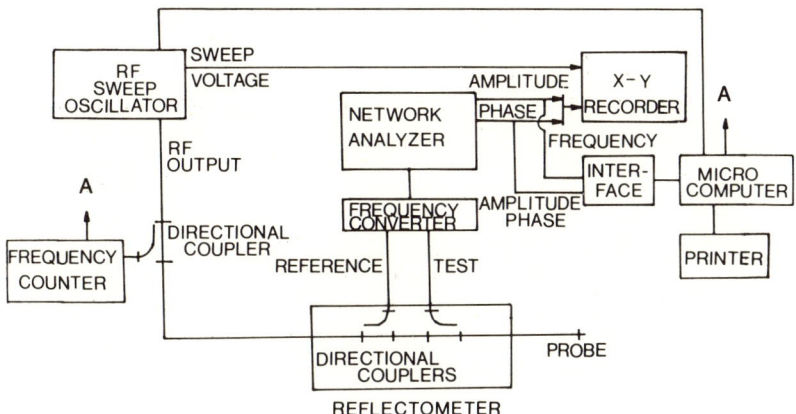

FIGURE 4-16. Block diagram of *in vivo* dielectric property measurement system consisting of probe, network analyzer, and associated instrumentation (Burdette *et al.*, 1980).

continuous measurements throughout the above frequency range and the capability to do so very rapidly.

4.5. PERMITTIVITY OF WATER

Water is by far the most abundant constituent of animals, and constitutes approximately 60% of the total body mass in humans. For example, water makes up 93% of the blood, about 80% of skeletal muscle, somewhat less than 9% of fat, and approximately 70% of white matter (Altman and Dittner, 1964; Schepps and Foster, 1980). The fluid nature of water allows both the dissolved electrolytes and the suspended substances to diffuse to different parts of the cell or tissue. When the cell or tissue loses its water, life is endangered or extinguished.

Of the total body water, about 62% is in the intracellular space and about 38% in the extracellular space (Guyton, 1969). One may thus expect water to exert major influences on the permittivity properties (i.e., dielectric constant and conductivity) of biological materials. We will therefore briefly consider the dielectric properties of water as a function of frequency and temperature.

It is well known that the permittivity of water shows a characteristic dispersion at microwave frequencies (Eisenberg and Kauzmann, 1969; Franks, 1972; Hasted, 1973; Hasted and El Sabeh, 1953). A graph showing the frequency dependence of the dielectric constant and conductivity of water at 37°C is given in Fig. 4-17. It is seen that water has a

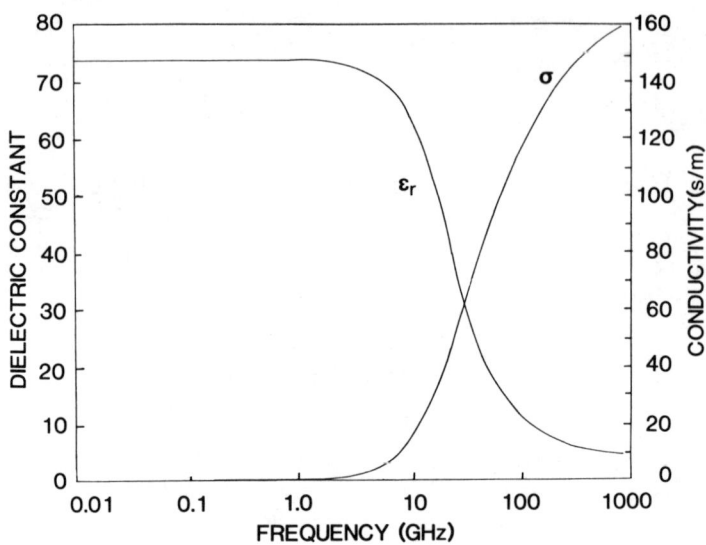

FIGURE 4-17. Dielectric constant and conductivity of free water at 37°C.

relaxation frequency of about 32 GHz at 37°C. Both the dielectric constant and the conductivity are invariant with frequency from dc to 1.0 GHz. At frequencies above 3–5 GHz, water starts to disperse. The dielectric constant falls from a static value of 74 to about 28 at 35 GHz before reaching a lower bound near 4.5. Conversely, the conductivity increases almost monotonically for frequencies up to and beyond the microwave range. Clearly, the dielectric behavior of water is characterized by a single relaxation process between dc and microwave frequencies, which is governed by the rotation of individual water molecules as dipoles in a viscous fluid. Moreover, they can be approximated by the simple Debye equations (Schwan et al., 1976):

$$\varepsilon = \varepsilon(\infty) + \frac{\varepsilon(0) - \varepsilon(\infty)}{1 + (\omega/\omega_s)^2} \qquad (4.36)$$

$$\sigma = \sigma(0) + |\varepsilon(0) - \varepsilon(\infty)| \frac{\varepsilon_r(\omega/\omega_s)^2}{1 + (\omega/\omega_s)^2} \qquad (4.37)$$

where $\sigma(0)$ is the dc conductivity and is essentially zero for water. The other constants were discussed earlier.

The temperature relations of the dielectric properties of water for six frequencies are illustrated in Fig. 4-18. These graphs show that the dielectric constants and conductivities of water at 0.577, 1.74, and

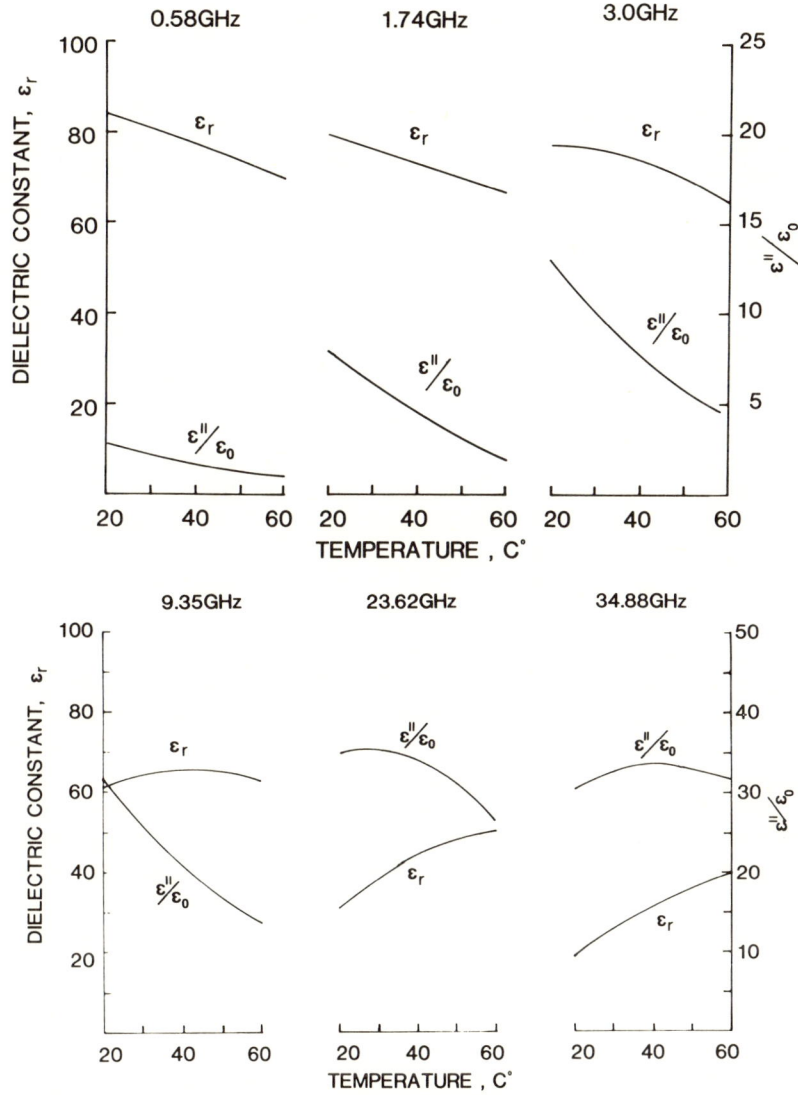

FIGURE 4-18. Temperature dependence of dielectric properties at six microwave frequencies.

3.00 GHz decrease with increasing temperature, while those at 9.4, 23.7, and 34.9 GHz may increase, peak, and decrease with increasing temperature. These subtleties in the temperature behavior of water at higher frequencies probably stem from the fact that water starts to disperse above 5 GHz.

It is interesting to note that the relaxation frequency of water increases with increasing temperature in an exponential fashion (Grant et al., 1978). In particular, the relaxation frequency at 0°C is 8.84 GHz and becomes 39.8 GHz at 60°C. Furthermore, in the presence of polar solute molecules the relaxation frequency shifts to lower frequencies because the dispersion of the solute molecules takes place at frequencies far below that for water. This will give rise to second or third regions of dispersion, which is usually well separated from that of water.

4.6. DIELECTRIC PROPERTIES OF BIOLOGICAL MATERIALS

Biological materials may be classified into three major groups according to their water content. The first group is of high water content (90% or more) and consists of fluids containing electrolytes, macromolecules, and other cellular materials, and includes blood, vitreous humor, and cerebrospinal fluid. The second is of moderate water content (less than 80%) and consists of skin, muscle, brain, and internal organs. The last group is made up of tissues with low water content (about 40%) such as bone, fat, and tendon (Lin, 1978).

This section will summarize the measured dielectric constants and conductivities of tissue materials as a function of frequency and temperature. Representative data for each group are given separately. It will be seen that the electrical properties of biological materials are indeed described by the relaxation phenomenon detailed in Section 4.2 and

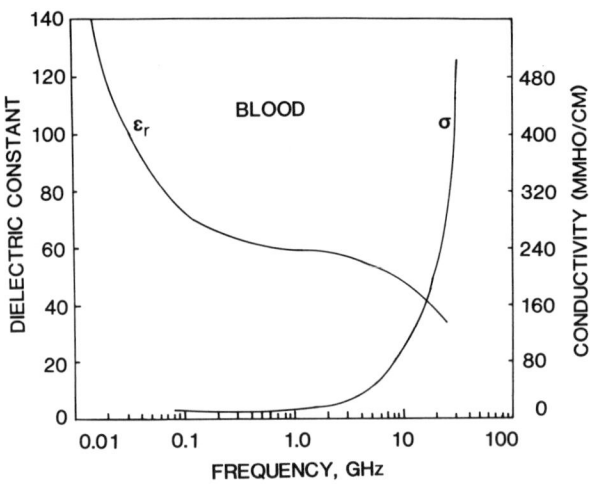

FIGURE 4-19. Dielectric constant and conductivity of blood at 37°C.

illustrated in Fig. 4-4. The dielectric constants and conductivities of many other types of tissue materials will also be presented in this section.

The dielectric constant ε_r and conductivity σ for blood in the frequency range 10 MHz to 10 GHz at 37°C are shown in Fig. 4-19. It can be seen that the changes in ε_r and σ are quite large and are in opposite directions. For example, ε_r decreases from greater than 200 to less than 50 as the frequency increases from 10 MHz to 10 GHz, while σ increases from 1.5 to 8.0 S/m. Note that the *in vitro* data are in close agreement with recent *in vivo* measurements (Burdette *et al.*, 1980).

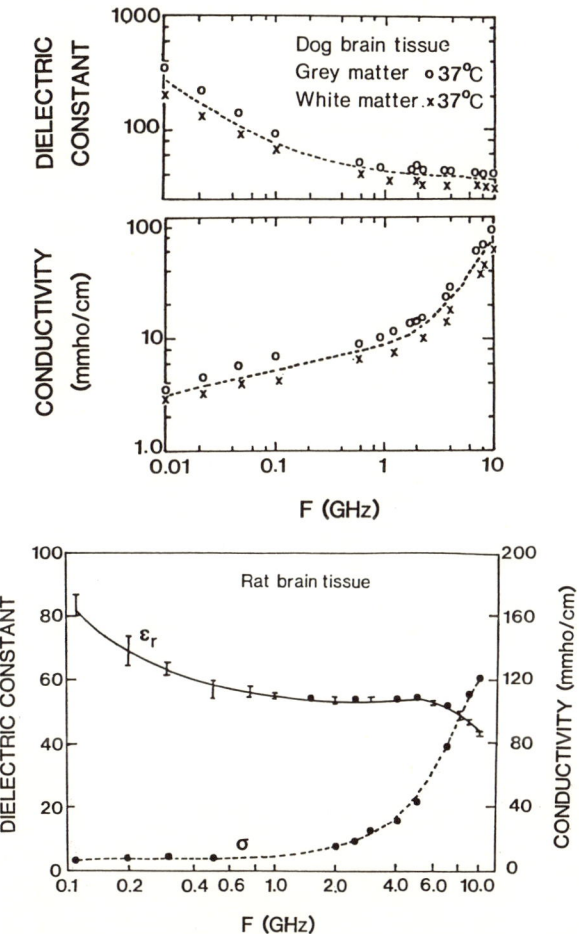

FIGURE 4-20. (a) Dielectric properties of canine brain tissue at 37°C. Dashed line represents the "average" dielectric properties (Foster *et al.*, 1979). (b) Relative dielectric constant and conductivity of *in vivo* rat brain at 32°C (Burdette *et al.*, 1980).

The frequency dependence of the dielectric constants and conductivities for *in vitro* brain, muscle, and skin at 37°C are presented in Figs. 4-20a, 4-21, and 4-22, respectively. It is seen from Fig. 4-20 that the dielectric constant for brain tissue slowly decreases from 80 to 44 as the frequency varies from 100 MHz to 10 GHz. On the other hand, the conductivity is almost frequency independent until 2 GHz is reached; it then abruptly rises from 2.5 to greater than 12 S/m. Recent measurements on *in vivo* rat brain tissue at 32°C yielded 25% higher values than the "average" *in vitro* data shown in Fig. 4-20a. The differences in permittivity of white and gray matter, and in *in vivo* and *in vitro* measurements most probably result from the differences in water content. The dielectric constants and conductivities for skin and muscle are almost identical (Cook, 1951) and have values between that for blood and brain, reflecting their intermediate water content. Note that the dielectric constants decrease and the conductivities increase with increasing frequency.

Because microwave frequencies are situated between the two principal dispersion regions (β and γ dispersions), the dielectric constants for tissues with higher water contents are nearly constant for frequencies between 100 MHz and 10 GHz. Cell membranes have high capacitance and become short-circuited for frequencies above the γ dispersion, permitting the intracellular fluid to participate in current conduction. This causes the conductivity to increase as the frequency increases. Similarly, at these frequencies there is insufficient time during each cycle to allow

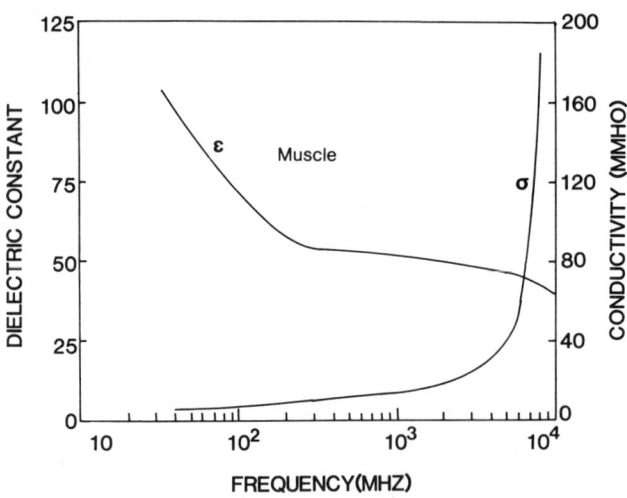

FIGURE 4-21. Dielectric constant and conductivity of *in vitro* muscle tissue at 37°C.

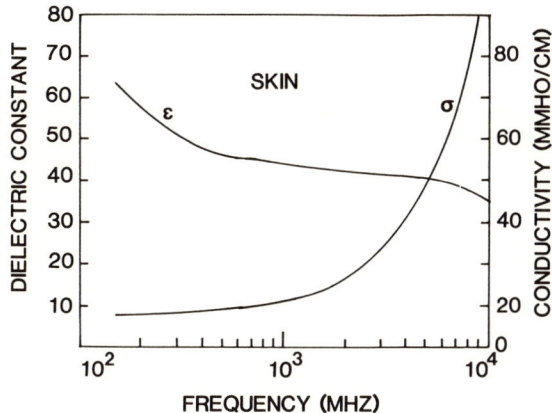

FIGURE 4-22. Dielectric constant and conductivity of *in vitro* skin tissue at 37°C.

complete charging of the cell membranes. The total charge per cycle must decrease along with the membrane capacitance as the frequency is increased. This is manifested as a decrease in the dielectric constant. As the frequency increases still further, both current flow and membrane capacitance reach plateaus until the polar properties of water become important and cause the γ dispersion.

The data presented above for 37°C can be summarized by sums of power series and Debye equations (Schepps and Foster, 1980):

$$\varepsilon_r = 4 + 1.71^{-1.13} + \frac{\varepsilon_s^m - 4}{1 + (f/25)^2} \quad (4.38)$$

$$\sigma = 1.35 f^{0.23} \sigma_{0.1} + 0.0222 f^2 \frac{\varepsilon_s^m - 4}{1 + (f/25)^2} \quad (4.39)$$

where f is the frequency (GHz), σ is the conductivity (mS/cm), and the parameters ε_s^m and $\sigma_{0.1}$ are tabulated in Table 4-2 for several tissues. These equations apply for the entire frequency range of interest in this book, and are used to predict the dielectric properties of other soft tissues containing over 60% water by volume.

The electrical properties of bone, fatty tissue, and other tissues with low water content have not been extensively investigated. The precise mechanism involved in their dielectric behavior is not well understood and there are also large variations in the measured dielectric constant and conductivity (see Figs. 4-23 and 4-24). This is partially caused by the difficulty in handling fatty tissues *in vitro* without changing the fat and

TABLE 4-2
Microwave Dielectric Parameters for Equations (4.38) and (4.39) at 37°C[a]

	Volume fraction of water	Extrapolated microwave permittivity, ε_s^m	Conductivity at 1 GHz, $\sigma_{0.1}$ (mS/cm)	Extrapolated microwave conductivity, σ_s^m (mS/cm)
Brain				
Gray matter	0.84	44	7.0	11.3
White matter	0.74	34	4.8	7.5
Skeletal muscle	0.80	47	7.0	24.0
Liver	0.80	43	6.7	23.0
Fat	0.09	10	0.5	1.0

[a] Modified from Schepps and Foster (1980).

water content. In general, the dielectric constant and conductivity of tissues with low water content are an order of magnitude lower than the corresponding values for tissues with higher water content. The upper conductivity curve in Fig. 4-24 is for wet fat representing horse fat, with somewhat higher water content. The lower curve is for dry fat, which has been found to be more characteristic of pork fat. Human fat values lie somewhere in between (Schwan and Li, 1956).

In vivo measurement techniques have only more recently advanced to the useful stage (Guy *et al.*, 1974; Toler and Seals, 1977; Burdette *et al.*, 1980). Results of *in vivo* canine fat measurements are shown in Fig. 4-25. Compared to the *in vitro* data of Fig. 4-24, the former yield dielectric constant values a factor of approximately 1.5 to 2 times greater

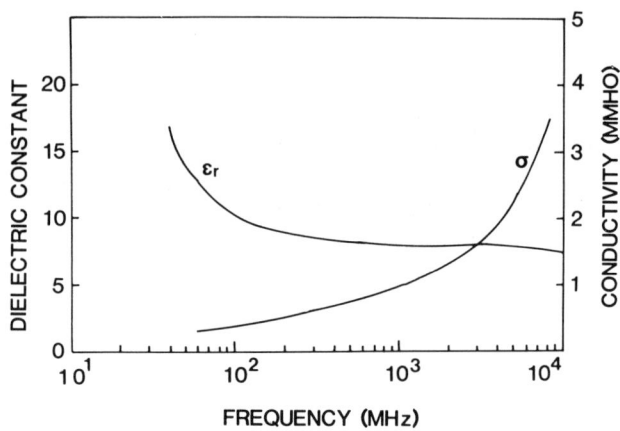

FIGURE 4-23. Dielectric constant and conductivity of *in vitro* bone at 37°C.

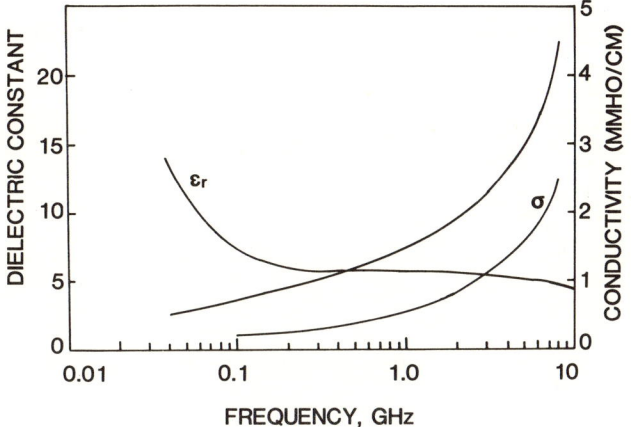

FIGURE 4-24. Dielectric constant and conductivity of *in vitro* fatty tissue at 37°C.

than the *in vitro* results at frequencies from 50 MHz to 2.0 GHz. These differences in dielectric constants are most likely related to the difference in water content between *in vivo* and *in vitro* measurement conditions.

The dielectric constants and conductivities for some other tissues with high water content are listed in Table 4-3. Values for normal saline solution also are listed owing to its importance in biological investigations involving microwave radiation. It is seen that the electrical properties of

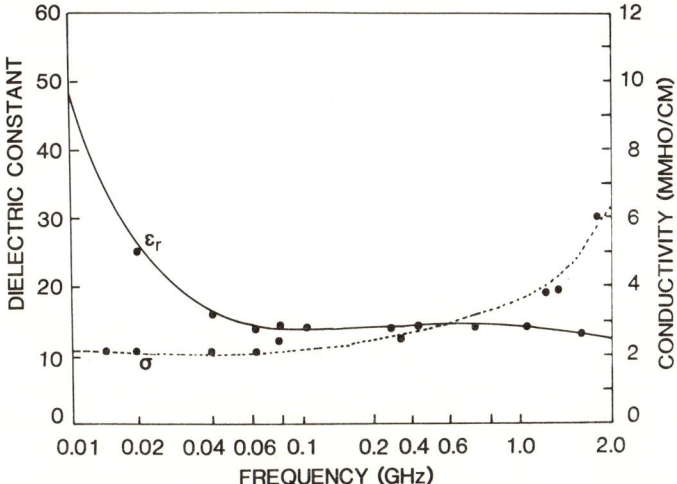

FIGURE 4-25. Relative dielectric constant and conductivity of *in vivo* canine fat tissue at 37°C (Burdette et al., 1980).

TABLE 4-3
Relative Dielectric Constants and Conductivities (S/m) for Selected Tissues with High Water Content[a]

Frequency (MHz)	Wavelength in air (m)	Blood serum		Vitreous humor[b]		0.9% saline	
		ε_r	σ	ε_r	σ	ε_r	σ
100	3.0	73.3[c]	1.17[c]	70	1.6	78	1.67
200	1.5	69.3[c]	1.11[c]	70	1.6	78	1.68
400	0.75	68.5[c]	1.23[c]	70	1.6	74[d]	1.72[d]
500	0.60	68.7[c]	1.38[c]	70	1.6	78	1.72
700	0.43			70	1.6	77[d]	1.85[d]
1,000	0.30	69[c]	1.85[e]	70	1.6	77	1.88
2,500	0.12	71[g]	1.55[g]	70	2.7		
3,000	0.10	70[f]	3.76[f]	70	3.2		
5,000	0.06			69	5.4		
10,000	0.03	57.5[f]	12.6[f]	62	15.3	66[e]	11.1[c]
24.000	0.012	45[f]	38.0[f]	40	46.0		

[a] Values of the dielectric constant ε_r and conductivity σ are for 37°C and are adapted from Schwan (1957), unless otherwise indicated.
[b] Schwan (1958).
[c] Zore et al. (1967), 23°C.
[d] Schwan and Li (1953).
[e] Presman (1970).
[f] England (1950).
[g] Cook (1951), 2.36 GHz.

the vitreous humor are the higher of the two tissues examined. The dielectric constant and conductivity are independent of frequency between 100 and 1000 MHz, the values being 70 and 1.6 S/m, respectively. Above 1000 MHz, the conductivity increases and the dielectric constant decreases with increasing frequency.

The dielectric properties for various tissues with intermediate water content are given in Table 4-4. Note that the dielectric constants and conductivities are reduced by about 30 to 40% from the respective values for high-water-content tissues. For example, a value of 50 is close to the dielectric constants of all the tissues listed at 1000 MHz, and a value of 1.0 S/m is typical for all tissues with intermediate water content. It is apparent from the table that the electrical properties for a large number of tissue materials remain to be measured.

It should be noted that although the dielectric constants and conductivities in this section have been derived from tissues of many species, there is very little variation among the measured values for a given tissue type. An exception is fatty tissue, which is characterized by low dielectric constant and conductivity and by low electrolyte content. The water content of fatty tissues ranges from a few percent to more than

TABLE 4-4
Relative Dielectric Constants and Conductivities (S/m) for Representative Tissues with Intermediate Water Content[a]

Frequency (MHz)	Wavelength in air (m)	Eye lens[b] ε_r	Eye lens[b] σ	Heart muscle ε_r	Heart muscle σ	Kidney ε_r	Kidney σ	Liver ε_r	Liver σ	Lung ε_r	Lung σ
10	30.0	100[c]	0.38[c]			220[d]	0.88[g]	143[d]	0.88[d]		0.67[e]
25	12.0	65[c]	0.4[c]			200	1.0[d]	137	0.51		
50	6.00	60[c]	0.4[c]			126	0.9	91	0.55		0.54[d]
100	3.00	48	0.4			90	1.0	78	0.59		0.71
200	1.50	40	0.4	61	0.96	62	1.11	53	0.79	35	0.63
400	0.75	34	0.4	54	1.09	54	1.18	48	0.86	35	0.71
500	0.60	33	0.4					47	0.88		
700	0.43	32	0.5	53	1.17	52	1.31	47	0.93	34	0.77
1,000	0.3	31	0.5	53[f]	1.19[f]	53[e]	1.23[e]	46	0.98	35[e]	0.73[e]
2,500	0.12	30	1.1			51[g]	2.28[g]				
3,000	0.10	30	1.3			49[g]	2.71[g]	43	2.02		
5,000	0.06	29	3.0			46[g]	5.43[g]				
8,500	0.04	28	6.7			39[g]	9.22[g]	36	6.28		
10,000	0.03	27	8.0			36[g]	11.60[g]	36[e]	6.67[e]		

[a] Values of the dielectric constant ε_r and conductivity σ are for 37°C and are adapted from Schwan (1957), unless otherwise indicated.
[b] Schwan (1958).
[c] Pauly and Schwan (1964).
[d] Schwan (1965), 20–23°C.
[e] Schwan (1963).
[f] Schwan and Li (1953).
[g] Burdette et al. (1980).

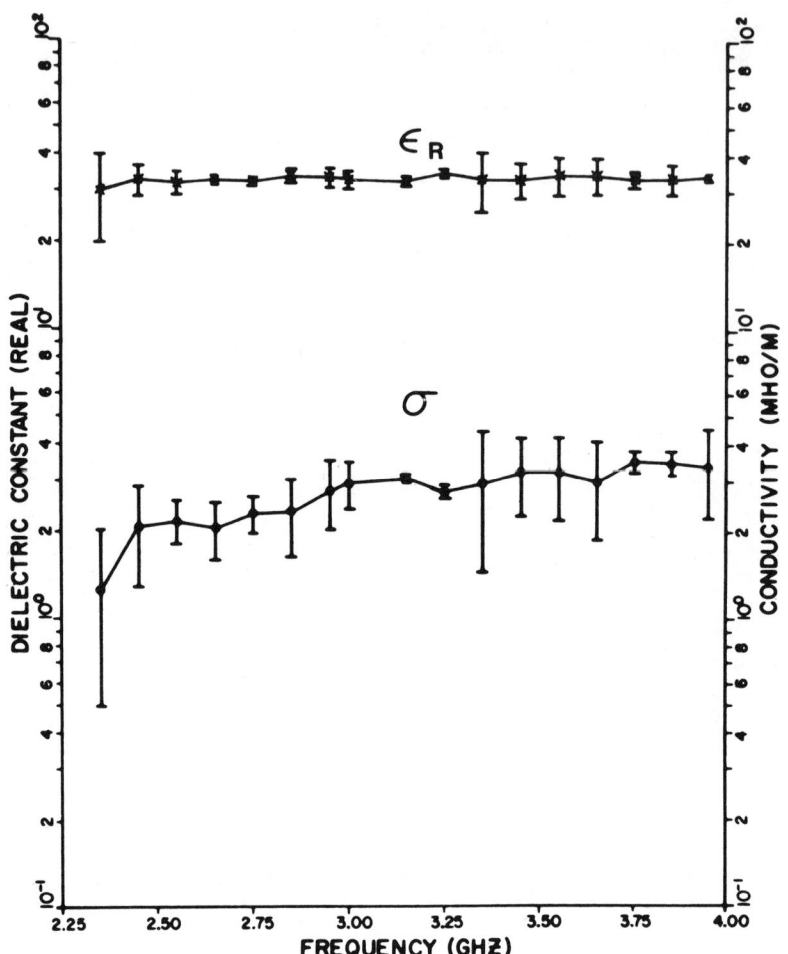

FIGURE 4-26. Dielectric properties of homogenized brain tissue at 37°C in the frequency range 2.25–4 GHz. (a) Human data; (b) combined primate, canine, ovine, swine, and human data.

40%, depending on the animal species (Schwan, 1958). Since the dielectric constant and conductivity of water are very high, the electrical properties of fatty materials differ significantly with differences in water content.

A comparison of the dielectric properties for human brain tissue with those for primate, canine, ovine, and swine brain tissues at 37°C in the frequency range 2.25–4 GHz is given in Fig. 4-26. Within this frequency range the dielectric constant remains unaltered for all species, while the conductivity increases with increasing frequency. Moreover, the similarity

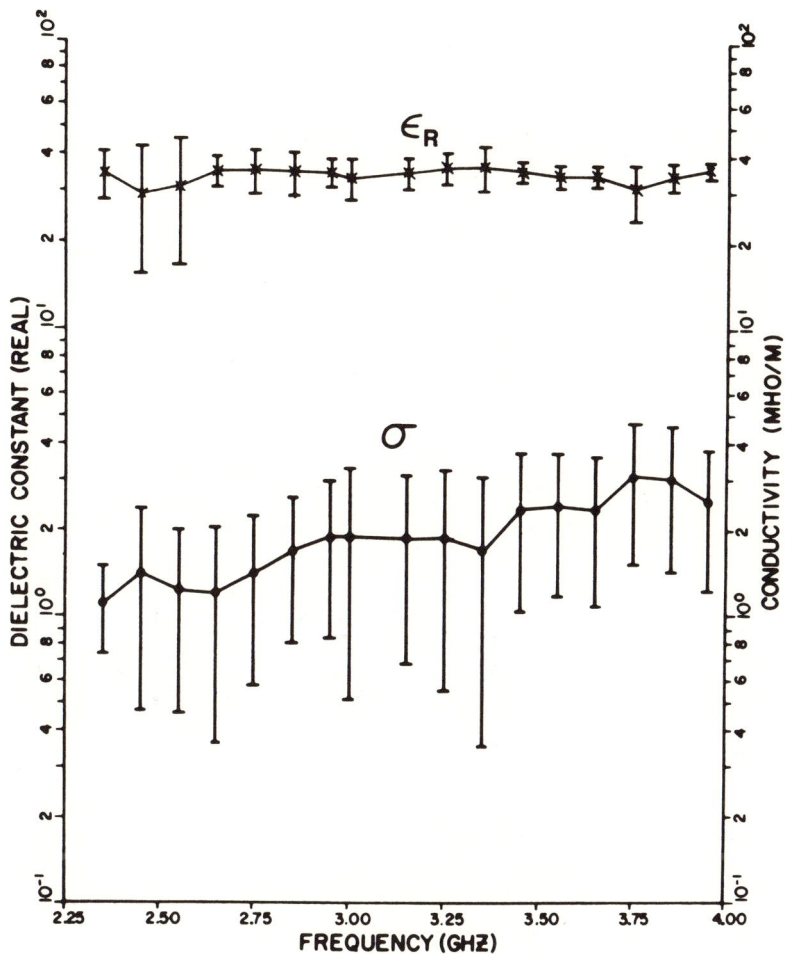

FIGURE 4-26. (continued)

between the human data and the composite representation of all brain tissue data indicates, within the accuracy of these data, that the dielectric properties of brain tissue from different mammalian species are identical (Lin, 1973).

The temperature coefficients for selected tissues with high, intermediate, and low water contents are summarized in Table 4-5. It is to be noted that although the temperature coefficients of the dielectric constants are quite small, they range from negative (-0.4% per °C) to positive (1.3% per °C) values and are frequency dependent. The

TABLE 4-5
Temperature Coefficients of Dielectric Constant and Conductivity of Tissue Materials[a]

	\multicolumn{8}{c}{Frequency (MHz)}							
	50	100	200	400	900	3000	7000	10,000
				$100\, \Delta\varepsilon_r/\varepsilon_r$ per °C				
				Tissues with high water content				
Blood	0.3							
Serum and 0.9% saline	−0.4		−0.4	−0.4	−0.4	−0.34[b]		
				Tissues with intermediate water content				
Brain	1.1(2.0)[c]	1.3[d]	0.0[c]	0.0[c]	0.0[c]	0.0[c]	0.0[c]	0.2[c]
Kidney	0.5		0.2	−0.2	−0.4			
Liver	0.3		0.2	−0.2	−0.4			
Muscle	0.3			−0.2 (0.25)[d]	−0.4 (0.36)[d]	−0.10[d,e]		
				Tissues with low water content				
Fat		0.0[f]		0.0[f]	1.1	0.0[f]		0.0[f]

			100 Δσ/σ per °C					
			Tissues with high water content					
Blood	2.7		1.7	1.6	1.3		−0.7[b]	
Serum and 0.9% saline	2.0							
			Tissues with intermediate water content					
Brain	1.4	1.5[d]	2.0	2.0	1.3(1.0)[c]		−1.0[c]	1.6[d]
Kidney	1.6		1.8	1.8	1.4			
Liver	2.0		1.5	1.3	1.0			
Muscle	2.5			2.5[d]	1.0[d]	0.56[d,e]		
			Tissues with low water content					
Fat	1.7–4.3	3.5[f]	4.9	4.0[f]	4.2	6.30[f]		14.0[f]

[a] Modified from Schwan (1957).
[b] Cook (1952).
[c] Foster et al. (1979).
[d] Schepps and Foster (1981).
[e] 2450 MHz.
[f] Schwan and Li (1956).

temperature dependence of the dielectric constant is related to the temperature coefficients of cell membrane capacitance, macromolecules, and water. The temperature dependence of conductivity is considerably larger, with values of -1.0 to 14% per °C, and is most likely controlled by electrolytes and water (Schwan, 1965).

4.7. DIELECTRIC PROPERTIES OF TUMOR TISSUE

There has been increasing interest in recent years in the use of controlled local hyperthermia as an adjunct in tumor therapy. Radio and microwave energy may be used to produce the required heating. But in order to couple the energy into the tissue efficiently or to predict the subsequent microwave absorption in the heated region of tissue, its dielectric properties must be known. Moreover, microwave radiometry has been used to detect subcutaneous tumors. The success of this modality also will depend on accurate knowledge of the dielectric properties of tumors. The dielectric constant and conductivity data from 3 to 300 MHz for rat sarcoma, and from 10 MHz to 17 GHz for three other representative tumor tissues are shown in Figs. 4-27 and 4-28, respectively. The data for normal muscle are included for comparison. It is seen that the dielectric properties of muscle and soft tissue tumors are similar at frequencies of about 100 MHz, but significantly different for frequencies below 100 MHz, except for hemangiopericytoma. As in all soft tissues, the dielectric constant rises rapidly at frequencies below 100 MHz, but much more so for tumor tissues. Similarly, the conductivity for tumor tissue is higher than for muscle at frequencies below 100 MHz. Thus, from the dielectric property standpoint, frequencies below 100 MHz will be best suited for differential detection and treatment of tumors. The data presented in Fig. 4-28 can be summarized by equations (4.38) and (4.39) with the parameters $\sigma_{0.1}$ and ε_s^m as given in Table 4-6, which also includes values for a variety of other tumor tissues. These empirical results apply for the entire radio and microwave frequency range. Moreover, they allow prediction of the dielectric properties of other soft tissues, most reliably those containing over 60% water by volume (Schepps and Foster, 1980). The contributions from dielectric relaxation of tissue water and from ionic conductivity are relatively constant in different mammalian soft tissues with a given water content. In contrast, the dielectric properties of tissues below 100 MHz mirror interfacial polarization effects involving cellular membranes and other ultrastructures that are more variable among different tissues and thus give rise to the observed differences at these frequencies. Since the volume fraction of water (and blood) was generally higher for the tumors

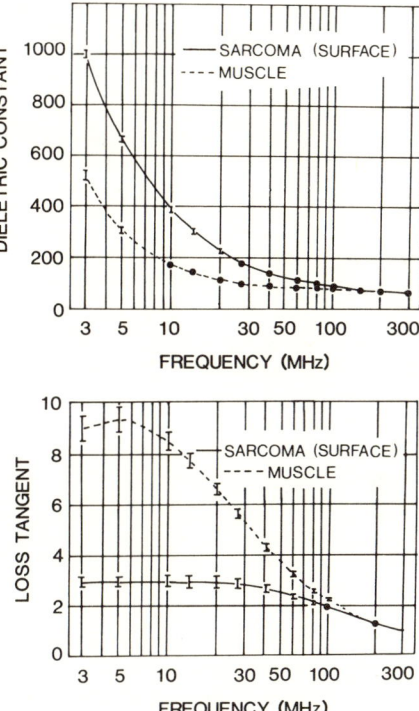

FIGURE 4-27. Dielectric properties of normal rat muscle and rat sarcoma (tumor) tissue at 28°C (Burdette et al., 1980).

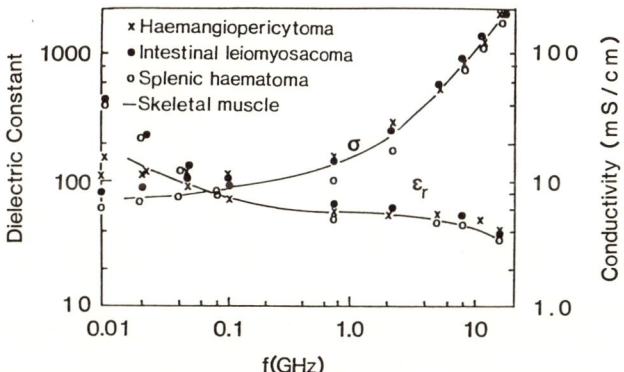

FIGURE 4-28. Dielectric constant and conductivity data for three representative tumor tissues at 37°C with the locus of the data for dog skeletal muscle shown for comparison (Schepps and Foster, 1980).

TABLE 4-6
Dielectric Data $\sigma_{0.1}$ and ε_s^m for Tumor Tissues[a]

	Volume fraction of water	Extrapolated microwave permittivity, ε_s^m	Conductivity at 0.1 GHz $\varepsilon_{0.1}$ (mS/cm)	Extrapolated microwave conductivity, σ_s^m (mS/cm)
Splenic hematoma	0.86	56	9.2	16
	0.795	47	8.5	13
Skeletal muscle	0.795	47	7.0	24
Hemangiopericytoma	0.91	53	11.6	29
	0.92	58	13.7	36
Intestinal leiomyosarcoma	0.87	53	10.5	23
Vaginal fibroleiomyoma	0.87	59	—	18
Pulmonary papillary adenosarcoma	0.84	51	—	14
Lipoma	0.28	20	—	4
Renal tubular adenosarcoma	0.84	50	—	24

[a] Modified from Schepps and Foster (1980).

listed in Table 4-6 than for skeletal muscle, dielectric constants, and conductivities for these tumors were somewhat higher than for skeletal muscle. Tumor tissues have, on the average, 83% water content versus 75% for normal tissue. Correspondingly, the tumor tissues, as a group, showed a 67% higher conductivity and a 25% higher dielectric constant than normal tissues, as indicated by the parameters σ_s^m and ε_s^m, respectively. However, many tumors actually have reduced blood flow (Song *et al.*, 1980); one would expect the dielectric values to be somewhat lower in these cases.

REFERENCES

Altman, P. L., and D. S. Dittmer (eds.) (1964) *The Biology Data Book*. Fed. Am. Soc. Exp. Biol., Washington, D.C., pp. 392–396.

Boettcher, C. J. F. (1952) *Theory of Electric Polarization*. Elsevier, Amsterdam.

Burdette, E. C., F. L. Cain, and J. Seals (1980) In vivo probe measurement technique for determining dielectric properties of VHF through microwave frequencies. *IEEE Trans. Microwave Theory Tech.* **MTT-28**:414.

Cole, K. S. (1968) *Membranes, Ions, and Impulses*. University of California Press, Berkeley.

Cook, H. F. (1951) Dielectric behavior of some types of human tissues at microwave frequencies. *Br. J. Appl. Phys.* **2**:295.

Cook, H. F. (1952) A comparison of dielectric behavior of pure water and human blood at microwave frequencies. *Br. J. Appl. Phys.* **3**:249.

Cook, H. F. (1951) Dielectric behavior of human blood at microwave frequencies. *Nature* **168**:247.

Daniel, V. V. (1967) *Dielectric Relaxation.* Academic Press, New York.
Debye, P. (1929) *Polar Molecules.* Reinhold, New York.
Eisenberg, D., and W. Kauzmann (1969) *The Structure and Properties of Water.* Clarendon Press, Oxford.
England, T. S. (1950) Dielectric properties of human body for wavelengths in the 1–10 cm range. *Nature* **166**:480.
Foster, K. R., J. L. Schepps, R. D. Story, and H. P. Schwan (1979) Dielectric properties of brain tissue between 0.01 and 10 GHz. *Phys. Med. Biol.* **24**:1177.
Franks, F. (1972) *Water—A Comprehensive Treatise,* Vol. 1. Plenum Press, New York.
Fröhlich, H. (1958) *Theory of Dielectrics.* Clarendon Press, Oxford.
Grant, E. H., R. J. Sheppard, and G. P. South (1978) *Dielectric Behavior of Biological Molecules in Solution.* Clarendon Press, Oxford.
Guy, A. W., M. D. Webb, A. F. Emery, R. H. Willard, and J. C. Lin (1974) High frequency EM fields phantom models of man and measured electrical properties of tissues materials. Science Report No. 3, Bioelectromagnetics Research Laboratories, University of Washington.
Guyton, A. C. (1969) *Function of the Human Body.* Saunders, Philadelphia.
Hasted, J. B. (1973) *Aqueous Dielectric.* Chapman & Hall, London.
Hasted, J. B., and S. H. M. El Sabeh (1953) The dielectric properties of water in solution. *Trans. Faraday Soc.* **49**:1003.
Hill, N. E., W. E. Vaughan, A. H. Price, and M. Davies (1969) *Dielectric Properties and Molecular Behavior.* Van Nostrand, Prenceton, N.J.
Jordan, E. C., and K. G. Balmain (1968). *Electromagnetic Waves and Radiating Systems.* McGraw-Hill, New York.
Lin, J. C. (1975) Microwave properties of fresh mammalian brain tissues at body temperature. *IEEE Trans. Biomed. Eng.* **BME-22**:74.
Lin, J. C. (1978) Microwave biophysics. In *Microwave Bioeffects and Radiation Safety,* M. Stuchly (ed.). International Microwave Power Institute, Alberta, Canada, pp. 15–54.
Lin, J. C., and J. H. Jacobi (1975) Computer-controlled measurement of microwave properties of biomaterials. *Int. Microwave Power Symp. Digest,* pp. 265–271.
Pauly, H., and H. P. Schwan (1964) The dielectric properties of the bovine eye lens. *IEEE Trans. Biomed. Eng.* **BME-11**:103.
Presman, A. S. (1970) *Electromagnetic Fields and Life.* Plenum Press, New York.
Roberts, S., and A. R. von Hippel (1946) A new method for measuring dielectric constant and loss in the range of centimeter waves. *J. Appl. Phys.* **17**:610.
Schepps, J. L., and K. R. Foster (1980) The UHF and microwave dielectric properties of normal and tumor tissues: variation in dielectric properties with tissue water content. *Phys. Med. Biol.* **25**:1149.
Schepps, J. L., and K. R. Foster (1981) UHF and microwave dielectric properties of normal and tumor tissues. *Digest Microwave Power Inst.,* Toronto, Canada, pp. 34–36.
Schwan, H. P. (1957) Electrical properties of tissues and cell suspensions. *Adv. Biol. Med. Phys.* **4**:147.
Schwan, H. P. (1958) Survey of microwave absorption characteristics of body tissues. In: *Proceedings of the Second Annual Tri-Service Conference on Biological Effects of Microwave Energy,* E. G. Pattishall and F. W. Banghart (eds.). University of Virginia, Charlottesville, pp. 126–145.
Schwan, H. P. (1963). Electric characteristics of tissues. *Biophysik* **1**:198.
Schwan, H. P. (1965) Biophysics of diathermy. In: *Therapeutic Heat and Cold,* S. Licht (ed.). Waverly Press, Baltimore, pp. 63–125.
Schwan, H. P. (1975) Dielectric properties of biological materials and interaction of microwave fields at the cellular and molecular level. In: *Fundamental and Applied*

Aspects of Nonionizing Radiation, S. M. Michaelson, M. W. Miller, R. Magin, and E. L. Carstensen (eds.). Plenum Press, New York, p. 3.

Schwan, H. P. (1977) Field interaction with biological matter. *Ann. N.Y. Acad. Sci.* **303**:198.

Schwan, H. P., and K. R. Foster (1980) RF-field interaction with biological systems: electrical properties and biophysical mechanisms. *Proc. IEEE* **68**:104.

Schwan, H. P., and K. Li (1953) Capacity and conductivity of body tissues at ultrahigh frequencies. *Proc. IRE* **41**:1735.

Schwan, H. P., and K. Li (1956) Hazard due to total body irradiation by radar. *Proc. IRE* **44**:1572.

Schwan, H. P., R. J. Sheppard, and E. H. Grant (1976) Complex permittivity of water. *J. Chem. Phys.* **64**:2257.

Song, C. W., M. S. Kang, J. G. Rhee, and S. H. Levitt (1980) Effect of hyperthermia on vascular function in normal and neoplastic tissues. *Ann. N.Y. Acad. Sci.* **335**:35.

Tai, C. T. (1961) Characteristics of linear antennas. In: *Antenna Engineering Handbook,* H. Jasik (ed.). McGraw-Hill, New York, p. 3.2.

Toler, J., and J. Seals (1977) RF Dielectric Properties Measurement System: Human and Animal Data. NIOSH Research Dep., Cincinnati, Ohio.

von Hippel, A. R. (1954) *Dielectric and Applications.* MIT Press, Cambridge, Mass.

Westman, H. P. (ed.) (1968). *Reference Data for Radio Engineers.* Sams, Indianapolis, Ind.

Wind, M., and H. Rapaport (1955) *Handbook of Microwave Measurements.* Polytechnic Press, New York.

Zore, V. A., D. D. Kimerfield, V. V. Sudzdaleva, and Y. S. Genkins (1967) Complex dielectric permeability in the frequency range 100–500 Mcs of human blood serum in normal conditions and in certain diseases, *Biophysik* **12**:142.

5

Propagation and Absorption in Tissue Media

The propagation of electromagnetic waves in biological materials is governed by the dielectric constant, conductivity, source configuration, and the geometrical factors that describe the tissue structure. These parameters also determine the quantity of energy a given biological body extracts from the propagating wave. When the radius of curvature of the body surface is large compared to the wavelength and beam width of the impinging radiation, planar tissue models may be used to estimate the absorbed energy and its distribution inside the body. Otherwise, the absorbed energy will be dictated by the size of the body, the curvature of its surface, the ratio of body size to wavelength, and the source characteristics.

The purpose of this chapter is to present a concise account of electromagnetic wave propagation in biological media, with special emphasis on the energy coupling and distribution characteristics in models of biological structures. Such information is essential for analyzing the interrelationships among various observed biological effects, for separating known and substantiated effects from those that are speculative and unsubstantiated, for assessing therapeutic effectiveness of electromagnetic waves, and for extracting diagnostic information from field effects.

It should be noted that the whole-body absorption of electromagnetic energy by humans and laboratory animals is of interest because it is related to the energy required to alter the thermoregulatory system of the exposed subject, and because it may serve as an index for extrapolating experimental results to human exposures. The distribution of absorbed electromagnetic waves within an irradiated body is important because it relates to specific responses of the body, because it facilitates understanding of phenomena, and because it contributes to definition of mechanisms of interaction.

5.1. PLANAR TISSUE GEOMETRIES

5.1.1. Reflection and Transmission

The fate of plane waves at a planar tissue interface depends on the frequency, polarization, and angle of incidence of the wave, and on the dielectric constant and conductivity of the tissue. For a linearly polarized plane wave impinging normally on a boundary separating two semi-infinite media, the reflection and transmission coefficients are respectively given by equations (2.55) and (2.56). When the dielectric properties of the media are approximately equal, there is no reflection and the transmission is maximum. In contrast, there is complete reflection if the second medium is perfectly conductive.

Table 5-1 summarizes the magnitude of the reflection coefficient at the boundary separating various tissues. The fraction of normal incident power reflected by the discontinuity is given by R^2. Clearly, about one-half of the incident power is reflected at these boundaries. Further, the reflection coefficients for tissue–tissue interfaces range from a low of about 5 for muscle–blood to high of about 50 for bone–biological fluid interfaces. This suggests that the closer the dielectric properties on both sides of the interface, the smaller is the power reflection.

The fraction of transmitted power is related to the power transmission coefficient $(1 - R^2)$. It is readily apparent from Table 5-1 that the transmitted power at air–tissue interfaces is quite substantial at radio and microwave frequencies. Moreover, Fig. 5-1 shows that the power transmission coefficient is highly frequency dependent, especially at lower frequencies, while the transmitted power for an air–fat interface is about twice as great as for an air–muscle boundary (about 40% at 1 GHz); it is nearly the same as that for a fat–muscle interface. Clearly, power transmission is highest when the dielectric properties of the adjacent media are similar.

As the transmitted wave propagates in the tissue medium, energy is extracted from the wave and absorbed by the medium. This absorption will result in a progressive reduction of the wave's power density as it advances in the tissue. This reduction is quantified by the depth of penetration δ, which is the distance in which the power density decreases by a factor of e^{-2}. Table 5-2 presents the calculated depth of penetration in selected tissues using typical dielectric constants and conductivities provided in Chapter 4. A graphical representation of penetration depth versus frequency for blood, muscle, and fat is given in Fig. 5-2. It is seen that δ is frequency dependent and takes on different values for different tissues. In particular, the penetration depth for fat and bone is nearly five times greater than for higher-water-content tissues, and has values that range from a few millimeters to several centimeters.

TABLE 5-1
Reflection Coefficient (Magnitude in Percent) between Biological Tissues at 37°C

	Frequency (MHz)	Air	Fat (bone)	Lung	Muscle (skin)	Blood	Saline
Air	433	0	46	76	82	81	83
	915	0	43	73	78	79	80
	2,450	0	41	71	76	77	79
	5,800	0	39	70	75	76	78
	10,000	0	37	70	74	76	78
Fat	433		0	46	56	56	60
(bone)	915		0	43	52	54	57
	2,450		0	42	50	53	57
	5,800		0	42	50	53	56
	10,000		0	45	52	54	58
Lung	433			0	14	13	19
	915			0	12	14	18
	2,450			0	10	15	19
	5,800			0	10	14	19
	10,000			0	10	13	18
Muscle	433				0	4	6
(skin)	915				0	4	7
	2,450				0	5	10
	5,800				0	4	9
	10,000				0	3	9
Blood	433					0	6
	915					0	4
	2,450					0	5
	5,800					0	5
	10,000					0	6
Saline	433						0
	915						0
	2,450						0
	5,800						0
	10,000						0

A wave of general polarization usually is decomposed into its orthogonal linearly polarized components whose electric or magnetic field is parallel to the interface. These components can be treated separately and combined afterward. Figures 5-3 and 5-4 illustrate the magnitude and phase of the reflection coefficients of representative tissue interfaces at a temperature of 37°C for irradiation at 2450 MHz. These figures clearly show the difference between E and H polarization. E polarization, also

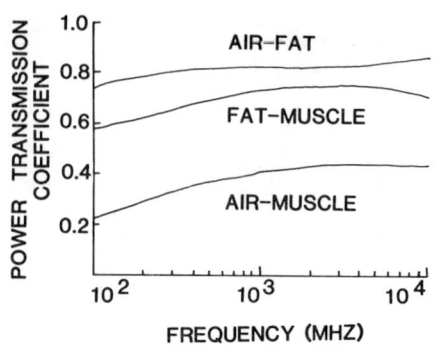

FIGURE 5-1. Power transmission coefficient at three tissue interfaces as a function of frequency.

TABLE 5-2
Depth of Electromagnetic Wave's Penetration into Biological Tissues as a Function of Frequency

Frequency (MHz)	Depth of penetration (cm) into				
	Saline	Blood	Muscle (skin)	Lung	Fat (bone)
433	2.8	3.7	3.0	4.7	16.3
915	2.5	3.0	2.5	4.5	12.8
2,450	1.3	1.9	1.7	2.3	7.9
5,800	0.7	0.7	0.8	0.7	4.7
10,000	0.2	0.3	0.3	0.3	2.5

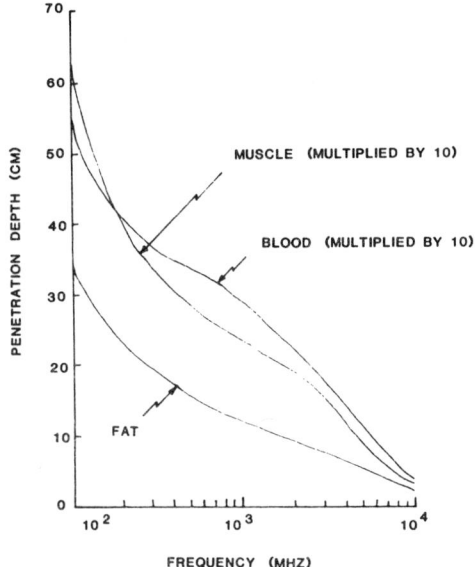

FIGURE 5-2. Depth of penetration for blood, muscle, and fat as a function of frequency.

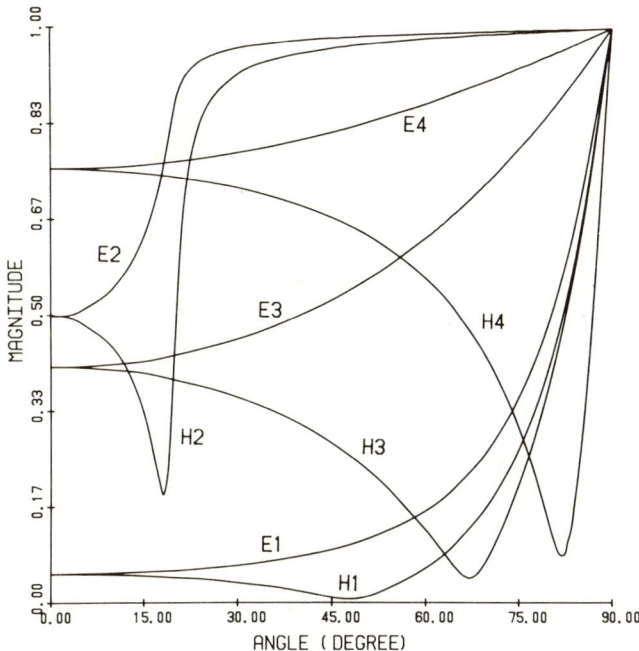

FIGURE 5-3. Magnitude of reflection coefficient for E and H polarized plane waves at 2450 MHz. 1, Muscle–blood; 2, fat–muscle; 3, air–fat; 4, air–muscle.

called perpendicular polarization, and H polarization, also referred to as parallel polarization, are defined in Fig. 2-2. For E polarization, there is only a slight variation in magnitude and phase of the reflection coefficient with incidence angle. For H polarization, however, there is a pronounced dependence on incidence angle. The reflection coefficient reaches a minimum magnitude and has a phase angle of 90° at the Brewster angle. Thus, the H-polarized wave is totally transmitted into the muscle medium at the Brewster angle.

5.1.2. Multiple Layers of Tissue

When there are several layers of different tissues, the reflection and transmission characteristics become more complicated. Multiple reflections can occur between the skin and subcutaneous tissue boundaries, with a resulting modification of the reflection and transmission coefficients (Schwan and Piersol, 1954; Johnson and Guy, 1972). In

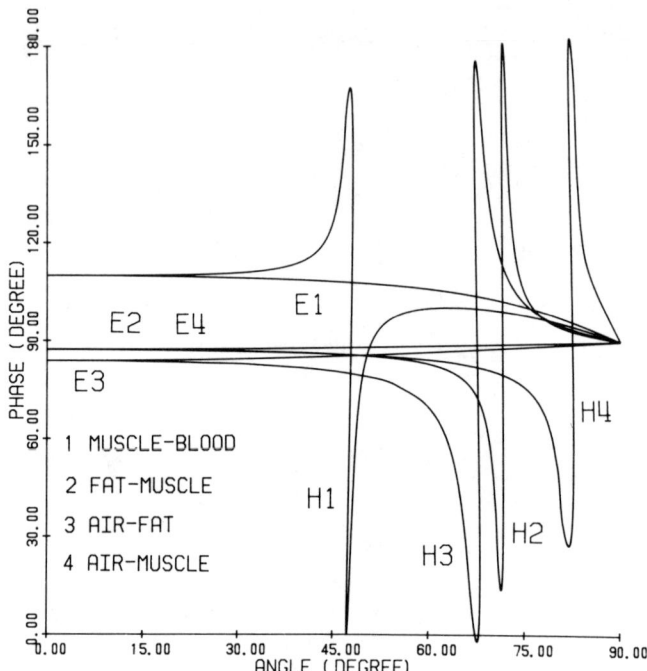

FIGURE 5-4. Phase of reflection coefficient for E- and H-polarized 2450-MHz plane waves.

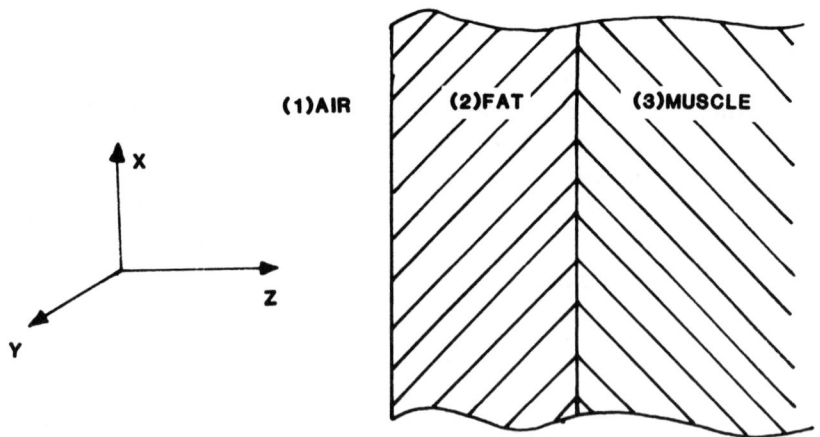

FIGURE 5-5. Plane wave impinging on a composite fat–muscle layer.

general, the transmitted wave will combine with the reflected wave to form standing waves in each layer. This phenomenon becomes especially pronounced if the thickness of each layer is less than the penetration depth for that tissue medium. Plane waves impinging on the human body considered as consisting of parallel layers of subcutaneous fat and more deeply lying muscle have been studied in detail by Schwan and Li (1956).

For the situation depicted in Fig. 5-5, the electric field strength in the fat layer is given by

$$E_f = F_l E_0 [e^{-(\alpha_2+j\beta_2)z} + R_{32} e^{(\alpha_2+j\beta_2)z}] \quad (5.1)$$

and the electric field in the underlying musle tissue is given by

$$E_m = F_t E_0 e^{-(\alpha_3+j\beta_3)z} \quad (5.2)$$

where α_2, β_2 and α_3, β_3 are the attenuation and propagation coefficients in fat and muscle, respectively. The layer function F_l and the transmission function F_t are given by

$$F_l = T_{12}/[e^{-(\alpha_2+j\beta_2)l} + R_{21}R_{32} e^{-(\alpha_2+j\beta_2)l}] \quad (5.3)$$

$$F_t = T_{12}T_{23}/[e^{(\alpha_2+j\beta_2)l} + R_{21}R_{32} e^{-(\alpha_2+j\beta_2)l}] \quad (5.4)$$

where T_{12} and T_{23} are the transmission coefficients at the air–fat and fat–muscle boundaries, respectively. R_{21} and R_{32} denote, respectively, the reflection coefficients at these boundaries; l is the thickness of the fat layer. The power absorption in a given layer can be obtained from equation (2.32).

Figure 5-6 shows the numerical results obtained using the above equations and the dielectric data given in Chapter 4. The values are normalized to the SAR in muscle at the fat–muscle boundary. Note that the absorbed energy is much lower in fat than in muscle. The standing wave maximum becomes greater in fat and the penetration into muscle becomes smaller as the frequency increases.

The absorbed microwave energy in models composed of planar layers of skin, fat, and muscle can be analyzed in a similar manner (Schwan and Li, 1956) except that the distribution of absorbed energy becomes more complex. Figure 5-7 shows that in addition to frequency dependence, the peak SARs exhibit considerable fluctuation with thickness of subcutaneous fatty layer. The incident power density is, in this case, 10 W/m^2 and the skin layer is 0.2 cm thick. Note that the peak SARs are always higher in the skin layer for planar models at microwave frequencies. The depth of penetration for 10-GHz radiation in skin is less

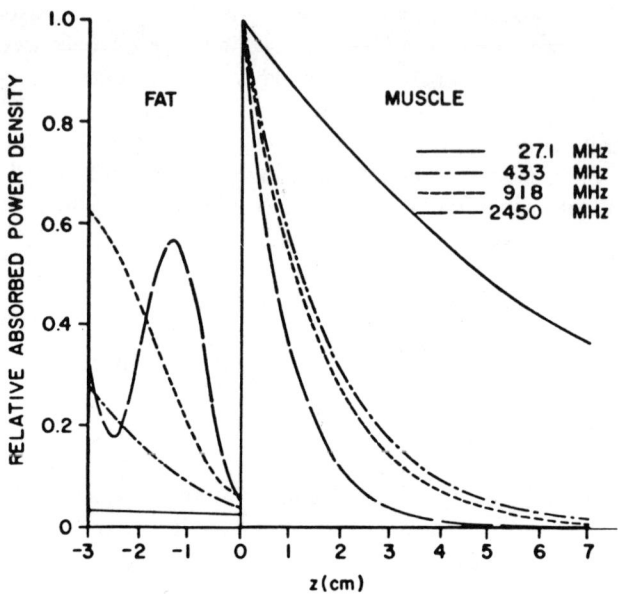

FIGURE 5-6. SAR distribution (absorbed power density) in planar fat–muscle layers (Johnson and Guy, 1972).

than 0.05 cm; thus, the transmitted energy is almost completely absorbed in the skin and the SAR is rather unaffected by changing fatty layer thickness. The fact that the SAR is highest in skin is very significant since skin is populated with thermosensitive free nerve endings that may be excited along with cutaneous pain receptors when the absorbed energy exceeds the normal range that can be handled by thermoregulation.

Figure 5-8 shows the distribution of induced electric field strength in a layer of muscle beneath layers of fat, muscle, and bone for two frequencies (Johnson and Guy, 1972). It is seen that in addition to frequency dependence, the electric fields exhibit considerable fluctuation within each tissue layer. While the standing-wave oscillations become greater at 2450 MHz than at 915 MHz, microwave energy at both frequencies can penetrate into more deeply situated tissues. This result, together with Figs. 5-6 and 5-7, implies that at frequencies between 300 and 3000 MHz, sufficient energy may be transmitted and reflected to allow investigation of organs within the body. Furthermore, at these frequencies, electromagnetic energy can penetrate into more deeply situated tissues, making it most hazardous to humans in an uncontrolled situation.

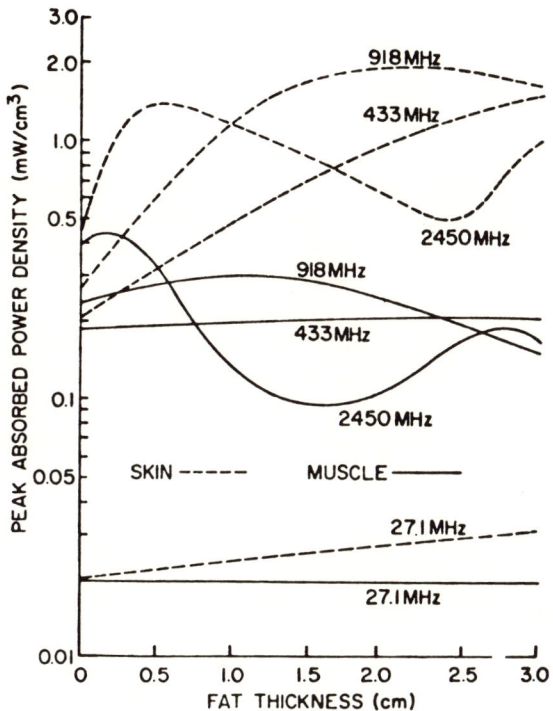

FIGURE 5-7. Peak SAR (absorbed power density) in models composed of skin–fat–muscle layers (Johnson and Guy, 1972).

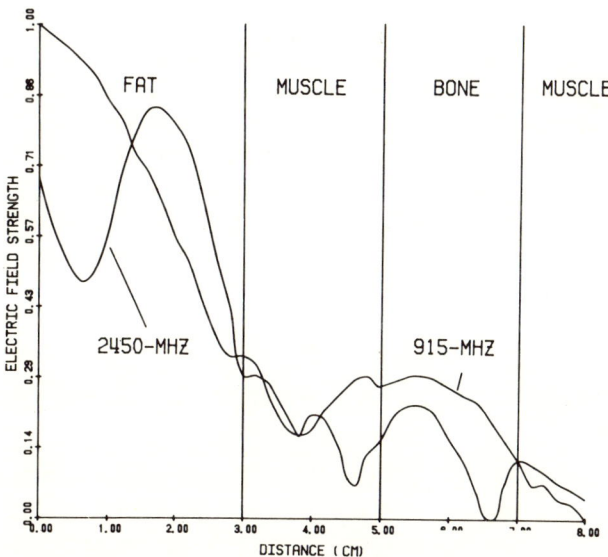

FIGURE 5-8. Distribution of electric field strength in planar layers of fat–muscle–bone–muscle tissue model.

5.2. BODIES OF REVOLUTION

Although depth of penetration and reflection and transmission data for planar tissue structures provide considerable physical insight into coupling and distribution of radio and microwave energy, biological bodies generally are more complex in form and exhibit substantial curvature that can modify radio and microwave energy transmission and reflection. For bodies with complex shape, the propagation characteristics depend critically on polarization and on orientation of the incident wave with respect to the body, as well as the ratio of body size to wavelength. These complications place severe limitations on reflection and transmission calculations for bodies of arbitrary shape and complex permittivity. This section presents a summary of analytical/numerical results that have been obtained for homogeneous and multilayered models based on bodies of revolution that approximate mammalian tissue structures.

5.2.1. Spherical Tissue Models

The distribution of the electric field induced inside a homogeneous dielectric sphere by a plane wave propagating in the positive z direction and polarized along the x axis is given by

$$E = E_0 e^{j\omega t} \sum_{n=1}^{\infty} (-j)^n \frac{2n+1}{n(n+1)} [a_n^t m_{o1n}^{(1)} + j b_n^t n_{e1n}^{(1)}] \quad (5.5)$$

where a_n^t and b_n^t denote the magnetic and electric modes of oscillations inside the sphere, respectively, and m_{o1n} and n_{e1n} are two independent solutions called vector spherical wave functions (Stratton, 1941). They are all functions of the wavelength, dielectric constant, conductivity, and size of the sphere. The infinite series of equation (5.5) is readily adapable for computer calculation using the numerical values of dielectric permittivity and conductivity given in Chapter 4. The absorbed power is once again given by equation (2.32) and the total time rate of energy absorption is obtained from

$$W_a = W_t - W_s \quad (5.6)$$

with the time rate of total energy derived from the incident waves and the energy scattered by the sphere given by

$$W_t = \frac{E_0^2}{120 k_0^2} \operatorname{Re} \sum_{n=1}^{\infty} (2n+1)(a_n^r + b_n^r) \quad (5.7)$$

$$W_s = \frac{E_0^2}{120 k_0^2} \sum_{n=1}^{\infty} (2n+1)(|a_n^r|^2 + |b_n^r|^2) \quad (5.8)$$

and

$$a_n^r = a_n^t \left[\frac{j_n(Nk_0a)}{h_n(k_0a)} - \frac{j_n(k_0a)}{h_n(k_0a)} \right] \quad (5.9)$$

$$b_n^r = b_n^t \left[\frac{Nj_n(Nk_0a)}{h_n(k_0a)} - \frac{j_n(k_0a)}{h_n(k_0a)} \right] \quad (5.10)$$

where $N^2 = \varepsilon_r$, $k_0 = 2\pi/\lambda_0$, and μ_0 and λ_0 are the permittivity and wavelength in a vacuum, respectively; j_n and h_n are the spherical Bessel functions and a is the radius of the sphere.

Some representative calculations of the SAR are shown in Fig. 5-9 for two models at 918 and 2450 MHz (Johnson and Guy, 1972; Lin et al., 1973b). The 6-cm-diameter sphere approximates in size that of a cat or rhesus monkey brain while the 14-cm-diameter sphere is more typical of a human adult brain. Figure 5-9 plots the SAR distribution along the three rectangular coordinate axes whose origin coincides with the center of the sphere. An incident plane wave power density of 10 W/m^2 is assumed. It is seen that at 918 MHz, maximum absorption occurs near the center of both spheres. When the frequency is increased to 2450 MHz, the location of peak SAR for the cat-size brain sphere remains near the center, whereas for the human-size brain sphere peak SAR is now at an anterior location.

In general, standing wave patterns with many oscillations are observed. Note that at 918 MHz, peak SARs in the cat-size brain are larger by a factor of two than in the human-size brain, the peak absorption is four times greater in the cat-size brain than in the human-size brain for 2450 MHz. A comparison of available studies (Shapiro et al., 1971; Kritikos and Schwan, 1972; Lin et al., 1973b; Ho and Guy, 1975) indicates that the peak absorption may be as much as five times greater than the average, and the enhanced absorption near the center of these brain models may be two to three orders of magnitude greater than that expected from the planar tissue models. The increased absorptions are due to a combination of high dielectric constant and curvature of the model, which produce a strong focusing of energy toward the interior of the sphere that more than compensates for the transmission losses through the tissue (Lin, 1978).

The peak absorption per unit volume, average absorption per unit volume, and average absorption per unit surface area as a function of frequency and radius of spherical brain model are illustrated in Fig. 5-10. It can be seen that the absorbed energy varies widely with sphere size and frequency. In general, the absorption initially increases rapidly with increasing radius and is then followed by some resonant behavior. The

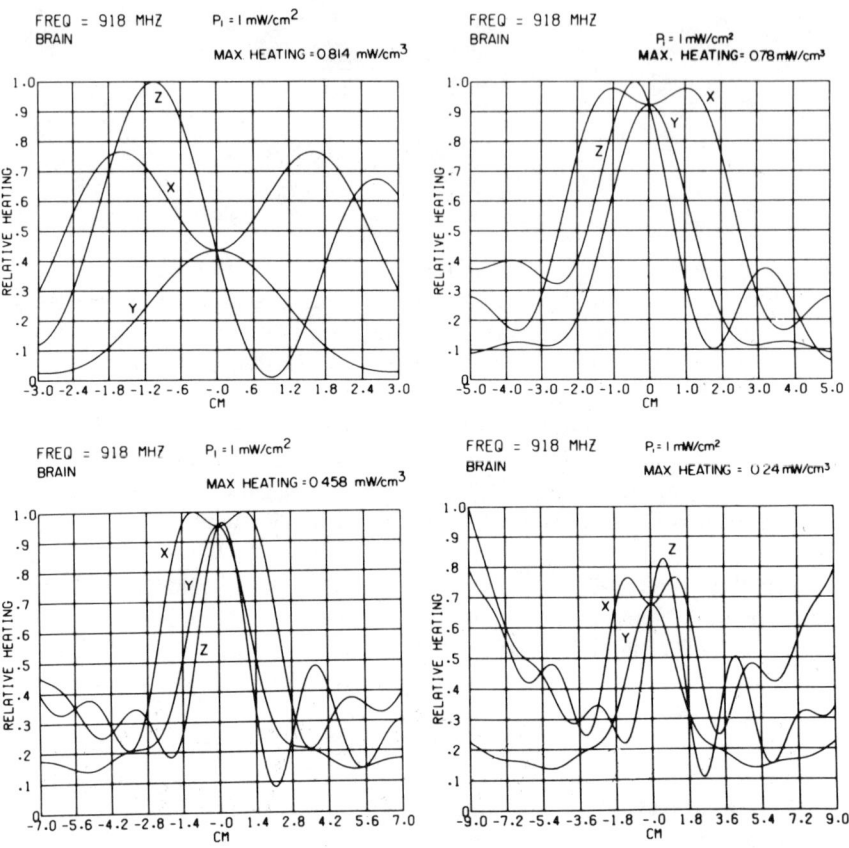

FIGURE 5-9. Predicted SAR distribution (heating pattern) along the three rectangular axes of spherical models of brain exposed to plane waves (Lin *et al.*, 1973b).

peaks of these resonant oscillations are related to the maxima, or hot spots, in the distribution of absorbed energy inside the head model, as shown in Fig. 5-9. For $(2\pi a/\lambda_0) < 0.4$, where a is the sphere radius and λ_0 is the wavelength in a vacuum, in general, hot spots do not occur inside the sphere. However, for some combinations of irradiation frequency and radius, hot spots will occur, for example, in spheres with radii between 2 and 8 cm at 918 MHz and between 0.9 and 5 cm at 2450 MHz. For spheres whose radii exceed the size ranges mentioned above, the maximum absorption appears at the anterior portion (exposed surface) of the sphere, and the penetration depth at the surface becomes a dominating factor. The planar model discussed in Section 5.1 may be applied to obtain a theoretical estimate of the absorbed energy in this case.

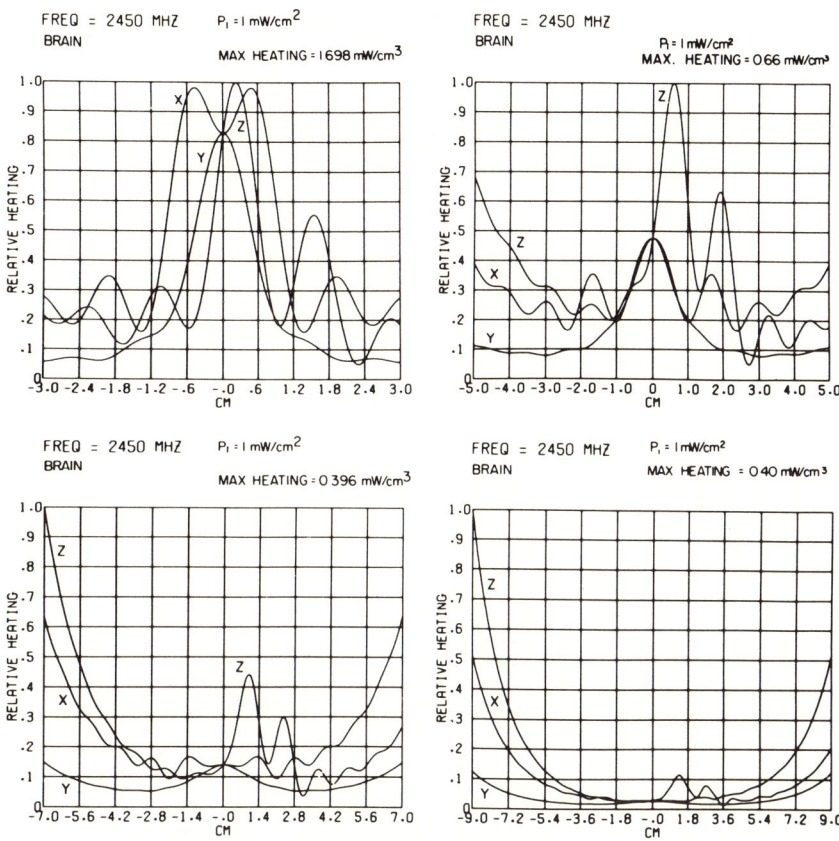

FIGURE 5-9. (continued)

The frequency dependence of energy absorption is illustrated in the upper graphs in Fig. 5-10 for the head of a small animal, such as a cat or rhesus monkey, and a human head-size sphere. In addition to the resonant peak, at these frequencies, increased energy is absorbed in a decreasingly smaller volume as a result of shortened penetration depth.

The effects of skin, fat, bone, dura, and cerebrospinal fluid on the absorption of radio and microwaves by the brain have been investigated in several laboratories (Shapiro et al., 1971; Weil, 1975; Guy et al., 1975; Joines and Spiegel, 1975; Lin, 1976), using more complex spherical structures where the spherical core of brain is surrounded by five concentric shells of tissues (see Table 5-3). It is interesting to note that if brain sizes remain unchanged, but the overall sphere diameter is

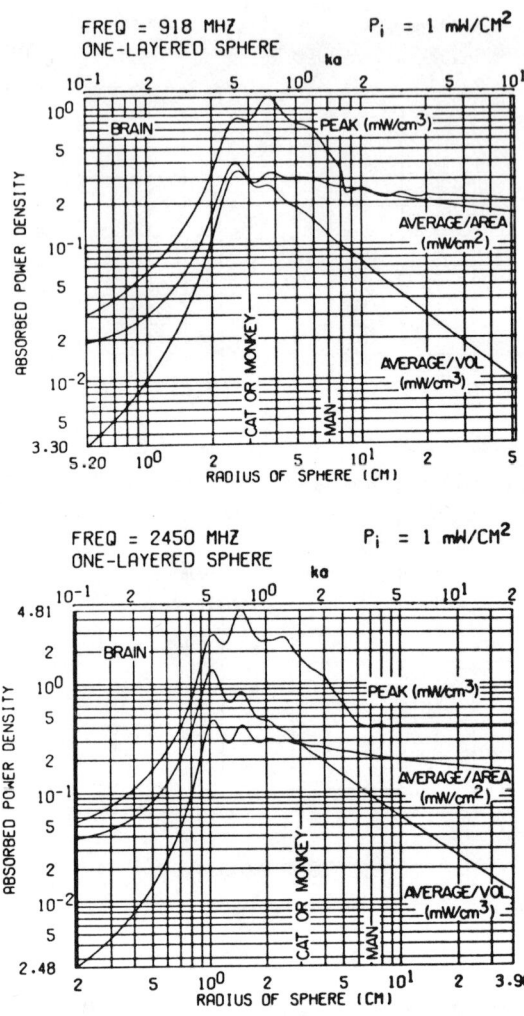

FIGURE 5-10. Electromagnetic energy absorption characteristics for spherical models of the brain.

increased to account for the outer tissue layers, absorption in brain tissues may be increased by 25% for human- and cat-size heads at 918 MHz or decreased by 70% or more in the case of 2450 MHz (see Figs. 5-11 and 5-12). Moreover, surface absorption is greatly increased in the case of layered models, while fat and bone always absorb the least amount of energy.

If the outer diameter of the sphere remains the same, while the composition of the tissue layers is allowed to be either layered or

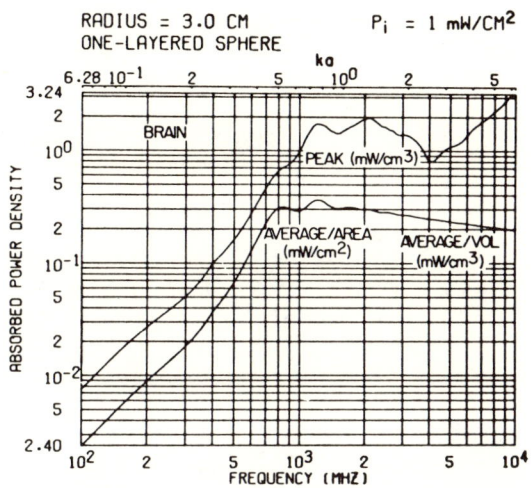

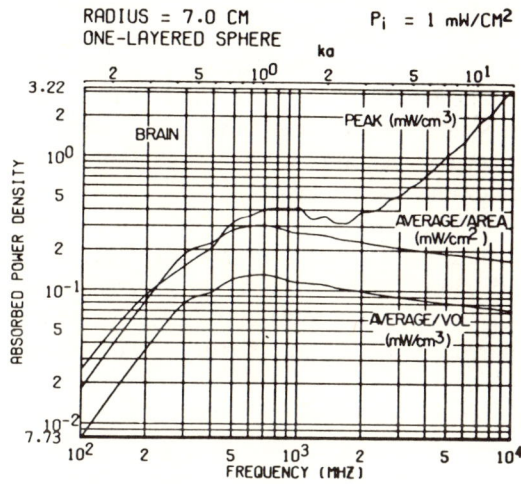

FIGURE 5-10. (continued)

homogeneous, the peak and average SARs show very little change except when the radius of the spherical head is between 0.1 and 1.0 times the wavelength in air. The peak and average SARs for layered models may be several times as great as for homogeneous models. Enhancement is apparently the result of resonant coupling of energy into the sphere by the outer tissue layers.

It should be mentioned that the computed absorption characteristics are highly sensitive to the dielectric constant and conductivity. There are

TABLE 5-3
Composition of a Six-Layer Model of a Mammalian Head

	Dielectric constant		Thickness (cm)	
	918 MHz	2450 MHz	3.5 cm	10 cm
Brain	34.42-j 15.49	32.78-j 15.37	2.88	6.98
CSF	80.85-j 14.05	77.0 -j 13.94	0.20	1.10
Dura	51.40-j 25.08	47.52-j 11.42	0.05	0.8
Bone	5.56-j 0.856	5.0 -j 0.857	0.20	0.7
Fat	5.56-j 0.856	5.0 -j 0.857	0.07	0.27
Skin	51.40-j 25.08	47.52-j 11.42	0.10	0.15

two divergent sets of brain dielectric constant and conductivity in the literature (Johnson and Guy, 1972; Kritikos and Schwan, 1972; Joines and Spiegel, 1975; Schwan, 1957, 1958). Depending on the particular values chosen for these quantities, the interpretation of the relative hazard at 2450 MHz has varied from least to most hazardous (Shapiro *et al.*, 1971; Weil, 1975; Joines and Spiegel, 1975; Lin, 1976). The conclusion that 2450 MHz represents a highly hazardous frequency for humans most likely stems from the fact that inordinately high (as much as a factor of 2) dielectric constant used in their computation (Lin, 1975; Lin *et al.*, 1975; Schwan and Foster, 1980).

A study also has been made of the interaction of circularly polarized plane electromagnetic waves with six-layered spherical models of the mammalian head (Lin, 1976). The approach is a classic one; Mie equations as given in equations (5.5) and (5.10) are modified to account for the two polarizations that are orthogonal in space. Two sets of representative calculations are shown in Figs. 5-13 and 5-14 for 918 and 2450 MHz, respectively. The 7-cm-diameter sphere represents a cat- or monkey-size head while the 20-cm-diameter sphere is typical of an adult human-size head. In each case, the absorbed power distribution is normalized to the maximum along the z axis. An incident power density of 10 W/m^2 is again assumed.

As for the case of linearly polarized plane waves, the maximum absorption at 918 MHz occurs near the center of a cat-size head, whereas that for a human-size head is at the surface. At 2450 MHz, the location of maximum absorption for both spheres shifts to the leading surface. The distribution of absorbed energy for circularly polarized waves is more uniform compared with the linearly polarized case. In fact, the absorbed energy distribution in the planes transverse to the direction of propagation is rotationally symmetric, i.e., it is independent of angular variation (see curves B). Note also that the maximum energy absorbed in the

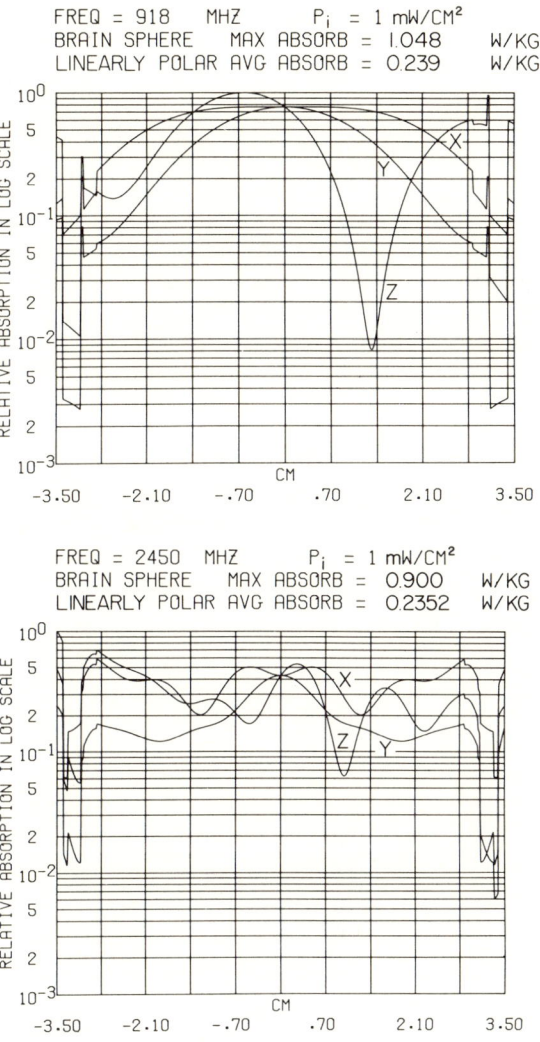

FIGURE 5-11. Distribution of absorbed energy in a six-layered spherical model of the cat head (Lin, 1976).

spherical head models varies only slightly between the two frequencies studied. However, a greater quantity of energy is deposited in the inner sphere (representing the brain of a human head) for 918-MHz than for 2450-MHz radiation.

A number of investigations (Schwan, 1968; Johnson and Guy, 1972; Lin *et al.*, 1973a; Kritikos and Schwan, 1975) have used muscle spheres as

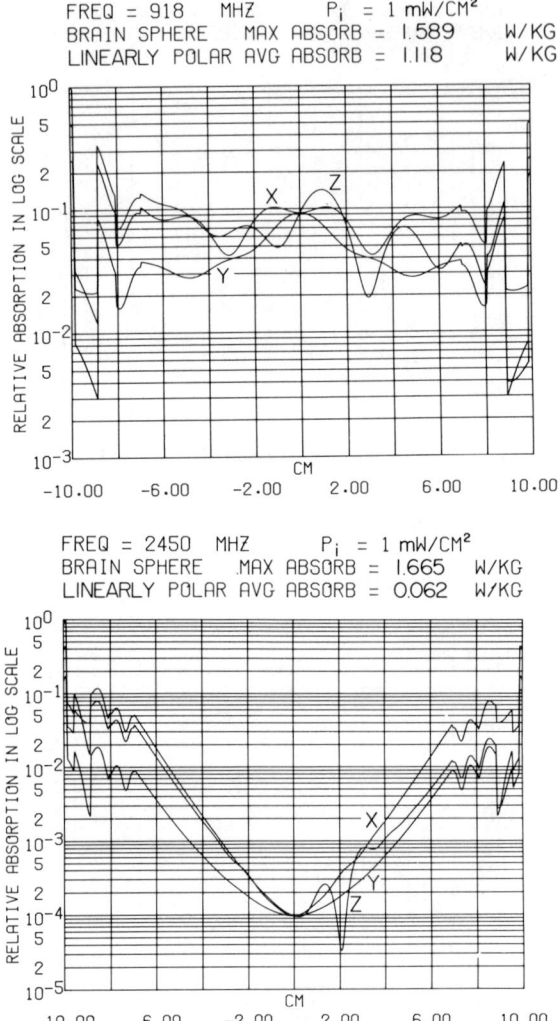

FIGURE 5-12. SAR distribution in a six-layered spherical model of the adult human head (Lin, 1976).

a first-order approximation for the extrapolation to humans of results obtained from laboratory animals and as an index to whole-body absorption of electromagnetic energy as a function of frequency. The spherical model is attractive since exact solutions for absorbed energy can be obtained for all frequencies and body sizes. The absorptions for homogeneous muscle spheres, whose volumes correspond to small

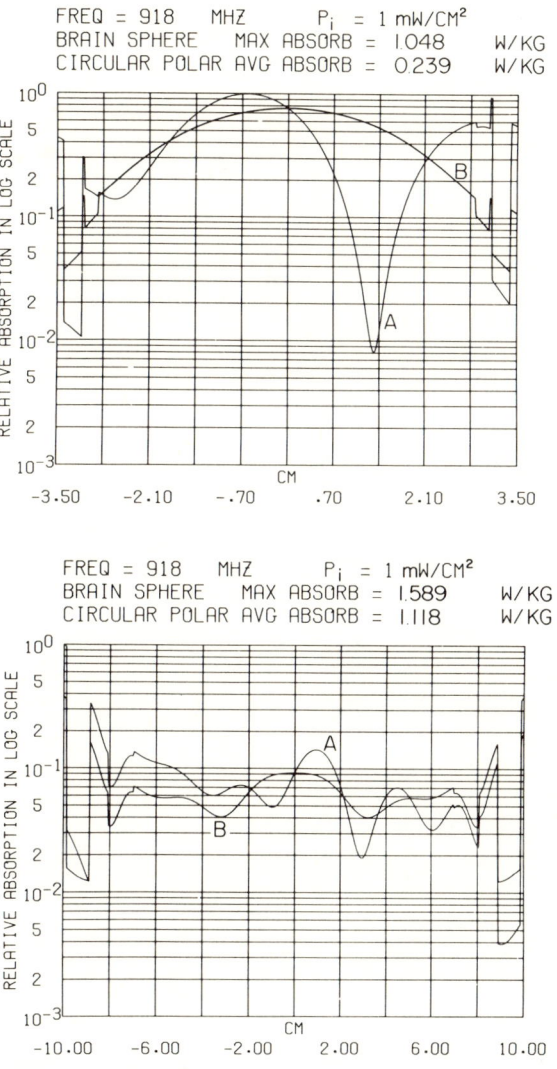

FIGURE 5-13. Relative absorption of circularly polarized 918-MHz radiation in spherical models of the mammalian head (Lin, 1976).

animals such as a rat, and a standard man, computed as a function of frequency, are shown in Fig. 5-15. While in this case the peak absorption is of very limited utility, the average absorption per unit surface area is related to the time and power required to overload the thermoregulatory capacity of an exposed object. Note that the average absorption for the rat model is at least ten times higher than for a muscle sphere

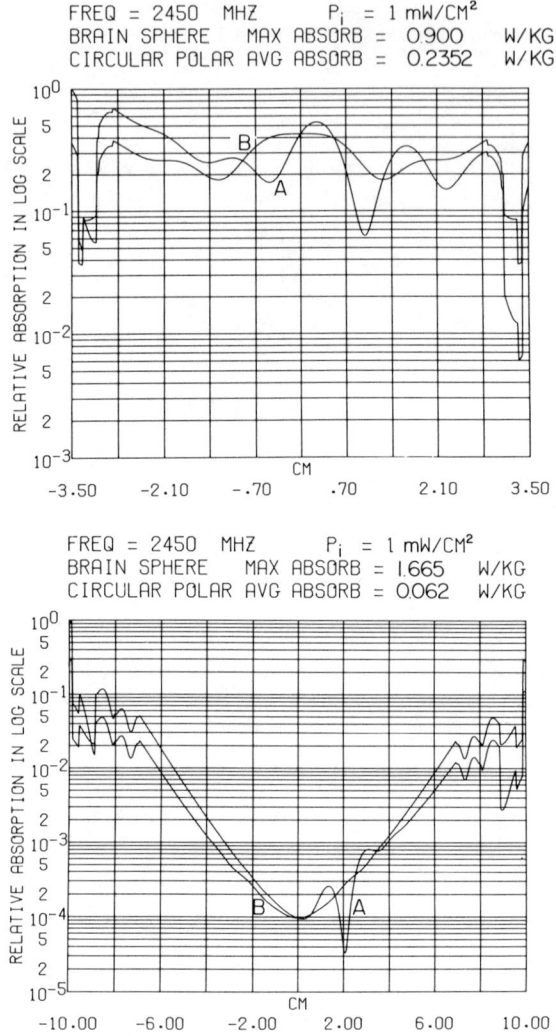

FIGURE 5-14. Circularly polarized 2450-MHz microwave-induced SAR distribution in spherical models of the mammalian head (Lin, 1976).

representing a human body at frequencies greater than 500 MHz. Absorptions in both cases increase rapidly with frequency until the sphere diameter approaches the free space wavelength of impinging radiation. A number of resonant oscillations appear that tend to increase the amount and nonuniformity of absorbed energy. Above this range the absorption falls off slowly, indicating details of body surface curvature are of little significance.

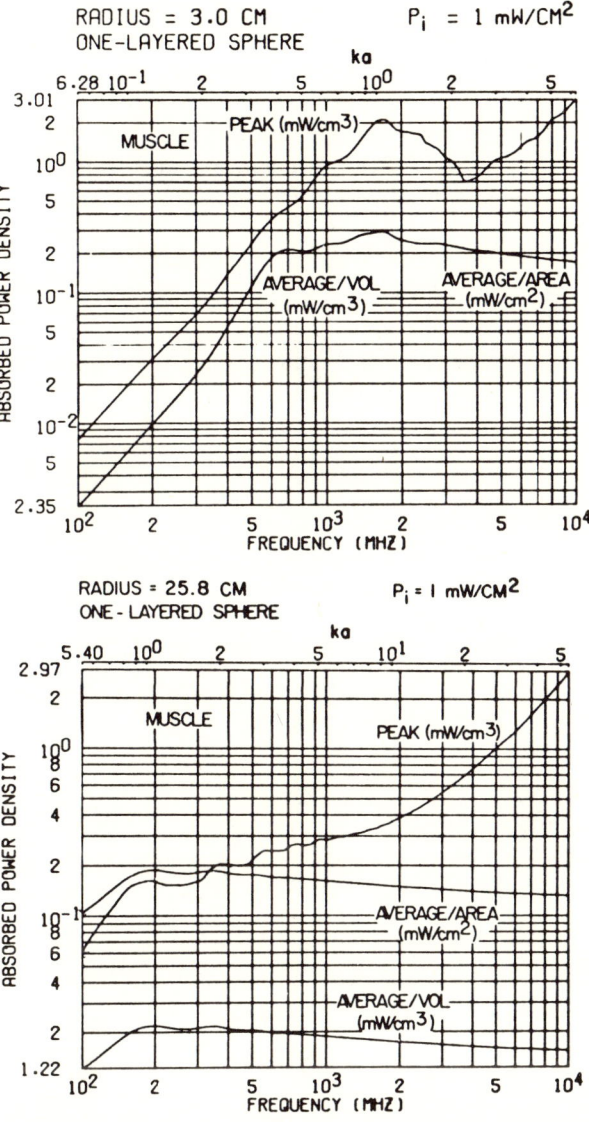

FIGURE 5-15. Absorption characteristics of spherical body models.

We have thus far dealt mainly with situations where the diameter of the sphere is comparable to or larger than a wavelength in air. When the sphere is small compared with a wavelength, the absorbed energy distribution varies almost as the square of the radius or distance from the magnetic axis (the axis parallel to the direction of the magnetic field vector) as shown in Fig. 5-16. If the sphere is extremely small compared with a wavelength, the absorbed energy distribution becomes nearly uniform in the x and y directions but decreases continuously with distance from the exposed surface (see Fig. 5-17). This behavior can be explained by a quasi-static field theory (Lin et al., 1973a). Accordingly, for a plane wave polarized in the x direction that propagates in the z direction, the induced electric field inside a dielectric sphere is given by

$$E_t = E_0 e^{j\omega t}\left[\frac{3}{\varepsilon}\hat{x} - j\frac{kr}{2}(\cos\phi\hat{\theta} - \cos\theta\sin\phi\hat{\phi})\right] \quad (5\text{-}11)$$

where E_0 is the strength of the incident electric field and r is the radial variable. The whole-body absorption rate is given by

$$P_a = \frac{1}{2}\sigma E_0^2 V\left[\frac{9}{|\varepsilon|^2} + \frac{1}{10}(ka)^2\right] \quad (5\text{-}12)$$

where V and a are respectively the volume and radius of the spherical model.

The electric field component of the incident plane wave couples to the object in the same fashion as an electrostatic field. This gives rise to a

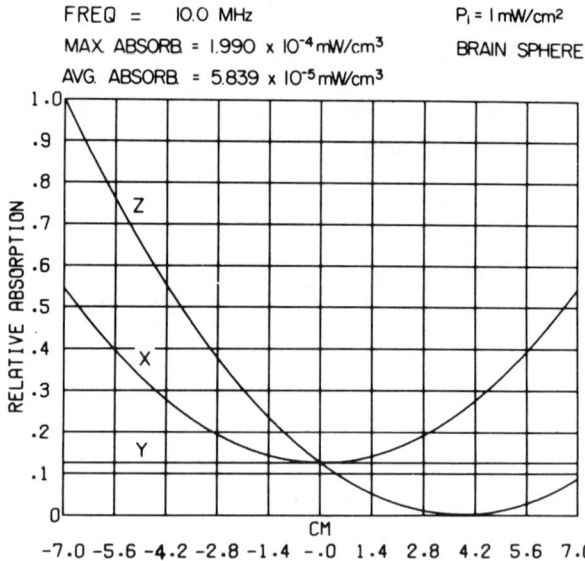

FIGURE 5-16. SAR distribution along the x, y, and z axes of a small brain sphere (Lin et al., 1973a).

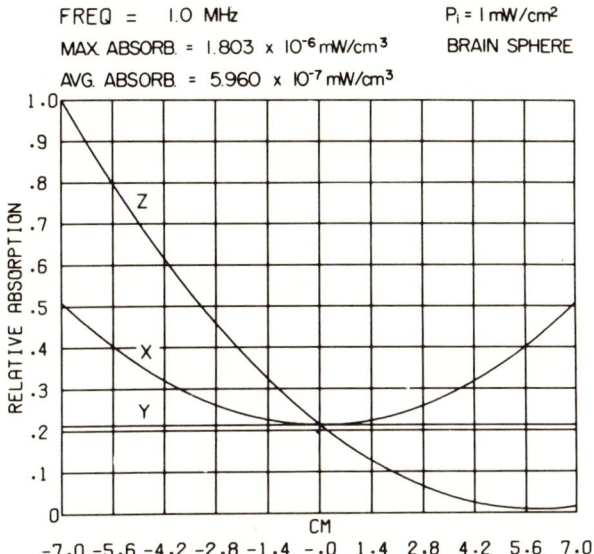

FIGURE 5-17. Predicted SAR distribution in a sphere whose size is extremely small compared to the wavelength. x, y, and z are the orthogonal coordinates of a rectangular system (Lin et al., 1973a).

constant induced electric field inside the sphere that has the same direction but is reduced by $3/\varepsilon$ from the applied electric field for biological materials and is independent of sphere size. Similarly, the magnetically induced electric field inside the body is identical to the quasi-static solution whose magnitude is given by $E = \pi f \mu r H$, where f is the frequency, μ is the permeability, r is the radius, and H is the magnetic field component. Thus, the magnetic field component of the incident plane wave produces an internal electric field that varies directly with distance away from the axis and in proportion to the frequency.

Figure 5-18 depicts how the induced electric fields combined inside the sphere. The magnetically induced electric field encircles the y axis (magnetic axis) and gives rise to an eddy current whose magnitude increases with distance away from the y axis. This indicates that while the H-induced energy absorption in a mouse or larger animal is much greater than the E-induced component, electrically and magnetically induced absorption may be equally significant in even smaller animals at lower frequencies (below 30 MHz). Moreover, for a small insect or pupa the electric field will be the predominant factor.

The variation of average and maximum energy absorption with frequency for a human-size sphere is illustrated in Fig. 5-19. In the

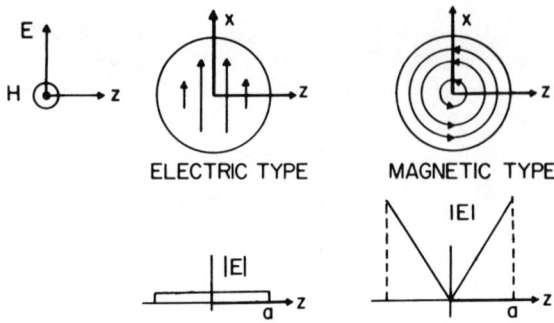

FIGURE 5-18. Diagrammatic representation of the behavior of electric and magnetic fields under quasi-static conditions of irradiation (Lin *et al.*, 1973a).

frequency range 1–10,000 MHz, the maximum absorption rate is only 10^{-6} to 10^{-3} W/kg per W/m² of incident power. Inspection of the maximum absorption rate induced by a plane wave, a quasi-static electric field, and a quasi-static magnetic field shows that absorption in the frequency range 1–20 MHz is primarily due to the magnetic induction and is characterized by a square-of-frequency dependence. The approximate frequency dependence of average or total energy absorption throughout the frequency range 1 MHz–10 GHz is indicated by the dashed line. For frequencies between 1 and 20 MHz, the average absorption varies as the square of the frequency. In the frequency range 20–200 MHz, the average absorption increases directly in proportion to frequency and reaches a maximum of about 2×10^{-3} W/kg per W/m² of incident power at 200 MHz. The average absorption rate remains fairly constant with increasing frequency. (It actually is inversely proportional to frequency for higher frequencies.) There is thus little doubt that electromagnetic energy absorption varies both with frequency and with body size, and in a predictable manner.

5.2.2. Prolate Spheroidal Tissue Models

Since the bodies of humans and experimental animals are seldom spherical, we need a more appropriate model to analytically and numerically describe the induced fields and absorbed energy inside experimental subjects. A prolate spheroid approaches more closely the shape of mammalian bodies, but most analyses have been restricted to homogeneous models for humans and experimental animals (Johnson *et al.*, 1975; Durney *et al.*, 1975, 1979; Massoudi *et al.*, 1977; Wu and Lin,

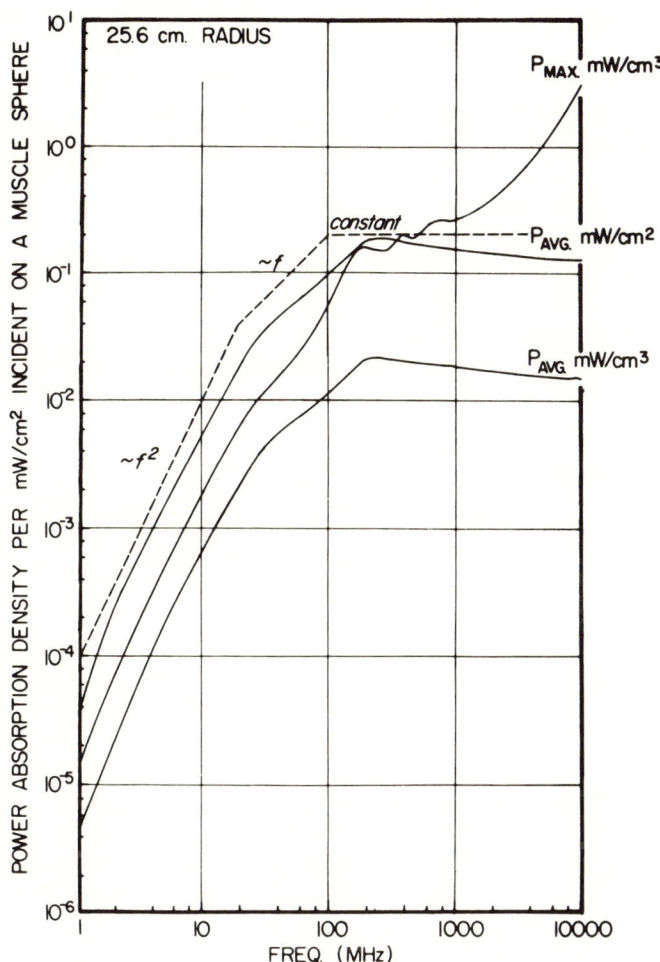

FIGURE 5-19. Frequency dependence of absorption in a spherical model of the human body (Lin et al., 1973a).

1977; Barber, 1977a,b; Rowlandson and Barber, 1979). The basic approach (Asano and Yamamoto, 1975) is to expand the incident, scattered, and transmitted electric fields in terms of vector wave functions in spheroidal coordinates. The expansion coefficients are determined from the boundary conditions requiring that the tangential components of the fields be continuous across the surface of the spheroid. The absorbed power is obtained from equation (2.32) and the average absorptions are found from relationships similar to those of equations (5.9)–(5.13).

In addition, for frequencies below resonance (resonance is defined as the condition of maximum absorption), long-wavelength formulations (Durney *et al.*, 1975; Massoudi *et al.*, 1977) and quasi-static approximations (Lin, 1980) have been used to obtain absorption information. More recently, geometric-optics approximations have been developed for computation of absorption characteristics of prolate spheroidal models of humans, at frequencies whose wavelengths are short compared with body size (Rowlandson and Barber, 1979).

Three orientations of the impinging plane wave with respect to the body must be distinguished (see Fig. 5-20): E polarization in which the electric field is parallel to the major axis of the spheroid, H polarization in which the magnetic field vector is parallel to the major axis, and K polarization in which both electric and magnetic field vectors are

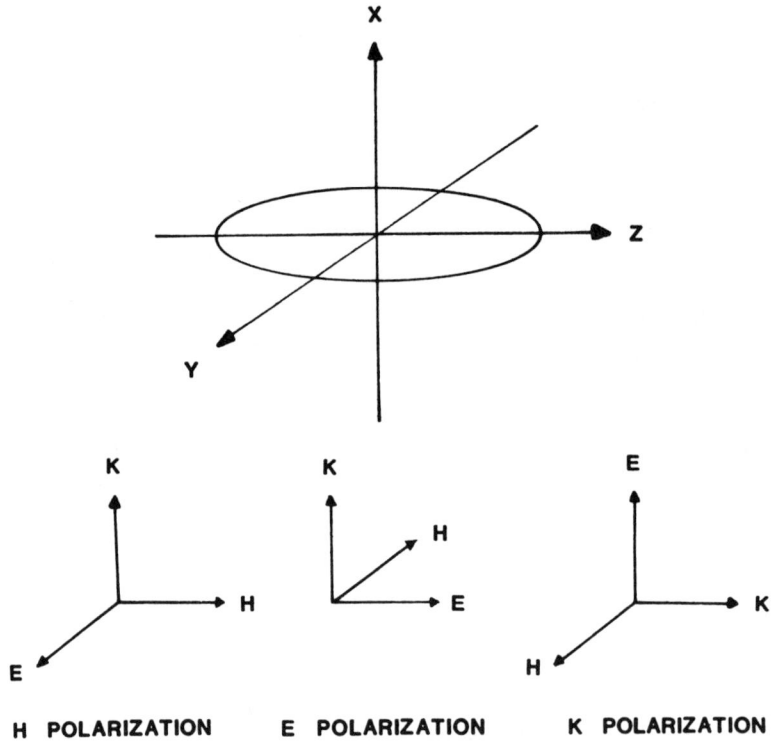

FIGURE 5-20. Polarization states of a plane wave impinging on a prolate spheroidal body model.

perpendicular to the major axis of the spheroid. In general, E polarization produces the highest energy absorption for frequencies up to and slightly beyond the resonance region.

The induced electric fields inside a dielectric prolate spheroid (a, semimajor axis; b, semiminor axis) in a plane wave electromagnetic field with long wavelength ($\lambda > a$) may be represented by

$$E_e = \frac{E_0}{C_1}\hat{z} - j\tfrac{1}{2}E_0\frac{\omega\mu_0}{377}(z\cos\phi\hat{\rho} - z\sin\phi\hat{\phi} - \rho\cos\phi\hat{z}) \quad (5.13)$$

for E polarization and

$$E_h = \frac{-E_0\hat{y}}{C_2} + \tfrac{1}{2}E_0\frac{\omega\mu_0\rho\hat{\phi}}{377} \quad (5.14)$$

for H polarization. The whole-body energy absorption rate is generally given by

$$P_a = \tfrac{1}{2}\sigma\int_{\text{volume}} \mathbf{E}\cdot\mathbf{E}^*\,dv \quad (5.15)$$

where $\sigma = \omega\varepsilon_0\varepsilon''$ is the electrical conductivity and E^* denotes the complex conjugate of the induced field E inside the body. The whole-body rates of absorbed energy by substituting equations (5.13) and (5.14) into (5.15) are

$$P_{ae} = \tfrac{1}{2}\sigma E_0^2(\tfrac{4}{3}\pi ab^2)\left[\frac{1}{C_1^2} + \frac{1}{20}\left(\frac{\omega\mu_0}{377}\right)^2(a^2+b^2)\right] \quad (5.16)$$

for E polarization and

$$P_{ah} = \tfrac{1}{2}\sigma E_0^2(\tfrac{4}{3}\pi ab^2)\left[\frac{1}{C_2^2} + \frac{1}{10}\left(\frac{\omega\mu_0}{377}\right)^2 b^2\right] \quad (5.17)$$

for H polarization (Lin, 1980). The constants C_1 and C_2 are given by

$$C_1 = (1-\varepsilon)\eta_0[(1-\eta_0^2)\coth^{-1}\eta_0 + \eta_0] + \varepsilon \quad (5.18)$$

$$C_2 = 1 + \tfrac{1}{2}(\varepsilon-1)\eta_0[(1-\eta_0^2)\coth^{-1}\eta_0 + \eta_0] \quad (5.19)$$

where $\varepsilon = \varepsilon' - j\varepsilon''$ is the complex relative permittivity and η_0 is the eccentricity given by

$$\eta_0 = a/(a^2 - b^2)^{1/2} \qquad (5.20)$$

Since C_1 and C_2 do not depend on spatial variables, the induced fields within the spheroid are uniform and independent of size when the external field is uniform. For $\varepsilon > 1$, the field inside the spheroid is weaker than the applied field. Moreover, the whole-body energy absorption depends not only on the strength of impressed fields, but also on the orientation of the field with respect to the major axis of the body.

As in the case of spherical models, the absorption is produced by an electrically induced current in the direction of the applied E-field vector, combined with a circulating current induced by the incident H field. One would therefore expect the electrically induced absorption to be uniform, whereas the absorption due to the circulating eddy current would be zero at the center and increase as the square of the distance from the center.

Computations for the absorbed energy as a function of frequency and body size have been made using homogeneous muscle material both as an index of SARs in mammals and as a guide for extrapolating data from experimental animals to humans, particularly with regard to averages of absorbed energy (Durney et al., 1980). Figure 5-21 shows the theoretically projected frequency dependence of absorbed energy for humans and for laboratory rats. Note that for a given incident field orientation, the average SAR for humans may be either higher or lower than for rats, depending on the frequency. For example, at 70 MHz, the average SAR is higher for humans, having a value of 0.25 W/kg for an incident power density of 10 W/m^2; the rat's average SAR is only 0.0125 W/kg. In contrast, the average SAR of 0.8 W/kg at 700 MHz is higher for rats; the corresponding value for humans is less than 1/25th of this. It is thus extremely important to take into account the body size and operating frequency when drawing any relationship between the biological effects that arise in the laboratory and corresponding effects that might occur in humans at a given incident power density.

The frequency for maximal absorption (resonance frequency) depends on the subject and its orientation with respect to the incident field. In general, the shorter the subject, the higher is the resonance frequency and vice versa. Further, the frequency dependence of whole-body or average absorption may be partitioned into three regions. This may be illustrated using the orientation that is most efficient in energy coupling, E polarization. Figure 5-22 gives the whole-body absorption data for a prolate spheroidal model of the rat irradiated with plane waves in free space. For frequencies well below resonance such that the ratio of the longest body dimension (L) to the free-space wavelength (λ) is less than

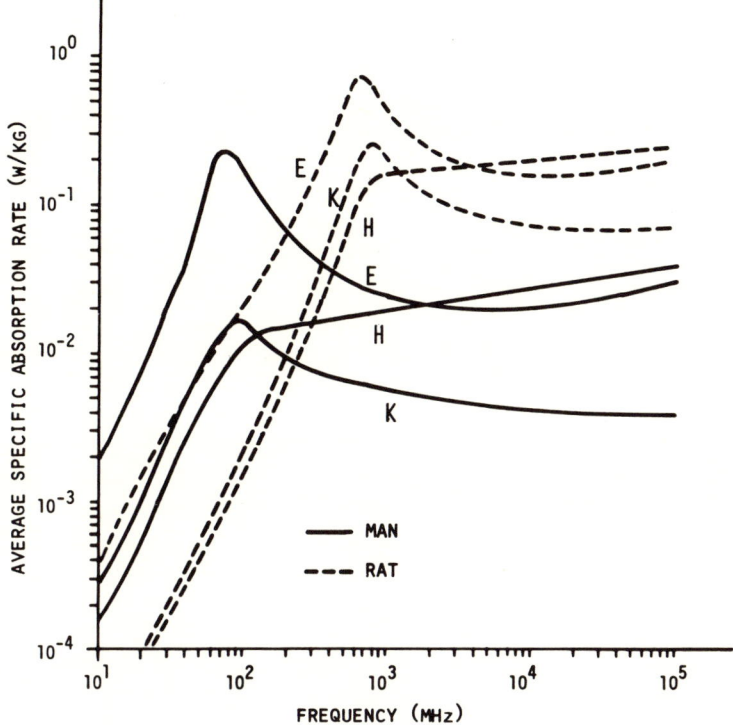

FIGURE 5-21. Predicted frequency dependence of absorbed energy in spheroidal models of biological bodies.

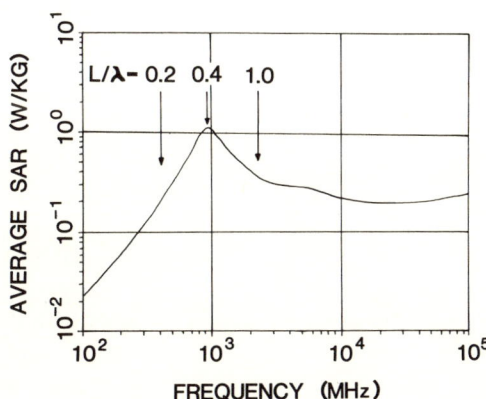

FIGURE 5-22. The three distinct regions of absorption as a function of frequency.

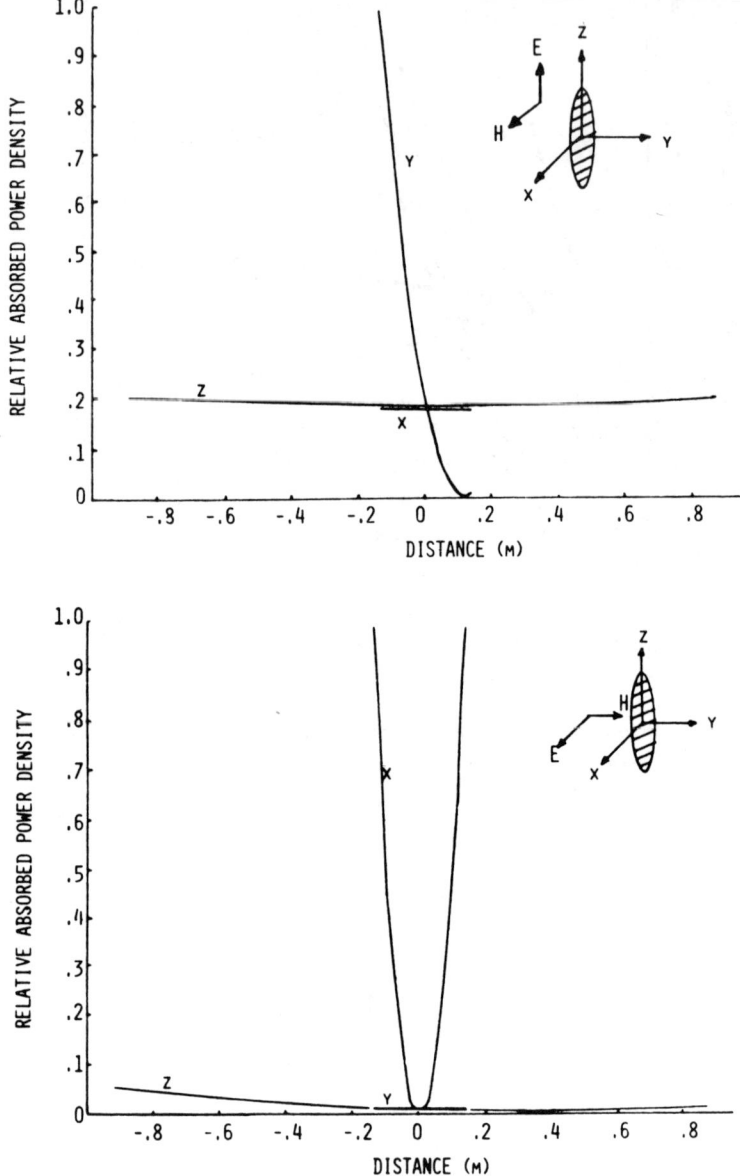

FIGURE 5-23. SAR distributions along the x, y, and z axes of a prolate spheroidal model of man. The maximum absorptions are 6.14, 1.93, and 0.64 mW/kg for E, K, and H polarizations, respectively. The incident power density is 1 mW/cm^2 (Durney et al., 1980).

PROPAGATION AND ABSORPTION IN TISSUE MEDIA 167

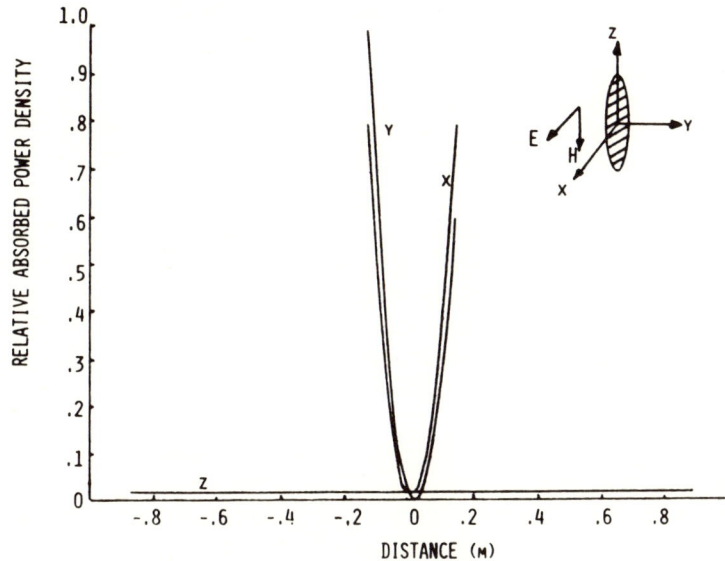

FIGURE 5-23. (*continued*)

0.2, the average SAR is characterized by an f^2 dependence. The average absorption goes through a resonance in the region where $0.2 < L/\lambda < 1.0$. In this case, the average SAR rapidly increases to a maximum near $L/\lambda = 0.4$ and then falls off as $1/f$. At frequencies for which $L/\lambda > 1.0$, the whole-body absorption decreases slightly but approaches asymptotically the geometrical optics limit of about one-half of the incident power (1 − power reflection coefficient).

It should be noted that the resonant absorption length of 0.4λ is in good agreement with results from antenna analysis (see Chapter 2). In addition, whole-body absorptions for H and K polarizations are totally different. The resonances are not nearly as well defined as for E polarization. In fact, the whole-body absorption curve for H polarization gradually reaches a plateau and stays at the plateau for higher frequencies.

The distribution of absorbed energy in a prolate spheroidal model whose size is small compared with wavelength is shown in Fig. 5-23 for the three distinct polarizations. The height of the prolate spheroid equals 1.75 m with a major-to-minor axis ratio of 6.34 and 70-kg mass corresponding to a human body. The dielectric constant and conductivity are those for muscle tissue at 10 MHz. These graphs are qualitatively similar to those for spherical models. As expected, the absorbed energy is highest for E polarization. In fact, there is approximately an order of magnitude difference in the peak rate of absorbed energy, depending on the polarization.

For E polarization, the eddy current is zero on the x axis; thus, a low relative absorption is seen along the x axis, which is only due to the electrically induced current. The absorption rate is elevated considerably, however, indicating a strong coupling of the impressed electric field into the interior of the prolate spheroid. The slender spheroid forces the internal electric field to more closely correspond to the incident field because of the boundary condition that requires continuity of tangential fields. The relatively flat energy distribution along the z axis again shows the strong coupling of impressed electric field and relatively weak eddy-current contribution due to a smaller cross section for intercepting the magnetic flux. The distribution, along the y axis, indicates that the electrically and magnetically induced field components are nearly equal. The electric polarization field and the circulating eddy current add at the front side and subtract on the back side of the spheroid to render an absorption pattern that peaks at the front surface and is reduced to almost zero deeper inside the spheroid.

For H polarization, the electrically induced current flows along the x axis (direction of incident E field) and the eddy-current field encircles the z axis (direction of incident H fiedl). The relatively low power on the z axis comes solely from the incident electric field. The combination of E- and H-induced components generates a displaced parabolic energy absorption pattern along both x and y axes. Clearly, magnetically induced eddy current predominates in this case and the absorption is highest along the transverse circumference at the middle of the prolate spheroid. For K polarization, both electric and magnetic components of the incident field are again along the minor axes of the spheroid. The electrically induced current flows along the x axis. The incident magnetic field induces an eddy-current electric field that encircles the y axis and the absorption is lowest on the axis. Whereas in both E- and H-polarization cases, the peak absorption occurs at the front surface of the spheroid (the surface of the spheroid encountered first by the incident plane wave), this is not the case for K polarization. Maximum absorption appears at $x = \pm b$ and the absorbed energy varies parabolically along the x axis. This results from the large quantity of magnetic flux intercepted by the broad cross section (and resulting concentration of eddy current). It should be noted that the results illustrated in Fig. 5-23 match very well with experimental measurements (Guy et al., 1976). Moreover, the peak absorptions may be two orders of magnitude higher than those for dielectric spheres of equal mass.

Contours of absorbed energy distribution in prolate spheroidal models close to resonance are illustrated in Figs. 5-24 and 5-25 for small

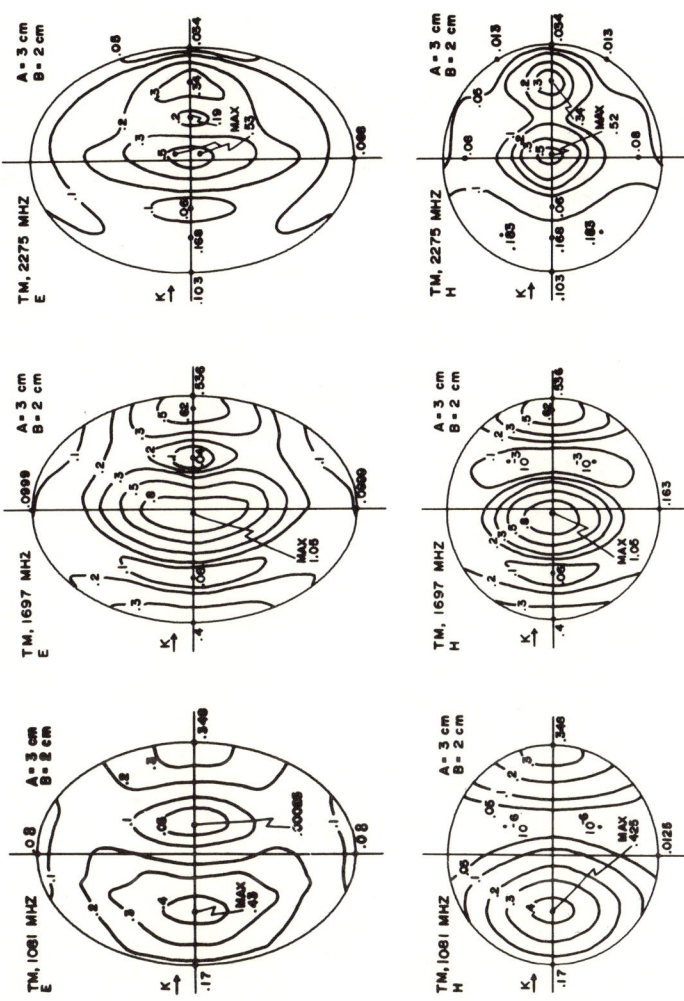

FIGURE 5-24. SAR (square of induced electric field) contours in a prolate spheroidal model of a small animal body (mouse) in an E-polarized plane wave field of 1 V/m at three resonance frequencies.

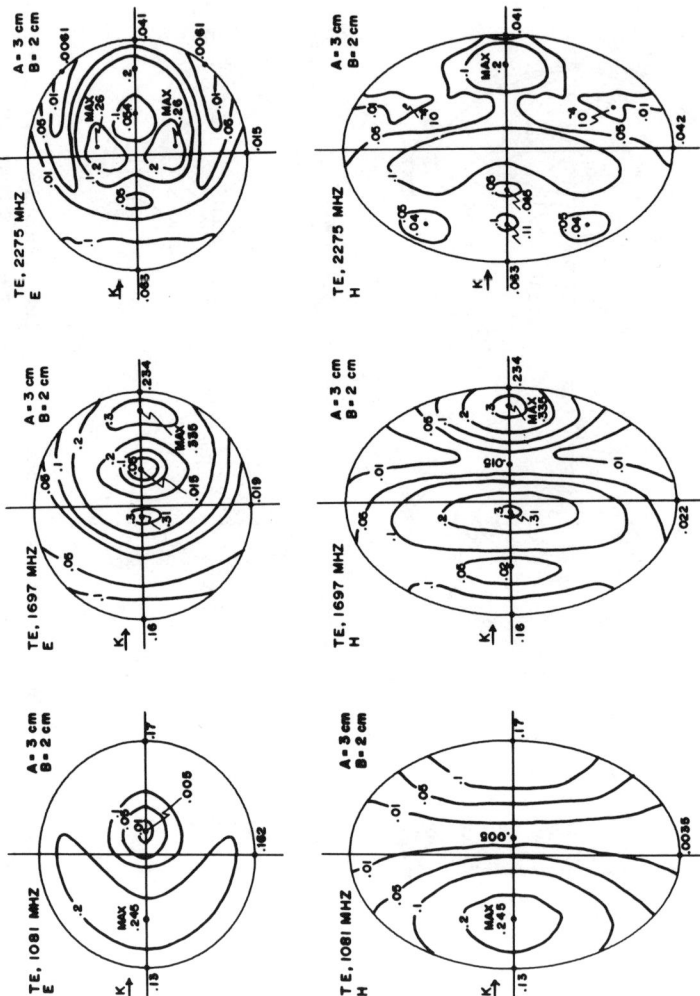

FIGURE 5-25. Distribution contours for induced electric field inside a prolate spheroidal model of a small animal body (mouse) in an H-polarized plane wave field of 1 V/m. The frequencies are for the first, second, and third resonances.

animals. In this case, the square of induced electric fields are shown; the SARs can be easily calculated using equation (2.32) and the dielectric properties for muscle. The top graphs show the distribution over the plane parallel to the electric field vector through the center. The lower graphs give the distribution over the plane parallel to the magnetic field vector through the middle of the spheroid. The nonuniform nature of the distribution is apparent in all cases; each graph shows several absorption peaks. The intense fields in the prolate spheroidal models are about 30% higher than those predicted using a sphere. The corresponding curve for a spheroidal object usually falls just above the curves for H and K polarizations and well below the curve for E polarizations, as one would expect from symmetry considerations.

5.3. COMPLEX TISSUE MODELS

We have summarized above some of the analytical approaches for quantifying the absorbed energy in biological objects. It should be recognized that while spheres and spheroids are good models of some animal bodies and certain body parts, they may not always suffice for humans and experimental animals under a variety of exposure situations. More realistic models, such as models of human bodies formed from cubes, have been developed to account for the irregular shapes (Liversay and Chen, 1974; Guru and Chen, 1976; Chen and Guru, 1977; Hagman *et al.*, 1979a,b; Chen, 1980; Durney, 1980; Gandhi, 1982). These models, based on numerical techniques, hold great promise for accurately predicting energy absorption and its distribution in biological objects exposed to radio and microwave radiation. In what follows, we will summarize a number of computer techniques that have been applied with some success to solving electromagnetic energy absorption and distribution problems. We will also describe some results obtained using the volume integral equation method for human bodies exposed to plane waves in free space, and to near-zone fields.

5.3.1. Computational Schemes

The methods used to treat biological bodies of realistic shapes include the volume integral equation method (Liversay and Chen, 1974; Guru and Chen, 1976; Chen and Guru, 1977; Hagman *et al.*, 1979a,b) and the surface integral equation method (Wu and Tsai, 1977a,b; Wu, 1979). The method of moments (Harrington, 1968) is used in both approaches for finding solutions to the unknown fields inside the body. The approaches differ, however, in specifics, in that the surface integral equation method finds the unknown currents on the body surface and calculates the interior fields from the surface currents, the reciprocity theorem, and a "measurement matrix." In contrast, the volume integral equation method requires determination of unknown fields throughout the volume of the body, using the volume equivalence principle and the method of moments.

Several studies have shown that the calculated whole-body-averaged SAR increases with the number of cells employed in the moment method computation (Hagman, 1978; Chen, 1980; Deford *et al.*, 1983). This is attributable to the insufficient number of cells used to represent field variations inside the body. In general, moment method algorithms using a pulse function basis require that the field be approximately constant throughout each cell. The upper bound on usable cell size is given by

$$l/\lambda' < 0.39 \quad \text{and} \quad 0.27 \tag{5.21}$$

for high- and low-conductivity dielectrics, respectively (Lin, 1986). In this case, for tissues with high and low conductivities, l is the length of the side of a square cell and λ' is the wavelength in tissue. Thus, there must be at least three cells per wavelength, if not four. Otherwise, the magnitude and phase resolutions would be such that even with convergence, the reliability of the computed SAR would be questionable.

To acheive sufficiently fine sampling throughout the entire volume of the model and to permit more accurate geometric representation of the model, a reasonable cell size would be $l < 0.1\lambda'$. Such fine discretization implies human models with 10,000 to 100,000 cells at microwave frequencies. Since, for moment method algorithms, the required computer storage is proportional to N^2 and the computation time rises as N^3, moment method solutions would be impractical with presently available computational resources. Clearly, new approaches based on different principles are needed to acquire precise information on the distribution of absorbed microwave energy inside biological bodies.

Presently, there exist two alternative methods that promise to provide highly efficient procedures for field intensity calculations using a large number of cells in a finely discretized model. One technique involves the use of finite difference algorithms for the time-dependent Maxwell equations (Taflove and Brodwin, 1975a,b; Hagman, 1978; Taflove, 1980; Taflove and Lin, 1981; Taflove and Umashankar, 1982) and the other employs a fast-Fourier-transform (FFT) procedure (Borup and Gandhi, 1984) to solve the electric field integral equation.

The numerical technique that has been adopted for most of the field intensity computations is the *volume integral equation method* employing the volume equivalence principle (Schelkunoff, 1951; Lin and Wu, 1976;

Chen and Guru, 1977; Lin et al., 1977; Hagman et al., 1979a,b). The method of moments is used to transform the integral equation into a matrix equation by subdividing the body into N simple shaped cells. This is accomplished with the aid of an appropriate set of expansion functions chosen to satisfy the boundary conditions and a set of weighting (testing) functions to reduce the matrix fill-in time. The total electric field at each of the N cells is given by matrix inversion.

According to the method of moments, a biological body may be partitioned into N cubic subvolumes or cells that are sufficiently small for the electric field and dielectric permittivity to be constant within each cell. The integral equation is then transformed into a system of $3N$ simultaneous linear equations for the three orthogonal components of the electric field at the center of each cell. The simultaneous equations may be written in matrix form. Each matrix can be evaluated as shown in Liversay and Chen (1974) and Chen (1980). In particular, the diagonal elements of the matrix may be evaluated exactly by approximating each subvolume with a sphere of equal volume centered at the position of an interior point. If the actual shape of the subvolume differs appreciably from that of a sphere, this approximation may lead to unsatisfactory numerical results. In such cases, a small cylindrical volume may be created around an interior point. It may also be necessary to evaluate these terms by numerical integration throughout the cubic subvolume for increased accuracy. The evaluation of off-diagonal elements of the matrix is considerably simplified since it does not involve principal value operations.

Several computer programs have been developed to implement this numerical procedure. Factors that influence the computational accuracy include frequency, body size, cell dimensions, and computer memory. It has been found that reliable numerical results can be obtained if the linear dimensions of the cell do not exceed a quarter free-space wavelength (Liversay and Chen, 1974). For a computer with sufficient capacity to invert a 120×120 matrix, the maximum number of cells is limited to 40. If we assume, for simplicity, symmetries between the right and the left half and the front and the back of a 1.7-m-tall adult human body, this computer would handle approximately a cell size around $10^{-2}\,m^3$. Once the $10^{-2}\,m^3$ cell size is adopted, 750 MHz would be the highest frequency considered for field intensity calculation without violating the criterion that the linear dimension of the cell not exceed a quarter free-space wavelength.

The computational resources needed are quite extensive. A relatively full complex matrix, $3N \times 3N$ in dimensions, is required for a model with N cells. The requisite computation time for a noniterative solution of the matrix equation is therefore proportional to N^2 to N^3, which increases rapidly as N increases. The faithfulness with which a cubic cell model approximates the detailed structure of a biological body and the maximum usable frequency both increase with the number of cells.

Thus, a fundamental limitation of this method is the use of full or nearly full matrices and, therefore, the requirement of extensive computer storage and long running time. Even with the availability of larger and faster computers, this difficulty may not be completely resolved. The need for excessively large numbers of mathematical cells to render a more accurate representation of the body will give rise to an equally large and full matrix. The inversion of large, full matrices often leads to numerical instabilities in the solution. Nevertheless, the method does allow the use of nonhomogeneous models with up to 180 cells and is the only one available at present for computing field intensity distributions. In fact, this method has been employed, successfully, to calculate whole-body-averaged absorption and to obtain the regional distribution of absorbed radio and microwave energy using nonhomogeneous block models composed of rectangular cells (Chen and Guru, 1977; Hagman *et al.*, 1979a,b; Gandhi *et al.*, 1979; Chen, 1980; Gandhi, 1982). This method also has been used to study the interaction of the near-zone field with biological bodies (Chen, 1980; Karimullah *et al.*, 1980; Chatterjee *et al.*, 1980).

Another approach for predicting the distribution of absorbed electromagnetic energy is the *surface integral equation method* (Wu and Tsai, 1977a,b; Poggio and Miller, 1973; Massoudi *et al.*, 1982). This method makes use of two coupled integral equations, i.e., the electric field and magnetic field integral equations for the tangential components of the field on the surface separating the biological body from air. The unknown surface currents are found by Fourier decomposition and the moment method. The fields inside the biological body are calculated using the previously computed surface currents, the reciprocity theorem, and the concept of measurement matrix (Mautz and Harrington, 1969; Harrington and Mautz, 1972; Wu and Tsai, 1977b; Wu, 1979).

The method begins with the matrix representation of the coupled integral equations. If the body is assumed to be rotationally symmetric, the incident wave and the induced current could then be expanded in a Fourier series expansion in the angle of rotation. This reduces the problem to that of solving a system of orthogonal modes. The method further expands the surface components in terms of triangular expansion or basis functions and allows the testing functions to be the complex conjugate of the basis functions taking advantage of the orthogonality property. Thus, the major advantage of introducing the Fourier series is to enable each mode to be treated completely independently of all other modes. This results in a much smaller size, manageable matrix equation to be evaluated for the unknown expansion coefficients that determine the surface currents. It should be noted that for biological bodies, triangular expansion and testing functions are preferred over flat pulse expansion functions (Wu and Tsai, 1977b). In fact, an expansion function with a continuous first derivative may constitute an even better choice for the expansion basis function. In any event, once the surface currents are obtained, the fields everywhere, or specific absorption rate at each point inside the body, can be calculated using the reciprocity theorem (Mautz and Harrington, 1969; Harrington and Mautz, 1972). The total absorption can be found by integrating the surface Poynting vector.

The validity of this surface integral equation method has been substantiated by using a dielectric sphere (Wu and Tsai, 1977b). Calculations for a human torso modeled by a homogeneous muscle body of revolution with a height of 1.78 m at 30, 80, and 300 MHz showed enhanced absorption in the neck region for all three frequencies and both vertical and horizontal polarization (Wu, 1979). Note that the vertical direction is aligned with the long dimension of the torso and serves as the axis of symmetry. The strongest absorption in the torso model was found to occur with vertical polarization and near the first resonance frequency of the torso (80 MHz). In general, the surface integral equation method is applicable to any arbitrarily shaped homogeneous body of revolution. This method can be used not only with incident plane waves, but also with a wide variety of other field exposure conditions, including direct contact situations and near-zone sources.

Since both surface and volume integral equation methods for field intensity prediction rely on the method of moments, it is instructive to compare the relative advantages of these two techniques. For simplicity, consider a homogeneous cube with N samples on each side: the computer storage requirements are $24N^2$ and $3N^3$ for the surface and volume integral equation methods, respectively (Wu and Tsai, 1977b). For sufficient sampling to ensure accurate description of field variations, N is usually a large number. Thus, the surface integral equation method requires significantly less unknowns for homogeneous models. Moreover, in cases where permittivity and conductivity values are large, such as in biological bodies, the wavelength becomes contracted inside the body, and a much larger number of cells than that indicated above may actually be needed. If the model is nonhomogeneous, then the volume integral equation method would prove to be more suitable. It is possible, however, to generalize the surface integral equation technique to account for nonhomogeneities by employing the invariant embedding procedure (Pogorzelski and Wu, 1977).

An alternate surface integral equation method for computing the distribution of absorbed electromagnetic energy in realistic models of a biological body is the *extended boundary condition method* (Waterman, 1965). This method employs analytical continuation, spherical harmonics, and the equivalence theorem to calculate fields inside the body. Specifically, the fields induced inside the body are replaced by equivalent surface currents. These surface currents are such that they reduce the total fields inside the body to zero. Thus, upon applying the boundary conditions at the surface of the body, an integral equation results that relates the incident field to the surface currents. This equation is then cast in a form suitable for numerical computation by expansion of the various field quantities in vector spherical harmonics (Barber and Yeh, 1975). It should be noted that the expansion coefficients for the incident field are known; only the coefficients for the surface currents need to be determined. This is accomplished by applying the orthogonality properties of vector spherical harmonics, giving rise to a set of simultaneous equations that can be solved for the unknown coefficients. The induced fields are then determined in terms of the surface currents through the equivalence theorem.

This technique thus far has been applied to treat axisymmetric models such as spherical, spheroidal, and finite cylindrical bodies (Barber and Yeh, 1975; Barber, 1977a,b) with limited success. Because the complex arguments associated with vector spherical harmonics, especially the spherical Bessel functions, tend to be singular for large conductivities, the application of the technique is severely restricted. It appears that this method is amenable predominantly for predicting fields at high frequencies (i.e., frequencies well above the resonance region). The technique fails to yield convergent induced field distributions in lossy biological bodies in the resonance region for models of large aspect ratio in which the long dimension is very large compared with the short dimension of the body. In this case, an ill-conditioned set of matrix equations results from the large number of terms required to fit the vector spherical harmonic expansion to a nonspherical body.

A number of attempts have been made to formulate computational schemes by which the ill-conditioned matrix obtained in the resonance region could be avoided. Among them the iterative techniques (Lakhtakia *et al.,* 1983) proposed to overcome the convergence-related stability problem appear to have merit. This iterative procedure has the unique feature of approximating the interior of the body with several overlapping subregions, each represented by an expansion appropriate to its geometry. These subregional expansions are linked to each other by explicit matching in the appropriate overlapping zones. Since all the subregional field expansions are simultaneously solved, continuous and convergent field values are assured throughout the interior of the body.

In this method a noniterative procedure is used first to obtain the initial estimate of the tangential fields on the body surface. This is done by replacing the biological model with a perfectly conducting one of the same size and shape. Therefore, for subsequent iterations, the incident field and the results of the previous iteration for the surface fields are used to obtain the unknown coefficients that determine the surface fields for the current iteration. This is done by applying the orthogonality properties of vector spherical harmonics and solving the resultant system of simultaneous equations. To determine the unknown internal field expansion coefficients, the boundary condition is satisfied at an appropriate number of points on each of the subregional surfaces and, in addition, the continuity of internal fields is enforced at an appropriate number of points in each of the overlapping zones. The set of equations developed through these manipulations are simultaneously solved for the unknown coefficients of the subregional internal field expansions. The iterative procedure outlined above is continued until a preset convergence criterion is fulfilled. This may be satisfied by requiring the incremental surface electric current density to approach zero. Once the internal field distribution is known, and thus the SAR distribution, the whole-body-averaged SAR can be obtained by averaging the SAR distribution over the entire model volume.

This method has been applied to calculate the distribution of absorbed energy in two body models exposed to plane wave irradiation in the resonance and postresonance frequency ranges (Lakhtakia *et al.*, 1983). The calculated results for homogeneous prolate spheroidal and capped cylindrical models of the human body showed applicability for frequencies up to 300 MHz, whereas the simple extended boundary conditions method was restricted to frequencies less than 70 MHz for similar models. It was found that the number of iterations required to obtain a convergent solution did not change with various schemes for subdividing the volume. From the perspective of computational efficiency, however, subregional geometries and expansion functions with appropriate geometric conformation are found to be advantageous.

5.3.2. Models of the Human Body

This section will present some results obtained for both plane wave and near-field exposure conditions using the volume integral equation technique (Hagman *et al.*, 1979a,b; Chen, 1980). The accuracy of the numerical procedure has been verified by comparison with known results from exact analytic solutions based on well-defined geometries such as spheres. It should be noted that perfect agreement between the exact solution and numerical approximation based on the volume integral equation is not expected unless a very large number of cells are used. Nevertheless, for a brain sphere constructed from 40 cubic cells at a frequency of 918 MHz, the computed maximum field deviated from the exact solution by less than 9% (Rukspollmuang and Chen, 1979).

A model of a human body consisting of 180 cubic cells that accounts for the anatomic and biometric characteristics of humans is shown in Fig. 5-26. The model is 1.75-m tall and can be made either homogeneous or nonhomogeneous by using an equivalent or a volume-weighted complex permittivity for each cell (Hagman *et al.*, 1979a,b). The distributions of absorbed energy inside the model in free space at 80 MHz (near resonance) for homogeneous and nonhomogeneous tissue properties are shown in Figs. 5-27 and 5-28, respectively. The electric field vector is oriented along the height of the model and the plane wave propagates from the front to the back of the body. It is interesting to observe that the absorbed energy in the upper torso is higher in the middle and back layers than in the front layer on which the plane wave impinges; the highest absorption in the transverse dimension occurs generally near the center of the torso. Energy deposition along the height of the body shows several peaks, which appear in the neck, the thoracic region, the pelvic/thigh region, and the calf for the homogeneous model. The SARs for 10 W/m^2 of incident power density are 86 W/kg for the pelvic/thigh region, 79 W/kg for the calf, 47 W/kg for the thorax, and 34 W/kg for the neck. It should be noted that the distribution of absorbed energy in

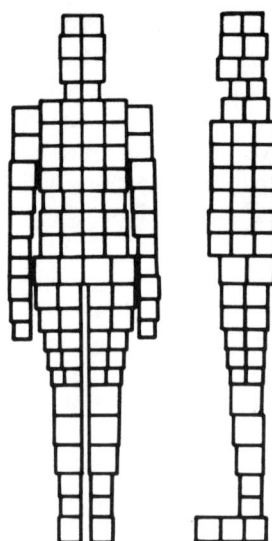

FIGURE 5-26. A cubic-cell representation of the human body (Gandhi *et al.*, 1979).

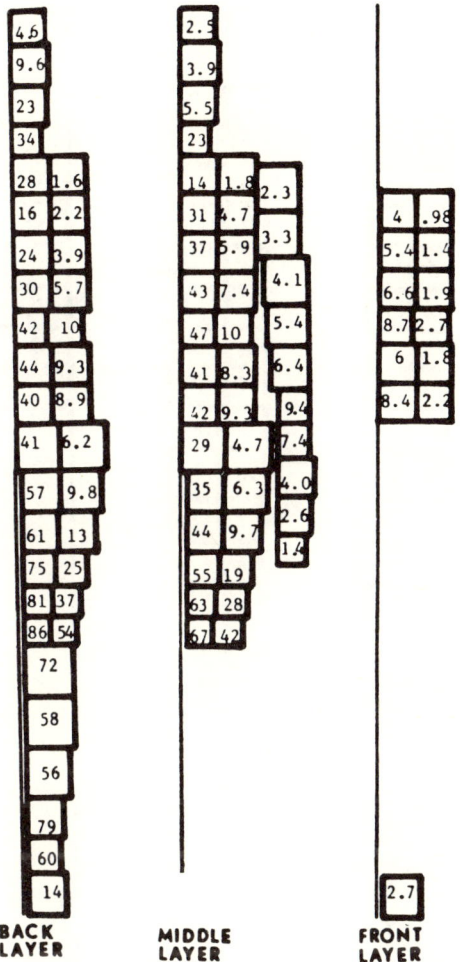

FIGURE 5-27. SARs for a homogeneous 180-cell model of man exposed to vertically polarized, 80-MHz plane waves (Hagman *et al.*, 1979a). Values are W/kg per mW/cm^2 × 100.

the homogeneous model is close to that measured using scaled models (Hagman *et al.*, 1979a,b; Chen, 1980).

The effect of nonhomogeneity produced by volume-weighted cell complex permittivity is mostly revealed in the relative strength of absorbed energy in different regions of the body. The general distribution of the absorbed energy shows very little difference between homogeneous and nonhomogeneous models. That is, enhanced absorptions occur in the

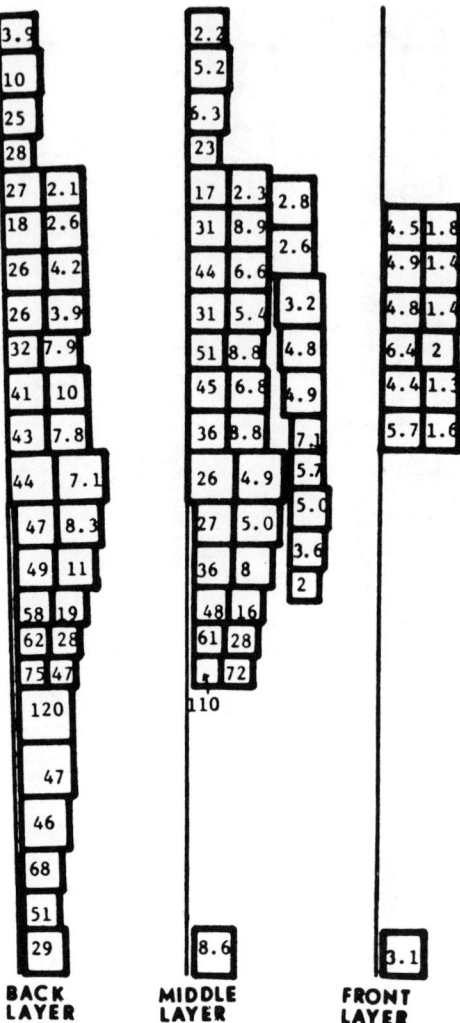

FIGURE 5-28. SARs for a nonhomogeneous 180-cell model of human body exposed to vertically polarized, 80-MHz plane waves (Hagman *et al.*, 1979a). Values are W/kg per mW/cm^2 × 100.

same region, but the SAR in the pelvic/thigh and thoracic regions is now, respectively, 12 and 5.1 W/kg per W/m^2 incident power density. The SAR in the neck and the calf, however, is reduced to 2.8 and 6.8 W/kg, respectively. Since the heart and the pelvic/thigh regions are characterized by tissues with high water content, whereas the neck and the calf are composed largely of tissues with low water content, this suggests that energy absorption in the body is increased in regions with a larger quantity of muscle tissue and is decreased in regions that consist mainly of bone tissue. Changes in coupling characteristics that stem from the nonhomogeneity, however, may also have contributed to the difference in absorbed energy distribution.

The average absorption or whole-body SAR for the model of the human body shown in Fig. 5-26 as a function of frequency is given in Fig. 5-29. Again, the electric field vector is along the height of the body and the plane wave propagates from the front to the back of the model with a power density of 10 W/m^2. A homogeneous complex permittivity approximately two-thirds of that for muscle is used in the calculations. Note that the whole-body SAR increases with frequency until it reaches a maximum of about 0.23 W/kg at 77 MHz (resonance frequency) and then decreases according to 1/frequency. The experimental data shown in Fig. 5-30 were obtained from a saline-filled scale model of the human body. It is seen that the calculated absorption is in good agreement with that found experimentally (Gandhi *et al.*, 1977; Hagman *et al.*, 1979a,b), except for the resonance frequency, which is somewhat lower (70 MHz) in the experimental case. It should be mentioned that the whole-body SAR given in Fig. 5-29 is typically within 10% of that estimated from prolate spheroidal models of the same height and dielectric property. Further, when nonhomogeneous complex permittitivities are used with the model, the whole-body SAR changes less than 2% from that given in Fig. 5-29. Thus, if one is primarily concerned with average absorption over the body, a homogeneous prolate spheroidal model may be quite adequate.

The method of moments based on the volume integral equation also can be invoked to determine the resonance frequency for the head region of the human model shown in Fig. 5-26. To provide a SAR distribution of sufficient resolution, the number of cells is increased from 12 to 144 in the head region and from 4 to 32 in the neck region for a whole-body total of 340 homogeneous cells (Hagman *et al.*, 1979a,b). The head and whole-body average absorption rates for this model in free space, exposed to plane waves having two different polarizations, are shown in Figs. 5-31 and 5-32. Observe that the average absorption rate of 0.02 W/kg per W/m^2 for the head, when the propagation vector is parallel to the body axis, for a plane wave propagating from head to toe, is higher by approximately 70% at 350 MHz than it is when the electric field vector is parallel to the body axis. The comparable whole-body average absorption is about 0.006 W/kg per W/m^2 of incident plane wave power density. This result shows that resonance absorption in the head of the human model occurs at a frequency near 350 MHz. In contrast, the data shown in Fig. 5-10 indicate a much higher resonance frequency for a

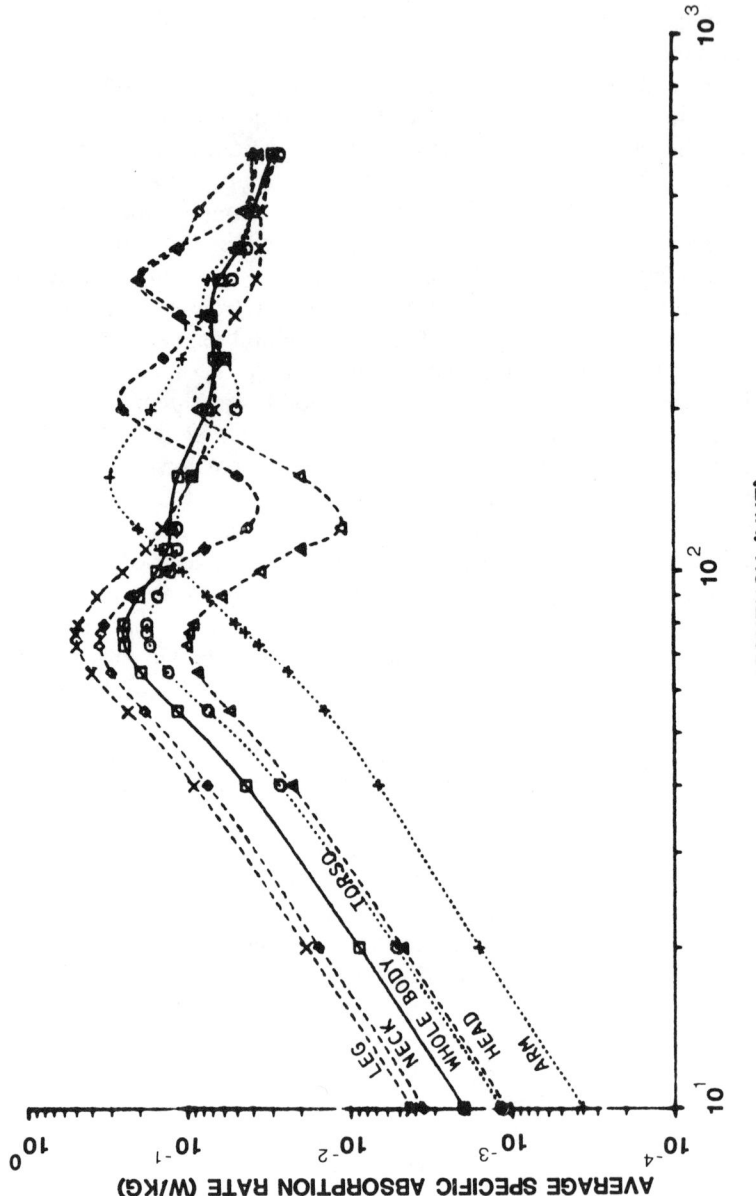

FIGURE 5-29. Average SARs for a homogeneous 180-cell model of human body exposed to vertically polarized plane waves in free space (Gandhi et al., 1979). The incident power density is 1 mW/cm².

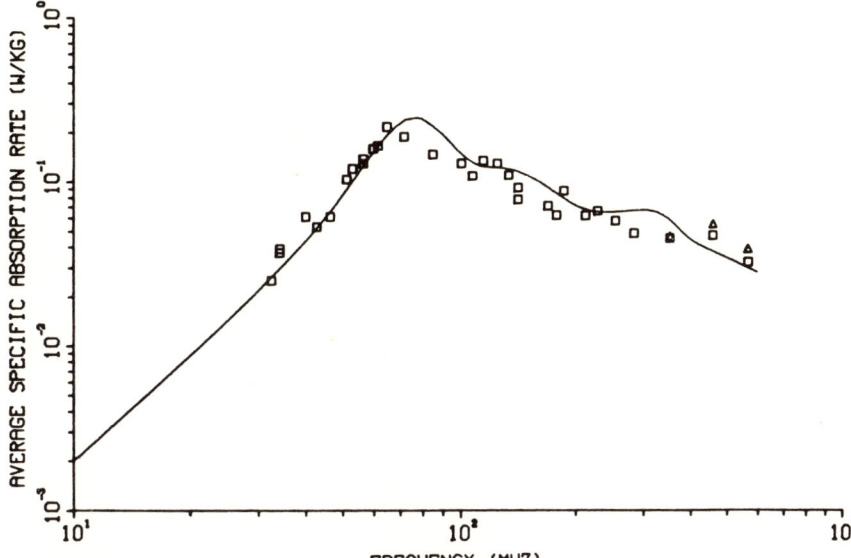

FIGURE 5-30. Whole-body-averaged absorption for a homogeneous cubic-cell model of man exposed to vertically polarized plane waves in free space. Squares and triangles represent measured values for normal saline and phantom mixture filled figurines (Hagman et al., 1979a). The incident power density is 1 mW/cm^2.

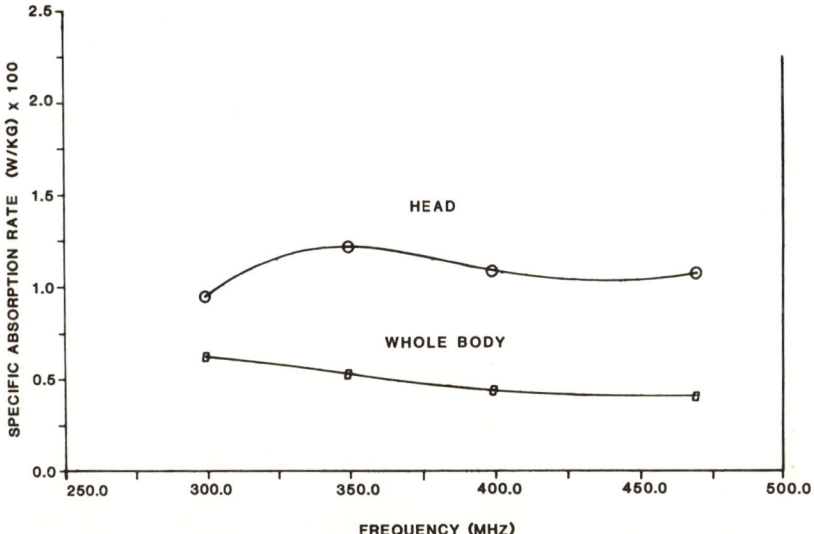

FIGURE 5-31. Head and whole-body absorption for E polarization, propagation from front to back (Hagman et al., 1979). The incident power density is 1 W/m^2.

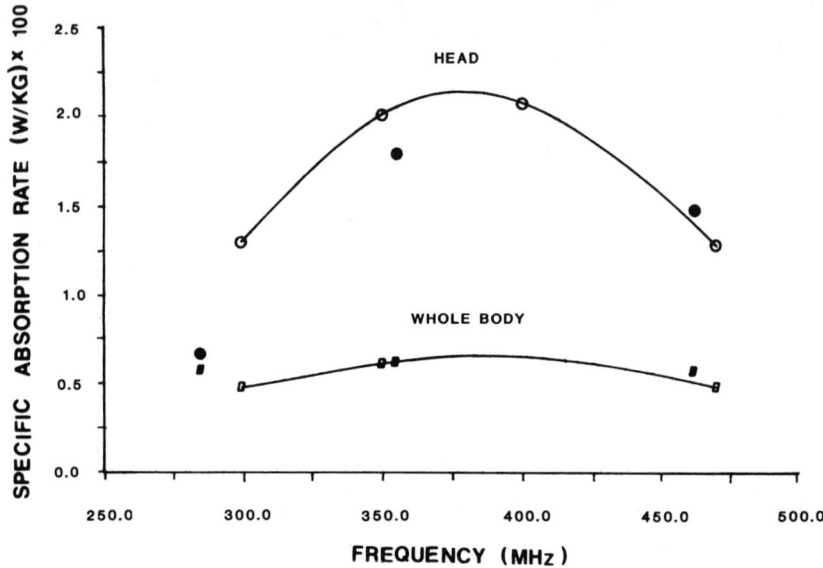

FIGURE 5-32. Head and whole-body absorption for wave propagation from head to toe, E front to back; incident power density = 1 W/m². Solid symbols are for phantom models of man (Hagman *et al.*, 1979a).

spherical model of an isolated human-size head. Clearly, the absorption in the head region is strongly influenced by the rest of the body.

The result of calorimetric measurements using accurately scaled figurines filled with phantom mixtures is shown by solid symbols in Fig. 5-32. Note the good agreement between the numerical solutions and experiments with phantom models.

Distributions of absorbed energy in the head region at 350 MHz are illustrated in Fig. 5-33. Note the presence of peak absorptions not only near the center of the head, but also in the neck region. The hot spot near the center of the head has been predicted by using spherical models (see Figs. 5-9–5-13).

Near-zone exposures often are encountered in the operation of equipment using electromagnetic energy for radar, communication, industrial, and biomedical applications. It has been generally known that the interaction of biological bodies with near-zone fields differs from that of plane wave exposures and varies with several source–body parameters. Systematic studies, however, have become available only in recent years.

The interaction of a near field and a biological body depends on such factors as type and configuration of the source, geometric and dielectric properties of the body, and source–body spacing. In many near-zone

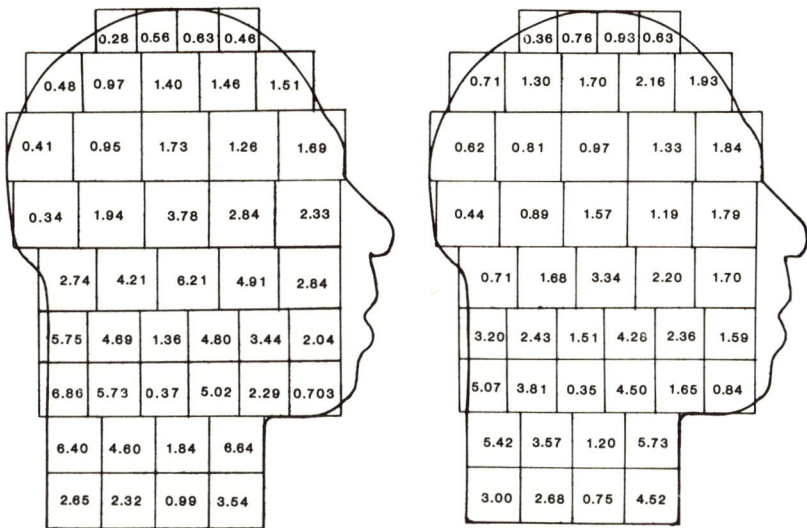

FIGURE 5-33. Local SAR values (W/kg per 100 W/m² incident field). (a) Inner layer of cells; (b) outer layer of cells. 350 MHz, K head to toe, E front to back, whole body average = 0.6132, head average = 2.014 (Hagman et al., 1979b).

exposure situations, mutual coupling between the body and the source complicates the quantification of induced field and absorbed energy inside the body. In practice, often the source is loosely coupled to the body such that the near-zone field is not altered by the presence of the body. Any direct coupling between the body and the source can be ignored. This approach is particularly suited for leakage-type near-zone fields. This section describes the numerically obtained electromagnetic energy absorption for a 180-cell model of the human body in a prescribed near-zone field where the coupling between the body and the source may be neglected. This is followed by a description of results that takes into account the mutual coupling between the body and the source.

Electromagnetic fields such as those found in close proximity to radiofrequency heat sealers are characterized by localized leakage-type near-zone fields that roll off monotonically to negligible values in the plane transverse to the source–body axis (connecting the source and body of the operator). Moreover, it has been shown that a half-cosine function is a good approximation to the leakage field distribution (Chatterjee et al., 1980), and gives whole-body absorption rates that are within 5–10% of values that would be obtained from measured electric field values. The phase variation of the prescribed field is an important consideration, especially at higher frequencies, if exact calculations are desired. Figure

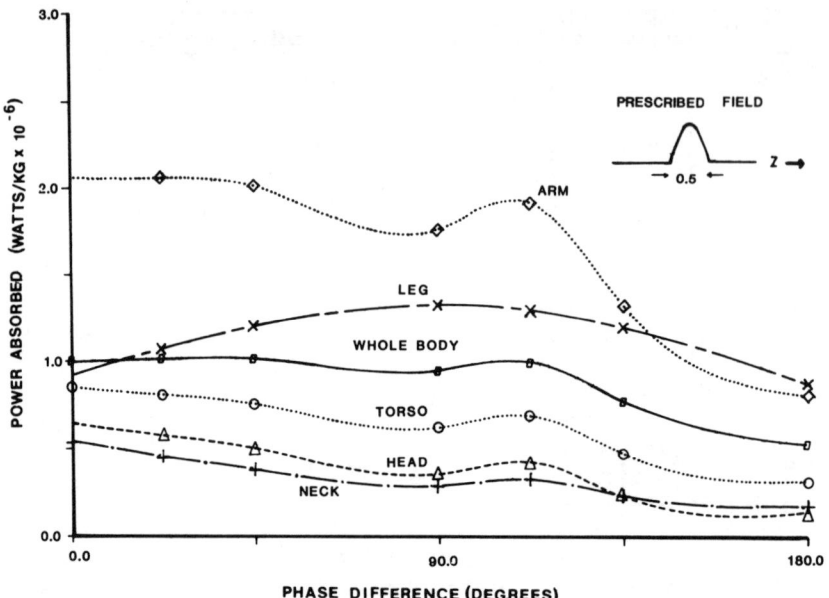

FIGURE 5-34. Average whole- and part-body SAR in a 180-cell model of human body placed in front of a prescribed field distribution with half-cycle cosine amplitude variation and a linear antisymmetric phase variation in the z direction; frequency = 350 MHz, field width = 0.5 wavelength, peak electric field = 1 V/m (Chatterjee *et al.*, 1980).

5-34 presents the average whole- and part-body absorption in the model placed in front of the near-zone field with a linear phase variation in the direction along the long axis of the body. The plane of the prescribed field distribution is tangential to the toes, and the polarization is such that no component of the electric field is directed from arm to arm. Observe that the whole-body-averaged SAR is highest when there is zero phase variation. At this frequency (350 MHz), there are large variations in energy deposition in the arm. At lower frequencies, changes in energy deposition as a function of phase variation are smooth and gradual. This is attributable to the large wavelength in comparison to the height of the model. It is noted that the above field configuration represents the most effective near-zone polarization from the whole-body energy deposition perspective at frequencies below 100 MHz (Chatterjee *et al.*, 1980).

The whole-body-averaged SAR and its distribution in the 180-cell model are shown in Figs. 5-35 and 5-36 for 27.12 and 77 MHz, respectively. The field configuration is the same as that adopted for Fig. 5-34. The frequency of 27.12 MHz is commonly used for RF sealers in the United States (Conover *et al.*, 1980) and 77 MHz is near the resonance frequency of the body model. It should be noted that 350 MHz

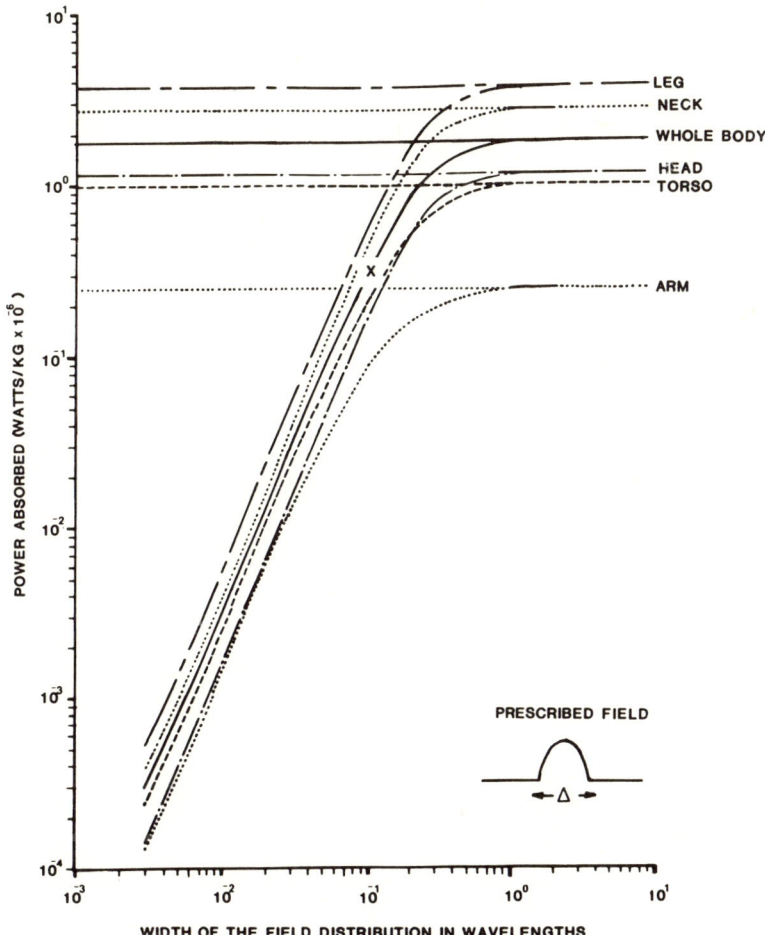

FIGURE 5-35. Average whole- and part-body SAR in a 180-cell model of human body placed in front of a half-cycle cosine field; frequency = 27.12 MHz, $E_{z\,max} = 1$ V/m (Chatterjee et al., 1980).

is the resonance frequency predicted for the head of the model, as mentioned previously. For both frequencies, the whole-body-averaged SAR as well as that in various parts of the model, increases approximately as the square of the width of the field distribution expressed in wavelengths to the asymptotic plane wave values indicated by the straight lines. Moreover, values of energy absorption for field widths on the order of 1.5 to 1.8 times the model height are nearly identical to the plane wave

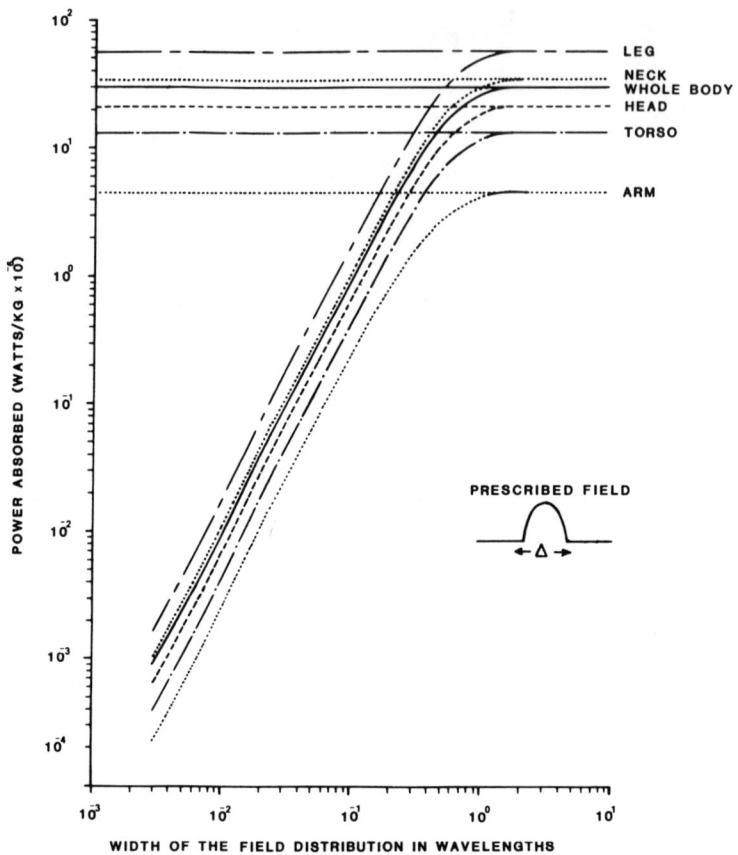

FIGURE 5-36. Average whole- and part-body SAR in a 180-cell model of human body placed in front of a half-cycle cosine field; frequency = 77 MHz, $E_{z\,max}$ = 1 V/m (Chatterjee et al., 1980).

results. This stems from the fact that the half-cycle cosine field distribution is fairly constant over the height of the model and closely resembles a plane wave. The "x" in Fig. 5-35 indicates the whole-body-averaged SAR obtained for the cosine approximation of a real-life near-zone exposure situation with a field width of 1.0 m and field strength of 827 V/m. The value of 0.18 compares favorably with 0.16 W/kg obtained by calculation using the measured electric field distribution shown in Fig. 5-37.

The whole-body-averaged rates of energy absorption and its distribution for the measured field shown in Fig. 5-37 are given in Fig. 5-38. Again, the plane of field is tangential to the toes, in front of the model.

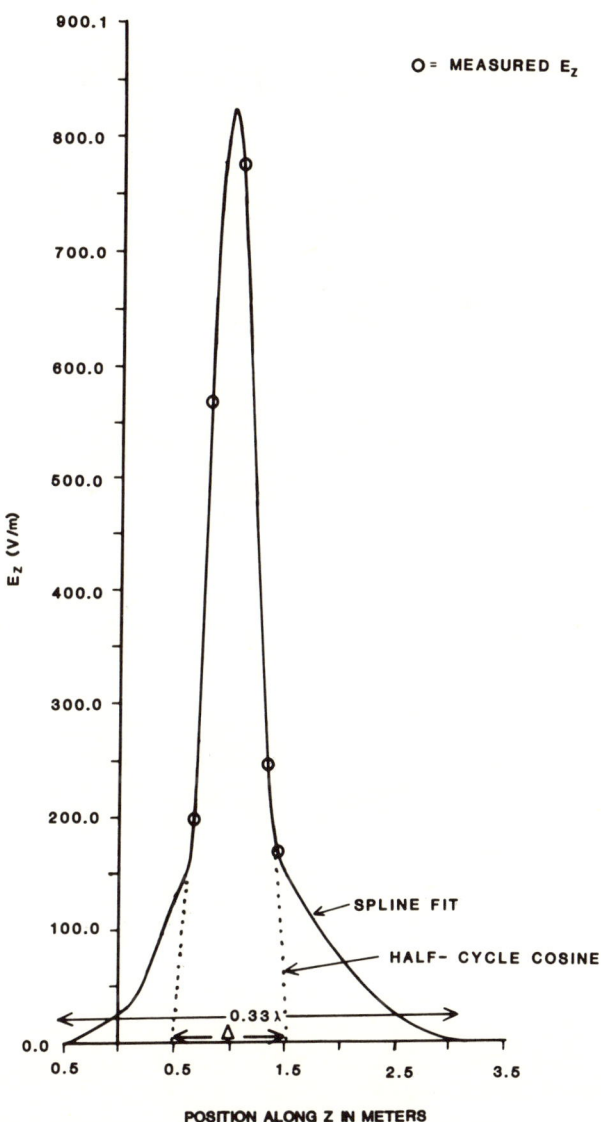

FIGURE 5-37. Measured and half-cosine prescription of leakage electric field (Chatterjee et al., 1980).

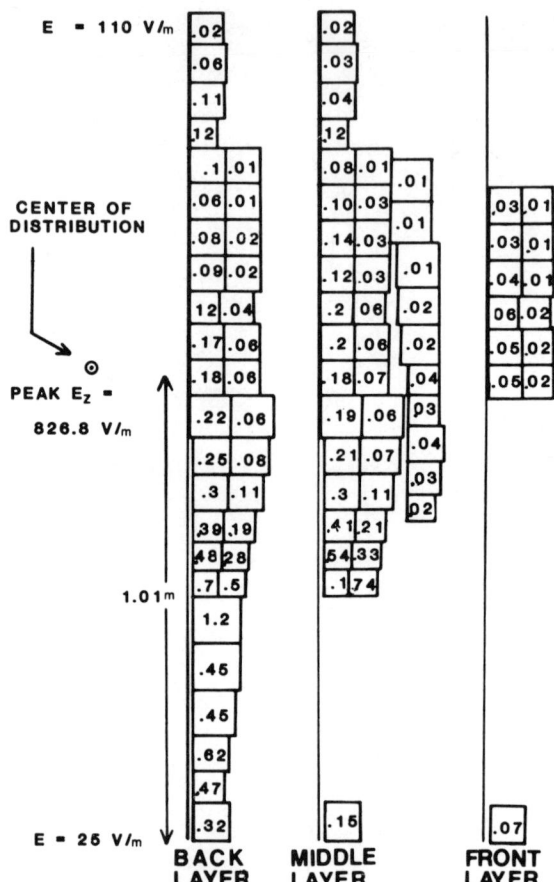

FIGURE 5-38. SAR distribution in a 180-cell model of human body placed in the leakage field of a 27.23-MHz RF sealer, zero phase difference, peak E_z = 826.8 V/m (Chatterjee et al., 1980).

The absorption rates for a ventrally incident plane wave with a peak electric field of 827 V/m, corresponding to the maximum value measured from the RF sealer, are included in this figure for comparison. It is seen that the lower body has a higher absorption than the rest of the model with maxima occurring in the abdominal and calf regions. Moreover, a whole-body SAR of only about 13% of the corresponding plane wave value is obtained for the leakage field. Other studies have shown that the SARs for a leakage-type, near-zone field exposure in general are nearly an order of magnitude smaller than those for plane-wave irradiation conditions (Chatterjee et al., 1980).

In some near-field situations, such as a biological body in the near zone of a radiating antenna, the source is strongly coupled to the body. Both the near-zone electromagnetic field and the current on the antenna are altered by the presence of the body. The body and source need to be treated as a coupled system to take into account effects of mutual coupling. One such approach involves use of the method of moments and coupled integral equations (Karimullah et al., 1980). In this case, the induced electric field inside the body and the induced current on the antenna must be considered as unknown quantities to be determined from two coupled integral equations.

One configuration adopted to study the effect of mutual coupling is shown in Fig. 5-39. The configuration is simple in that it consists of a homogeneous, rectangular cylinder of finite dimensions and a half-wave dipole isolated in free space, but it is possible to extract from it some rather pertinent information concerning source–body interaction in the near-zone field. The height and mass of the cylinder are chosen to approximate those of a human adult weighing 68 kg and having the dimensions of $170 \times 20 \times 20$ cm. The total length of the antenna $(2h)$ is 5.54 m at an operating frequency of 27 MHz, and is maintained at an antenna–body spacing of 20 cm. The cylindrical body is partitioned into 60 homogeneous square cells of equal volume, each having a dielectric constant of 113 and a conductivity of 0.62 S/m. For an input power of 1 W to the antenna, the system exhibits a rate of 6.44 mW of absorbed energy. The corresponding distribution of absorbed energy is indicated in Fig. 5-39, showing a peak rate of absorption near the center of the cylindrical body exposed to a center-fed dipole. If, instead, the body is in direct contact with an infinitely large conductive ground and the antenna is replaced by a quarter-wave monopole over ground, the rate at which energy is absorbed by the body would increase by 14 times to 0.084 W for the same amount of input power. That is, about 8.5% of the antenna input power is deposited in the cylindrical body when it is in direct contact with ground. Moreover, the peak SAR is now shifted to the bottom of the model in accordance with the relocation of the driving point of the antenna (Karimullah et al., 1980).

The effect of mutual coupling on absorption is illustrated in Fig. 5.40, where the antenna–body spacing is varied from 0.25 m to distances equivalent to a dipole in free space. The antenna input power has been adjusted in this case to that needed to produce an incident power density of 100 W/m^2 at a distance of 100 m from the dipole antenna in free space. The graph shows results for three source–body configurations: isolated antenna–body model, monopole–body model, and monopole–body with a 5-cm air–insulation gap between body and ground. As previously discussed, the isolated antenna–body configuration provides the least

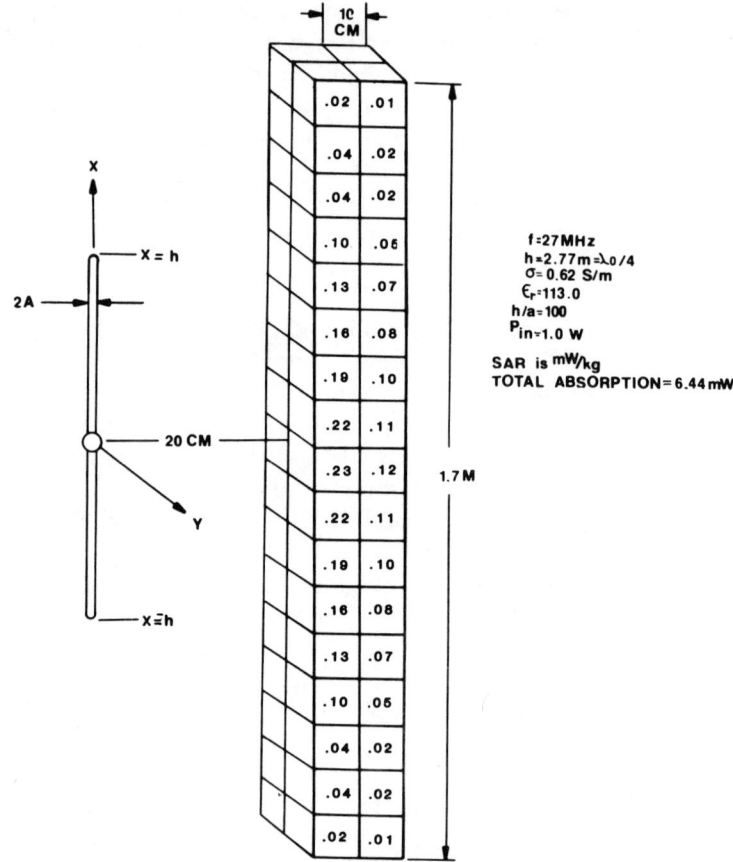

FIGURE 5-39. Total rate of absorption and its distribution at the central location of each cell of the body for an isolated antenna–body system. The antenna input power is 1 W (Karimullah *et al.*, 1980).

amount of power deposition, while the monopole–body configuration gives the highest. In all cases, the absorption values decreased with increasing antenna–body spacing, suggesting a diminishing influence at direct coupling. It should be noted that the absorption values at 100 m agree well with those predicted for a body of similar dimensions illuminated by a uniform plane wave of equivalent incident power density (Massoudi *et al.*, 1977; Karimullah *et al.*, 1980).

The distribution of absorbed energy in a 94-cell model of a human adult in contact with ground is presented in Fig. 5-41 for a 90-MHz quarter-wave monopole antenna spaced at a distance of 20 cm from the

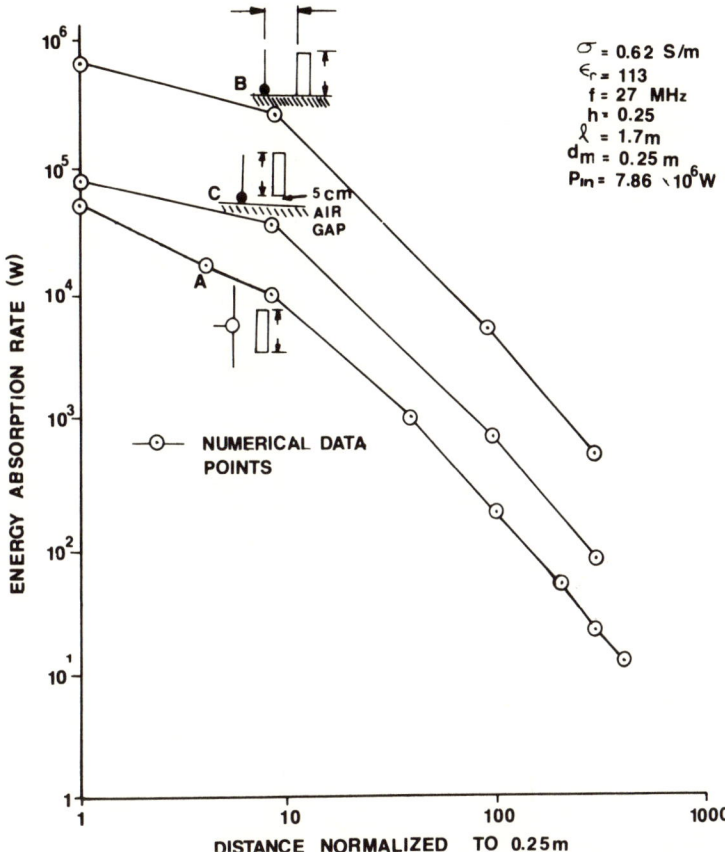

FIGURE 5-40. Rate of energy absorption in the body versus the antenna–body spacing for 27-MHz antenna–body systems. The height of the body is 1.7 m and its mass is approximately 68 kg (Karimullah et al., 1980).

body. The model is subdivided into homogeneous cells of different size with dielectric constant and conductivity of 76 and 0.85 S/m, respectively, and overall height and weight of 1.7 cm and 81 kg, respectively. Note that the greatest absorption occurs in the legs, which are in contact with the conductive ground. The absorption decreases monotonically to a minimum at the top of the head, an observation in agreement with the monopole–body configuration described earlier. The total rate of energy absorption of 0.52 W is more than 50% of the antenna input power. In contrast, the absorption for 27 MHz is only 8.5%. This is because the body is electrically much larger at 90 than at 27 MHz. Moreover, at 90

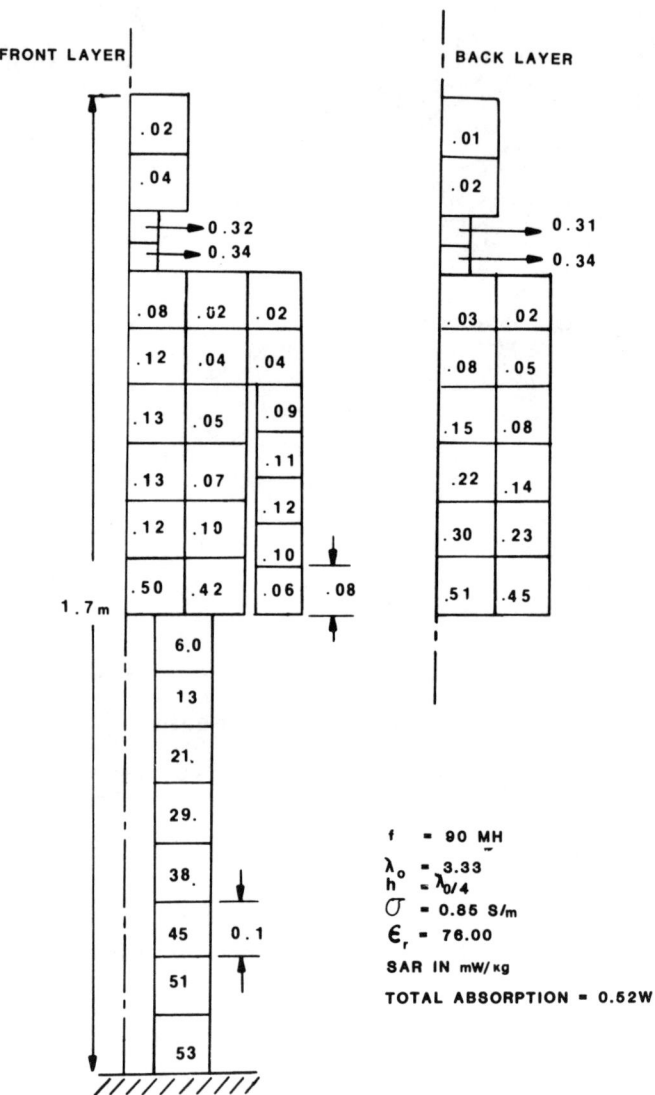

FIGURE 5-41. SAR distribution inside a 94-cell model of human body located in the immediate vicinity of a grounded quarter-wave monopole antenna. Values are based on input power of 1 W and antenna–body spacing of 20 cm (Karimullah *et al.*, 1980).

MHz, the body is nearly a resonant structure that enhances energy deposition or absorption.

5.4. SCALED DIELECTRIC BODIES

This section will outline a number of experimental models that have been successfully employed to analyze the propagation and absorption characteristics of radio and microwave radiation in tissue structures. These results are very useful in analyzing electromagnetic energy coupling to animal and human bodies, which are difficult, if not impossible, to analyze theoretically.

There are two common approaches: one involves the use of thermography and tissue modeling materials and the other relies on temperature probes and saline-filled proportionate models. As mentioned in Chapter 3, the thermographic procedure is most suited for analyzing distribution of absorbed energy in reduced- as well as full-scale models. While the probe method can also be used to map absorbed energy, it is a very time-intensive procedure. Recent developments in nonperturbing temperature sensors and automated data acquisition techniques may alleviate some of this problem. For whole-body absorption, the twin-well or dewar calorimeter described in Chapter 3 may be used.

The advantages of using reduced-scale models include smaller mass, which facilitates handling and requires less power, and not as much working space. The approach, however, is limited to simple models and does not lend itself easily to nonhomogeneous tissue structures or organ-specific absorption phenomena. It involves the use of synthetic tissue materials with the same dielectric constant of actual tissue, but with the electrical conductivity and source frequency increased by the scale factor. If L denotes the height of the subject, f the frequency of interest, ε_r the tissue dielectric constant, σ the actual electrical conductivity of the tissue, s the scaling factor, and P_a the specific absorption rate, the relationships among the subject and its equivalent model denoted by primed parameters are

$$L = sL' \qquad (5.22)$$

$$f = f'/s \qquad (5.23)$$

$$\varepsilon_r = \varepsilon_r' \qquad (5.24)$$

$$\sigma = \sigma'/s \qquad (5.25)$$

$$P_a = P_a'/s \qquad (5.26)$$

Clearly, the distribution of absorbed energy in the subject irradiated at a given frequency of interest is the same as that of its reduced-scale model except that the magnitude of the absorbed energy is increased by a quantity equaling the scale factor at a given incident field strength.

5.4.1. Thermographic Measurements

Examples of results obtained using the thermographic and reduced-scale-model technique are given in Fig. 5-42 through 5-47 for a 1.74-m-tall, 70-kg man. Figure 5-42 illustrates thermograms taken from a midfrontal section irradiated with a 31-MHz electric field oriented parallel to the long axis of the body. The line profiles were scanned through regions of maximal absorption where the body boundaries are marked by white vertical lines. The arrows indicate points at which the maximal SARs were calculated. The reduced-scale model was 0.38-m-

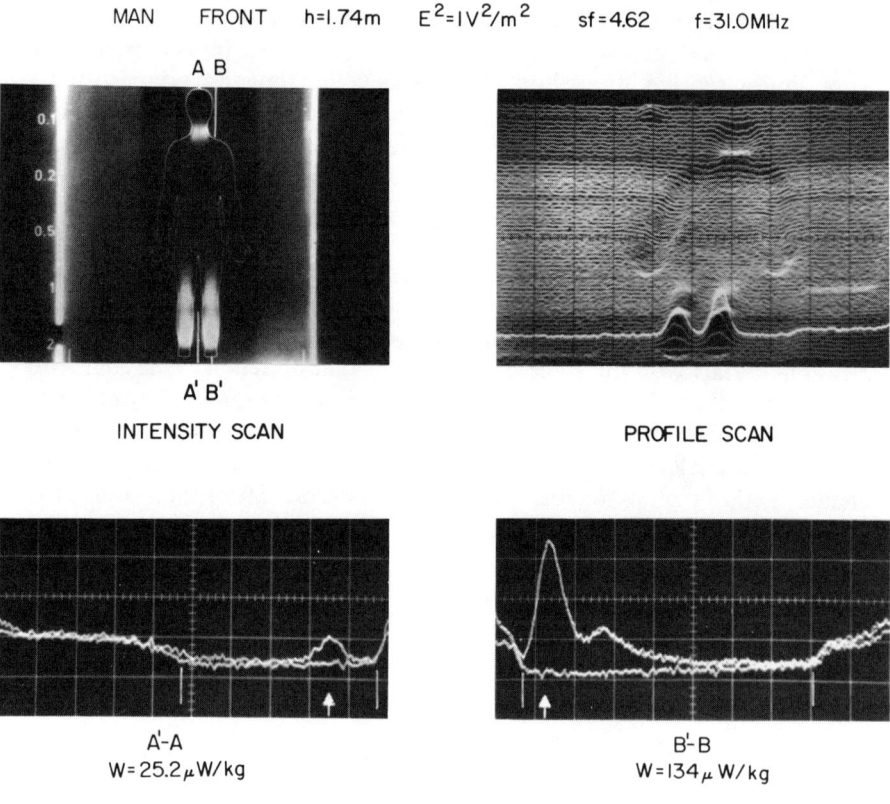

FIGURE 5-42. Absorbed energy distribution in a scaled model of man exposed to a 31-MHz electric field parallel to the long axis of the body.

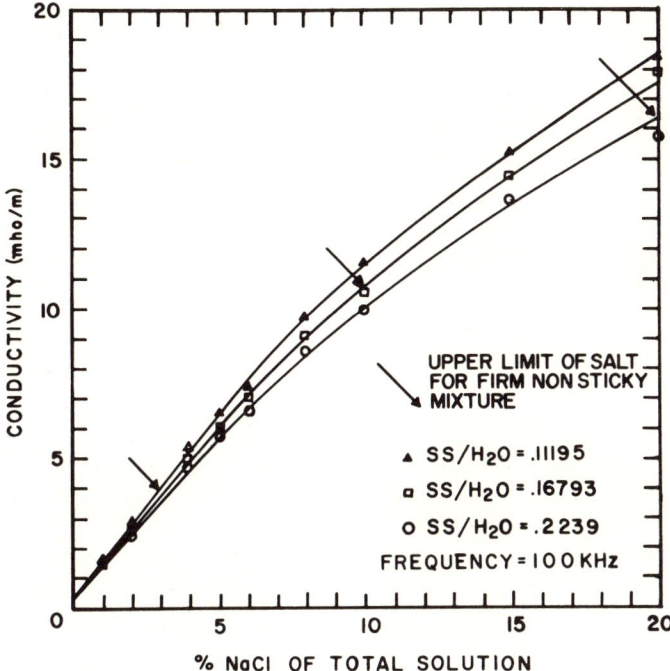

FIGURE 5-43. The electrical conductivity of muscle-equivalent modeling material.

long, the operating frequency was 144 MHz, and the scaling factor was 4.62. The electrical conductivity of the synthetic muscle material is given in Fig. 5-43.

It can be seen that maximum absorption occurs in the neck, knees, and ankles, i.e., in regions with narrow cross sections. The highest SAR of 134 m W/g per V/m in the ankles of the model is over one order of magnitude greater than that for an equivalent volume spheroid (Guy et al., 1976). The enhanced absorption in body regions with reduced cross sections stems from constriction of the induced longitudinal current at these body parts, thereby increasing the current density and electric field in these areas. The arms are not affected since they are parallel to the body trunk, whose large cross section shunts most of the induced current.

Figure 5-44 shows the absorbed energy distribution in the same reduced-scale model of man in a 31-MHz magnetic field oriented perpendicular to the frontal plane. As expected, circulating eddy-current-induced absorption predominates in this case. The absorption away from the center of the body increases proportionately with distance and attains maximal value near the surface. The highest absorption appears in the

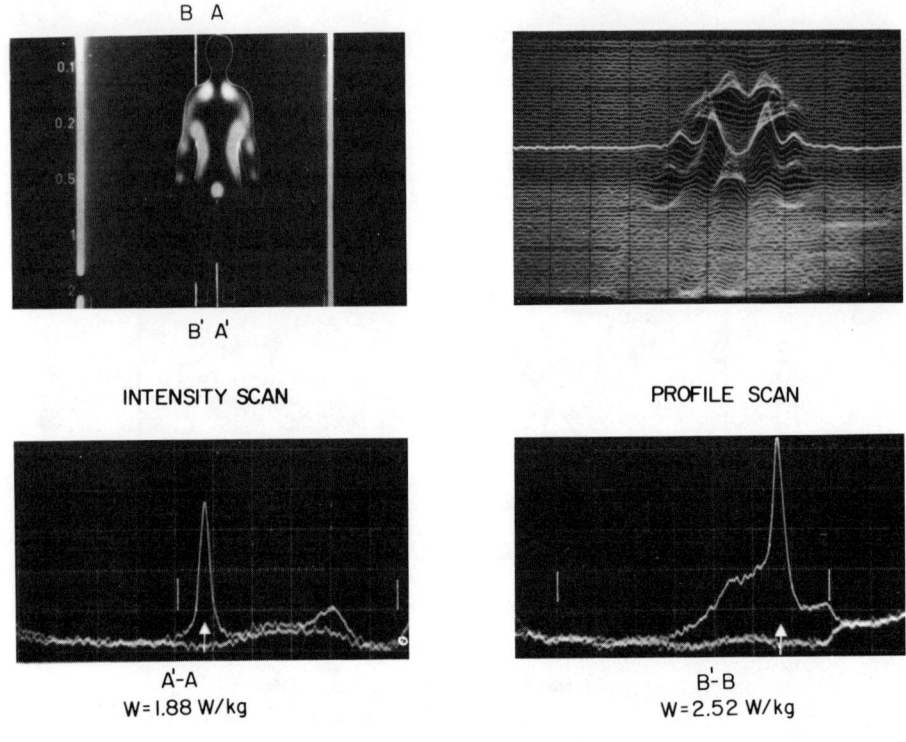

FIGURE 5-44. Absorbed energy distribution in a scaled model of man exposed to a 31-MHz magnetic field oriented perpendicular to the frontal plane.

axilla, which is about 2.52 W/kg for 1 A/m of applied magnetic field strength. It should be noted that enhanced absorption also occurs in the perineum, waist, and arms. These areas are characterized by abrupt changed in geometry, which tend to concentrate the induced eddy current.

A comparison of Figs. 5-42 and 5-44 shows that maxima of electric and magnetic field-induced absorptions appear in different regions of the body. In fact, electrically induced maximum absorption occurs at points where the magnetically induced absorption is minimal and vice versa. One may therefore predict the maximum SAR for any combination of electric and magnetic field parameters, including that of a plane wave, from the results given in these figures.

If the external electric field is applied from one side of the body but polarized along the long axis of the body, the induced energy absorption is similar to that shown in Fig. 5.42. The maximum absorption occurs again in the neck area and has a value of 24.1 mW/g. For a laterally applied magnetic field (directed from one side of the body to the other) such that the magnetic field is perpendicular to the median plane (midsagittal section), the peak absorption becomes 0.724 W/kg for 1 A/m of applied magnetic field strength (see Fig. 5.45). These SARs are lower than the corresponding values given in Figs. 5-42 and 5-44. In the electric case, the difference between the cross-sectional areas of the neck and trunk in this orientation is smaller; thus, the induced longitudinal current density at the neck is smaller. Similarly, the magnetically induced eddy current is related to the cross-sectional area. Since the side profile presents a smaller cross section, the induced circulating current is reduced by as much as two-thirds from the values for the frontal plane irradiation.

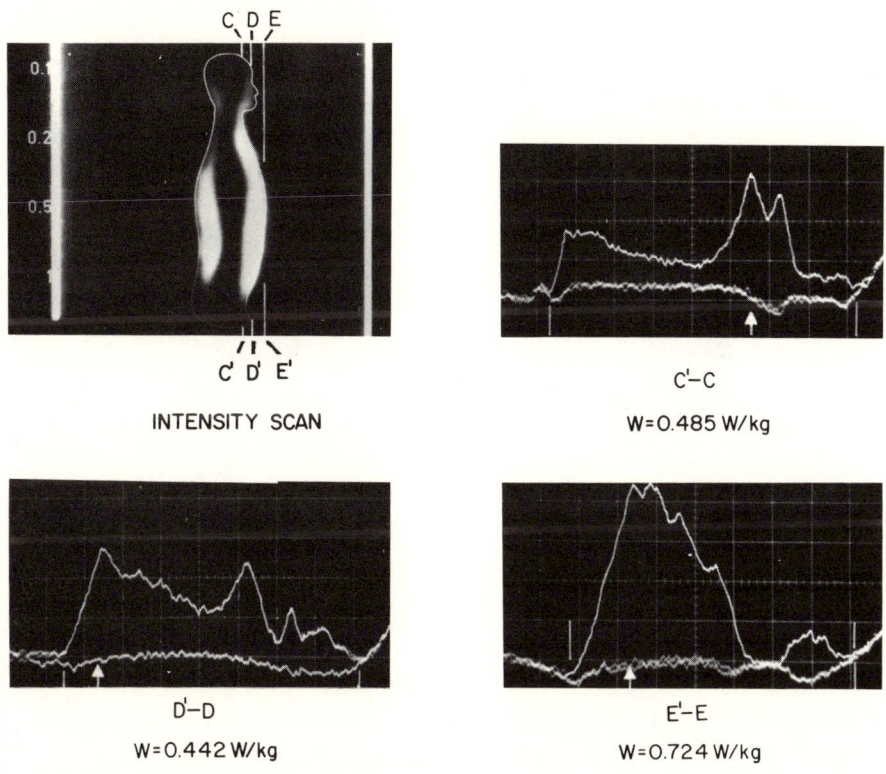

FIGURE 5-45. Absorbed energy distribution in a scaled model of man exposed to a 31-MHz magnetic field directed from one side of the body to the other.

By increasing the operating frequency to 915 MHz and irradiating the model in a microwave anechoic chamber, the same reduced-scale models (with proper conductivity adjustment) can be used to determine the SAR distribution in a 70-kg, 1.74-m-tall man exposed to 198-MHz plane waves. Figure 5-46 illustrates results obtained from an E-polarized plane wave impinging frontally on the model. Note that the enhanced SAR occurs in the neck, wrist, and ankle regions near the exposed side of the body with the right and left limbs absorbing the same amount. A high SAR of 0.087 W/kg per W/m^2 appears in the neck, which is more than an order of magnitude greater than the average SAR calculated from a prolate spheroidal model (Durney *et al.*, 1979). It is interesting to note that regions of high absorption correspond to body areas with narrowed cross sections, suggesting that the enhancement is due to longitudinal currents induced throughout the body that are forced to flow through comparatively narrow areas.

The distribution of absorbed energy is also highly dependent on the

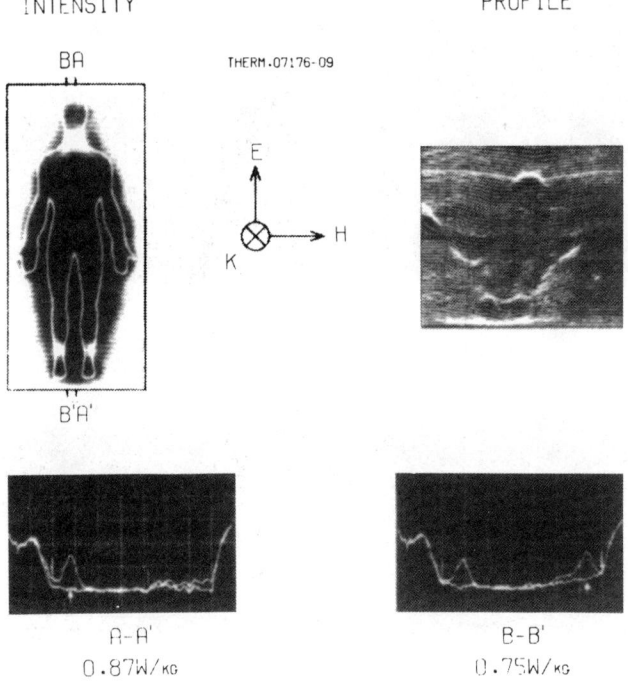

FIGURE 5-46. Power deposition patterns in a scaled model of man exposed to a 198-MHz E-polarized plane wave impinging frontally. (Courtesy of A. W. Guy, University of Washington, Seattle.)

orientation of the model with respect to the source. In general, H polarization gives the lowest SARs and E polarization, the highest SARs (Guy and Chou, 1978). Further, an E-polarized plane wave impinging laterally on the model produces a higher SAR than the same plane wave impinging frontally. This is because in humans the sagittal cross section is considerably smaller than the frontal cross section. Thus, the longitudinal electric currents, induced along the height of the body by the parallel electric fields, are constrained to flow through a smaller cross section. This phenomenon is illustrated in Fig. 5-47. It is seen that the highest SARs occur only in the neck, wrist, and ankle regions on the ipsilateral side of the exposed body. The peak SAR of 1.83 W/kg measured in the wrist area is more than twice the value given in Fig. 5-46.

These results indicate that care must be exercised in using average SAR values to define thresholds of biological effects in humans exposed to radio and microwave radiation. Even though the average SAR might be small over the total body mass, the absorbed energy could be distributed in such a manner that most of the energy is absorbed in a

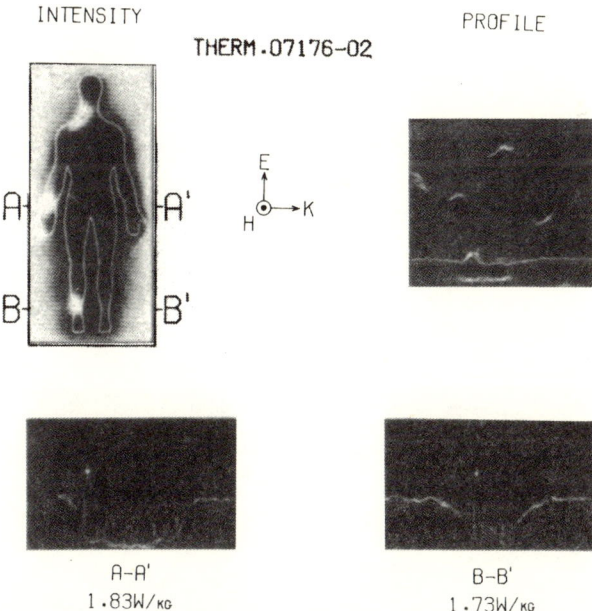

FIGURE 5-47. Power deposition patterns in a scaled model of man exposed to a 198-MHz E-polarized plane wave impinging laterally.

5.4.2. Probe Measurements

Some results of probe-measured SAR distributions in saline-filled models of humans are given in Figs. 5-48 and 5-49 for free space and grounded conditions, respectively (Gandhi, 1980). The electric field vectors in both cases are directed along the height of the body and the waves impinge laterally as indicated. Moreover, these SAR distributions correspond to conditions of maximal absorption. This occurs at about 68 MHz for the same subject in direct contact with a ground plane. Note that in the case of free-space irradiation, there are three localized regions with increased energy deposition: the neck, legs, and the arm on the exposed side of the body. The highest absorption occurs in the knee region, and is almost an order of magnitude higher than the whole-body average of 0.02 W/kg per W/m^2 of incident power density. The nearly symmetric pattern of energy deposition in the lower extremities at

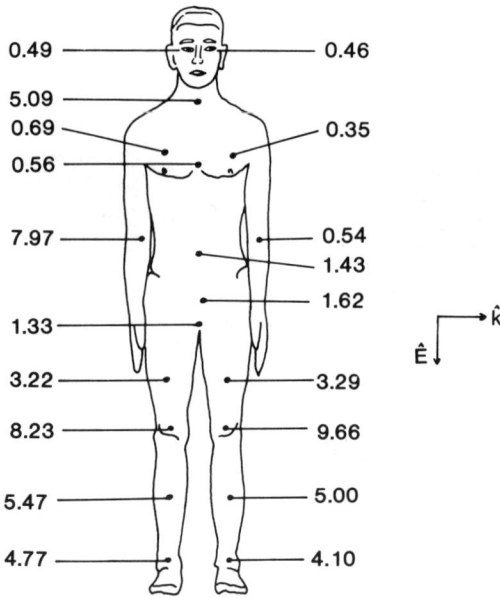

FIGURE 5-48. Sampled SAR distribution in a human model exposed to free-space plane-wave irradiation. The values are normalized to a whole-body average of 0.02 W/kg per W/m^2 of incident power (Gandhi, 1980).

PROPAGATION AND ABSORPTION IN TISSUE MEDIA

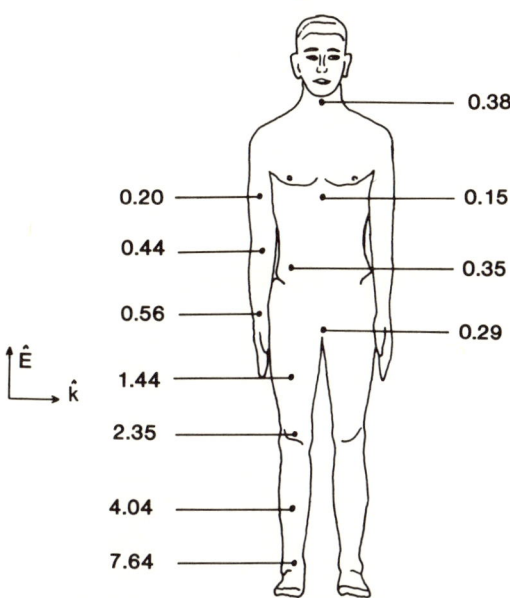

FIGURE 5-49. Sampled SAR distribution in a human model whose feet are in electrical contact with the ground. The values are relative to a whole-body average of 0.04 W/kg per W/m² of incident power (Gandhi, 1980).

resonance is different from results obtained at other frequencies using thermographic procedures (see Figs. 5-46 and 5-47). In contrast, the appearance of higher SARs in body parts with narrow cross sections is similar to that observed in previous cases.

The effect of a human body whose feet are in conductive contact with a ground (the earth or a highly conductive metallic sheet of large extent) is to increase the apparent height of the subject to the incident radiation. Consequently, the resonance frequency for a 1.75-m-tall man whose feet are in electrical contact with the ground is reduced by a factor of 2 to approximately 34 MHz. Furthermore, the distribution of absorbed energy also departs from the free-space situation such that the highest SAR in this case occurs in the ankles. It can be seen from Fig. 5-49 that a peak SAR of 0.3 W/kg per W/m² of incident power is found in the ankle, and is nearly ten times higher than the average whole-body absorption. In addition, the peak SAR is twice the value obtained in the same subject exposed under resonant conditions in free space. In general, the maximum energy deposition under grounded conditions occurs at a frequency about one-half of that occurring under free-space conditions. In a similar fashion, the absorbed energy also increases by a factor of two. This is consistent with the antenna theory discussed in Chapter 2.

It is interesting to note that for the cases just described, the grounding effect may be eliminated or substantially reduced by a small separation between the feet and the ground. In fact, for separations greater than 7 cm, the whole-body energy absorption and its distribution are identical to those for free-space irradiation conditions (Gandhi, 1980).

5.5. LABORATORY ANIMAL MODELS

In the laboratory, small animals are irradiated to study the biological responses to radio and microwave radiation. The whole-body absorption and its distribution can be directly quantified using the animal carcass. In addition, partially as a result of some of the difficulties with measurement in animals, tissue-equivalent synthetic materials are commonly used to measure whole-body absorption and its distribution in models of biological bodies.

The whole-body absorption of microwave energy by humans and experimental animals is of interest because it is related to the energy required to alter the thermoregulatory system of the exposed subject, and because it may serve as an index for extrapolating experimental results to human exposures. Several techniques may be called upon to provide this information, depending on whether the exposure is done in a closed space or open space system (see Chapter 3). The distribution of absorbed microwaves within an irradiated body is important because it relates to specific responses of the body. Internal distribution can be determined by thermographic procedures. Small non-field-perturbing temperature probes or field sensors also can be implanted in the tissues to measure the temperature rise or field strength either at a particular spot or in some small volume. A series of these measurements can be used to determine the distribution of absorbed electromagnetic energy within an irradiated body.

5.5.1. Whole-Body Absorption

Many factors influence the whole-body absorption when an animal is irradiated with microwave energy. The previous sections have discussed these factors in detail. Clearly, frequency, body size and orientation must influence the absorption. Table 5-4 lists the whole-body SAR for rodents irradiated in the far field of a 2450-MHz source as a function of body mass. The second and third rows relate to mice (Kinn, 1977) and Chinese hamsters (Huang *et al.*, 1977), respectively. The remainder are for Sprague–Dawley rats (Kinn, 1977). Twin-well calorimeters were used for

TABLE 5-4
Whole-Body Absorption by Rodents Irradiated with E-Polarized 2450-MHz Plane Waves[a]

Body mass (g)	Average SAR (mW/g) (mean ± S.D.)
6–10	0.94 ± 0.27
20–35[b]	0.42 ± 0.09
35–40[c]	0.46 ± 0.08
40–60	0.49 ± 0.26
70–110	0.32 ± 0.18
110–220	0.18 ± 0.07
310–350	0.14 ± 0.04
430–440	0.09 ± 0.08

[a] Values are for rats (Kinn, 1977) unless otherwise indicated.
[b] Mice (Kinn, 1977).
[c] Chinese hamsters (Huang et al., 1977).

all measurements. The data for rats are normalized to 1 mW/cm^2 and are for animals at birth to 92 days of age. The body mass of these animals ranges from 6 g at birth to in excess of 400 g. It is seen that the whole-body SAR decreases as the body mass increases as a function of age, conforming to earlier theoretical observations. Some measured average SAR values for mice at frequencies between 200 and 2600 MHz are given in Table 5-5. The data are derived from either small anechoic chambers or TEM exposure systems that provide a close approximation to plane-wave irradiation environments. The whole-body-averaged SAR slowly increases from 0.12 to 0.42 mW/g per mW/cm^2 at 2450 MHz. It jumps to a high value of 1.15 mW/g at 2600 MHz, clearly indicating a resonance absorption peak in the vicinity of 2600 MHz. It is interesting to note that acrylic restraining cages may cause the average SAR to be a

TABLE 5-5
Whole-Body Absorption by Mice Exposed to Quasi-Plane Waves of E Polarization

Frequency (MHz)	Body mass (g)	SAR (mW/g) (mean ± S.D.)
200	20–30	0.12[a]
300	20–30	0.18[a]
400	20–30	0.20[a]
2450	20–35	0.42[b]
2600	20–35	1.15[c]

[a] Marshall and Brown (1983).
[b] Kinn (1977).
[c] Allen and Hurt (1979).

factor of 1.34 higher than that obtained for uncaged animals (Marshall and Brown, 1983). This appears to stem from local field enhancement caused by the acrylic material (Lin and Wu, 1976; Lin et al., 1979).

The whole-body SARs for small and medium-sized rats in the frequency range 300 to 3000 MHz and 1000 to 3000 MHz, respectively, are shown in Figs. 5-50 and 5-51, which also include theoretical calculations based on prolate spheroidal models of animals for comparison (Durney et al., 1978, 1980). The data shown in Fig. 5-50 for K polarization and frequency between 300 and 500 MHz are for 150- to 170-g Syrian hamsters in a TEM chamber (Segal, 1981). The results between 600 and 3000 MHz are for a 158-g Wistar rate in a parallel plate transmission line (Gandhi, 1975). It is interesting to note that values for the former group are higher, while those for the latter group are lower than the values predicted by the theoretical model. The difference most likely stems from the infidelity of the model and variations in animal shapes and experimental protocol. The large discrepancy, about six fold greater SAR values for hamsters, is attributable to the fact that the configuration of a hamster is different from that of a rat, even though their body masses are equivalent. Further, the irradiation system and experimental protocol undoubtedly have an influence on the final outcome. However, the important features, such as the frequency

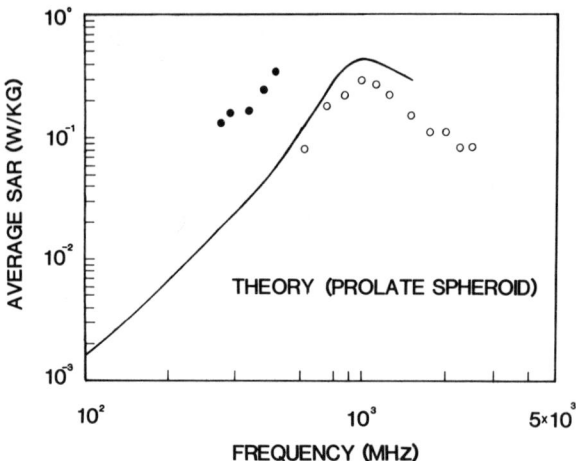

FIGURE 5-50. The whole-body-averaged SAR for a small rat. The point entries are measured values compared with prediction based on a 158-g rat exposed to 1 mW/cm^2.

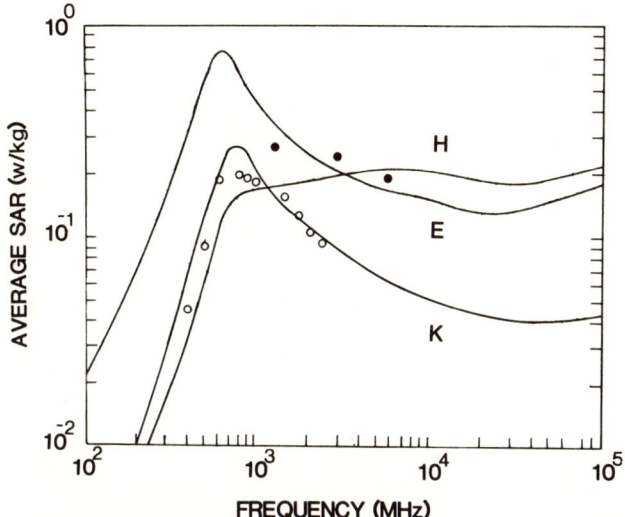

FIGURE 5-51. The whole-body-averaged SAR for a medium-sized (320-g) rat. The solid curves are calculated values using a prolate spheroidal model exposed to 1 mW/cm².

dependence and resonance absorption, are clearly demonstrated. Data for a medium-sized rat (Fig. 5-51) show, for E polarization at three postresonance frequencies, that the measured SARs confirm the general behavior of the model calculations for both E and K polarization. The SARs of 0.25, 0.23, and 0.19 W/kg for E-polarized 1.28-, 2.88-, and 5.62-GHz microwaves (Phillips *et al.*, 1975; de Lorge, 1984), even though pertaining only to the postresonance region, indicate close agreement between measured data and predictions based on prolate spheroids of equal mass.

The whole-body absorbed energy in rats exposed to 2450-MHz microwaves has been measured using tissue-equivalent models in a rectangular waveguide irradiation chamber. Figure 5-52 shows sagittal sections of models of rats in a rectangular waveguide system (Leicher-Preka and Ho, 1976). The models correspond to 1-, 4-, 10-, 23-, 30-, and 60-day-old animals. These models of rats were individually irradiated in the center of the waveguide with either the head (dorsal irradiation) or the tail (frontal irradiation) oriented in the direction of propagation of the incident microwaves. Figure 5-53 illustrates the average whole-body SAR as a function of size of the rat model. It can be seen that the absorption drops precipitously at first, and then gradually decreases as the mass of the rat model increases. This indicates that the model sizes

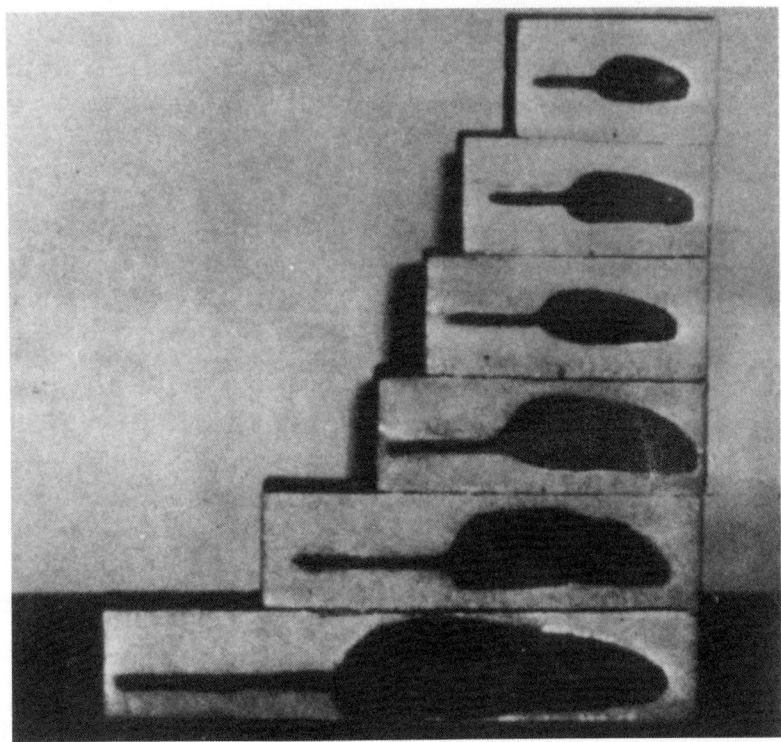

FIGURE 5-52. Sagittal sections of rat phantoms corresponding to 1-, 4-, 10-, 23-, 30-, and 60-day-old animals. The masses of these models are 7.8, 14.3, 17.0, 40.0, 52.4, and 111.3 g, respectively. (Courtesy of H. S. Ho, Center for Devices and Radiological Health, Washington, D.C.)

are in the near- and post-resonance regions of the absorption curve at this frequency, and is consistent with the results described previously.

The averaged absorption data for a sitting rhesus monkey are shown in Fig. 5-54 and indicate reasonable agreement between measured and predicted results. The data at 275 MHz are for a live monkey in a circularly polarized waveguide exposure chamber (Olsen *et al.*, 1984), and all others are for phantom models filled with muscle-simulating materials exposed to plane waves with E polarization (Olsen *et al.*, 1980; de Lorge, 1984). The SARs of 0.40 and 0.33 W/kg at 225 and 275 MHz are considerably higher than at the other three frequencies, since they are close to the peak of energy absorption. Note that except for the value of 0.032 W/kg at 5.62 GHz, higher values are shown for the measured than the predicted SARs. This disparity appears to arise from a higher SAR in the arms relative to the trunk and from the fact that prolate spheroidal models do not have arms.

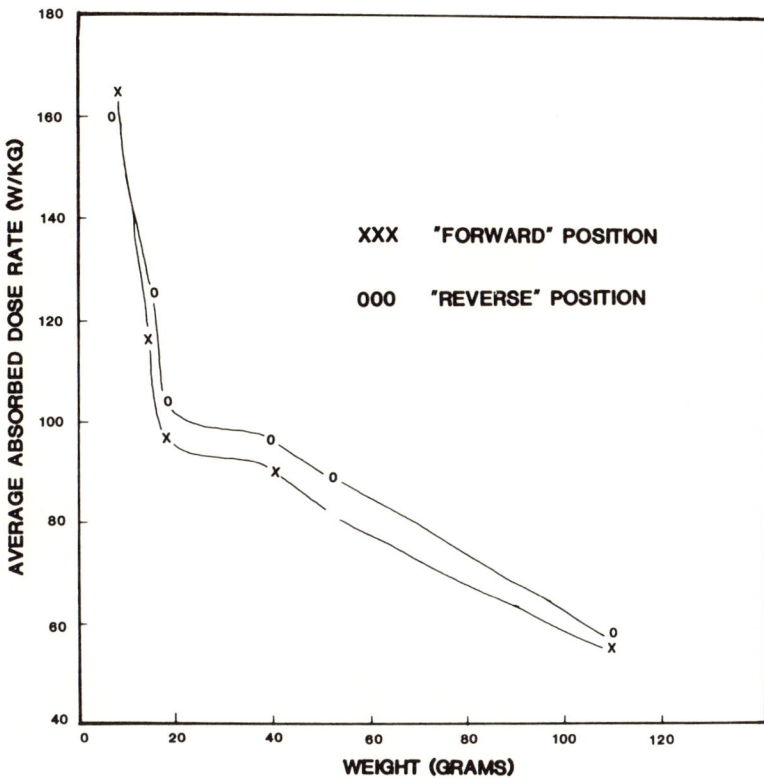

FIGURE 5-53. Whole-body-averaged SAR in a rat phantom as a function of body mass (Leicher-Preka and Ho, 1976).

There is a paucity of data for specific rates of energy absorption for humans. Table 5-6 gives the whole-body absorption rates of three male subjects in a TEM chamber at 18.5 MHz (Hill, 1982). These human volunteers were exposed to 11 $\mu W/cm^2$, and the rate of energy absorption was limited to 1 W. Note that the measured average SARs are highest for the two principal E orientations (EHK and EKH) and they exceed calculations based on dielectric ellipsoidal models by a factor of 2.0 or 2.9. The "ABC" designation is for the orientation of field vectors. In this case, A is aligned with the direction of body length, B with the side-to-side direction, and C with the front-to-back direction. It is interesting to note that the wearing of clothing and metal accessories by the subjects did not cause detectable changes in the whole-body absorption rate. The absorption of 1.29- and 2.0-GHz plane waves by a full-sized model of a standing man filled with muscle-equivalent material

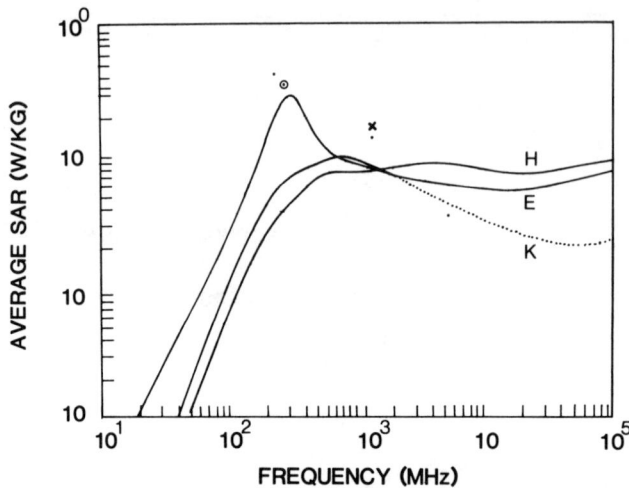

FIGURE 5-54. Whole-body absorption values for a rhesus monkey exposed to 1 mW/cm^2. The calculated values are based on a prolate spheroid having dimensions of 0.2 and 0.0646 m.

is smaller by two orders of magnitude than at 18.5 MHz. The SAR of 0.031 W/kg at 1.29 GHz compared well with that predicted for this frequency in a prolate spheroidal model of man (Olsen, 1979). There is, however, a rather wide disparity at 2.0 GHz. The SAR value of 0.094 W/kg per mW/cm^2 is about three times higher than that estimated

TABLE 5-6
Specific Absorption Rates (W/g per mW/cm^2) [± S.E. (N = 6-9)] for Three Male Subjects Exposed to 18.50-MHz Radiation in a TEM Chamber[a]

Body orientation	Human subject			Ellipsoid model	
	F	I	K	Calculated SAR	Human average Calculation
EKH	22.3 ± 3.1	18.4 ± 3.7	26.8 ± 2.2	7.77	2.9
EHK	11.5 ± 5.5	12.3 ± 2.7	15.8 ± 1.9	6.56	2.0
KEH	3.5 ± 2.9	2.8 ± 0.9	3.7 ± 0.7	1.74	2.0
KHE	0.9 ± 1.5	−0.4 ± 1.6	2.3 ± 1.1	0.45	—[b]
HEK	1.7 ± 1.4	0.0 ± 1.6	3.0 ± 1.0	0.44	—[b]
HKE	0.3 ± 0.9	−0.7 ± 1.5	−1.7 ± 2.3	0.37	—[b]
Height (cm)	175.3	178.2	179.5	175	
Mass (kg)	84.6	77.7	73.2	70	

[a] Hill (1982).
[b] Comparisons would be meaningless because SE > mean.

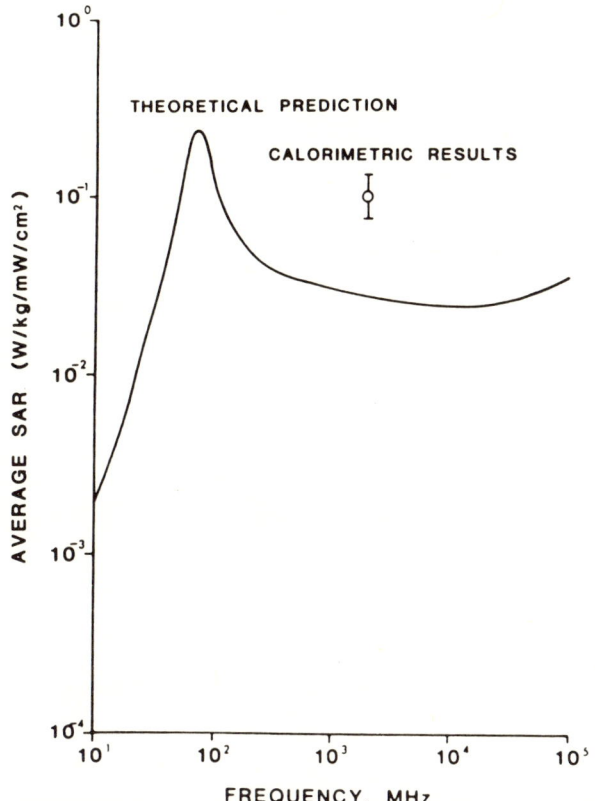

FIGURE 5-55. Averaged whole-body absorption in a prolate spheroidal model of man and results of calorimetric measurement at 2.0 GHz (Olsen, 1982).

theoretically for a prolate spheroidal model of man (Olsen, 1982). This disparity arises perhaps because prolate spheroids do not have arms to allow higher partial body absorption in relation to the torso (see Fig. 5-55).

5.5.2. Distribution of Absorbed Energy

The distribution of absorbed energy in animal bodies is important not only in the interpretation of observed biological responses, but also in the understanding of the nature and mode of microwave interaction with biological systems. In many situations, large differences in SAR distribution may exist in an irradiated animal even though the whole-body SAR shows only slight variations. Figure 5-56 qualitatively illustrates the

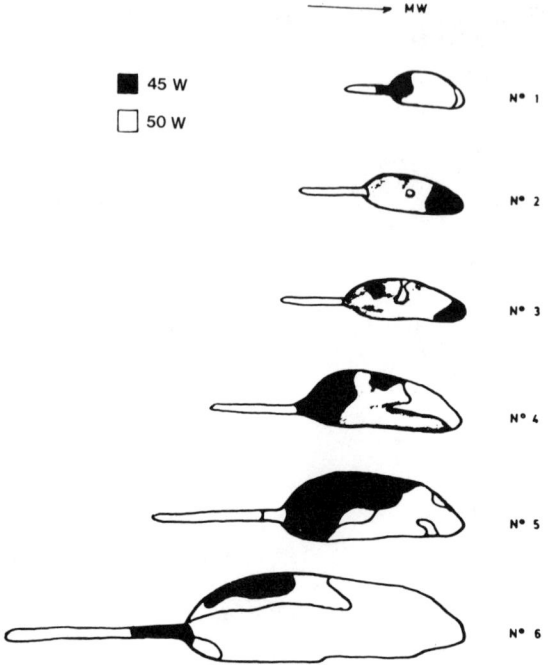

FIGURE 5-56. Qualitative distribution of absorbed microwave energy in midsagittal planes of rat phantoms subjected to dorsal irradiation (see Fig. 5-52).

distribution of absorbed microwave energy in the midsagittal planes of the model of rats described above. The models were subjected to dorsal irradiation in a 2450-MHz rectangular waveguide (Leicher-Preka and Ho, 1976). Most of the models irradiated in this orientation have the highest absorption in the dorsal portions of the body, i.e., the tail and abdominal regions shown in black. The single thermographic line scan through the head and tail regions clearly shows the areas of enhanced absorption. The distribution of absorbed energy for the frontal irradiation position is depicted in Fig. 5-57. The highest absorption, in this case, occurs in the head region, with the same spread of absorbed energy as for the larger models. Recall that the average whole-body SAR for these models of the rat changes only slightly for the two irradiation postures. In contrast, we have just seen that the distribution of the absorbed energy may change drastically. In fact, the whole-body absorption may be concentrated in a small portion of the body that migrates around as the irradiation parameters are altered. Thus, it is important to ascertain the distributed SAR for meaningful interpretation of observed biological responses to microwave radiation.

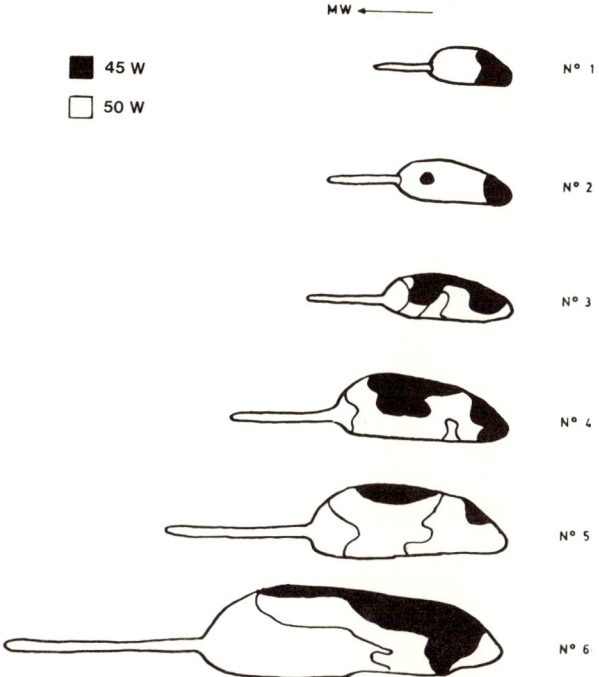

FIGURE 5-57. Qualitative SAR distribution in midsagittal planes of rat phantoms subjected to frontal irradiation (see Fig. 5-52).

Quantitative SAR distributions in small animal cadavers have been determined using the cylindrical waveguide chambers described in Chapter 3. These chambers, when properly excited, can support circularly polarized, guided waves that deliver relatively constant microwave energy to the animal at either 915 or 2450 MHz (Guy and Chou, 1976; Guy et al., 1979). Figure 5-58 depicts the SAR distribution along the sagittal section of a 388-g rat cadaver using thermographic methods (Guy and Chou, 1976). The thermograms were digitally processed to present equal SAR lines induced by 1 W of 915-MHz power input to the chamber. The 1-W input gives rise to a space-averaged power density of 3.13 mW/cm^2 over the cross section of the waveguide. Two different orientations of the rat cadaver, with respect to the incident field, are shown: frontal irradiation—axial position with head exposure; dorsal irradiation—axial position with rear exposure. It is seen that the distributed SAR varies considerably with orientation. Maximum SARs of 1.92 and 1.68 mW/g are observed in the neck and back regions, respectively, for frontal and dorsal irradiation. Similarly, the total absorption is higher for the frontal irradiation configuration.

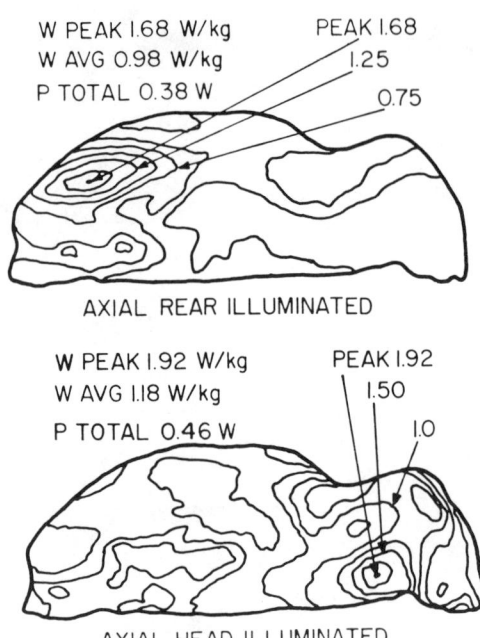

FIGURE 5-58. Patterns of SAR distribution along the sagittal section of a rat in a 915-MHz cylindrical waveguide chamber as a function of orientation (Guy and Chou, 1978).

Results for 2450-MHz irradiation are shown in Fig. 5-59. These processed thermographic recordings are for the cadaver of a 324-g rat, irradiated in the frontal and dorsal orientations (Guy *et al.*, 1979). The spaced-averaged power density is 3.13 mW/cm^2. As for the case of 915-MHz irradiation, the distributed SAR varies widely with orientation. However, unlike at 915 MHz, irradiation in the 2450-MHz chamber usually results in two peak SARs with nearly equal magnitudes. Moreover, the total absorption is somewhat diffused. The peak SARs are respectively 4.39 and 6.08 mW/g for the frontal and dorsal postures, with corresponding whole-body-averaged SARs of 2.47 and 2.43 mW/g. These data illustrate further the complicated nature of absorbed energy and its distribution inside biological bodies exposed to microwave radiation. This situation prevails even though the animal is irradiated uniformly by a propagating wave.

It would be of interest to compare the above results to those observed under plane-wave irradiation conditions. Unfortunately, there is a paucity of experimental data. Moreover, available data often refer to animals of different size and configuration, making comparison difficult.

Irradiation of a rat model by a 918-MHz aperture source at a

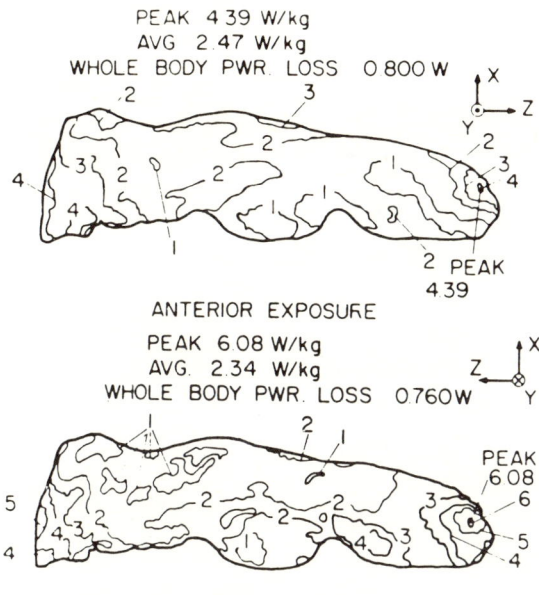

FIGURE 5-59. SAR distribution in a rat (324 g) as a function of orientation in a 2450-MHz cylindrical waveguide chamber (Guy et al., 1979).

distance of 8 cm shows that the tail of the rat has tremendous influence on the distribution of absorbed energy (Guy, 1974). Figure 5-60 shows peak SARs occurring in both the body and the tail. The enhanced SAR at the base of the tail is undoubtedly due to an increased current density as a result of abrupt change in cross sections of the adjoining body members. The low SAR observed in the pelvic region stems most likely from a standing wave null created by the body resonance condition. The rat model is approximately one wavelength at 918 MHz.

If a rabbit is irradiated by a 2450-MHz plane wave polarized along the long axis of the body, one would expect the absorbed energy to be concentrated near the surface of the exposed side of the body. Figure 5-61 illustrates this situation with the exception that instead of a true plane wave, the illuminating field is a close approximation, being formed by a standard-gain horn located 1 m from the dorsal surface of the rabbit (Guy and Chou, 1978; Chou et al., 1983). It can be seen that the SAR distribution along the midsagittal section is indeed concentrated near the body surface. Interestingly, high SARs occur in both the head and the dorsal surface, indicating partial resonance in the head region. This observation reinforces our earlier emphasis on the importance of

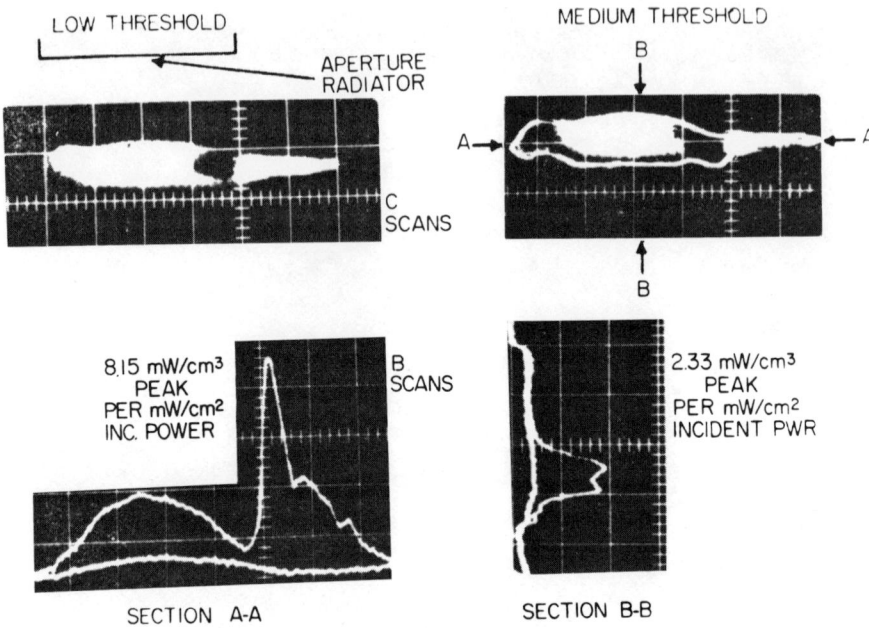

FIGURE 5-60. Thermograms of a rat phantom exposed in the near field of a 918-MHz aperture source (Guy, 1974).

distributed SAR and its contribution toward understanding microwave interaction with biological systems.

SAR data at nine locations of a full-size model of man filled with muscle-equivalent material, irradiated with 2.0-GHz plane waves, are shown in Fig. 5-62 as a function of distance from the front surface (Olsen, 1982). While SARs at each location exhibit the expected monotonic decay function of distance, they reveal great variability among locations. The extremities tend to show higher absorption rates than the torso. This selective absorption, perhaps as a result of resonance phenomena, may have contributed to the wide disparity between these measured SARs and those predicted by simple prolate spheroidal models in both man and rhesus monkey.

This chapter has summarized the rate of microwave energy absorption and its distribution in both simple and complex models of biological bodies as well as live subjects. Available information, however, is far from complete and is insufficient for understanding the biological interactions of radio and microwave radiation. Clearly, there exists a need for whole-body as well as distributive SAR measurements in a large number of species of laboratory animals and humans, and throughout the radio and microwave frequency range.

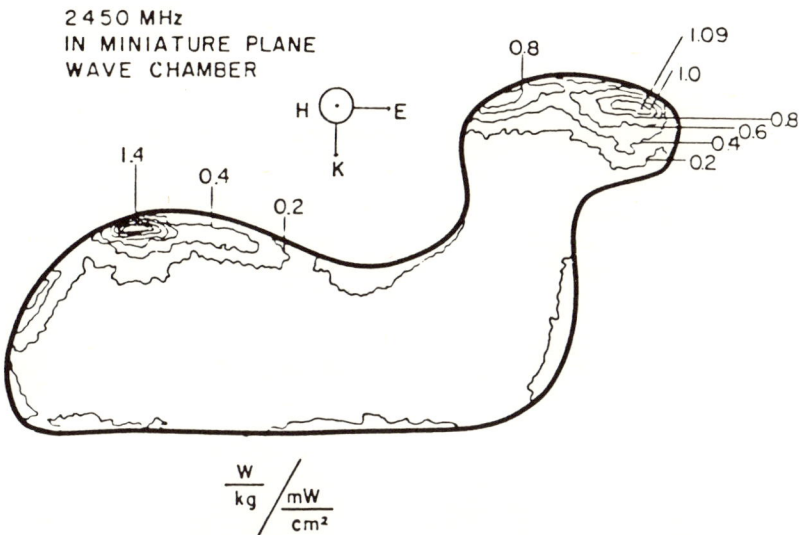

FIGURE 5-61. Absorption pattern in a rabbit (3.5 kg) exposed to 2450-MHz microwaves from a standard-gain horn located 1 m from the dorsal surface (Chou *et al.*, 1983).

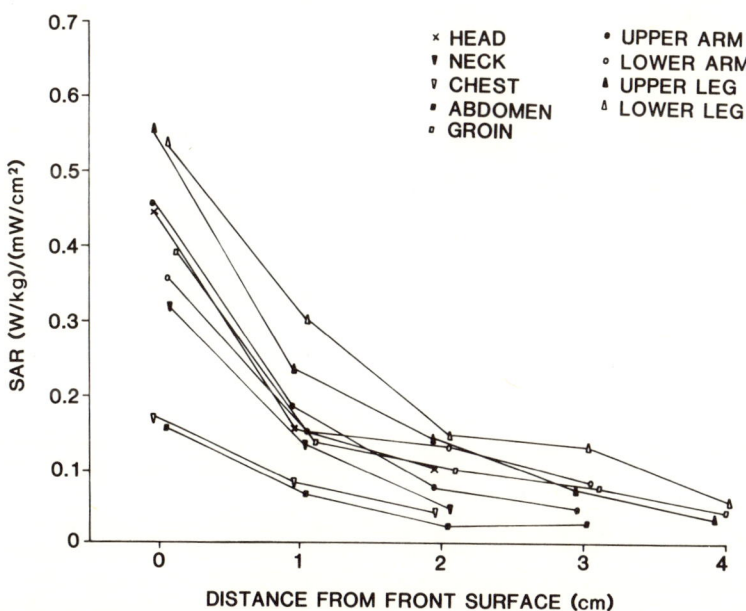

FIGURE 5-62. Microwave absorption profiles in a model of man exposed to 2.0-GHz plane waves (Olsen, 1982).

REFERENCES

Allen, S. J., and W. D. Hurt (1979) Calorimetric measurements of microwave energy absorption by mice after simultaneous exposure of 18 animals. *Radio Sci.* **14**:1S.

Asano, A., and G. Yamamoto (1975) Light scattering by spheroidal particles. *Appl. Opt.* **14**:29.

Barber, P. (1977a) Electromagnetic power absorption in prolate spheroidal models of man and animals at resonance. *IEEE Trans. Biomed. Eng.* **BME-24**:513.

Barber, P. W. (1977b) Resonance electromagnetic absorption by nonspherical dielectric objects. *IEEE Trans. Microwave Theory Tech.* **MTT-25**:373.

Barber, P. W., and C. Yeh (1975) Scattering of electromagnetic waves by arbitrary shaped dielectric bodies. *Appl. Opt.* **14**:2864.

Borup, D. T., and O. P. Gandhi (1984) Fast-Fourier transform method for calculation of SAR distributions in finely discretized inhomogeneous models of biological bodies. *IEEE Trans. Microwave Theory Tech.* **MTT-32**:355.

Chatterjee, I., M. J. Hagman, and O. P. Gandhi (1980) Electromagnetic energy deposition in an inhomogeneous block model for near-field irradiation conditions. *IEEE Trans. Microwave Theory Tech.* **MTT-28**:1452.

Chen, K. M. (1980) Interaction of electromagnetic fields with biological bodies. In: *Research Topics in Electromagnetic Theory*, J. A. Kong (ed.). Wiley, New York, p. 290.

Chen, K. M., and B. S. Guru (1977) Internal EM field and absorbed power density in human torsos induced by 1–500 MHz EM waves. *IEEE Trans. Microwave Theory Tech.* **MTT-25**:746.

Chou, C. K., A. W. Guy, L. E. Borneman, L. L. Kunz, and P. Kramar (1983) Chronic exposure of rabbits to 0.5 and 5 mW/cm^2 2450-MHz CW microwave radiation. *Bioelectromagnetics* **4**:63.

Conover, D. L., W. E. Murray, Jr., E. D. Foley, J. M. Lary, and W. H. Parr (1980) Measurement of electric and magnetic field strengths from industrial radio frequency (6–38 MHz) plastic sealers. *Proc. IEEE* **68**:17.

Deford, J. F., O. P. Gandhi, and M. J. Hagman (1983) Moment-method solutions and SAR calculations for inhomogeneous models of man with large number of cells. *IEEE Trans. Microwave Theory Tech.* **MTT-31**:848.

de Lorge, J. O. (1984) Operant behavior and colonic temperature of *Macaca mulatta* exposed to RF fields at and above resonance frequencies. *Bioelectromagnetics* **5**:233.

Durney, C. H. (1980) Electromagnetic dosimetry for models of humans and animals: A review of theoretical and numerical techniques. *Proc. IEEE* **68**:22.

Durney, C. H., C. C. Johnson, and H. Massoudi (1975) Long wave-length analysis of plane wave irradiation of a prolate spheroidal model of man. *IEEE Trans. Microwave Theory Tech.* **MTT-23**:246.

Durney, C. H., C. C. Johnson, P. W. Barber, H. Massoudi, M. F. Iskander, J. L. Lords, D. K. Ryser, S. J. Allen, and J. C. Mitchell (1978) Radiofrequency Radiation Dosimetry Handbook, 2nd ed. Rep. SAM-TR-28-22/32, USAF School of Aerospace Medicine, Brooks AFB, Texas.

Durney, C. H., M. F. Iskander, H. Massoudi, and C. C. Johnson (1979) An empirical formula for broadband SAR calculations of prolate spheroidal models of humans and animals. *IEEE Trans. Microwave Theory Tech.* **MTT-27**:758.

Durney, C. H., M. F. Iskander, H. Massoudi, S. J. Allen, and J. C. Mitchell (1980) Radio Frequency Radiation Dosimetry Handbook, 3rd ed. Brooks AFB, Texas.

Gandhi, O. P. (1975) Frequency and orientation effects on whole animal absorption of electromagnetic waves. *IEEE Trans. Biomed. Eng.* **BME-22**:536.

Gandhi, O. P. (1980) State of the knowledge for electromagnetic absorbed dose in man and animals. *Proc. IEEE* **68**:24.

Gandhi, O. P. (1982) Electromagnetic absorption in inhomogeneous model of man for realistic exposure conditions. *Bioelectromagnetics* **3**:81.

Gandhi, O. P., E. L. Hunt, and J. A. D'Andrea (1977) Deposition of EM energy in animals and in models of man with and without grounding and reflector effects. *Radio Sci.* **12**:39S.

Gandhi, O. P., M. J. Hagman, and J. A. D'Andrea (1979) Part-body and multi-body effects on absorption of radio frequency electromagnetic energy by animals and by models of man. *Radio Sci.* **14**:15S.

Guru, B. S., and K. M. Chen (1976) Experimental and theoretical studies in electromagnetic field induced inside finite biological bodies. *IEEE Trans. Microwave Theory Tech.* **MTT-24**:433.

Guy, A. W. (1974) Quantitation of induced electromagnetic field patterns in tissue and associated biological effects. In: *Biological Effects and Health Hazards of Microwave Radiation*, P. Czerski (ed.). Polish Medical Publishers, Warsaw, pp. 203–216.

Guy, A. W., and C. K. Chou (1976) System for quantitative chronic exposure of a population of rodents to UHF fields. In: *Biological Effects of Electromagnetic Waves*, Vol. II, C. C. Johnson and M. L. Shore (eds.). HEW Publ. (FDA) 77-8011, pp. 389–410.

Guy, A. W., and C. K. Chou (1978) Microwave and RF dosimetry. In: *The Physical Basis of Electromagnetic Interaction with Biological Systems*, L. S. Taylor, and A. Y. Cheung (eds.). HEW Publ. (FDA) 78-8055, pp. 165–216.

Guy, A. W., J. C. Lin, and C. K. Chou (1975) Electrophysiologic effects of electromagnetic fields on animals. In: *Fundamental and Applied Aspects of Nonionizing Radiation*, S. M. Michaelson, M. W. Miller, R. Magin, and E. L. Carstensen (eds.). Plenum Press, New York, p. 167.

Guy, A. W., M. D. Webb, and C. C. Sorensen (1976) Determination of power absorption in man exposed to HF electromagnetic fields by thermographic measurements on scale models. *IEEE Trans. Biomed. Eng.* **BME-23**:361.

Guy, A. W., J. Wallace, and J. A. McDougall (1979) Circularly polarized 2450-MHz waveguide system for chronic exposure of small animals to microwaves. *Radio Sci.* **14**:63S.

Hagman, M. J. (1978) Numerical Studies of Absorption of Electromagnetic Energy by Man. Ph.D. dissertation, Department of Electrical Engineering, University of Utah.

Hagman, M. J., O. P. Gandhi, and C. H. Durney (1979a) Numerical calculation of electromagnetic energy deposition for a realistic model of man. *IEEE Trans. Microwave Theory Tech.* **MTT-27**:804.

Hagman, M. J., O. P. Gandhi, J. A. D'Andrea, and I. Chatterjee (1979b) Head resonance: Numerical solutions and experimental results. *IEEE Trans. Microwave Theory Tech.* **MTT-27**:809.

Harrington, R. F. (1968) *Field Computation by Moment Methods*. McGraw-Hill, New York.

Harrington, R. F., and J. R. Mautz (1972) Green's function for surfaces of revolution. *Radio Sci.* **7**:603.

Hill, D. A. (1982) Human whole-body RF absorption studies using a TEM cell exposure system. *IEEE Trans. Microwave Theory Tech.* **MTT-30**:1847.

Ho, H. S., and A. W. Guy (1975) Development of dosimetry for RF and microwave radiation. *Health Phys.* **29**:317.

Huang, A. T., M. E. Engle, J. A. Elder, J. B. Kinn, and T. R. Ward (1977) The effects of microwave radiation (2450 MHz) on the morphology and chromosomes of lymphocytes. *Radio Sci.* **12**:173S.

Johnson, C. C., and A. W. Guy (1972) Nonionizing electromagnetic wave effects in biological materials and systems. *Proc. IEEE* **60**:692.

Johnson, C. C., C. H. Durney, and H. Massoudi (1975) Long-wavelength electromagnetic power absorption in prolate spheroidal models of man and animals. *IEEE Trans. Microwave Theory Tech.* **MTT-23**:739.

Joines, W. T., and R. J. Spiegel (1975) Resonance absorption of microwaves by the human skull. *IEEE Trans. Biomed. Eng.* **BME-21**: 46.

Karimullah, K., K. M. Chen, and D. P. Nyquist (1980) Electromagnetic coupling between a thin-wire antenna and a neighboring biological body. *IEEE Trans. Microwave Theory Tech.* **MTT-28**:1218.

Kinn, J. B. (1977) Whole-body dosimetry of microwave radiation in small animals: The effect of body mass and exposure geometry. *Radio Sci.* **12**:61S.

Kritikos, H. N., and H. P. Schwan (1972) Hot spot generated in conduction spheres by EM waves and biological implications. *IEEE Trans. Biomed. Eng.* **BME-19**:53.

Kritikos, H. N., and H. P. Schwan (1975) The distribution of heating potential inside lossy spheres. *IEEE Trans. Biomed. Eng.* **BME-22**:457.

Lakhtakia, A., M. F. Iskander, and C. H. Durney (1983) An iterative extended boundary condition method for solving the absorption characteristics of lossy dielectric objects of large aspect ratios. *IEEE Trans. Microwave Theory Tech.* **MTT-32**:640.

Leicher-Preka, A., and H. S. Ho (1976) Dependence of total and distributed absorbed microwave energy upon size and orientation of rat phantoms in waveguide. In: *Biological Effects of Electromagnetic Waves*, Vol. II, C. C. Johnson and M. L. Shore (eds.). HEW Publ. (FDA) 77-8011, pp. 158–168.

Lin, J. C. (1975) Microwave properties of fresh mammalian brain tissues at body temperature. *IEEE Trans. Biomed. Eng.* **BME-22**:74.

Lin, J. C. (1976) Interaction of two cross-polarized electromagnetic waves with mammalian cranial structures. *IEEE Trans. Biomed. Eng.* **BME-23**:371.

Lin, J. C. (1978) Microwave biophysics. In: *Microwave Bioeffects and Radiation Safety*, M. A. Stuchly (ed.). IMPI, Edmonton, Canada, pp. 15–54.

Lin, J. C. (1980) Whole-body exposure in the near zone of HF electromagnetic fields. *Int. Electromagnetic Waves and Biology Symposium*, Jouy en Josas, France.

Lin, J. C. (1986) Computer methods for field intensity predictions. In: *Handbook of Biological Effects of Electromagnetic Fields*, C. Polk and E. Postow (eds.). CRC Press, Boca Raton, Fla, pp. 273–314.

Lin, J. C., and C. L. Wu (1976) Scattering of microwaves by dielectric materials used in laboratory animal restrainers. *IEEE Trans. Microwave Theory Tech.* **MTT-24**:219.

Lin, J. C., A. W. Guy, and C. C. Johnson (1973a) Power deposition in a spherical model of man exposed to 1–20 MHz electromagnetic fields. *IEEE Trans. Microwave Theory Tech.* **MTT-21**:791.

Lin, J. C., A. W. Guy, and G. H. Kraft (1973b) Microwave selective brain heating. *J. Microwave Power* **8**:275.

Lin, J. C., H. M. Grove, and J. C. Sharp (1975) Comparative measurement of dielectric properites of fresh mammalian tissues. *Proc. Conference Proc. Electromagnetic Meas.*, p. 246.

Lin, J. C., H. J. Bassen, and C. L. Wu (1977) Perturbation effects of animal restraining materials on microwave exposure. *IEEE Trans. Biomed. Eng.* **BME-24**:80.

Liversay, D. E., and K. M. Chen (1974) Electromagnetic fields induced inside arbitrary shaped biological bodies. *IEEE Trans. Microwave Theory Tech.* **MTT-22**:1273.

Marshall, S. V., and R. F. Brown (1983) Experimental determination of whole body average SAR of mice exposed to 200–400 MHz CW. *Bioelectromagnetics* **4**:267.

Massoudi, H., C. H. Durney, and C. C. Johnson (1977) Long wavelength electromagnetic power absorption in ellipsoidal models of man and animals. *IEEE Trans. Microwave Theory Tech.* **MTT-25**:41.

Massoudi, H., C. H. Durney, P. W. Barber, and M. F. Iskander (1982) Post resonance EM absorption by man and animals. *Bioelectromagnetics* **3**:333.

Mautz, J. R., and R. F. Harrington (1969) Radiation and scattering from bodies of revolution. *Appl. Sci. Res.* **20**:405.

Olsen, R. G. (1979) Preliminary studies: Far-field microwave dosimetric measurements in a full-sized model of man. *J. Microwave Power* **14**:383.

Olsen, R. G. (1982) Far-field dosimetric measurements in a full-sized man model at 2 GHz. *Bioelectromagnetics* **3**:433.

Olsen, R. G., T. A. Griner, and G. D. Prettyman (1980) Far-field microwave dosimetry in a rhesus monkey model. *Bioelectromagnetics* **1**:149.

Olsen, R. G., J. O. de Lorge, J. R. Forstall, and C. S. Ezell (1984) A circular waveguide irradiation system for nonhuman primates: Design and dosimetry. *Bioelectromagnetics* **5**:79.

Phillips, R. D., E. L. Hunt, and N. W. King (1975) Field measurements, absorbed dose, and biological dosimetry of microwaves. *Ann. N.Y. Acad. Sci.* **247**:499.

Poggio, A. J., and E. K. Miller (1973) Integral equation solution of three-dimensional scattering problems. In: *Computer Techniques for Electromagnetics,* R. Mittra (ed.). Pergamon Press, New York, p. 159.

Pogorzelski, R. J., and T. K. Wu (1977) Computations of scattering from inhomogeneous penetrable elliptic cylinders by means of invariant imbedding. *URSI Symp. Electromagnetic Wave Theory,* Stanford, p. 323.

Rowlandson, G. I., and P. W. Barber (1979) Absorption of high frequency RF energy by biological models: Calculations based on geometrical optics. *Radio Sci.* **14**:43S.

Rukspollmuang, S., and K. M. Chen (1979) Heating of spherical vs. realistic models of human and infrahuman heads by electromagnetic waves. *Radio Sci.* **14**:51.

Schelkunoff, S. A. (1951) Field equivalence theorems. *Commun. Pure Appl. Math.* **4**:43.

Schwan, H. P. (1957) Electrical properties of tissues and cell suspensions. *Adv. Biol. Med. Phys.* **4**:147.

Schwan, H. P. (1958) Survey of microwave absorption characteristics of body tissues. In: *Proceedings of the Second Annual Tri-service Conference on Biological Effects of Microwave Energy,* E. G. Pattishall and F. W. Banghart (eds.). University of Virginia, Charlottesville, p. 126.

Schwan, H. P. (1968) Microwave biophysics. In: *Microwave Power Engineering,* E. C. Okress (ed.). Academic Press, New York, p. 213.

Schwan, H. P., and K. R. Foster (1980) RF-field interaction with biological systems: Electrical properties and biophysical mechanisms. *Proc. IEEE* **68**:104.

Schwan, H. P., and K. Li (1956) Hazards due to total body irradiation by radar. *Proc. IRE* **44**:1572.

Schwan, H. P., and G. M. Piersol (1954) The absorption of electromagnetic energy in body tissues, a review and critical analysis. Part I. Biophysical aspects. *Am. J. Phys. Med.* **33**:371.

Segal, A. S. (1981) The Design and Characterization of a Crawford Cell Animal Exposure Facility for Dosimetric Measurements Between 225 and 500 MHz. M.S., E.E. thesis, University of Illinois, Urbana–Champaign.

Shapiro, A. R., R. F. Lutomirski, and H. T. Yura (1971) Induced fields and heating within a cranial structure irradiated by an electromagnetic plane wave. *IEEE Trans. Microwave Theory Tech.* **MTT-19**:187.

Stratton, J. A. (1941) *Electromagnetic Theory.* McGraw–Hill, New York.

Taflove, A. (1980) Application of the finite-difference time domain method to sinusoidal steady-state electromagnetic-penetration problems. *IEEE Trans. Electromagn. Compat.* **22**:191.

Taflove, A., and M. E. Brodwin (1975a) Numerical solution of steady-state EM scattering problems using the time dependent Maxwell's equation. *IEEE Trans. Microwave Theory Tech.* **MTT-23**:623.

Taflove, A., and M. E. Brodwin (1975b) Computation of the electromagnetic fields and induced temperatures within a model of the microwave-irradiated human eye. *IEEE Trans. Microwave Theory Tech.* **MTT-23**:888.

Taflove, A., and J. C. Lin (1981) Finite difference time domain computation of microwave absorption in models of biological bodies. *Abstracts of Bioelectromagnetics Society Annual Meeting,* Washington, D.C., p. 62.

Taflove, A., and K. Umashankar (1982) A hybrid moment method/finite difference time domain approach to electromagnetic coupling and aperture penetration into complex geometries. *IEEE Trans. Antennas Propag.* **30**:617.

Waterman, P. C. (1965) Matrix formulation of electromagnetic scattering. *Proc. IEEE* **53**:805.

Weil, C. M. (1975) Absorption characteristics of multi-layered sphere models exposed to UHF/microwave radiation. *IEEE Trans. Biomed. Eng.* **BME-22**:468.

Wu, C. L., and J. C. Lin (1977) Absorption and scattering of EM waves by prolate spheroidal models of biological structures. *IEEE AP-S Int. Symp.,* Stanford, Calif., p. 142.

Wu, T. K. (1979) Electromagnetic fields and power deposition in body of revolution models of man. *IEEE Trans. Microwave Theory Tech.* **MTT-27**:279.

Wu, T. K., and L. L. Tsai (1977a) Scattering from arbitrary-shaped lossy dielectric bodies of revolution. *Radio Sci.* **12**:709.

Wu, T. K., and L. L. Tsai (1977b) Electromagnetic fields induced inside arbitrary cylinders of biological tissue. *IEEE Trans. Microwave Theory Tech.* **MTT-25**:61.

6

Criteria for Evaluation of Biological Literature

6.1. PRINCIPLES OF ANIMAL EXPERIMENTATION

Most of the research on biological effects of microwave/radiofrequency (MW/RF) energies has been done with small rodents having coefficients of heat absorption, field concentration effects, body surface areas, and thermoregulatory mechanisms significantly different from those of man. Even closely related species can differ widely in their responses. The literature is replete with "anomalous" reactions. Thus, results of exposure of common laboratory animals cannot be readily extrapolated to man unless a comparative biology approach and some form of "scaling" among different animal species, and from animal to man, is used in an appropriate manner to obtain quantitatively valid extrapolation relationships from the observed data.

Even by using approaches where absorbed energy patterns in test animals closely approximate those that may exist in man under certain exposure conditions, the intrinsic physical and physiological dissimilarities between species further confound the problem of extrapolating between animals and man. In addition to the obvious external geometric differences, physiological differences are important for MW/RF exposures. Body size and orientation are critical in such studies.

Biological experiments using human subjects have either been few in number or inapplicable to the specific biological indicator one desires to study. It is often important, therefore, to use data obtained from experiments using other organisms, such as small animals, to predict the human response to a specific stimulus. There are general principles that allow the results of experiments on one organism (an animal) to be extrapolated to predict the biological responses in organisms different from those tested (i.e., a human).

In making such extrapolations, we must be particularly mindful of the limitations and pitfalls in the use of animal experimentation data. Many factors must be considered in the design of experiments using organisms other than man as a test subject. These include the species, strain, sex, and age of the animal, the methods of caring for the test animals, the animals' feeding patterns, the roles of seasonal and circadian rhythms, temperature, and humidity.

The reliability of laboratory studies using experimental animal models may depend on the following considerations: (1) the selection of the animal model with consideration of its cognitive limits, (2) use of appropriate scaling factors in association with the nature of the field in laboratory investigations of biological processes using animal models, and (3) the method by which the extrapolation of data from the animal models relates to human studies.

The cognitive value of the animal model increases sharply in relation to the physiological and biochemical similarities of the experimental animal to man. Regrettably, criteria for assessing similarity are not always available or apparent. Concomitantly, with physiological and biological similarities, the investigator must recognize (1) the biological parameters of systems reacting on exposure to the selected stimulus, (2) the quantitative indices of response in relation to the energy intensity–time effect relations, and (3) the characteristics of the physiology and biochemistry involved.

In any review of experiments concerned with possible electromagnetic field (EMF) effects, one has to be acutely aware of the critical importance of how experiments are designed and executed and how results are interpreted. Even in experiments that appear to be impeccably planned, it is easy to come to incorrect conclusions. There are a number of cases where a claimed EMF effect was very likely an effect of something else in the experiments. We have also seen cases where no effect was found, but where the design of the experiment was such that probably none could have been found even if it did exist. Any experiment is subject to pitfalls. But this is especially true in many investigations of possible weak EMF effects on organisms, because in some cases no mechanism is known or even postulated by which such fields could produce some of the reported or looked-for effects.

Standard laboratory stressors can easily be found in the experimental procedures that are used in biomedical studies. Such commonplace procedures as handling, novelty of the experimental environment and procedures, extreme environmental temperatures, forced muscular exercise, immobilization, transportation, noise, electrical shock, ether anesthesia, and so on can act as stressors under certain conditions. Great care must thus be exercised to ensure that observed changes are the response to the specific stressor in question (i.e., the EMF) rather than to some extraneous factor. Therefore, investigations must be carefully designed and controlled, and should be conducted on animals properly adapted to environmental conditions. For rats, the adaptation period should be at least 14 days (Grant *et al.*, 1971). Unless these factors are taken into consideration, it is not possible to eliminate stress reactions due to extraneous factors in experiments designed to investigate physiological function in relation to microwave exposure. This is of paramount importance if one is interested in studying subtle indicators of microwave exposure, especially at lower intensities applied for long periods of time.

Some of the criteria used for assessing the results of research on MW/RF biological effects are:

1. The techniques used should be such that possible effects of intervening factors, i.e., changes in ambient temperature, noise, vibration, and chemicals in the environment such as air, bedding, and so on, are avoided.
2. The sensitivity of the experiment should be adequate to ensure a reasonable probability that an effect would be detected if indeed any existed.
3. The experiment and observational techniques, methods, and conditions should be objective. Wherever there is a possibility of investigator bias, special safeguards such as double-blind techniques, blind scoring, or codes should be employed. Appropriate controls for the experimental subjects and quality control of experimental procedures are mandatory.
4. All data analyses should be objective and subjected to acceptable analytical methods with no relevant data deleted from consideration.
5. If an effect is claimed, the results should demonstrate it at an acceptable level of statistical significance by application of appropriate tests.
6. A given experiment should be internally consistent with respect to the effect of interest.
7. Finally, the results should be quantifiable and susceptible to confirmation by other investigators.

6.2. ANALYSIS OF SCIENTIFIC LITERATURE

There are a number of general principles that should be applied in the evaluation of the scientific literature to determine the probability of biological effects caused by exposure to an unknown situation or known factors. In many cases, the reports and information come from recent experiments, and thus are often not confirmed or throughly understood. The publication of preliminary results or incomplete studies, by their very nature, may stimulate misinterpretation by individuals who in turn influence public opinion. In contrast, properly designed and completed experimental studies will only benefit from being subjected to appropriate, scientific criticism. It thus is essential to define the conditions under which experimental data may be seriously considered as significant. Before reported effects in the scientific literature may be used as a basis for concluding that a factor would cause biological effects, certain minimum criteria for the evaluation of this literature should be met.

Before the claims of positive effects in an individual report are accepted into the body of established scientific knowledge, that report should meet the following criteria: (1) The experimental and observational techniques, methods, and conditions should be as completely objective as possible; (2) the published description of the methods should be given in sufficient detail that a critical reader would be convinced that all reasonable precautions were taken to meet requirement 1; (3) all data analyses should be fully and completely objective, no relevant data deleted from consideration, and uniform analytical methods used; (4) the published description of methods should be given in sufficient detail that a critical reviewer would be convinced that all reasonable precautions were taken to meet requirement 3; (5) the results should demonstrate an effect of the relevant variable at a high level of statistical significance using appropriate tests; the effects of interest should ordinarily be shown by a majority of test organisms and the responses found should be consistent; and (6) the results should be quantifiable and susceptible to confirmation by independent researchers.

Once an individual report has been reviewed to assure its reliability, the results of that report must then be considered in light of existing scientific principles and the results of other studies of the parameter under investigation. The results of an individual report should be compared to the rest of the literature being reviewed using the following criteria: (1) The experimental results should be consistent with results of similar experiments; (2) the biological systems involved should be comparable; (3) the claimed effects should be consistent; and (4) the results should be viewed with respect to previously accepted scientific principles before ascribing them to new ones.

Without any attempt to conduct such a review in perspective, broad conclusions, which are based simply upon the existence of a number of studies reporting diverse and inconsistent (as well as incompatible) results, are not scientifically justifiable.

In an analysis of the scientific literature to determine the probability of a biological response from exposure to a noxious agent, we must consider the consistency of experimental results claimed, both the nature of the response and the biological system involved, the ability to consistently replicate the results of studies, and whether the results claimed and observations reported can be explained by previously accepted biological principles or must be explained only on the basis of new, untested hypotheses.

Effect versus Hazard

Experiments with small animals, such as mice and rats, that are undertaken to evaluate the potential effects of a stressor, such as an EMF must be carefully designed and performed. The reported observations may be the result of another, unrelated stressor inadvertently introduced into the experimental design rather than the stressor intended to be studied. That an organism responds to many stimuli is a fact of life; such responses are examples of biological "effects." Since organisms do have adaptive, compensatory ability and tolerance to change, these "effects" may be well within the capability of the organism to maintain a normal equilibrium or condition of homeostasis. If, on the other hand, an effect is of such an intense nature that it compromises the individual's ability to function properly or overcomes the recovery capability of the individual, then the "effect" may be considered a "hazard." In any discussion of the potential for biological "effects" from exposure to electromagnetic energies, we must first determine whether any "effect" can be shown, and then determine whether such an observed "effect" is "hazardous."

The reason for discussing this distinction is to note that while many biological "effects" have been claimed as a result of EMF exposure, it is highly questionable whether such effects, even if substantiated, can be considered to be hazardous, simply because we do not unequivocally understand the mechanisms by which they are caused.

If a specified electromagnetic environment produces a characterizable biological effect, the effect must be evaluated as a potential hazard to man. Since initial experiments are usually performed on animal models, this necessitates an extrapolation from the experimental animal to man. The fact that a biological change is observed or suspected to occur in humans does not by itself indicate that the environment that produces the change is hazardous.

As noted previously, the body responds to many stimuli as part of the process of living and such responses are examples of biological effects. Since the body has considerable redundancy, these effects are within the capability of the body to maintain normal homeostasis. Homeostasis can be defined as the ability of the body to maintain stability in the face of perturbing influences. On the other hand, if the stimulus is of such an intense nature that it overcomes the recovery capability of the body, the stimulus becomes a hazard. For example, a drug such as aspirin when taken in small amounts, i.e., 650 mg every 4 hr, has a biological effect: it alleviates a headache or the pain of arthritis. If, however, the dose of aspirin were increased by a factor of 10 or 100, then the drug could be toxic, i.e., a hazard.

6.3. THE NATURE OF CAUSALITY

Contrary to widespread belief, evaluation of the causal nature of an observed association is a statistical problem, and does not involve the concept of "proof" in any definitive sense. Attention should primarily be focused not on whether the association is "proven," but on the limitations, the adequacy of the data, the lack of design and corresponding artifacts, and finally the choice of appropriate "controls" for the situation.

In the absence of experimental evidence, three types of consideration are useful:

1. *Time sequence.* For the field to be considered the cause of a particular disease, it is clear that the exposure must precede the appearance of the disease.
2. *Strength of the association.* The higher the ratio of the incidence of the disease following a given exposure to the agent in question (i.e., the EMF) to the incidence of the disease at lower exposure or in the absence of exposure, the more likely is the association to be causal.
3. *Consonance with existing knowledge.* Belief in the causal nature of an association is supported by knowledge of a cellular or subcellular mechanism that makes a causal relationship reasonable in the light of existing knowledge in relevant sciences, by analogy from experimental work in other species, and by evidence that the distribution of the disease in populations follows the distribution of the supposed cause. Evidence obtained through exclusion may also be pertinent—the more extensive the efforts that have been made to identify noncausal explanations of an association, the more one is likely to believe, if these efforts have been unsuccessful, that the association is causal.

To review rationally the publications and assess the implications of the reported results of exposure to microwaves, it is essential to consider fundamental principles and concepts related to biomedical research in the laboratory and extrapolation to man.

Experimental animal models are used extensively to study physical factors in the environment in an attempt to ensure human health and safety. The best we can do experimentally is to create an arbitrary set of conditions that we consider to be as relevant as possible for the purpose of the study. Many factors such as methods of animal care, the role of seasonal and circadian rhythms, temperature, humidity, and so on, as well as psychosocial interactions, must be considered in experimental design and analysis of results. Reliability of laboratory studies depends on the following:

1. Selection of the animal model with consideration of its cognitive limits
2. Application of methods developed for investigation of biological processes in animals
3. Extrapolation of data from animals to man

Direct extrapolation from animal experiments to man cannot always be performed *a priori*. This is due not only to the physiological differences, but also to differences in physical dimensions and shape among animals and man.

Meticulous care must be used in defining the experimental conditions. One of the general problems in studying biological effects is the selection of the most appropriate animal species for extrapolation to man. Animals are quite often selected on the basis of convenience, economy, or familiarity and without regard to their suitability for the problem under study. Results obtained in small laboratory animals should not be extrapolated to larger animals or man without consideration of size distributions as well as metabolic and physiological differences.

Proper investigation of the biological effects of EMFs requires an understanding and appreciation of biophysical principles and "comparative medicine." Such studies require interspecies "scaling," selection of biomedical parameters that consider basic physiological functions, identification of specific and nonspecific reactions, and differentiation of adaptational or compensatory changes from pathological manifestations. In comparing results of experiments performed in the same or different laboratories, standardization of conditions is mandatory.

The investigator must determine whether an observed difference can be attributed to the factor being tested, or whether it may simply have occurred spontaneously. In cases in which no difference is observed, the question is whether any conclusion is warranted, and if so, what confidence should be placed in it. For guidance the investigator often turns to statistical analysis; statistics, however, cannot decide what is true and what is not. Statistical analysis should be considered only as an adjunct to, and an integral part of, experiment and observation. But as

TABLE 6-1
Factors That Affect Microwave/Radiofrequency Absorption

Physical parameters of the electromagnetic source
  Frequency
  Polarization
  Modulation (AM, FM, pulse, CW)
  Power density
  Field pattern (near, intermediate, or far field: uniformity)
  Measuring technique
  Calibration technique
  Power
  Transmitting and radiating equipment
  Chamber material and dimensions
Biological parameters
  Tissue dielectric properties
  Size, geometry
  Relation to polarizations
  Spatial relations of animals
Artifacts
  Ground or conductor plate
  Container (material, size)
  Metal implants
  Shielding materials
  Metal or nonmetallic objects in the field

---

with any tool, its usefulness will be enhanced only if its inherent limitations are properly recognized.

The parameters and criteria listed in Tables 6-1 and 6-2 should be recognized and noted when reporting and analyzing biological effects of RF energies.

6.4. SCALING

The need for proper dosimetry in experimental procedures and the importance of realistic scaling factors for extrapolation of data obtained with small laboratory animals to man are clear. Detailed discussions that serve as the basis for scaling have been published (Guy *et al.*, 1975; Massoudi, 1976; Massoudi *et al.*, 1977; Gandhi, 1980).

For the most part, research on the biological effects of microwaves relates to the problem of hazard assessment regarding microwave exposure of man. Two complex, integrative tasks must be systematically accomplished to reach an objective, scientifically valid solution to the

TABLE 6-2
Factors That Influence Biological Responses to the
Same Specific Absorption Rate

Subject variables
  Species
    Sex
    Age
    Weight
  Sensitivity
  Number of subjects
  Interventions (anesthetics; drugs; electrodes; lesions)
  Animal husbandry
Environmental variables
  Temperature; humidity; air flow
  Lighting
  Time of day of exposure
  Noise; odor
Concomitant variables
  Genetic predisposition
  Baseline of the response
  Functional and metabolic disorders
Experimental variables
  Acclimation procedures
  Duration of exposure
  Number and schedule of exposures
  Mode of exposure (partial- or whole-body)
  Sampling technique
  Time between exposure and sampling
  Restraint devices
  Investigator–animal interaction

hazard assessment problem. One of these tasks is the determination of the exposure required to cause deleterious changes in the bodily functions of experimental animals. This determination requires a quantitative evaluation and comparison of the many experiments that have been conducted. The second complex task is the extrapolation of the results of animal experiments to man, a process that will be referred to as "scaling."

There are many factors that complicate these two tasks. Different bodily functions may be affected at different levels of microwave exposure. The most sensitive function could be taken as the determinant of a hazard level, but the possible differentiation between an effect and a deleterious change in function is an important question in hazard assessment. Different conditions of exposure, including microwave frequency, waveform, exposure facility (cavity, free space, waveguide, and so on), and orientation of the exposure target to the E and H vectors of the field may all lead to differences in the effect of the exposure on biological systems. A major underlying factor in all these variants, however, is the absolute need for information in the reporting of an experiment, which will make possible the quantitative comparison of experiments and effects.

Much of the research on the biological effects of microwaves has been done with small rodents that have coefficients of heat absorption, field concentration effects, body surface areas, and thermoregulatory mechanisms significantly different from those of man. Thus, these results cannot be readily extrapolated to man unless some form of "scaling" among different animal species, and from animal to man, can be invoked in an accurate way to obtain a quantitatively valid extrapolation from the actual data observed. The process of scaling in microwave biological effects research is a very complex one. The physical factors that must be considered include: wavelength of energy, intensity, orientation of the animal with respect to the source, size of the animal with respect to the wavelength, portion of the body irradiated, exposure time–intensity factors, environmental conditions (temperature, humidity, air flow), and absorbed energy distribution in the body. In addition, biological variables such as state of health, restraints, medication, metabolic rate, body volume/surface area ratio, and thermoregulatory mechanisms may affect the biological response to microwaves.

Many of the above-mentioned physical variables have been extensively studied by Schwan (1960, 1968, 1971, 1974, 1975) and his associates (Schwan and Piersol, 1954, 1955; Anne *et al.,* 1961, 1962; Anne, 1963) using a "model" approach. The experimental work of Guy and Lehmann and their associates (Guy, 1971a,b; Guy and Lehmann, 1966; Guy *et al.,* 1968; Lehmann, 1965; Lehmann *et al.,* 1962a,b, 1964, 1965, 1966) has demonstrated that the model approach of Schwan and his associates agrees qualitatively and semiquantitatively with measured temperature values. The problem of uneven heat distribution in the body may be of particular significance to the scaling problem.

Schaffer (1962) reviewed experimental data involving microwave heating of small animals and proposed experiments to equate temperature–time responses to microwave exposure. These data reveal wavelength, animal species, competence of the thermoregulatory mechanisms, thermal peculiarities, and environmental conditions to be important factors affecting the thermal threshold.

Hoeft (1965) pointed out that extrapolating the results of microwave heating experiments from various species of animals to man has been done frequently without regard for the interspecies differences in mass and size. He described an analysis to derive a theoretical basis for extrapolation and to suggest ways to improve experiments. The exposure times required to produce a 5°C temperature rise in man and experimental animals were calculated as a function of the microwave intensity, using a simplified model. These calculations show that, while the intensity for which infinitely long exposures are permitted is approximately the same for all species, higher intensities will elevate temperatures quicker in small animals than in larger ones.

As noted by Lowrance (1976), adverse reaction in animals does not prove adverse effect in man, and lack of reaction in animals does not prove that man will not be affected. Even closely related species can differ widely in their responses. The literature is replete with "anomalous" reactions. In an extreme case, common table salt is, in massive amounts, teratogenic to mice: when injected under the skin (at 2500 mg/kg body w) of 11-day-pregnant mice, it produced malformed digits, feet, and wrist and ankle joints in many of the offspring (Nishimura and Miyamoto, 1969). Clearly, drawing implications from any such tests requires care. There is absolutely no evidence that salt at low doses causes human birth defects.

In toxicology, extrapolation of results from animals to man is based on the establishment of a linear relationship between toxicity indices of compounds for various animal species and their body weight. These relations have the characteristics of a general biological regularity (allometric correlations) intrinsic to higher species of animals.

Indices of the relative weight of the internal organs of mammals decrease regularly, starting with small animals and proceeding to large ones. Physiological constants of mammals (pulse rate, breathing rate, and the consumption of oxygen, food, water, and air) also decrease linearly as a function of increasing size of the animal. The linear relationship with body weight is also characteristic of the indices of the microsomal activity of the liver enzymes.

Using the straight line equation, it is possible to describe adequately the changes of many of the constants of the blood (methionine, glutathione, glucose content, and cholinesterase activity among others) as a function of increase in body weight of mammals. This trend also holds for the duraction of pregnancy, the number of simultaneously born offspring, latent period of tumor manifestation, nerve and muscle cell dimension, maturation time of bone marrow cellular elements, extent of erythrocyte life, and a number of other physiological constants that refer to the respiratory and cardiovascular systems (Krasovskii, 1976).

The metabolic activities of mammals show a constant proportional relationship to body mass. Heat production is proportional to $W^{0.75}$ for animals ranging in size from mice to elephants (McMahon, 1973). Many other constant proportionalities in physiological processes have also been documented. Adolph (1949) analyzed the interrelations of physiological processes within and among species, using the heterogonic equation $Y = aX^k$. The interrelations found, imply quantitative orderliness among many diverse characteristics. These interrelations apply not only to rates of physiological processes, but also to sizes of organs, numbers of reduplicated structures, and biochemical compositions.

A linear logarithmic relationship to body weight has been established for more than 100 of the most diverse mammalian parameters. These observations are in agreement with other research results. It was noted in these works that the parameters of energy and water exchange, the dimensions of the blood vessels, and the body length to width ratio were linearly correlated to mammalian body weight.

The average life span of the rat ($\sim 2\frac{1}{2}$ years) corresponds to 65–75 years of a human life. For this reason, in order to find the smallest threshold dose, a complex of the most suitable research methods with respect to the disturbed functions of an organism must be used in conjunction with integrated (nonspecific) tests. The disproportionality in the life spans of animals and man must be considered in the experimental study of the long-term effects of substances and in the substantitation of extrapolation of the results to man.

The problem of hazard assessment cannot be solved with qualitative information, because the objective is the establishment of a quantitative limit for safe exposure. The lack of quantitative information regarding exposure conditions which exists in much of the bioeffects research literature, has already been discussed. Johnson (1975) listed recommendations for specifying electromagnetic wave exposure conditions in bioeffects research.

The extrapolation theories to which Johnson (1975) refers seem to be physical ones regarding the interaction of an animal (including man) with an EMF and the absorption of energy that results in a particular tissue value of watts per kilogram. This absorption is dependent on the size and geometry of the animal with respect to the wavelength of the energy. This wavelength-to-animal-size (λ to a, where a is one-half the longest axis dimension of the body) relationship is also a critical factor in the relative absorption cross section, the ratio of the absorbed energy per second to the power incident on the geometrical cross-sectional area of the animal (Anne *et al.*, 1961). At longer wavelengths, the orientation of the animal with respect to the E and H vectors also affects the relative absorption cross section (Gandhi, 1975).

The question of scaling in electromagnetic bioeffects research is not, however, only one of extrapolation of the physical absorption of the energy, but includes the problems of quantitatively comparing the relative efficiency of various biological processes in different experimental animals to each other and to those processes in man. The same biological processes in different animals are not necessarily affected by the same local tissue value of watts per kilogram. It is also possible that the absorbed energy in a particular area or tissue may not be the most useful indicator in the comparison of disturbances of some biological functions, if those functions are perturbed by a systemic stimulus, instead of a localized stimulus. The need for proper dosimetry in experimental procedures and the importance of realistic scaling factors for extrapolation of data obtained with small laboratory animals to man, are thus clearly indicated.

From the results of theoretical analysis of a simple physical model and considerations of comparative aspects of size, metabolism, and thermal tolerance, some general conclusions can be made on the validity of scaling results from one species of animal to another, particularly man. Energy absorption from a plane wave depends on frequency and object geometry, orientation, and electrical properties. For a given object and orientation, there is a typical frequency for maximum energy absorption. Since this frequency varies greatly with the size of the animal, one cannot extrapolate results *at the same frequency* to animals greatly different in size. It is of practical importance to realize that experiments on the biological effects at 2450 MHz on small animals, like mice and rats, do not scale to man at 2450 MHz, but rather more to effects on man at $\sim$ VHF frequencies ($\sim$ 100 MHz), an important broadcast region of the spectrum.

To extrapolate observations in animals to predict results that might occur during human exposure, some method of scaling must be used. The best method available at present, albeit fraught with oversimplifications, is frequency scaling. This approach assumes the use of shorter wavelengths (higher frequencies) for smaller animals and longer wavelengths (lower frequencies) for larger animals. Approximating the bodies of all animals and man as prolate spheroids, an attempt has been made to ascertain what maximum absorption of lower-frequency energy is required for larger animals if the total absorbed dose rate (at the same plane-wave exposure field intensity) is to be the same as that obtained at a higher frequency for a smaller animal (Durney *et al.*, 1978).

Where absorbed energy patterns in a test animal are used to approximate the pattern that may exist in man under certain conditions of exposure, the intrinsic physical and physiological dissimilarities between species further confound the problem of extrapolating from animals to man. In addition to the obvious external geometric differences, the differences in internal vascular anatomy and mechanisms of heat dissipation in fur-bearing animals compared to man, allow only limited conclusions from such frequency scaling.

Durney et al. (1978) have made calculations of the specific absorption rate (SAR) as a function of frequency for different sizes of laboratory animals and man. This concept is useful to allow limited extrapolation from one species to another, but it should be used cautiously in view of its limitations. Except for spherical models, the bodies studied had uniform properties. Because of the very different properties of bone and muscle, for instance, energy distribution may be much more uneven in animals than the models predict.

Responses induced by exposure to MW/RF energies depend on the amount of energy absorbed, which is a function of the wavelength, and on the geometry, orientation, and electrical properties of the object(s) being irradiated (Durney et al., 1978). Maximum absorption (maximum SAR) during whole-body irradiation of small animals apparently occurs at frequencies between approximately 0.5 and 3 GHz, and for man, at around 60–100 MHz with a peak at about 80 MHz. At frequencies below 30 MHz, absorption drops off rapidly and is also much less at frequencies above 500 MHz.

MW/RF energy, the absorption of which is dependent on polarization, frequency, and the immediate physical environment, is rapidly converted to thermal energy. This thermal energy is then rapidly redistributed by conduction, convection (e.g., blood flow) within, and, to a lesser extent, radiation from the biological target. The tissue heat capacity and heat transfer processes influence the dose and dose distribution within the body.

An effort is being made to standardize dosimetric measures of MW/RF exposure by employing the SAR. The unit-mass, time-averaged rate of MW/RF energy absorption is specified in SI units of watts per kilogram (NCRP, 1981). The SAR depends on a finite period of exposure to yield the amount of energy absorbed by a given mass of material, which is termed specific absorption (SA), i.e., joules per kilogram. Thus, the *specific absorption* rate is the time rate at which radiofrequency energy is imparted to a component or mass of a biological body. The SAR is applicable to any tissue or organ of interest, or is expressed as a whole-body average.

Whole-body absorption rates approach maximal values when the long axis of a body is parallel to the E-field vector and is four-tenths the wavelength of the incident field. At 2450 MHz ($\lambda = 12.5$ cm) for example, "standard man" (long axis 175 cm) will absorb about half of the incident energy. If the human whole-body SAR is divided by the basal metabolic rate (BMR) for man, a ratio is obtained that provides a measure of the thermal load incurred due to a known incident power density (Stuchly, 1978). Table 6-3 illustrates the variation of this ratio with frequency at two incident power densities. In the region of human whole-body resonance (60–80 MHz), this ratio reaches a maximum value (about 0.16 for an incident far-field power density of $1\,\text{mW/cm}^2$). The ratio drops off rapidly on either side of this peak, and at 10 MHz and below, the ratio is less than 0.001 (Johnson et al., 1976).

At frequencies that result in maximal absorption, which defines whole-body resonance, the electrical cross section of an exposed body increases in area. This increase occurs at a frequency near 70 MHz for "standard man" and results, as shown in Table 6-4, in an approximate eightfold increase in absorption relative to that in a 2450-MHz field.

Although most of the experimental data indicate that the effects of microwave exposure are primarily a response to local or general hyperthermia, the total picture is not completely resolved. Unfortunately, large areas of confusion, uncertainty, and actual misinformation now exist and hence detract from valid scientific inquiry. To put the question of MW/RF bioeffects in its proper perspective, a critical analysis of the published literature is essential to differentiate the known and substantiated from the speculative and unsubstantiated. In addition, an appreciation of the nature of EMFs and the possible effects of exposure

TABLE 6-3
Ratio of Specific Absorption Rate to Basal Metabolic Rate for an Average Man Exposed to Far-Field Incident Power Densities of 1 and 5 mW/cm²[a]

Frequency (MHz)	Average SAR/BMR (%)	
	$1\,\text{mW/cm}^2$	$5\,\text{mW/cm}^2$
10	0.13	0.65
20	0.60	3.00
50	5.80	29.00
60	10.00	50.00
80	16.00	80.00
100	12.00	60.00
200	5.20	26.00
500	3.70	18.50
1,000	2.90	14.50
2,000	2.50	12.50
5,000	2.50	12.50
10,000	2.50	12.50
20,000		

[a] Based on Stuchly (1978).

TABLE 6-4
Specific Absorption Rate for Animals and Man (W/kg for 1 mW/cm² Incident Power Density)[a]

	Maximum absorption (MHz)	Frequency (MHz)						
		20–30	70	300	1000	2450	3000	10,000
Mouse	2000	8×10^{-4}	0.008	0.06	0.4	1.00	0.965	0.322
		(0.05)	(0.04)	(1.50)	(13)	(36)	(36.60)	(12.40)
Rat	600	1.8×10^{-3}	0.0125	0.3	0.6	0.23	0.26	0.25
		(0.12)	(0.06)	(7.50)	(20)	(8)	(9.60)	(9.60)
Rabbit	320	5×10^{-3}	0.050	0.80	0.250	0.15	0.08	0.07
		(0.33)	(0.22)	(20)	(8.30)	(5.40)	(2.96)	(2.69)
Rhesus	300	1.7×10^{-3}	0.0125	0.195	0.10	0.07	0.065	0.060
		(0.01)	(0.06)	(5.00)	(3.33)	(2.50)	(2.41)	(2.30)
Dog	200	1.5×10^{-3}	0.010	0.100	0.050	0.040	0.037	0.030
		(0.10)	(0.04)	(2.50)	(1.67)	(1.40)	(1.40)	(1.15)
Human								
1 year	150	0.004	0.040	0.15	0.065	0.055	0.050	0.042
Average	70	0.015	0.225	0.04	0.03	0.028	0.027	0.026

[a] Values in parentheses are SARs relative to average man.

to their energies is required to preclude unnecessary restrictions that may hinder the development of the beneficial applications of these energies.

REFERENCES

Adolph, E. F. (1949) Quantitative relations in the physiological constitutions of mammals. *Science* **109**:579.

Anne, A. (1963) Scattering and Absorption of Microwaves by Dissipative Dielectric Objects: The Biological Significance and Hazard to Mankind. Ph.D. thesis, University of Pennsylvania, Philadelphia.

Anne, A., M. Saito, O. M. Salati, and H. P. Schwan (1961) Relative microwave absorption cross sections of biological significance. In: *Proceedings of the 4th Annual Tri-Service Conference on Biological Effects of Microwave Radiating Equipments*, M. F. Peyton (ed.). Plenum Press, New York, p. 153.

Anne, A., M. Saito, O. M. Salati, and H. P. Schwan (1962) Penetration and Thermal Dissipation of Microwaves in Tissues. RADC-TDR-62-244. Contract AF 30 (602)-2344 (ASTIA 284 981). University of Pennsylvania, Philadelphia.

Durney, C. H., C. C. Johnson, P. W. Barber, H. Massoudi, M. F. Iskander, J. L. Lords, D. J. Ryser, S. J. Allen, and J. C. Mitchell (1978) Radiofrequency Radiation Dosimetry Handbook, 2nd ed. Report SAM-TR-78-22, USAF School of Aerospace Medicine, Brooks AFB, Texas.

Gandhi, O. P. (1975) Conditions of strongest electromagnetic power deposition in man and animals. *IEEE Trans. Microwave Theory Tech.* **MTT-23**:1021

Gandhi, O.P. (1980) State of knowledge for electromagnetic absorbed dose in man and animals. *Proc. IEEE* **68**:24.

Grant, L., P. Hopkinson, G. Jennings, and F. A. Jennre (1971) Period of adjustment of rats used for experimental studies. *Nature (London)* **232:**135.

Guy, A. W. (1971a) Analyses of electromagnetic fields induced in biological tissues by thermographic studies on equivalent phantom models. *IEEE Trans. Microwave Theory Tech.* **MTT-19:**205.

Guy, A. W. (1971b) Electromagnetic fields and relative heating patterns due to a rectangular aperture source in direct contact with bilayered biological tissue. *IEEE Trans. Microwave Theory Tech.* **MTT-19:**214.

Guy, A. W., and J. F. Lehmann (1966) On the determination of an optimum microwave diathermy frequency for a direct contact applicator. *IEEE Trans. Biomed. Eng.* **BME-13:**76.

Guy, A. W., J. F. Lehmann, J. A. McDougall, and C. C. Sorensen (1968) Studies on therapeutic heating by electromagnetic energy. In: *Thermal Problems in Biotechnology*. American Society of Mechanical Engineers, United Engineering Center, New York, p. 26.

Guy, A. W., J. C. Lin, and C. K. Chou (1975) Electrophysiological effects of electromagnetic fields on animals. In: *Fundamental and Applied Aspects of Nonionizing Radiation*, S. M. Michaelson, M. W. Miller, R. Magin, and E. L. Carstensen (eds.). Plenum Press, New York, p. 167.

Hoeft, L. O. (1965) Microwave heating: A study of the critical exposure variables for man and experimental animals. *Aerosp. Med.* **37:**621.

Johnson, C. C. (1975) Recommendations for specifying EM wave irradiation conditions in bioeffects research. *J. Microwave Power* **10:**249.

Johnson, C. C., C. H. Durney, P. W. Barber, H. Massoudi, S. J. Allen, and J. C. Mitchell (1976) Radiofrequency Radiation Dosimetry Handbook. SAM-TR-76-35. Brooks AFB, AFSC, AMD, SAM.

Krasovskii, G. N. (1976) Extrapolation of experimental data from animals to man. *Environ. Health Perspect.* **13:**51.

Lehmann, J. F. (1965) Diathermy. In: *Handbook of Physical Medicine and Rehabilitation*, F. H. Krusen, F. J. Kottke, and P. Ellwood (eds.). Saunders, Philadelphia, p. 244.

Lehmann, J. F., A. W. Guy, V. C. Johnston, G. D. Brunner, and J. W. Bell (1962a) Comparison of relative heating patterns produced in tissues by exposure to microwave energy at frequencies of 2450 and 900 megacycles. *Arch. Phys. Med.* **43:**69.

Lehmann, J. F., J. A. McMillan, G. D. Brunner, and A. W. Guy (1962b) A comparative evaluation of temperature distributions produced by microwaves at 2456 and 900 megacycles in geometrically complex specimens. *Arch. Phys. Med.* **43:**502.

Lehmann, J. F., J. A. McMillan, G. D. Brunner, D. R. Silverman, and V. C. Johnston (1964) Modification of heating patterns produced by microwaves at the frequencies of 2456 and 900 mc. by physiologic factors in the human. *Arch. Phys. Med.* **45:**555.

Lehmann, J. F., V. C. Johnston, J. A. McMillan, D. R. Silverman, G. D. Brunner, and L. A. Rathbun (1965) Comparison of deep heating by microwaves at frequencies of 2456 and 900 megacycles. *Arch. Phys. Med.* **46:**307.

Lehmann, J. F., D. R. Silverman, B. A. Baum, N. L. Kirk, and V. C. Johnston (1966) Temperature distributions in the human thigh, produced by infrared, hot pack and microwave applications. *Arch. Phys. Med. Rehabil.* **47:**291.

Lowrance, W. W. (1976) *Of Acceptable Risk: Science and the Determination of Safety*. Kaufmann, Los Altos, Calif.

McMahon, T. (1973) Size and shape in biology. *Science* **179:**1201.

Massoudi, H. (1976) Long Wavelength Analysis of Electromagnetic Power Absorption by Prolate Spheroidal and Ellipsoidal Models of Man. Ph.D. thesis, University of Utah, Salt Lake City.

Massoudi, H., C. H. Durney, and C. C. Johnson (1977) Long-wavelength electromagnetic power absorption in ellipsoidal models of man and animals. *IEEE Trans. Microwave Theory Tech.* **MTT-25:**47.

National Council on Radiation Protection and Measurements (1981) Radiofrequency Electromagnetic Fields. NCRP Report No. 67. Washington, D.C.

Nishimura, H., and S. Miyamoto (1969) Teratogenic effects of sodium chloride in mice. *Acta Anat.* **74:**121.

Schaffer, M. B. (1962) The Thermal Response of Small Animals to Microwave Radiation. The Rand Corporation (Rep. Rand-P-2558-1), Santa Monica, Calif.

Schwan, H. P. (1960) Characteristics of absorption and energy transfer of microwaves and ultrasound in tissues. In: *Medical Physics,* Vol. 3, O. Glasser (ed.). Year Book Medical, Chicago, pp. 1–7.

Schwan, H. P. (1968) Radiation biology, medical applications and radiation hazards. In: *Microwave Power Engineering,* Vol. 2, E. C. Okress (ed.). Academic Press, New York, p. 213.

Schwan, H. P. (1971) Interaction of microwave and radiofrequency radiation with biological systems. *IEEE Trans. Microwave Theory Tech.* **MTT-19:**146.

Schwan, H. P. (1974) Principles of interaction of microwave fields at the cellular and molecular level. In: *Biological Effects and Health Hazards of Microwave Radiation,* P. Czerski, K. Ostrowski, M. L. Shore, C. Silverman, M. J. Suess, and B. Waldeskog (eds.). Polish Medical Publishers, Warsaw, p. 152.

Schwan, H. P. (1975) Dielectric properties of biological materials and interaction of microwave fields at the cellular and molecular level. In: *Fundamental and Applied Aspects of Nonionizing Radiation,* S. M. Michaelson, M. W. Miller, R. Magin, and E. L. Cartensen (eds.). Plenum Press, New York, p. 3.

Schwan, H. P., and G. M. Piersol (1954) The absorption of electromagnetic energy in body tissues, a review and critical analysis. Part I. Biophysical aspects. *Am. J. Phys. Med.* **33:**371.

Schwan, H. P., and G. M. Piersol (1955) The absorption of electromagnetic energy in body tissues, a review and critical analysis. Part II. Physiological and clinical aspects. *Am. J. Phys. Med.* **34:**425.

Stuchly, M. A. (1978) Health Aspects of Radiofrequency and Microwave Radiation Exposure, Part 2. Department of National Health and Welfare, Ottawa.

7

Molecular, Cellular, Invertebrate Biology

7.1. MACROMOLECULES

To determine if microwaves disrupt the hydrogen bonding between DNA strands of the double helix, Hamrick (1973) constructed DNA melting curves after exposure of DNA to continuous-wave (CW) 2.45-GHz microwaves at 67 W/kg for 16 hr and up to 160 W/kg for 1 hr. Temperature was controlled, usually at 37°C, but for some experiments at 40°C, 45°C, and 50°C. All melting curves were virtually identical to those for unexposed, temperature-matched controls.

To examine macromolecular structure, Allis (1975) exposed bovine serum albumin to 1.70- and 2.45-GHz CW microwaves with SARs ranging from 30 to 100 W/kg in an exposure apparatus where UV and visible spectrophotometric measurements could be made during exposure. The temperature of the exposed samples was controlled during exposure, and equaled the temperature of the control samples. Temperatures ranged from 24 to 32°C depending upon the SAR. Spectra were measured immediately upon initiation of exposure and 30 min later (with continuous exposure). The study concluded that no changes in the UV spectrum could be found over a variety of structural states of the protein. Thus, no changes in the structure of the protein due to exposure to microwaves could be inferred.

Kerova (1964) reported changes in nucleic acid metabolism in the skin and internal organs of rats exposed to 10,000 MHz, 100–500 mW/cm^2, for 6 min. An increase in RNA and a decrease in DNA in the skin and internal organs were noted.

A decrease in skin and increase in spleen RNA and DNA have been noted in white rats exposed to 10,000 MHz, 200 mW/cm^2, for 30 min. A more significant increase in DNA content was observed on the day following irradiation. The RNA content remained practically unchanged in the liver on the day of treatment, while the DNA decreased (Syngayevskaya, 1970).

Repeated exposures to 3000–10,000 MHz, for 10–20 min daily for 21–22 days, amplified or maintained the changes observed after a single exposure. The deviations in nucleic acid content were different in different organs and tissues (liver, spleen, skin) of the irradiated animal, which were apparently related to wavelength and the degree of absorption of the energy by these organs and tissues. The fact that the changes in nucleic acid content either persisted or were even slightly greater on the day following exposure, suggested to the author that disturbances arising during irradiation persist for a certain time after it is terminated. More pronounced changes were observed in the intact organism after exposure at higher intensities, and were accompanied by an increase in colonic temperature. According to Kerova (1964), the changes in nucleoprotein metabolism are the same under the thermal effects of 10,000-MHz microwaves as under ordinary infrared heating of the body surface.

Kamat and Laskey (1970) attempted to determine if the heat-resistant bacterial α-amylase (*Bacillus subtilis*) could be inactivated with 2450-MHz microwaves under conditions that maintained the temperature below the thermocritical temperature for this enzyme. The results of *in vitro* microwave irradiation at 2450 MHz, 100 mW/cm^2, clearly indicate a thermal effect. The inactivation of the bacterial α-amylase depended on the temperature increase during irradiation. There was no significant inactivation of the enzyme in samples that did not exceed 38°C. Significant inactivation (62.78%) as compared with controls occurred only when the temperature of the samples was raised to about 65°C or maintained at 63.7 ± 11.1°C for 15 min during irradiation. The temperature-dependent inactivation of the bacterial enzyme with 2450-MHz microwaves is supported by the significant inactivation of the enzyme (96.51%) by heating at 72.0 ± 1.6°C for 15 min.

Ward *et al.* (1975) examined three enzymes, glucose-6-phosphate dehydrogenase, adenylate kinase, and NADPH-cytochrome reductase, exposed to 2.45-GHz CW microwaves at an SAR of 42 W/kg for about 5 min during which the enzyme activity was measured. All exposed and control samples were maintained at 25°C. No differences between exposed and control samples were found. Bini *et al.* (1978) followed the activity of lactic acid dehydrogenase exposed to 3.0-GHz CW microwaves at SAR values between 33 and 960 W/kg. They demonstrated that the changes found in the enzyme activity were entirely consistent with calculations of thermal inactivation of the enzyme at the temperatures attained. The sample exposed at 33 W/kg was not different from the unexposed control; all other exposures (165–960 W/kg) showed evidence of enzyme inactivation.

The effects of 2.8-GHz with 1-kHz square wave modulated microwaves at SAR levels of 200 to 500 W/kg on enzyme preparations (glucose-6-phosphate dehydrogenase, lactic acid dehydrogenase, acid phosphatase, and alkaline phosphatase) were analyzed by Belkhode *et al.* (1974a,b). Exposures were conducted at 37, 46.7, and 49.7°C, and enzyme activities were compared to heat-treated controls. Activities of the exposed enzymes at each temperature were indistinguishable from those of the controls.

Henderson *et al.* (1975) reported a change in enzyme activity that was interpreted as being indicative of a direct action of microwaves on the enzyme. In this experiment, horseradish peroxidase was exposed to 2.45 GHz CW at levels between 62,500 and 375,000 W/kg in a tube (4.7-mm ID) protruding through a waveguide. The sample tube was surrounded by a concentric cooling jacket through which an organic coolant was pumped continuously to maintain the temperature at 25°C. Total sample exposed was about 0.8 ml. A marked decrease in enzyme activity was found at 62,500 W/kg after 30 min of exposure and at 187,500 W/kg after 20 min of exposure, even though the temperature was reported never to exceed 35°C. At these extremely high dose rates, however, it appears likely that very high local heating occurred in the sample and that this was responsible for the enzyme inactivation. This likelihood was substantiated by the work of Harrison *et al.* (1980), who performed liquid-crystal thermography for a similar exposure situation. Temperature rises of as much as 0.3°C were recorded within a micropipette suspended in a waveguide and cooled with water circulating through the waveguide.

UV absorption spectra were determined during exposure to CW microwaves at 1.70 and 2.45 GHz with an SAR of 39 W/kg to determine if the binding relationship between an enzyme and substrate could be affected by microwaves (Allis and Fromme, 1976). Measurements were performed immediately upon beginning irradiation and after 30 min of exposure. Neither structural change in the enzyme–substrate complex nor change in the binding constants was found.

Allis and Fromme (1979) also studied ATPase in RBC membranes and cytochrome oxidase in the inner mitochondrial membrane of rat liver cells. The dose rate was 26 W/kg, and the 2.45-GHz microwaves were sinusoidally modulated at 16, 30, 90, and 120 Hz. The enzyme activity was not measurably affected by these exposures.

Tyazhelov *et al.* (1979) exposed a phospholipid membrane formed between two chambers containing solutions of NaCl or KCl. An antibiotic was added to facilitate passage of Na^+ or K^+. Conductance was measured across the membrane as a function of exposure from 125 to 280 V/m (internal field strength in the aqueous medium) at 900 MHz. Four-second pulses were delivered, during which conductance measurements were made. The results show a change in conductance under exposure that is consistent with a temperature rise of up to 12°C, but the temperature of the NaCl or KCl solutions did not vary by more than 0.5°C. However, information concerning the exposure setup is insufficient for judging whether serious nonhomogeneities in energy deposition and in the temperature distribution, were possible.

7.2. CELL MEMBRANES

Ismailov (1977) investigated the infrared absorption spectra of proteins in RBC membranes exposed to 1000 MHz at SAR levels of up to 45 W/kg with the temperature maintained at 25°C. The samples were exposed for 30 min in an aqueous suspension in a stripline, then dried to a thin film to obtain the infrared spectra. No change in α-helix or β-sheet content of the membrane proteins was noted. However, when D_2O was added to the suspension before initiation of exposure, application of microwaves was found to increase the degree to which strongly bound amide hydrogens were exchanged. This effect was pronounced at an SAR of 45 W/kg but disappeared when the SAR was below 10 W/kg.

Sheridan et al. (1979) reported results of Raman spectroscopy on single- and multilamellar synthetic phospholipid vesicles exposed to 2.45 GHz CW. No change was found in the Raman bands of single-layered vesicles. In contrast, the data for multilamellar vesicles indicate that the hydrocarbon tails of the phospholipids were undergoing a temperature-dependent phase transition at a point where the bulk temperature was too low for the transition to have begun. The change was reported to be equivalent to a temperature difference of about 2°C at an exposure of 25 mW/cm^2.

7.3. MITOCHONDRIA

Mitochondria function is indicative of cellular energy production and control. Studies by various Soviet investigators indicate that oxidative phosphorylation is uncoupled in liver mitochondria isolated from rats exposed to electromagnetic fields of low power density (≤ 1 mW/cm^2). Phosphorylation was decreased in rats exposed to electromagnetic fields of 7 kHz (Kolodub and Yevtushenko, 1972), 2.5 GHz (Dumansky and Rudichenko, 1976), and 10 GHz (Faitel'berg-Blank and Sivorinovs'kiy, 1972).

Elder and Ali (1975) and Elder et al. (1976) presented results of exposure of rat liver mitochondria to microwaves. They examined oxygen consumption of the mitochondria under various conditions. Elder and Ali (1975) tested mitochondria kept at 0°C during exposure in the far field at

2.45 GHz. The mitochondria functions were examined at 25°C after exposure. Exposures were conducted for up to $3\frac{1}{2}$ hr at SAR of 17.5 and 87.5 W/kg. No changes in mitochondria activity were seen. Elder *et al.* (1976) exposed samples to 2.45, 3.0, and 3.4 GHz CW at 41 W/kg and also to swept frequencies between 2 and 4 GHz with an SAR range of 1.6 to 2.3 W/kg. Again, no effect of the microwave exposure was detected under any condition. In general, a 5% change would have been sufficient for detection of a difference.

Straub and Carver (1975) reported that irradiation of isolated rat liver mitochondria at or near some of these frequencies at higher power densities did not alter oxidative phosphorylation.

Elder and Ali (1975) found no effect on oxidative phosphorylation of isolated liver mitochondria exposed to 2.5 GHz at power densities of 10 and 50 mW/cm^2. Straub and Carver (1975) found no effect on ADP/O$_2$ ratios of isolated rat liver mitochondria exposed to selected frequencies between 1 and 12 GHz at a power density of 2 mW/cm^2. Elder *et al.* (1976) also irradiated mitochondria at 2 to 4 GHz, and found no significant difference in oxidative phosphorylation between irradiated and control samples.

7.4. EFFECTS ON MICROORGANISMS

Studies on the effects of MW/RF exposure on microorganisms can be divided into two groups, according to the particular goals involved. First, and most common, studies have been made, systems proposed, and devices built to enhance or inhibit the growth of microorganisms. In some cases, the final devices have achieved some degree of commercial success. Second, studies have been made to relate effects observed in microorganisms to probable mechanisms for cellular and tissue damage, and hence to an understanding of the causes of responses in animals. The extrapolations involved have been neither theoretically nor experimentally substantiated, so such connections remain, at most, speculative.

7.4.1. Bacteria, Viruses, and Fungi

Studies on the effect of MW/RF energy on bacteria, viruses, fungi, and protozoa have been reported. In several of these studies, effects of higher power densities on bacteria were attributed to heating (Brown and Morrison, 1954; Epstein and Cook, 1951). Others have suggested nonthermal effects of microwaves on microorganisms (Chukhlovin, 1965, 1971; Nyrop, 1946) because lethal or altered growth effects were noted in the absence of a critical temperature rise in the surrounding medium.

Interpretation of these studies is difficult because the accuracy of determining the temperature rise within the culture receptacle during microwave exposure is unknown.

Nyrop (1946) reported effects on bacterial cultures that were ascribed to nonthermal interactions. Effects were observed on bacteria, viruses, and tissue cultures with the electromagnetic energy applied as low-repetition-frequency 20-MHz pulses, conditions that were considered to preclude thermal effects. Intestinal bacteria were destroyed in 5–10 sec when treated with these fields at 205 V/cm, the medium being heated to 40°C. However, with conductive heating this effect was obtained at 60°C in 10 min. Hoof-and-mouth disease virus was completely inactivated by a field intensity of 260 V/cm in 10 min, and in 2.4 sec at 480 V/cm. In studies in which RF energy of 10–100 kHz was applied to *Escherichia coli* in broth suspensions, 99.6% kill was achieved with a field strength of 205 V/cm in a 5-sec exposure and 99.8% kill in a 10-sec exposure. There was no marked difference in results when the treatments were made between 12–40°C and 40–60°C. Viruses inactivated by 20-MHz energy had no immunogenic capacity, suggesting action on the molecular structure of the virus. This is in contrast to evidence indicating that virus inactivated by heat has the capacity to induce an antibody response.

Webb and Dodds (1968) found that exposure to 136 GHz, 7 μW/cm^2, for up to a 4-hr duration appeared to affect cell metabolism in *E. coli*. If the washed cells were immediately exposed to the microwave energy, no cell division occurred. The radiation was not lethal, since the cell count showed no decrease during the 4-hr exposure. If the cells were incubated in nutrient broth for 90 min before exposure, inhibition of cell division was not immediate, and the number of cells per milliliter continued to increase until it approximately doubled. It was suggested that the radiation had two effects; retardation of cell division and specific inhibition of some metabolic process occurring during the early part of the cell's life span. In another study, Webb and Booth (1969) reported investigations of the absorption of 65- to 75-GHz microwave energy on isolated protein, RNA, and DNA and its effect on some metabolic processes. The bacterial cells were found to selectively absorb energy at specific frequencies, and the absorbed energy altered metabolic processes and cell growth. Temperature change did not seem to play a part in these phenomena. The authors suggested that apart from a possible value in cell identification, microwaves may prove useful in studies of *in vivo* macromolecular complexes and cell metabolism.

Blackman and Tell (1972) used 85–94 GHz to determine whether effects similar to those of Webb and Dodds (1968) and Webb and Booth (1969) could be obtained. The results essentially showed no reduction in the rate of cell doubling during exposure that could be attributed to the electromagnetic energy. The authors concluded that microwave energy in the frequency range 85–94 GHz under the exposure conditions used, does not inhibit growth of *E. coli* as had been cited for 136 GHz and 65–75 GHz. In a later study, Blackman *et al.* (1975), using 1.70 or 2.45 GHz CW, exposed *E. coli* to power densities of up to 50 mW/cm^2 (75 mW/g absorbed dose). In general, the results did not demonstrate microwave-induced cell growth inhibition. The data demonstrated growth enhancement attributed to the temperature rise in the test system.

Brown and Morrison (1954), studying the effect of RF energy at 50 Hz, 190 kHz, and 26 MHz on *E. coli*, observed many instances of destruction of the bacteria. However, a thermal effect was held responsible, as temperatures in the capsule reached 55°C. After repeating earlier work, it was concluded that there was no significant killing effect in most treatments unless the final temperature exceeded 50°C.

Fabian and Graham (1933) treated 30-cm^2 broth suspensions of *E. coli* with 7.5, 10, and 15 MHz in a heat exchanger apparatus that maintained the medium at about 19°C. Destruction of the bacteria occurred at the three frequencies with the lethal effect greatest at 10 MHz. About 88% destruction of *E. coli* occurred after 8 hr of treatment.

Jacobs *et al.* (1950) carried out many experiments on *E. coli* and *Staphylococcus aureus* at frequencies from 1.2 to 66 MHz. Six-milliliter aliquots of broth cultures of the organisms were exposed to the RF energy applied either by two flat electrodes or by a concentric coil electrode. In most of the experiments, no significant killing of the microorganisms was observed. The maximum temperature reached in the suspensions was about 23°C.

Fleming (1944) exposed *E. coli* at various frequencies from 11 to 350 MHz. A 10-W power input was used and the time of exposure for all treatments was 1 min. The maximum temperature reached during any treatment was 30°C. All frequencies tested had a lethal effect on the bacteria with the greatest effect, about 98% destruction, occurring at approximately 60 MHz.

Taking advantage of the thermal aspects of microwave exposure, the feasibility of using microwaves to destroy viable lyophilized microorganisms was investigated (Pederson and Blomquist, 1967). Samples of *Serratia marcescens* and *Bacillus subtilis* var. *niger* were exposed to power densities of 10, 15, and 20 W average power at a frequency of 1496 MHz. Parameters investigated included duration of exposure, power level, impedance, and moisture content. It was noted that a graphical plot of reduction at this frequency resembles classical thermal destruction, so it was postulated that heat is the primary destructive mechanism. It was suggested that microwave exposure is a feasible means of destroying resistant forms of microorganisms (spores) in a short period of time. Irradiation of fowl sarcoma viruses with 3000 MHz caused complete loss of activity, which was attributed to the heating of the medium (Epstein and Cook, 1951).

Olsen (1965) noted that bread mold fungal spores can be eliminated when treated in a 2450-MHz microwave conveyor of a simulated industrial process. The temperature of the bread was brought to 65°C in 2 min and cooled at room temperature. When spores of the same fungus were exposed to the same conditions by conductive heat, there was no reduction in spore viability. When *Penicillium* sp. spores on the microwave-treated bread were recovered and plated, counts showed only about 0.143 colony per plate, whereas samples from untreated bread yielded 1486 colonies per plate. A similar reduction in the number of viable spores of *Aspergillus niger,* recovered from microwave-treated bread, was noted. Temperature control below 65°C, however, was not achieved in these experiments and no conventionally heated controls were employed. Inhibition of bread mold is, in fact, the only effect of microwave energy upon microorganisms that has resulted in commercially viable systems: bread "sterilization" using microwave energy is in use in Japan (Suzuki and Oshima, 1973) and several countries in Europe (Meisel, 1973).

Olsen *et al.* (1966) found certain microorganism population reductions that could not be related to a time–temperature factor. They noted a substantial reduction in bacterial count on chicken parts during a 40-min steamcooking in which a temperature of 85°C was reached. When cooked by microwaves, however, the same reduction could be realized in about 10 min with the same final temperature.

Microwave energy has been used to reduce mesophilic bacteria by as much as 97–99% but thermophilic bacteria are more tolerant. Sterile food samples have been produced with a combination of microwave and infrared treatments. The infrared energy was used to preheat a microwave cavity prior to microwave irradiation. If the preheating phase was at least 65°C for 2 min followed by a treatment of 1 kW of available energy for 3 min, the spore-forming bacteria were killed (Olsen *et al.,* 1966).

Macrospores of *Fusarium solani* v. *phaseoli* were treated in water suspension in a microwave conveyor operating at 2450 MHz at various power densities and time durations. Similar techniques were applied to spores thermally treated in a water bath. The data plotted as cumulative spore germination curves revealed dissimilar shapes; the thermal treatment curves were conventional in shape but the microwave-treated spores (2 kW for 1 or 2 min) did not show any recovery in percent germination through the 7-day observation period (Olsen *et al.,* 1966).

During studies on soil sterilized with 915-, 2450-, and 5800-MHz microwaves, it was found that the microorganisms were killed at various temperatures depending on size. Root knot nematodes (*Meloidogyne javanica*) were killed with sufficient microwave energy to produce only a 4°C rise. A larger soil fungus, *Rhizoctonia soloni*, was killed at a temperature about 10°C below that of its normal thermal-death point. Bread mold fungal spores (relatively small spores) were killed at 3–5°C below the normal lethal temperature (Olsen, 1965). Non-spore-forming bacteria, however, are killed by microwave energy at a point as much as 10°C below their thermal-death point. Spore-forming bacteria require about the same temperature for kill regardless of the type of energy used (Olsen *et al.*, 1966).

Robe (1966) reported on a process for pasteurizing liquids with 27.12 MHz in a waveguide configuration surrounding a glass or plastic tube through which the liquid flows. Experiments were conducted on beer and wine inoculated with yeast. Sterilization of these products was brought about by heating them to 46.4–48.8°C with the RF energy. As 30 min at 60°C is usually required for sterilization using conventional heating, it was suggested that the RF energy had a synergistic killing effect with heat on the yeast.

Lechowich *et al.* (1969) investigated the effect of heat and 2450-MHz microwaves on the respiration rate of *Saccharomyces cerevisiae*, and on the viability of *Streptococcus faecalis* and *Saccharomyces cerevisiae*. The highest temperature attained by the *S. faecalis* suspension, after 30 min of microwave exposure, was 52°C, which produced approximately the same lethality as 30 min at 52°C from conventional heat. It was concluded that the death of *S. faecalis* cells upon exposure to microwaves is brought about by thermal rather than nonthermal effects.

Carpenter (1959) suggested that differentiation of *Neurospora* may be adversely affected by microwaves (2450 MHz CW, 400 mW/cm^2) through a nonthermal mechanism. Exposure of *Neurospora crassa* to 2450 MHz inhibited formation of conidiophores, thus showing interference with fungal cell differentiation without inhibiting growth.

Carroll and Lopez (1969) studied the lethality of 60-MHz energy upon *Saccharomyces cerevisiae*, *Escherichia coli*, and *Bacillus subtilis*. An aqueous buffer medium was used to suspend the microorganisms for treatment. No killing effect of the 60-MHz energy *per se* on the organism was observed at any of the various buffer pH values, nor was there any observable synergistic killing effect of RF energy and heat on the microorganisms in any of the buffers. However, a synergistic killing effect of ethanol and heat at 48.8°C was demonstrated on *S. cerevisiae*. Irradiating *S. cerevisiae* and *E. coli* in several liquid foods also failed to show a selective killing effect of RF energy. It was suggested that since most microbial cells carry an electrical charge, it is possible that cells may be caused to oscillate rapidly in the applied field. If these oscillations are rapid enough and/or of a large enough displacement, the elastic limits of the cell structure might be exceeded, thus causing the cell to rupture and die. It should be noted, however, that if RF energy of a given frequency is selectively absorbed by certain critical organic molecules of the microbial cell, such as essential protein or DNA molecules, these molecules could be irreversibly denatured and the microorganisms rendered nonviable at low-heating levels of the suspension medium.

Microwave ovens are used to heat precooked frozen foods. Because of the reported bactericidal action of microwave energy in such processes (Lechowich *et al.*, 1969; Baldwin *et al.*, 1968; Dessel *et al.*, 1960), the effect of freezing and 2450-MHz microwave heating of precooked frozen food deliberately contaminated with *E. coli* and *Streptococcus faecalis* was studied by Madson *et al.* (1970). The results suggest that microwave heating will satisfactorily kill or reduce incidental and introduced microorganisms to a safe level providing the microwave exposure time is correlated with the size and type of food substance being treated.

Pederson and Blomquist (1967) described several characteristics of microbial destruction by microwave energy, namely, (1) more energy is required to destroy bacterial spores than vegetative cells; (2) the destructive effect of microwaves is a direct function of the total joules delivered to the sample; (3) the decay rate for bacteria is very rapid at high power densities and remembles heat destruction curves at very high temperatures; (4) there is an increased decay rate in lyophilized bacteria as the proportion of moisture increases, suggesting that added moisture serves to enhance denaturation of cell proteins at high temperatures.

7.4.2. Mechanisms of Microbial Action

Bacteria have been used to study the mutagenic potential of microwaves because the single-cell systems are simple, easy to grow, quick to test, and relatively sensitive to the action of mutagenic agents. Blackman *et al.* (1976) exposed growing cultures of *E. coli* to either 1.7- or 2.45-GHz CW energy for 3 to 4 hr. Exposure to 1.7 GHz was in the near field at approximately 250 V/m, which corresponds to an SAR of 3 W/kg. The 2.45-GHz exposures were in the far field at either 10 or 50 mW/cm^2, corresponding to SAR values of 15 or 70 W/kg. No mutagenic activity was detected. UV light was used as a positive control to demonstrate the sensitivity of the assay method.

Dutta *et al.* (1979a) exposed growing cultures of various bacterial strains of *Salmonella typhimurium*, commonly used in the Ames's Test procedure to detect chemical mutagens (Ames *et al.*, 1975), to 2.45 GHz CW for 90 min at 20 mW/cm^2 (SAR = 40 W/kg) and to 8.6-,

8.8-, 9.0-, 9.2-, 9.4-, and 9.6-GHz pulsed energies [(1-μsec pulse width, 1-kHz Pulse Repetition Rate (PRR)] at 10 and 45 mW/cm^2 average, 10,000 and 45,000 mW/cm^2 peak power densities. (Estimated SAR at 45 mW/cm^2 is 80 W/kg.) No mutagenic activity was observed for any of these exposure conditions.

Another approach, which has been used with bacterial systems, is to test for radiation-induced alterations in genetic processes including cell death. Corelli et al. (1977) exposed cultures of E. coli to microwaves at frequencies between 2.6 and 4.0 GHz for 8 hr at an SAR of 19 W/kg. Although at 26°C these cultures were probably growing very slowly, no change was noted in the number of colony-forming units in the cultures following the exposure period, which indicates that no detectable lethal events occurred due to the irradiation. These workers also examined the infrared spectrum of these cells exposed to 3.2-GHz microwaves for 11 to 12 hr at an SAR of either 21 or 16 W/kg. There was no observable effect on the molecular or conformational structure of these cells, in contrast to results obtained using ionizing radiation, which constituted a positive control.

Two strains of E. coli, one deficient in an enzyme needed to repair damaged DNA, were tested by Dutta et al. (1979b) for survival following microwave exposure. The exposure conditions were 8.6 GHz pulsed (1-μsec pulse width, 1-kHz PRR) at 12 W/kg, for 1, 2, 4, or 7 hr. There were no significant changes in the relative growth patterns of these strains that could be attributed to microwave-induced DNA damage repairable in one strain but not in the other. Blackman et al. (1975) exposed a different strain of E. coli in log phase (actively dividing) and in lag phase (undergoing metabolic activities preparatory to division) at 32°C for 4 hr to 2.45 GHz at 0.05, 0.5, 5.0, or 50 mW/cm^2. (50 mW/cm^2 corresponds to an SAR of 75 W/kg.) Additional experiments were conducted at 5 mW/cm^2 and 25°C, to test for the influence of cold stress, and in two culture media at 30 and 35°C, to compare the relative influence of a rich medium versus a minimal medium, which requires greater utilization of the genetic apparatus of the cell for growth to occur. They found no change in the colony-forming ability of the cultures due to the exposure except for enhanced growth at 50 mW/cm^2, which was attributed to increased temperature in the exposed cultures.

Dutta et al. (1979a) exposed the yeast Saccharomyces cerevisiae, a primitive eukaryote, to 2.45 GHz CW for 2 hr at 20 mW/cm^2 (SAR = 40 W/kg). They found essentially no change in the number of mutations at either of two loci affecting the nutritional requirements for adenine or tryptophan. These investigators also did additional work at 8.4-, 8.6-, 8.8-, 9.0, 9.2, 9.4, and 9.6-GHz pulsed energies (1-μsec pulse width, 1-kHz PRR) for 2 hr at average power densities of 1, 5, 8.9, 10, 15, 30,

35, 40, and 45 mW/cm^2. Although no measurements of SAR were cited, thereby making comparisons with CW exposures difficult, the highest power density was reported to increase the temperature of the culture by 12°C, indicating substantial absorption of the energy. The estimated SAR at 45 mW/cm^2 is 80 W/kg. In no case did the exposures cause a change in the frequency of genetic events, altering the requirements for either adenine or tryptophan, in the treated population compared to the control population.

Some work has been done with bacterial and yeast cultures comparing the lethal and mutagenic effects of microwaves with those due to conventional heating. Dutta *et al.* (1980) examined the responses of various strains of the bacteria *Salmonella typhimurium* and *E. coli* and the yeast *Saccharomyces cerevisiae*, exposed to 8.6-, 8.8-, or 9.0-GHz microwaves (pulsed at 1-kHz PRR, with a 1-μsec pulse width) at average power densities of up to 45 mW/cm^2 (est. SAR up to 80 W/kg). The bacteria were exposed for 2 hr at 30°C. The results of these treatments were compared to those at temperatures elevated by conventional heating. Cellular damage leading to reduced survival was produced in both cases. Care must thus be exercised in evaluating genetic changes in microbial assay systems when elevated temperatures are induced during microwave exposure.

The emission of light by a photoactive bacterium, *Photobacterium fischeri*, has been used as the endpoint of one study (Barber, 1962), where the bacterial suspension was circulated through a waveguide. Bacteria were exposed at several frequencies between 2.6 and 3.0 GHz; assay was performed 24 hr later. In spite of extremely high dose rates (660 to 5300 W/kg), there were no differences between exposed samples and heated samples conducted in parallel.

Far-field exposures were made (Hamrick and Butler, 1973; Blackman *et al.*, 1975) on several strains or mutants of *E. coli* and on *Pseudomonas aeruginosa*. Samples were exposed in t-flasks or petri dishes principally at 2.45 GHz CW. Growth was measured by assaying for colony-forming units from exposure to 29 to 320 W/kg (60 to 600 mW/cm^2) (Hamrick and Butler, 1973) or 0.0075 to 75 W/kg (0.005 to 50 mW/cm^2) (Blackman *et al.*, 1975). In both experiments the duration of exposure was sufficiently long that the average cell divided at least once (12 and 4 hr). Blackman *et al.* (1975) examined several growth conditions such as lag, log, and stationary phases of growth, rich and minimal media, and a "normal" as well as a mutant amino-acid-requiring strain. In each case, no differences between the exposed samples and temperature-matched control samples were found.

Goldblith and Wang (1967) exposed *E. coli* and *B. subtilis* spores in a microwave oven (2.45 GHz) for up to 1 min. An SAR of about

400 W/kg can be estimated from their heating data. In this case, microwave heating and conventional heating were found to have identical effects on survival.

In an experiment conduced at 10 GHz, a transient effect was found in the virulence of *Agrobacterium tumefaciens* toward its normal hosts, potato and turnip disks (Moore et al., 1979). This bacterium produces a plasmid, which it injects into the host cells and which is responsible for turning these cells into uncontrolled tumor cells. In this experiment, a suspension of *A. tumefaciens* was exposed in a petri dish for 30, 60, or 230 min. The longer exposures produced a 60% decrease in virulence with no essential change in the number of viable cells. The effect was unchanged 6 hr postexposure, but virulence returned to normal 23 hr postexposure when the bacteria were maintained at 27°C or lower during irradiation. From the temperature data, cited in the paper, a dose rate of approximately 1 W/kg can be estimated. (Exposure was 0.58 mW/cm^2.) A possible explanation for this effect is that the plasmid DNA of the *A. tumefaciens* was incorporated into the major DNA of the bacteria during microwave exposure, preventing injection into the host. Normal growth may have subsequently allowed the plasmid to return to its original situation, restoring activity. The results of the experiments by Moore et al. (1979), in which the virulence of *A. tumefaciens* was decreased for more than 6 hr after exposure to microwaves, are suggestive of reversible functional change in the organism. In this case, the implications for cellular function after microwave exposure would be broad. However, no other worker has noted a similar effect with other unicellular organisms, and this experiment has not been independently replicated. Therefore, its significance is uncertain at this time.

Several investigators (Grundler et al., 1977; Keilmann, 1978; Grundler and Keilmann, 1980) have demonstrated that *S. cerevisiae* exhibits an enhanced or inhibited growth rate when exposed at certain closely spaced frequencies between 41.60 and 41.80 GHz. For example, they found a 10 to 15% increase in growth rate at 41.64 and 41.68 GHz, and a 20% decrease at 41.66 GHz. The experiments were conducted using a unique waveguide termination, which was dipped into a suspension of yeast cells. In a typical experiment, 24 W was dissipated in the yeast cell suspension, and the authors estimated a maximum exposure intensity of about 10 mW/cm^2; however, because of the unusual nature of the waveguide termination and the high attenuation of high-frequency energy by aqueous samples, SAR values are not available. Sample temperature was mentioned and was within 0.5°C of the desired 32°C. Temperature controls were performed, and the authors believe that changes of the observed magnitude are not temperature effects, since the growth rate increased or decreased at the same incident energy but at different frequencies. The decrease is difficult to explain, based on the authors' reports of no observable temperature rise. If, however, a localized temperature of greater than 37°C (more than 5°C above the controlled temperature) occurred close to the waveguide termination, then the decrease could be explained solely on the basis of temperature.

Averbeck et al. (1976), using microwaves of 70 and 75 GHz, at 5 to 100 mW/cm^2, studied the effects on bacterial growth and lethal and mutagenic effects in bacterial and yeast cells. A possible interaction between microwaves and X rays was tested as well. A growing culture of E. coli K12 (wild type) was exposed at a power density of ~ 10 mW/cm^2 in a temperature-controlled chamber. The number of cells in the growing culture was determined by plating cells on complete growth medium and counting the outgrowing colonies. No global thermal effects on E. coli were observed at the power density employed. The frequency was changed in steps of 0.5 GHz to permit detection of possible frequency-specific effects. In the neighborhood of 70.5 and 73 GHz, a decrease in cell growth was observed. The results were in good agreement with those reported by Webb and Booth (1969).

These authors (Averbeck et al., 1976) also reported that microwave irradiation for 30 min at frequencies between 70 and 75 GHz at power densities of up to 60 mW/cm^2 does not induce any killing in mutant and wild-type strains of E. coli and S. cerevisiae. Such exposure did not produce any DNA damage, which can be recognized by the known DNA repair systems. This was true for the prokaryotic as well as for the eukaryotic cell system. These results demonstrated that microwave irradiation does not produce mutagenic effects. Reversion rates observed after microwave treatment were always the same as the spontaneous mutation rates. The authors suggest that the effect of microwaves may be reversible. Simultaneous exposure to microwaves and X rays produced increased survival of X-irradiated E. coli, suggesting enhanced repair due to increased metabolism.

The effects of 9.4, 17, and 70–75 GHz were investigated in bacteria and yeast by Dardalhon et al. (1981). At power densities below 60 mW/cm^2 and SAR values not exceeding 28 mW/g, no significant effects on survival of repair-competent and -deficient strains were observed in E. coli and S. cerevisiae. In addition, 17 GHz did not induce mutations in E. coli B/r WP2 trp$^-$ uvr$^-$ above the spontaneous level, and the induction of nuclear reversions, cytoplasmic "petite" mutations, and mitotic recombination as well as the efficiency of sporulation was not affected in yeast.

The results of Dardalhon et al. (1981) indicate that microwaves at the frequencies and power densities used do not have appreciable effects on cell survival of the wild type and repair-deficient mutants and mutation induction in *E. coli* and *S. cerevisiae,* suggesting the absence of significant effects on DNA. In diploid yeast, the efficiency of sporulation and segregation of genes in meiosis does not appear to be significantly altered by the microwave treatment.

This is consistent with work performed at low power levels and at frequencies of 1.7, 2.45, 8.5–9.6, and 68–74 GHz in which there was an absence of lethal and mutagenic effects in several microorganisms (Blackman *et al.,* 1975, 1976; Dutta *et al.,* 1979a,b).

Studies on the effect of microwaves on viral multiplication in mammalian cells have been performed by Szmigielski *et al.* (1976) and Luczak *et al.* (1976). These investigators suggest that microwaves (3 GHz, 5–20 mW/cm^2) influence cell function and metabolism *in vitro,* leading to short-lasting stimulation of protein synthesis and glucose utilization (5 mW/cm^2) or temporary inhibition of the growth rate of cell cultures (20 mW/cm^2).

Experiments on viral multiplication *in vitro* were performed using WISH cells (continuous line of human embryonic cells) and myxovirus parainfluenza 3 (Luczak *et al.,* 1976). The cell cultures were irradiated with 3-GHz microwaves under far-field conditions in an anechoic chamber (30 min) at power densities of 5 or 20 mW/cm^2. Inoculation with viruses was performed 2 hr before, simultaneously, 2 hr after, or 24 hr after irradiation. Irradiation of cells at 5 mW/cm^2 resulted in increased viral multiplication in cultures inoculated 2 hr before, simultaneously, or 2 hr after inoculation, suggesting that the increased multiplication is due to stimulation of cell metabolism (protein and nucleic acid synthesis) and not to increased adsorption of viruses on the cell surface. On the other hand, irradiation of WISH cells at 20 mW/cm^2 resulted in lowered multiplication of viruses in cells irradiated at 2 hr before or 2 hr after inoculation, while in cultures irradiated 24 hr after inoculation normal viral multiplication was found.

In vivo experiments were performed on young (ca. 12-g bw) CFW mice infected with vaccinia or herpes viruses intravenously. The animals were irradiated 7 days after infection (3-GHz microwaves, far-field conditions, 40 mW/cm^2, 2 hr daily). The authors found that microwave heating of mice after viral infection produced virus block or decreased viral multiplication *in vitro.* Microwave hyperthermia produced a decrease in mortality in mice with nasally introduced virus. From this study it would appear that microwave hyperthermia may inhibit viral multiplication *in vivo* and *in vitro* if exposure is started immediately postinfection (Luczak *et al.,* 1976).

Baranski *et al.* (1976) studied the influence of microwaves on genetic processes of *Aspergillus nidulans*. Radiation was 2450 MHz, pulsed: power density not exceeding 10 mW/cm^2 for 1 hr at room temperature.

Spores of *A. nidulans* irradiated before or during germination did not show any changes in survival rate and, in addition, no increase in mutation frequency was noted.

7.5. EFFECTS ON PROTOZOA AND OTHER UNICELLULAR ORGANISMS

Marha *et al.* (1968) noted that unicellular organisms react in a variable manner to 30 to 300-kHz fields. The effect of pulsed 27-MHz energy was studied by Wildervanck *et al.* (1959), who found that dead and live nonmotile unicellular organisms behave exactly like colloidal solutions of inorganic or organic particles, i.e., they form chains. When motile microorganisms are exposed to fields, their spatial orientation is disturbed; they then move in a given direction. Organisms arrange themselves parallel to the lines of force of the field at low frequencies, whereas at higher frequencies they are sometimes transverse to the field. When the external forces cease, they usually resume their initial position. In some kinds of amoebae and a few larger microorganisms, changes in external and internal structures have been observed (orientation of subcellular particles). In the proper field, an amoeba can be made to divide and die.

The frequency at which the direction of movement changes and the minimum field intensity required for this phenomenon depend on the type of microorganism and can be dissimilar for two different strains of the same organism (Marha *et al.*, 1968). Attempts have been made to explain this phenomenon on the basis of nonhomogeneous dielectrics (Jaski and Susskind, 1961) as well as consideration of the time constant for pearl chain formation of colloid particles (Saito and Schwan, 1961).

The influence of 30 to 300-kHz fields on growth, viability, and other metabolic processes in unicellular organisms has been studied by several investigators (Frank-Kamenetskii, 1961; Gilles, 1944; Heller and Teixeira-Pinto, 1959; Lystsov and Frank-Kamenetskii, 1965). Dependence on frequency was found: growth is slow at low frequencies; at higher frequencies, growth is retarded and eventually halted so that the organism dies.

Presman and Rappeport (1965) studied the reaction of paramecia to pulsed and CW MW/RF energy. They found that irradiating a paramecium with a pulse or a series of pulses of direct or alternating current produces a so-called "electric shock" reaction, a sharp braking motion. For example, paramecia were exposed to pulsed or CW microwaves at 2450–3000 MHz, which produced an "electric shock" reaction similar to that when paramecia were exposed to ac or dc currents. The mean threshold values for eliciting the reaction were lower for CW than for pulsed microwaves. The threshold values of the power per pulse (or the mean power for the sequence of pulses) at which this reaction occurred were inversely proportional to the duration of the pulses or sequence of pulses. In addition, although microwaves did not elicit the "electric shock" reaction at subthreshold power values, there was a rise in the sensitivity of the paramecia to other stimuli.

Presman (1965) suggests that the "electric shock" reaction is a result of a nonthermal action of the RF fields, and that the nature of this reaction is independent of frequency. He described studies reported by Kulin and Morozov (1964, 1965) who showed that under the action of 2375-MHz microwaves, the phagocytic activity of *Infusoria* varies in two phases depending on the intensity; in the range from 1.5 to 275 mW/cm^2, there is at first an almost twofold increase in activity, and then a decrease to the normal level, and finally, a fall below the normal level.

Ismailov (1966) investigated the dynamics of the effect of RF energy on cells of the infusorian *Opalina ranarum*, a frog parasite. Capacitance of the cells was found to vary with cell size and at a frequency of 0.4 MHz it averaged 40–60 pF; it decreased with increasing exposure time until it finally disappeared when the cell died (at the 7th or 8th min). There was a definite relationship between the decrease in capacitance of the cells and the duration of exposure.

According to Mickey (1963), various organisms respond to specific ranges of frequencies. *Euglena* have been shown to align themselves parallel to an electric field of 6–7 MHz. At 27 to 30 MHz, however, the organisms orient themselves transverse to the electric field (Teixeira-Pinto *et al.*, 1960).

The observation that the main axis of paramecia or amoebae could be oriented in one direction at the same time that small asymetrical particles in their cytoplasm could be aligned at right angles suggested to Mickey (1963) that subcellular units of the cell would respond differently to RF fields; therefore, the mitotic mechanism could be modified to produce genetic changes. Presman (1965) suggests that the behavior of unicellular organisms when subjected to RF fields involves an excitable structure, a prototype of the neuromuscular system, that they are assumed to possess. On the basis of studies by Friend *et al.* (1975) in which they noticed perpendicular and parallel elongation of the giant amoeba *Chaos chaos* in alternating electric fields over a wide frequency range (from about 1 Hz to about 10 MHz), the authors suggest that simple dielectric forces may be important in the production of these effects. The changes were frequency dependent.

Conclusion

It is difficult to explain the killing effects of RF energy on microorganisms reported by various investigators other than on a thermal basis. Aside from the differences in frequencies employed, there is the possibility that localized overheating or some experimental artifact might be responsible for the observed lethality. Some authors feel that RF energies may lower the infective power of bacteria and inactivate certain viruses through some nonthermal mechanism (Pratt and Sheard, 1935; Presman et al., 1961). According to Nyrop (1946), such inactivated viruses do not possess the antigenic properties still present after usual heat inactivation.

Orientation effects that have been reported are no doubt caused by the change in potential electric energy that occurs when a nonspherical particle is turned with reference to the applied field (Schwan, 1968). Analysis by Schwan and Piersol (1954) has shown that selective RF effects are possible only if the particles are fairly large—no less than 1 mm in diameter. Hence, it seems doubtful that a selective effect on microorganisms exists in the absence of significant heating of the medium in which they are suspended. In the final analysis, no consistent biological effects of RF/MW exposure have yet been found with molecular and subcellular systems other than those effects resulting from general temperature increases.

7.6. CHROMOSOME–GENETIC EFFECTS

Some investigators have reported chromosomal changes in various plant and animal cells in tissue culture (Heller, 1970; Janes et al., 1969; Yao and Jiles, 1970). Other investigators have reported no changes (Huang et al., 1977). Reported chromosomal changes include structural aberrations, polyploidy, and stickiness (Yao and Jiles, 1970; Yao, 1976, 1978; Chen et al., 1974). Exposures range from $7\,\mathrm{mW/cm^2}$ to more than $200\,\mathrm{mW/cm^2}$.

Heller and Teixeira-Pinto (1959), using a 5-min exposure to 27-MHz pulsed (80–180 pulses/sec, pulse length $5 \times 10^{-5}\,\mathrm{sec}$) energy, reported various alterations in the chromosomes and mitosis of growing garlic root tip cells 24 hr postexposure. The field strength and other pertinent data, however, were not reported. The authors also failed to indicate any control groups or statistical analysis. To provide meaningful analysis of these data, one would need to know fixation time, aberration frequency, and spontaneous yield. This study must, therefore, be viewed with skepticism since heat-induced effects were not eliminated, leaving the possibility that the applied field caused biologically significant field-induced force effects. Although the authors describe their results as nonthermal, neither a description of the methods for measuring temperature nor actual measured temperature is given. This is a particularly important omission. Since the electrodes were separated by a distance of only a few millimeters, much of which was occupied by glass insulation, it is most likely that significant thermal effects were induced. Additionally, it is rather doubtful that one of the published photographs showing "linear shortening of chromomosomes" is any different from what one routinely sees when colchicine is used. The relative length of chromosomes also varies during mitosis; metaphase chromosomes are considerably "shorter" than anaphase chromosomes. In another report (Teixeira-Pinto et al., 1960), exposure of gladiolus bulbs to 21 MHz stimulated breaking dormancy and produced more vigorous plants. Because the dosimetry in these studies is vague and in serious question, it is possible that very high field strengths, probably much greater than 1 kV/m, were achieved.

Chinese hamster lung cells and human lympocytes were exposed in culture to pulsed RF fields at approximately 40–500 V/cm (Heller, 1970). At 15 MHz the chromosome aberration yield in the irradiated cultures was significantly greater than controls at postexposure fixiation periods of 24 and 30 hr. Cultures irradiated at 19 MHz had significantly greater aberration yields than controls. Results at 21 MHz were variable. At 25 MHz, significant increases in chromosome abnormalities in exposed cultures over controls appeared at 6, 18, and 48 hr postexposure. At 40 MHz, exposed cultures showed significant increases of chromosome breaks over controls at 18, 24, and 48 hr postexposure. The most effective frequency appeared to be 25 MHz. There was no difference in the amount of chromosome damage between 1 W/cm^2 and 50 mW/cm^2; the latter appeared to be the threshold for the observed effect.

The above reports restate the original conclusion of the authors (Heller and Teixeira-Pinto, 1959) that MW/RF exposure induces chromosome aberrations, but none offers any conclusive and statistically relevant data to support this conclusion. These investigators have attributed their findings to subthermal or nonthermal interactions of the energy and biological system. In the absence of reliable information, it is doubtful that the observed changes are nonthermal or even significant (Kalant, 1959).

These studies have been criticized by investigators who assert that the systems were subjected to thermal stress. The chosen parameters of the applied field caused biologically significant field-induced force effects and many of these experiments have not been independently replicated. Generally, in studies of the response of cells in culture, undetected temperature deviations between irradiated and control systems of no more than 1°C can lead to erroneous interpretations.

Subsequent studies have failed to confirm the findings of Heller and Teixeira-Pinto (1954) and Heller (1970). Coate and Hoo (1970) examined the tips of onion grown under 72-hr exposure to 45 and 75 Hz, 10 and 20 V/m electric fields and 1.0- and 2.0-G magnetic fields. For comparison, root tips were grown in only the earth's magnetic field (~ 0.6 G) and in an ambient 60-Hz electric field (about 0.05 V/m). They noted no chromosomal effects attributable to exposure to these fields.

Hamrick (1973) studied the thermal denaturation properties of isolated, dissolved DNA exposed *in vitro* at 37°C for 16 hr to 2450 MHz (SAR 94 W/kg). Using a series of buffer conditions and temperatures, he found no difference between control and exposed samples when the temperature of the exposed sample was identical to that of the control sample during treatment. Even elevated temperatures (up to 50°C) produced by microwaves (1 hr at an SAR ≤ 225 W/kg) did not cause a difference in the thermal denaturation profile of a DNA solution containing formaldehyde to enhance the sensitivity of the test to detect alterations in the pairing of the two strands of the DNA molecule when compared to a similar temperature elevation produced by conventional heating.

To investigate possible somatic consequences of exposure to RF energies, McLees and Finch (1971) and McLees *et al.* (1972) studied adult male rats that had been continuously irradiated with pulsed and CW fields at 13.12 MHz for up to 44 hr post partial hepatectomy. The experiment involved monitoring mitotic activity and chromosome aberrations in the regenerating liver. All experiments were conducted with radiation power levels just below the heating threshold. It is estimated that the absorbed dose was approximately 1 mW/g. Comparison of the results from control and experimental animals failed to reveal any statistically significant differences in mitotic activity or the number of chromosome aberrations. In addition, light and electron microscopy revealed no evidence of tissue damage.

Zufarov and Shnaivais (1970) have reported mitochondrial swelling and lysis following a 3-hr exposure to 1625 kHz and 2500 V/m RF energy. In the study by McLees *et al.* (1972), mitochondria from both kidney and liver showed no evidence of swelling. No giant mitochondria and no structure compatible with the myelinlike organelle described by Zufarov and Shnaivais (1970) were seen.

Yao and Jiles (1970) investigated the effects of microwave energy on cell proliferation and the induction of chromosome aberrations in cultured choroid and bone marrow cells derived from the kangaroo rat (*Potorous triadactylus apicalis*). The cells were exposed to 2450 MHz at power densities of 0.2, 1.0, and 5.0 W/cm^2. At 0.2 W/cm^2, a 10-min exposure increased cell proliferation; a 30-min exposure reduced cell proliferation. Cell proliferation was greatly reduced at 1 W/cm^2 for exposures of 20 min or longer. At 5 W/cm^2, cell proliferation was reduced and at the same time chromosome aberrations increased. The authors suggest that the types of chromosome aberrations observed in the cells were the same as those induced by X rays but the distribution of aberration types differed from that of X rays. Chromatid breaks were observed as late as 48 hr, and the peak aberration frequency was recorded at 48 and 72 hr postirradiation. This may be a reflection of cell proliferation delay, due possibly to the exposure regimens, culture conditions, and handling techniques. The very high field intensities and consequent heating are the critical factors in this study.

In X-irradiated cells, chromatid breaks are first observed about 6 hr postirradiation and are predominant among the aberrations (Chu et al., 1961). The peak frequency of aberrations occurs at 12 and 24 hr postirradiation. In the study by Yao and Jiles (1970), chromosome aberrations were observed only in the cells that were exposed to 5 W/cm^2 for more than 10 min but not longer than 20 min. Cultures that were exposed for longer than 20 min developed few or no mitotic cells.

Janes et al. (1969) reported an increased frequency of chromosome stickiness in cells obtained from bone marrow of Chinese hamsters 3, $4\frac{3}{4}$, and 5 hr after exposure to 2450 MHz. It should be noted, however, that the animals were irradiated in a field of unknown intensity for 15 min that caused 46% mortality with a mean lethal time of 15.4 min. The mean colonic temperature rise among survivors was 7.5°C. The data that were presented lack details. There is neither an indication of the number of animals used nor the number of metaphases scored per animal. The data appear inconsistent and highly variable. There are no calculations of the variability and confidence limits of the data. The authors' conclusions are not supported by statistical analyses. Furthermore, it is difficult to understand how the authors were able to score "chromosome stickiness" since they treated all their animals with colcemid, which "prevents" cells from proceeding to anaphase and telophase. This metaphase aberration can best be scored in the absence of any type of mitotic inhibitor since the "stickiness" becomes more apparent as the chromatids undergo separation at anaphase and telophase (Carlson and Harrington, 1965).

Prince et al. (1972) reported that in monkeys exposed to 10–27 MHz at power densities from 100 mW to 1.32 W/cm^2, karyotyping showed an increase in the number of visible "secondary characteristics" which appears to reach a peak at 96 hr postexposure. The incidence of cells with structurally altered chromosomes following RF exposure was 10.5% which is an increase of nearly three times that of the preexposure incidence. Sticky chromosomes were not found nor were rings and dicentrics. Monkeys exposed to 1.32 W/cm^2 at 10.5, 19.2, and 26.6 MHz for 30 min revealed a modification of peripheral blood lymphocyte growth potential. The most obvious effect was an apparent increase in the number of metaphase cells 70 hr postirradiation. There was a 9- to 15-fold increase in mitotic response, which could be partial synchronization.

Stodolnik-Baranska (1974) studied the influence of microwave energy on human lymphocytes unstimulated and stimulated to mitosis by phytohemagglutinin (PHA) treatment. Cultures were irradiated with pulsed 3000-MHz microwaves 15 min daily at 20 mW/cm^2 or 4 hr daily at 7 mW/cm^2 for 3–5 days. In addition, lymphocytes stimulated to mitosis by PHA treatment were exposed to microwaves for 5–30 min daily at 20 mW/cm^2 or 3–4 hr daily at 7 mW/cm^2. The results showed that untreated lymphocytes transform to blastoid forms and macrophagelike cells after microwave exposure. Microwave treatment was found to increase the mitotic index and to induce mitotic aberrations characterized by dicentric chromosomes and bridges between chromatids. Interphase cells were noted to have irregularly shaped or fragmented nuclei.

Other studies have used cytogenetic techniques to examine some physical and chemical properties of chromosomes in intact cells to determine if the relationship of various parts of the genetic material had been altered by microwave exposure. Huang et al. (1977) reported no RF-induced chromosome aberrations in white blood cells from Chinese hamsters exposed to 2450 MHz at up to 45 mW/cm^2 (SAR = 20.7 W/kg) for 15 min a day for 5 consecutive days. McRee et al. (1978) in a preliminary report found no sister chromatid exchanges in bone marrow cells of mice exposed to 2450 MHz at 20 mW/cm^2 (SAR = 15.4 W/kg) 8 hr daily for 28 days. Alam et al. (1978) showed that chromosome aberrations occur in a Chinese hamster cell line (CHO-K1) exposed for 30 min to 2450 MHz from a diathermy applicator only if the temperature of the culture is allowed to rise to 49°C during exposure. These authors demonstrated that high power densities exceeding 200 mW/cm^2 (est. SAR = 360 W/kg) could be used, under proper temperature control, without inducing cytogenetic effects. Thus, heating seems to account for the observed cytological changes.

Inferences of apparent genetic effects as a result of chromosome studies should be viewed with circumspection, since chromosome scoring techniques are tedious and require considerable skill (Savage, 1971). Such studies are very complex and conclusions made from only fragmentary data should be suspect. In general, results such as chromosome stickiness are interesting but unresolved phenomena. Stickiness has been attributed to a spatial dissociation and reorganization of the nucleoproteins and appears to be reversible.

Although studies of chromosome aberrations are potential early indicators of biological changes related to cancer or genetic effects, such effects in tissue culture may reflect total response of a specific tissue, but not neoplastic potential or genetic injury to the germinal epithelium where it is especially important. There are several sources of error in estimating chromosome aberration frequencies (Bender, 1967; Brooks and Lengemann, 1967; Evans, 1967) and in using these estimates to evaluate microwave exposure. When cells are cultured *in vitro*, aberration frequencies may vary with postexposure time in culture. A similar situation exists for whole organism responses. There are also many variables in the tissue culture techniques used in various laboratories, which must be considered when comparing and evaluating results. The possible influence of agents such as viruses, heat, chemicals, and so on, which are known to produce chromosome anomalies should not be ignored (Leonard and DeKnudt, 1967; Nichols, 1966; Wald et al., 1964). In short, numerical data representing the various types of chromosome lesions, like any other type of biological changes in any type of disease, are significant only in the context of all other available information about the exposed specimen. In evaluating studies on isolated cell systems, it is often possible to measure changes in cells when they are not a part of an integrated living system; it is not always correct, however, to extrapolate these findings to the intact organism where the cell may be in a different relationship to other cells with differing sensitivities or protective capacities (Ingram, 1969).

There have been some questions concerning the exact magnitude of the fields and temperatures within the receptacles containing cell culture, blood samples, and solutions during exposure. Often the samples are placed in fields of known strength and power density, but due to the complex shapes of the vessels holding the samples, the actual fields acting on the cells or organisms are unknown. Also, it is difficult in some cases to determine whether the effects are specifically due to the fields or simply due to a temperature rise. Attempts to measure the temperature of fields within the sample by conventional methods can produce perturbations that can significantly modify the results of the experiment (Guy, 1977).

Miro et al. (1974) exposed Swiss albino mice to pulsed 3105 MHz at 20 mW/cm^2 average power density (40 W/cm^2 peak) for 145 hr. Stimulation of splenic lymphopoiesis and increased [^{35}S]methionine incorporation in spleen, thymus, and liver were found. The authors interpret these results as a sign of stimulation of cells belonging to the reticuloendothelial system.

Both inhibitory and stimulatory effects on the expression of genetically regulated enzyme synthesis and on bacterial and mammalian cell growth were reported by Webb (1975) at 59 to 143 GHz, 10 to 50 mW/cm^2; a frequency-dependent periodicity of the effects was described. Hill et al. (1978) found no effect on growth of *E. coli* exposed to

$10-70 \, \text{mW/cm}^2$ at 65 to 75 GHz. Miro et al. (1974) also reported a "radioprotective" effect of exposure of bacteria to 3105 MHz, pulsed at a peak power of $39 \, \text{W/cm}^2$, temporal average $2 \, \text{mW/cm}^2$. Other reports show interference with genetically controlled synthesis in bacteria (Smolyanskaya and Vilenskaya, 1973; Zalyubovskaya, 1973). Blackman et al. (1975) reported no effect on bacterial growth at 68, 69, 70, 71, 72, 73, or 74 GHz at an incident power density estimated to be $0.3 \, \text{mW/cm}^2$, or at 1.70 or 2.45 GHz between 0.005 and $50 \, \text{mW/cm}^2$ (0.008 to 75 mW/g), nor was there any effect on mutagenesis in bacteria exposed to 2.45 GHz (10 and $50 \, \text{mW/cm}^2$, 15 and 70 W/kg) or to 1.70 GHz (88 V/m; 3 W/kg) (Blackman et al., 1976).

Baranski et al. (1976, 1978) were not able to attribute mutagenic effects or metabolic changes in *Physarum polycephalum* or *Aspergillus nidulans* to specific effects of $10 \, \text{mW/cm}^2$, 2450-MHz CW or pulsed microwaves. Corelli et al. (1977) also reported no mutagenesis after exposure to 2.6 to 4.0 GHz at 20 W/kg. They investigated the effects of RF energy on colony-forming ability (CFA) and molecular structure (determined by infrared spectroscopy) of *E. coli* B cells in aqueous suspension. Cells were exposed for 10 hr at SARs of 20 W/kg (equivalent to $50 \, \text{mW/cm}^2$). No RF-induced effects on either CFA or molecular structure were observed.

Sharp and Paperiello (1971) investigated the uptake of tritiated thymidine in female albino rats exposed to 2450-MHz microwaves. The results indicated that a 10-min exposure at $32 \, \text{mW/cm}^2$ decreased thymidine uptake in ovarian and intestinal tissues. At a power density of $16 \, \text{mW/cm}^2$ for 10 min of exposure, an increase in thymidine uptake in ovarian tissue was noted with no change in intestinal tissue uptake relative to controls. Little if any change in uptake by lung, liver, heart, or kidney was noticed. These tissues, it should be noted, are not normally proliferative; their cells are postmitotic and would not normally be expected to take up tritiated thymidine. The ovarian and intestinal cells are, however, normally proliferative. Presumably the changes in thymidine uptake in the intestinal and ovarian tissues reflect an alternation of cellular progression as a result of the microwave heating. It can be presumed that a rapid mitotic proliferation of the ovarian follicles was induced, although direct evidence is necessary to confirm this hypothesis. It would appear that subtle or gentle heating as in this study might have a stimulatory effect on partial cell synchronization on certain groupings of cellular systems. Pregnant rats were exposed to 2450 MHz at 50.67 to 63.82 mW/g and used for cytokinetic analysis by means of tritiated thymidine uptake. Rats were exposed to a total of 6 (1-hr) sessions at $5 \, \text{mW/cm}^2$, 12 (1-hr) sessions at $10 \, \text{mW/cm}^2$, 5 (1-hr) sessions at $20 \, \text{mW/cm}^2$, and 2 (1-hr) sessions at $30 \, \text{mW/cm}^2$. In examinations of the brain, it appeared that the G_2 (post DNA synthesis) interphase period was about twice as long in exposed fetuses as in controls. There was an increase in glial proliferation without affecting neurons. It is possible that the increased metabolic rate induced by the thermalizing radiation might have been associated with potentiation of mitotic activity.

Wiktor-Jedrzejczak *et al.* (1976) exposed adult male mice to 2450 MHz CW at an absorbed dose of 12–15 mW/g for 30 min in an environmentally controlled waveguide facility. Such exposure failed to produce any detectable increase in DNA, RNA, and protein synthesis, as measured by spontaneous incorporation of tritiated thymidine, uridine, and leucine by spleen, bone marrow, and peripheral blood lymphocytes *in vitro*. Results of this study, however, suggest that microwaves stimulate the maturation of B lymphocytes in the spleen of exposed mice.

The effects of 2450-MHz microwaves on the cellular elements in the peritoneal fluid and peripheral blood of the rat were investigated by Valtonen (1966). He reported the only pronounced change to be an increase in disrupted mast cells in rats exposed to microwaves. An electron microscopic examination of the fine structure of giant mast cells in the peritoneal fluid of the rat was also undertaken (Valtonen, 1967). The most obvious feature of the giant mast cell appeared to be an abundant swelling of the cytoplasm, which increased the distance between the granules, and the partial disappearance of the granules. Whether the formation of the giant mast cells is a reversible process could not be determined on the basis of this study.

Sawicki and Ostrowski (1968) performed an autoradiographic study of uptake of labeled sulfate by peritoneal mast cells exposed *in vitro* to 3000-MHz microwaves, 3 mW/cm^2 for 10 min. The dry mass of such cells and the intensity of metachromasia were determined. The irradiated mast cells remained alive, but their ability to be stained metachromatically was markedly reduced. The dry mass of mast cells, as well as their diameter, diminished by 50 to 65%. There was a two- to threefold reduction of sulfate uptake by the mast cells.

The mutagenic potential of microwave energy has been evaluated by various techniques, including the dominant lethal test in mammalian systems (Varma and Traboulay, 1976; Varma *et al.*, 1976; Berman and Carter, 1978), genetic transmission in *Drosophila* (Mittler, 1976; Pay *et al.*, 1972), and point mutations in bacterial assays (Blackman *et al.*, 1976), with inconsistent results.

Varma and Traboulay (1976, 1977) and Varma *et al.* (1976) reported increased mutagenesis, using the dominant lethal test with male mice exposed to 10 and 50 mW/cm^2, 1.7 GHz CW for 90 and 30 min, respectively. Mice exposed to 2.45 GHz CW at 100 mW/cm^2 for 10 min and at 50 mW/cm^2 three times, 10 min each within 1 day, also showed increased mutagenesis. Mice subjected to four exposures of $50\,mW/cm^2$, 10 min each over a period of 2 weeks, showed no increase of dominant lethality above control levels. These authors reported radiation-induced changes in thermal denaturation profiles as well as changes in the base composition of testicular DNA extracted from anesthetized mice whose testes were irradiated in the near field. Ten animals were exposed individually to either 1.7-GHz microwaves at $50\,mW/cm^2$ for 30 min (est. SAR in testes = 2.4 W/kg) or at $10\,mW/cm^2$ for 80 min (est. SAR in testes = 0.48 W/kg), or 0.985-GHz microwaves at $10\,mW/cm^2$ for 80 min (est. SAR in testes = 0.26 W/kg). The animals exposed to 1.7 GHz at $50\,mW/cm^2$ or to 0.985 GHz at $10\,mW/cm^2$ were used in another test for 8 weeks before they were sacrificed and the DNA was extracted. It is difficult to evaluate the results of these studies. Although the percent adenine/thymine is higher in the DNA extracted from the exposed animals, which could be responsible for the drop in the transition curve, the identical values cited for each measurement of the DNA extracted from the three groups of control animals are highly unlikely. Based on the variability normally inherent in these biochemical measures, a more probable explanation is that the control values were a pool of all the control groups or represent just one of those groups. Since the normal experimental variability in the measurements is not described—either for repeated measures on one DNA-extraction preparation, or between extraction preparations—it is impossible to conclude that the observed differences between control and exposed samples are significant and are due to the exposure directly, rather than to differences induced by the extraction procedures. Similarly, the crude SAR values estimated for testicular exposures appear to be too low to produce the types of damage cited by these authors. A more likely explanation is that the assumptions underlying either the SAR estimates or the exposure conditions are in error and that elevated temperatures produced by the exposures were the causative factor. In an anesthetized animal, exposed in the near field to 1.7 GHz at $50\,mW/cm^2$ for 30 min and shielded with loaded urethane foam except for the testes (est. SAR = 2.4 W/kg), a 1 to 2°C colonic temperature increase was recorded following exposure (Varma and Traboulay, 1977). In another report, animals were exposed under the same conditions, except that the exposure time varied between 30 and 40 min, and the testes were examined histologically (Varma and Traboulay, 1975). The lumens were empty with complete disintegration of spermatids, Sertoli cells, and the delicate connective tissue that surrounds the seminiferous tubules. In the same report, for animals exposed to 1.7 GHz at $10\,mW/cm^2$ there was little or no damage to the tests, except when the time of exposure was increased to 100 min, whereupon severe changes in morphology were observed. There was no explanation as to why little or no damage suddenly becomes severe changes at 100 min of exposure. It is probable that even at 10 mW/cm^2 there is sufficient energy deposition in these anesthetized animals to overcome any thermoregulatory function that may exist, and cause significant temperature elevation that results in many of the changes that are attributed to the microwave exposure directly. Thus, an evaluation of the existing evidence from physical studies on DNA indicates that low-to-moderate-intensity microwave radiation (1) does not cause changes in DNA bases, the fundamental unit of the genetic code, and (2) may cause disruptions in the pairing of the two complementary strands as well as other damage when substantial temperature elevations occur during exposure.

Manikowska et al. (1979) reported a non-dose-dependent increase in chromosome translocations and in chromosome pairs remaining as univalents at metaphase I in the sperm cells of mice exposed 1 hr/day, 5 days/week, for 2 weeks to 9.4 GHz pulsed at either 200, 1000, 2000, or 20,000 mW/cm^2 peak (pulse width 0.5 μsec; 1-kHz PRR; 0.1, 0.5, 1, and 10 mW/cm^2 average, respectively). A rough estimate of the SAR is 5 W/kg (average) and 9000 W/kg (peak), for the highest power density used. The authors do not describe the relationship of the animals' testes to the incident field, thereby raising the question of the actual exposure received by the target cells at 9.4 GHz, where the tissues exhibit large attenuation coefficients. A description of the environmental conditions during exposure is also not given. These omissions essentially prevent any critical assessment of the results. Furthermore, because of the small number of animals used in the study, the authors state that "the findings ... obviously need confirmation on larger number of animals ...."

Berman and Carter (1978) exposed male rats daily to 425 MHz CW (day 12 of gestation to 90 days of age, 10 mW/cm^2 4 hr/day) or 2450 MHz CW at 5, 10, or 28 mW/cm^2 from day 6 of gestation to 90 days of age, 4 or 5 hr/day. No significant evidence of germ cell mutagenesis or alteration in reproductive efficiency was detected.

Berman et al. (1980) exposed male mice to 2.45 GHz CW using three treatment regimens: 4 hr/day from day 6 of gestation to 90 days of age at 5 mW/cm^2 (SAR varied from 4.7 W/kg to ~ 0.9 W/kg at day 90 because of the growth of the animals), 5 hr/day for 5 days beginning on day 90 at 10 mW/cm^2 (est. SAR 2 W/kg), and 4 hr/day, 5 days/week, for 4 weeks beginning on day 90 at 28 mW/cm^2 (est. SAR 5.6 W/kg). At selected weekly periods after treatment, the exposed males were bred to untreated females that were examined in late pregnancy using the dominant lethal test. No significant germ-cell mutagenesis was detected for any treatment condition, even though significant increases in colonic and testicular temperature were observed during the 28 mW/cm^2 exposure with a concomitant decrease in pregnancies during some of the breeding periods, which indicates temporary sterility. In addition, these authors reexamined the data of Varma and Traboulay (1976) and Varma *et al.* (1976) and concluded that they had been incorrectly interpreted, because the effects of litter size on fetal mortality had been ignored and the differences between treated and control groups had been overemphasized when the control values were not representative of normal values. Thus, well-controlled experiments with biological systems having complex genomes similar to man's have not unequivocally demonstrated any mutagenic activity for microwave radiation.

There is no satisfactory evidence of microwave-induced genetic effects at low to modest power densities (Baranski and Czerski, 1976). It is known that the rate of induction of mutation increases with increasing temperature. It is possible, therefore, that artifacts or thermal stress could be factors in some of the reported studies.

Several studies on primitive organisms (Baranski *et al.*, 1976, 1978; Blackman *et al.*, 1976) and on rodents (Varma *et al.*, 1976; Varma and Traboulay, 1976; Leach, 1976) have confirmed earlier findings that microwave exposure at power densities below 10 mW/cm^2 is not mutagenic in these organisms.

Changes of cell membrane permeability have also been attributed to RF energy (Baranski *et al.*, 1974). Washed rabbit erythrocytes and isolated peritoneal granulocytes were irradiated with 3000-CW MHz microwaves at a power density of 1 mW/cm^2 for 15, 30, 60, 120, and 180 min. No increase in temperature of the suspensions was observed under these conditions. Irradiation at 1 mW/cm^2 for 15 and 30 min resulted in efflux of potassium from erythrocytes, followed by appearance of hemoglobin and lowering of osmotic resistance after 120 and 180 min of irradiation.

Hamrick (1973) examined the response of mammalian lymphocytes to 2450-MHz CW microwave exposure. Lymphocytes were exposed in cultures to 20 mW/cm^2 (7 mW/g) for 48 hr and examined for stimulation by changes in [^{3}H]thymidine uptake. Changes in the stimulation caused by PHA under control and exposed conditions were also tested. No effects of exposure were detected. No effect on DNA was found at power densities as high as 67 to 160 mW/g (~ 200–300 mW/cm^2). He concluded, therefore, that microwave energy (2450 MHz CW) "has very little, if any, effect other than the effect of heating on the secondary structure of DNA as determined by comparison of thermal denaturation curves." Others (Liu and Cleary, 1977) have failed to find effects different from those resulting from RF heating. Janiak and Szmigielski (1977) likewise reported no significant differences in the sequence and time course of cell membrane injury between cells treated in a water bath and those heated with 2450-MHz microwaves.

Chen and Lin (1978) exposed Chinese hamster lung cells, V79, in a waveguide fitted with a micropipette containing the cell suspension.

Temperature was regulated by circulating cooling water through the waveguide around the micropipette. Samples were exposed to 2450 MHz CW for 20 min and allowed to grow in cultures for 12 days after exposure. The exposed cells divided at a slower rate and exhibited a fibroblast type of growth, in contrast to the controls. These cells were exposed at 400 mW/cm^2 (1059 W/kg calculated SAR) under conditions very similar to those where Harrison et al. (1980) found temperature elevations in the sample that were up to 0.3°C higher than the cooling bath. Chen and Lin (1978) state that temperature-treated controls at 38°C (1°C higher than the coolant temperature during microwave exposure) did not display the changes observed in the microwave-exposed cells. It is not clear whether the changes in the microwave-treated cells are caused by heating inside the micropipette.

Carpenter (1965) and van Ummersen and Cogan (1970) have reportedly suppressed the maturation of lens epithelium. The right eyes of adult New Zealand white rabbits were exposed to cataractogenic levels (120 mW/cm^2) of 1450-MHz CW microwaves; the nonirradiated left eyes served as controls. At postexposure intervals varying from 6 hr to 1 month, the animals were sacrificed. One hour before sacrifice, tritiated thymidine, which is an indicator of cell cycle activity, was injected into the anterior chambers of both eyes. The irradiated lenses showed an initial pronounced suppression of both DNA synthesis and cell division. These effects gradually diminished during the ensuing 2 weeks, by which time cell progression had recovered and by 1 month postirradiation they were proceeding at a slightly accelerated rate. In several of the irradiated eyes, however, there was superimposed upon the usual course of recovery a precipitous rise in DNA synthesis occurring on the fourth to fifth day after exposure. This sharp rise in DNA synthesis is similar to that which is observed in galactose-fed rats when hydration of the lens occurs in the form of equatorial vesicles, which seem to stimulate the overlying epithelium to proliferate at a greatly accelerated rate. The metabolic stimulus of heat from this level of exposure should not be ignored.

It is thus reasonable to conclude that exposure to RF/MW energy does not appear to cause mutations or genetic changes in test systems unless temperatures well above the normal physiological range are produced. Similarly, no physical changes in chromosomes, DNA, or reproductive potential of animals have been reported in the absence of substantial temperature rises.

7.7. HYPERTHERMIA AND CELL KINETICS

Significant investigations on the effects of microwave-induced hyperthermia on cell kinetics have provided background information on the potential application of hyperthermia as an adjunct in cancer therapy. Moressi (1964) compared the influence of temperature and chronic 2450-MHz CW exposure on mouse sarcoma 180 cells. Tumor cell suspensions were irradiated with a field intensity of approximately 0.3 W/cm^2 at temperatures ranging from 43°C to 38°C. Cell mortality patterns were essentially identical for irradiated and nonirradiated cells when microwave-induced heat was dissipated at a rate that ensured comparable temperatures for both experimental and control systems. Rate of cell growth depression appeared to be highly temperature dependent as would be expected from the "spontaneous" destruction of cellular material.

Rats with hepatoma 223 were subjected to 3-GHz microwaves for 8–10 min by suspending the tumor-bearing limb in front of an open waveguide (Carter *et al.*, 1964). The tumor temperatures measured with a thermocouple ranged from 45 to 47°C. Little effect was evident, probably because of the short heating period. Other investigators, however, such as Overgaard and Overgaard (1972) treated mouse mammary adenocarcinoma locally with 27.12-MHz diathermy. A permanent cure was observed in approximately 25% of the treated mice when the degree of heating and duration of exposure were optimal. Other investigators such as Yerushalmi (1975) and Mendecki *et al.* (1976) have also used microwaves in experimental tumors with intriguing results.

Key and Charyulu (1976) exposed Chinese hamster cells to 2450 MHz raising the temperature to various levels between 34°C and 45°C for periods up to 5 hr. Several indices of cell damage were measured including inhibition of colony formation and vital dye exclusion. The therapeutic effect of the microwave exposure was assessed by using it to locally heat Ehrlich ascites cells grown intraperitoneally in mice. A temperature of 42.5°C for a period of 30 min repeated for several days generally produced extended survival times but very few total cures. Marmor *et al.* (1977) using 13.5 MHz for heating to 43–44°C were able to effect cures in mice with a large variety of transplanted tumors. The use of microwave-induced heating as an adjunct to other methods of cancer therapy is a fascinating area of investigation.

Overt thermal effects due to RF/MW energy absorption have been demonstrated and documented. The reports of effects that appear to depend on specific frequencies and amplitudes or "windows" (Bawin and Adey, 1977) would imply biological responses that may not always be due to a rise in temperature. Prohofsky and Lu (1979) have suggested that low-lying longitudinal vibrational modes of DNA molecules could be induced or enhanced by electromagnetic fields at microwave frequencies of 3 GHz or higher. Such induced modes could theoretically produce conformational changes in the DNA molecule and could result in biologically significant functional alterations. Fröhlich (1975) has similarly suggested microwave interactions with macromolecular biologically active complexes. Illinger (1976, 1978) has treated the problem of molecular interaction from a quantum mechanical approach. He suggests the possibility of field-induced quasi-resonant transitions occurring at frequencies higher than 10 GHz from the excitation of coherent vibrational modes. Although some experiments seem to provide results that support such a theory, it has been pointed out that great care must be exercised in differentiating between actual biological interactions and cyclic and multiple resonances in cavity, waveguide, and other exposure systems that have the capability of creating multiple reflections (Hershberger, 1978).

The principal technical problem in studying RF-induced effects on cells is that the studies are often conducted using conventional apparatus designed for cell studies—flasks, dishes, holders, agitators, water baths, incubators, and so on. Various elements of these apparatus may distort RF fields in such a way that the SAR in the cell cultures may be considerably higher or lower than field measurements would indicate. Some progress has been made in designing cell culture apparatus that will provide accurate, calibrated exposure to RF fields, but results of much of the earlier work on cell and tissue cultures must be questioned with regard to the actual absorbed RF energy in the cell culture media (Guy, 1977; Michaelson, 1970, 1978).

Our present knowledge of biophysical mechanisms underlying cell membrane function, and functional and structural properties of subcellular components is limited. Interpretation of studies of such phenomena and their biological significance, therefore, requires considerable circumspection. The anomalous behavior of the "bound water" of membranes as reported by Grant (1978) may help in providing explanations for such effects.

Conclusion

In investigations concerning the effects of MW/RF energies on biological systems, especially when some form of cellular response is involved, temperature control must be a major consideration.

Guy (1977) has noted that in analyzing the data from many experiments involving the effects of electromagnetic fields on cell cultures, blood samples, and solutions containing microorganisms, there have been some questions concerning the exact magnitude of the fields and temperature within the solutions during exposure. Often the samples are placed in fields of known strength and power density, but due to the complex shapes of the vessels holding the samples, the actual fields acting on the cells or organisms are unknown. Also, it is difficult in some cases to determine whether the effects are specifically due to the fields or simply due to a temperature rise. Attempts at measuring the temperature of fields within the sample by conventional methods can produce perturbations that may significantly modify the results of the experiment.

Because of the questionable techniques utilized, reports concerning the genetic implications of microwave exposure are highly suspect, especially since hyperthermia by itself has been shown to induce chromosome damage and gene mutations in a wide range of organisms (Lindegren, 1972).

It is known that hydrogen bond energy (perhaps the weakest bond of all) is nearly 5 kcal. Microwave energy is too low to produce nonthermal effects on the structure of DNA. Takashima (1966) using changes in optical density and viscosity as criteria for strand separation and, thus, structural change, failed to observe structural changes in DNA from exposure to pulsed energy (10 Hz–10 kHz and 100 kHz–10 MHz) at levels of 300 V (peak-to-peak) across the radiation cell.

The effects of RF/MW energies on cells and tissues should be investigated by reliable and carefully controlled techniques that are sufficiently sensitive to detect cellular damage in the absence of thermal influence. An essential element in the proof of mutagenicity is the establishment of a field intensity/time-related effect. Such studies should be free of interacting variables and should permit valid extrapolation to the whole organism with its multiple interdependent, integrated functions. In addition, testing must not be confined to one organism or cell type, but investigations must include a wide range of both *in vivo* and *in vitro* systems. If possible, testing should be done in parallel with recognized genetic tests, since only in this way will it be possible to decide which methods constitute a meaningful way of assessing genetic hazards from chromosomal aberration studies (Savage, 1971).

7.8. EFFECTS ON INVERTEBRATES

Historically, the effects of RF energy on insects were one of the earliest of the biological effects of nonionizing radiation to be studied: the possibilities for insect control using RF energy were explored in the 1930's (Ark and Parry, 1940). Insects at all metamorphic stages—egg, larva, pupa, and adult—have been the subject of RF radiation studies, both to evaluate the pertinent effects on invertebrates and, as in the earlier work, to hopefully arrive at inexpensive, effective schemes for insect control in the food and related industries.

7.8.1. Genetic Effects

It has been reported that when insects are exposed to RF fields, the first reaction is an attempt to escape; this is followed by disturbance of motor coordination, stiffening, immobility, and, after a certain interval, death, with the period of exposure required to kill depending on the type of insect. *Drosophila,* for example, survives longer than 30 min, while certain tropical species live only a few seconds at the same field intensity. Changes have also been noted in the concentrations of a great variety of metabolic products. Exposure to RF fields also affects embryogenesis: the period required for a butterfly to complete its metamorphosis is changed; gastrulation and the growth of larvae are accelerated (Marha *et al.,* 1968).

Drosophila melanogaster, the fruit fly, has been used in several studies to investigate possible genetic effects of microwave exposure since it has a well-described genetic system with a short generation time, large broods, ease of exposure, and minimal space requirements. Heller and Mickey (1961) and Mickey (1963) claim that somatic and genetic changes are produced in *D. melanogaster* by RF energy. In some experiments, flies were apparently exposed for 5 min to 1 hr to 5–40 MHz (15–30 μsec, 500–1000 pulses/sec, 250–6000 V/m peak). According to the authors, the number of lethal and externally manifested mutations increased approximately 13-fold as compared with the mean number of such mutations in control populations. The most effective frequency appeared to be 21 MHz, leading to the contention of frequency-specific effects. The genetic tests employed were not described nor were any data given with regard to the frequency of their observations. No temperature recordings were reported. From a careful analysis of these reports, it would appear that any response seen results from high E-field exposure under pulsed conditions. The authors did not determine thresholds, yet the lowest field value reported with damaging effects appears to correspond roughly to 53 W/cm^2.

The effects of chronic exposure of colonies of *D. melanogaster* larvae to 2450-MHz CW microwaves have been investigated by Imig and Searle (1962) and Searle *et al.* (1961). The larvae were exposed to power densities of up to ~ 1.0 W/cm^2. To eliminate the thermal effects of the exposure, the temperatures of the experimental and control groups were maintained at a constant 28°C. The larvae were exposed throughout their entire period of growth. Two experiments were conducted at approximately 0.3 W/cm^2. For an average $69\frac{1}{2}$ hr duration, the ratio of the exposed to control growth constants showed no significant difference from unity, having a value of 0.9 ± 0.058. Larvae were also irradiated for an average period of 48 hr at a power density of ~ 1.0 W/cm^2. In this case the ratio of the irradiated to control growth constants was 1.02 ± 0.025 and was also not significantly different from the control values of unity. Larvae were exposed to 0.3 W/cm^2 without the dissipation of heat. For irradiation periods of 20, 30, and 45 min, $\sim 95\%$ of the larvae survived. The equilibrium temperature noted was $\sim 30°C$, which is compatible with survival of these larvae. The results of these investigations seem to indicate the absence of specific or nonthermal effects upon *D. melanogaster*.

Beyer et al. (1970) also investigated the potential mutagenicity of 2450-MHz microwaves on *D. melanogaster*. Males were placed in an acrylic capsule 18 cm from the antenna and exposed to 2450-MHz CW energy generated at forward powers of 2.1, 2.75, and 3.0 kW. The 2.75-kW level was lethal to two of five flies. Each irradiated fly was serially placed with two virgin Muller-5 females at 24-hr intervals for a total of 15 days (30 females per male). Sham-exposed control flies at each radiation level were similarly mated. The F_1 generation times showed no effect. Total F_1 production and sex ratios (female/total) showed statistically significant daily deviations, but no trends were present. Sex-linked lethal mutations were not observed.

In contrast to the studies of Heller and Mickey (1961) and Mickey (1963) who reported a tenfold rise in sex-linked recessive mutations after pulsed radiation in the frequency range 30–60 MHz generated by capacitor plates, Beyer et al. (1970) did not find a rise in sex-linked recessive mutations after 2450-MHz CW radiation. No mutagenic effects were reported by Hamnerius et al. (1979) in embryos exposed in water at 24.5°C to 2450 MHz CW at 100 W/kg for 6 hr. Negative effects were also reported by Pay et al. (1972) who exposed adult males to 2450 MHz for 45 min at 4600, 5900, or 6500 mW/cm^2 (est. SARs 140, 190, and 210 W/kg, respectively) and mated the surviving males individually with two virgin females on each of 15 consecutive days. No changes were observed in the generation time or sex ratio pattern of the offspring, which were then mated and observed for possible sex-linked lethal mutations in their offspring. Such mutations were not found at frequencies greater than 1%, a detection limit based on the small number of chromosomes (less than 800) actually evaluated. Mittler (1976) exposed adult males from various strains of *D. melanogaster* to 29 MHz CW at 600 V/m (SAR ca. 0.024 W/kg) and to 146 MHz CW at 62.5 V/m (SAR ca. 0.015 W/kg) for 12 hr and mated them with virgin females for 12 hr every 2 days for four or five broods. There were no mutations induced by these treatments as evidenced by the lack of chromosome loss, nondisjunction, or sex-linked recessive lethals. In addition, Mittler (1977) observed no mutagenic effects (recessive lethals) when adult females were exposed to 98.5 MHz, frequency modulated with audio, at 0.3 V/m (est. SAR 0.0004 W/kg), 134 hr/week for 32 weeks.

Beyer et al. (1970) note that the extent of coupling between *Drosophila* and 2450-MHz microwave energy is in question because of the small size of the fly. Clustering of flies could account for the observed lethality. The number of flies may affect the observed lethality. It has been suggested that body dehydration during exposure could cause lethality. This idea was supported by microscopic examination, which revealed physical deformation of the thorax after receiving lethal microwave exposure (Tell, 1972).

While the results with *Drosophila* are difficult to extrapolate to humans, it is nevertheless worthy of note that this test system as a qualitative index was not able to detect any mutagenic alterations due to RF radiation over a wide frequency range.

In order to explain some of the results obtained with *Drosophila*, Tell (1972) exposed a group of 6-day-old, male, wild-type *D. melanogaster* to 2450 MHz for 55 min at an "intense" field. A dramatic change in body weight (about 65% reduction) resulted. To assess the absorption efficiency of the fruit flies, their absorption cross section to plane electromagnetic waves was computed. The important result of these calculations is that a fly presents an effective area for electromagnetic absorption of approximately 1/1000 of its geometric cross section. Clearly then, the fruit fly is a very inefficient test system with respect to imparting absorbed microwave energy at this frequency. It is possible, nevertheless, that the fruit fly might be reasonably responsive to absorbed energy provided adequate energy can be delivered and accurately measured. A rough estimate of the thermal dose–effect dependence from microwave exposure was made, based on the assumption that the fly is, for practical purposes, a black body radiator. If the fly is to be heated above the ambient temperature, it would take a power density of about 1.044×10^5 W/m^2 to raise the fly's temperature 1°C above an ambient of 25°C. This corresponds to a thermal flux of 0.562×10^{-3} cal (Tell, 1972).

7.8.2. Specific Effects: Insect Control

The response of insects to RF fields has been used to eradicate insect contaminants from grains (Baker et al., 1956; Frings, 1952; Whitney et al., 1961). It appears that the more specialized insects are the most susceptible to microwave exposure. It has been suggested that their more elaborate nervous system is less tolerant to exposure than are less highly specialized forms (Frings, 1952). The total temperature rise during treatment is thought to be important (Whitney et al., 1961). This indicates that thermal energy is the lethal factor since organisms incubated at low temperatures are less heat tolerant than are those incubated at higher levels. It has also been suggested that larvae are more tolerant than adults because of the absence of appendages, which act as conducting paths to the body, rather than their having a simpler nervous system (Frings, 1952).

Hirose et al. (1975) examined batch and conveyor 2450-MHz microwave exposure systems as alternatives to the conventional fumigation, spraying, and plant cleaning routinely used to control tobacco moths and cigarette beetles in manufacturing processes. Insects at all stages of metamorphosis were exposed to microwave energy at various power levels of up to 2 kW/kg tobacco, and for time durations adequate to produce final temperatures of 40°C to 60°C. Adult insects were found to be the most susceptible to exposure. Larvae surviving microwave exposure were found to produce adults identical to those from control populations, which ruled out genetic damage from the exposures. Mortality was found to approach 100% when the final temperature was 53°C or greater, The results observed were ascribed to: (1) differential absorption where the insects absorbed more power than their surroundings, (2) a possible inability of the insects to survive the thermal shock created by rapid turn-on of the microwave energy, and (3) a possible susceptibility to high electric field intensities. Differential absorption was partially confirmed through observations of lethality as a function of insect size. The thermal shock postulate was supported, but not confirmed, by exposure time tests. The electric field intensity postulate was checked by the authors by repeating the experiments at other frequencies, including 30 MHz, which suggested plausibility.

Larvae of the mealworm beetle, *Tenebrio molitor,* were exposed to two different intensities of 39 MHz (Kadoum et al., 1967a,b). An electrode voltage of 3.6 kV was used for one experiment, and 0.9 kV for another. Adults developing from larvae exposed at sublethal levels exhibited malformed and missing legs. It was concluded that the deformities most likely resulted from heat damage to the histoblasts that project into the legs of the sixth or last-instar larva. Mortality increased with exposure time and voltage applied across the holder. Mortality continued to increase over a 2-week period following exposure. Internal thoracic temperatures increased almost linearly with length of exposure. Temperatures in the thorax and last abdominal segment were significantly higher than temperatures in the cervical region or in the first and fourth abdominal segments, probably because the appendages in this region caused development of higher electric field intensities. Measured thoracic temperatures approached levels that were normally lethal, so that internal heating was suggested as the cause of death (Kadoum et al., 1967c).

Carpenter and Livstone (1971) studied the effects of 10-GHz CW microwaves on pupae of *T. molitor.* Each pupa was inserted into a waveguide and irradiated at 80 mW/cm^2 for either 20 or 30 min or at

$20\,mW/cm^2$ for 120 min, after which development was observed. In control groups, 90% metamorphosed to become normal adult beetles. In the exposed groups, only 24% developed normally; 25% died and 51% developed abnormally. When these thermal conditions within pupae were duplicated by radiant heating, subsequent development of pupae was normal in 80% of the experiments. The authors concluded that the abnormalities induced by microwave radiation were not a thermal effect.

Later studies by Lindauer et al. (1974) suggested that pulsed microwaves produced comparable effects as did CW microwaves at an equivalent "dosage", defined as energy level-exposure duration. Apparently total dose and not dose rate more nearly determines the extent of the morphological alteration (Liu et al., 1975). In experiments conducted by Olsen (1977) at 4.0 and 5.95 GHz and a calculated energy dose of 37.8 to 1526 J/g with exposures of 5 min to 6 hr, morphological alteration was found for both E-field and H-field exposures in both parallel and perpendicular polarization.

The probability of extremely high local fields created in exposures of *Tenebrio*, nutritional and health status of the organism, or the possibility of posthatching cannibalism were apparently not considered by many of these authors (Green et al., 1977). Olsen (1977) noted teratogenesis to be associated with a rise of pupal temperature in excess of 10°C.

REFERENCES

Alam, M. T., N. Barthakur, N. G. Lambert, and S. S. Kasatiya (1978) Cytological effects of microwave radiation in Chinese hamster cells in vitro. *Can. J. Genet. Cytol.* **20**:23.

Allis, J. W. (1975) Irradiation of bovine serum albumin with a crossed-beam exposure-detection system. *Ann. N.Y. Acad. Sci.* **247**:312.

Allis, J. W., and M. L. Fromme (1976) Pseudosubstrate binding to ribonuclease during exposure to microwave radiation at 1.70 and 2.45 GHz. In: *Biological Effects of Electromagnetic Waves*, Vol. I, C. C. Johnson and M. L. Shore (eds.). HEW Publ. (FDA) 77-80010, pp. 366–376.

Allis, J. W., and M. L. Fromme (1979) Activity of membrane-bound enzymes exposed to sinusoidally modulated 2450 MHz microwave radiation. *Radio Sci.* **14**(S):85.

Ames, B. N., J. McCann, and E. Yamasaki (1975) Methods for detecting carcinogens and mutagens with the *Salmonella* mammalian-microsome mutagenicity test. *Mutat. Res.* **31**:347.

Ark, P. A., and W. Parry (1940) Application of high-frequency electrostatic fields in agriculture. *Q. Rev. Biol.* **16**:172.

Averbeck, D., M. Dardalhon, and A. J. Berteaud (1976) Microwave action in procaryotic and eucaryotic cells and a possible interaction with X-rays. *J. Microwave Power* **11**:143.

Baker, V. H., D. E. Wiant, and O. Taboada (1956) Some effects of microwaves on certain insects which infest wheat and flour. *J. Econ. Entomol.* **49**:33.

Baldwin, R. E., M. Cloninger, and M. L. Fields (1968) Growth and destruction of *Salmonella typhimurium* in egg white foam products cooked by microwaves. *J. Appl. Microbiol.* **16**:1929.

Baranski, S., and P. Czerski (1976) *Biological Effects of Microwaves.* Dowden, Hutchinson & Ross, Stroudsburg, Pa.

Baranski, S., S. Szmigielski, and J. Moneta (1974) Effect of microwave irradiation in vitro on cell permeability. In: *Biological Effects and Health Hazards of Microwave Radiation,* P. Czerski, K. Ostrowski, M. L. Shore, C. Silverman, M. J. Suess, and B. Waldeskog (eds.). Polish Medical Publishers, Warsaw, p. 173.

Baranski, S., H. Debiec, K. Kwarecki, and T. Mezykowski (1976) Influence of microwaves on genetical processes of *Aspergillus nidulans. J. Microwave Power* **11**:146.

Baranski, S., J. Bal, H. Debiec, K. Kwarecki, and T. Mezykowski (1978) The influence of microwaves on genetic apparatus functions. *Proc. Biol. Eff. E.M. Waves.* XIX Gen. Assembly. Int. Union Radio Sci., Helsinki (Abstract).

Barber, D. E. (1962) The reaction of luminous bacteria to microwave radiation exposures in the frequency range of 2608.7–3082.3 Mc. *IRE Trans. Bio-Med. Electron.* **9**:77.

Bawin, S. M., and W. R. Adey (1977) Calcium binding in cerebral tissues. In: *Biological Effects and Measurement of Radiofrequency/Microwaves,* D. G. Hazzard (ed.). HEW Publ. (FDA) 77-8026, pp. 305–313.

Belkhode, M. L., D. L. Johnson, and A. M. Miro (1974a) Thermal and athermal effects of microwave radiation on the activity of glucose-6-phosphate dehydrogenase in human blood. *Health Phys.* **26**:45.

Belkhode, M. L., A. M. Miro, and D. L. Johnson (1974b) Thermal and athermal effects of 2.8 GHz microwaves on three human serum enzymes. *J. Microwave Power* **9**:23.

Bender, M. A. (1967) Effects of radiation on chromosomes. In: *Symposium on the Pacific Uses of Atomic Radiation.* Rio de Janeiro, ORNL-P-3201, Oak Ridge National Laboratory.

Berman, E., and H. Carter (1978) Mutagenic and reproductive tests in male rats exposed to 425 or 2450 MHz (CW) microwaves. *Proc. Biol. Eff. E.M. Waves.* XIX Gen. Assembly. Int. Union Radio Sci., Helsinki (Abstract).

Berman, E., H. B. Carter, and D. House (1980) Tests of mutagenesis, and reproduction in male rats exposed to 2450 MHz (CW) microwaves. *Bioelectromagnetics* **1**:65.

Beyer, E. C., T. L. Pay, and E. T. Irwin, Jr. (1970) Developmental and genetic testing of Drosophila with 2450 MHz microwave radiation. In: *Radiation Bio-effects Summary Report, January–December 1970,* D. M. Hodge (ed.). HEW, PHS, BRH Publ. BRH/DBE 70-7 (December), p. 45.

Bini, M., A. Checcucci, A. Ighesti, L. Millanta, N. Rubino, C. Camici, G. Marino, and G. Ramponi (1978) Analysis of the effects of microwave energy on enzymatic activity of lactate dehydrogenase (LDH). *J. Microwave Power* **13**:95.

Blackman, C. F., Jr., and R. Tell (1972) Biological response to microwave irradiation: Bacteria. In: Twinbrook Research Laboratory Annual Report 1971. U.S. Environmental Protection Agency, Washington, D.C., p. 106.

Blackman, C. F., S. G. Benane, C. M. Weil, and J. S. Ali (1975) Effects of nonionizing electromagnetic radiation on single-cell biologic systems. *Ann. N.Y. Acad. Sci.* **247**:352.

Blackman, C. F., M. C. Surles, and S. G. Benane (1976) The effects of microwave exposure on bacteria: Mutation induction. In: *Biological Effects of Electromagnetic Waves,* Vol. I, C. C. Johnson and M. L. Shore (eds.). HEW Publ. (FDA) 77-8010, pp. 406–413.

Brooks, A. L., and F. W. Lengemann (1967) Comparison of radiation-induced chromatid aberrations in the testes and bone marrow of the Chinese hamster. *Radiat. Res.* **32**:587.

Brown, G. H., and W. C. Morrison (1954) An exploration of the effects of strong radio-frequency fields on microorganisms in aqueous solutions. *Food Technol.* **8**:361.

Carlson, J. G., and N. G. Harrington (1965) X-ray induced "stickiness" of the chromo-

somes of the Chortophaga neuroblast in relation to dose and mitotic stage at treatment. *Radiat. Res.* **2**:84.
Carpenter, R. (1959) Inhibitory effect of microwave radiation on differentiation in Neurospora. In: *Proceedings of the Third Annual Tri-Service Conference on Biological Effects of Microwave Radiating Equipments,* C. Süsskind (ed.). University of California, Berkeley, p. 289.
Carpenter, R. L. (1965) Suppression of differentiation in living tissues exposed to microwave radiation. In: *Digest 6th Int. Conf. Med. Electron. Biomed. Eng.,* Tokyo, p. 573.
Carpenter, R. L., and E. M. Livstone (1971) Evidence for nonthermal effects of microwave radiation: Abnormal development of irradiated insect pupae. *IEEE Trans. Microwave Theory Tech.* **MTT-19**:173.
Carroll, D. E., and A. Lopez (1969) Lethality of radiofrequency energy upon microorganisms in liquid, buffered, and alcoholic food systems. *J. Food Sci.* **34**:320.
Cater, D. B., I. A. Silver, and D. A. Watkinson (1964) Combined therapy with 220 KV roentgen and 10 cm microwave heating in rat hepatoma. *Acta Radiol. Ther. Phys. Biol. (NS)* **2**:321.
Chen, K. C., and C. J. Lin (1978) A system for studying effects of microwaves on cells in culture. *J. Microwave Power* **13**:251.
Chen, K. M., A. Samuel, and R. Hoopingavner (1974) Chromosomal aberrations of living cells induced by microwave radiation. *Environ. Lett.* **6**:37.
Chu, E. H. Y., N. H. Giles, and K. Passano (1961) Types and frequencies of human chromosome aberrations induced by X rays. *Proc. Natl. Acad. Sci. USA* **47**:830.
Chukhlovin, B. A. (1965) The effect of SHF-UHF electromagnetic radiation on the immunobiological properties of the organism. *Voen. Med. Zh.* **7**:25.
Chukhlovin, B. A. (1971) Changes in immunologic reactivity of the organism and in the properties of bacteria, virus, and simple animals. In: *Influence of Microwave Radiation on the Organism of Man and Animals,* I. R. Petrov (ed.). Meditsina Press, Leningrad, 1970 (NASA TT F-708, p. 88).
Coate, W. H., and S. S. Hoo (1970) Plant cytogenetic study. In: *Project Sanguine Biological Effects Test Program Pilot Studies,* Hazelton Labs., Inc. Final report on Contract N0039-69-C-1572, AD 717408.
Corelli, J. C., R. J. Gutmann, S. Kohazi, and J. Levy (1977) Effects of 2.6–4.0 GHz microwave radiation on *E. coli* B. *J. Microwave Power* **12**:141.
Dardalhon, M., D. Averbeck, and A. J. Berteaud (1981) Studies on possible genetic effects of microwaves in procaryotic and eucaryotic cells. *Radiat. Environ. Biophys.* **20**:37.
Dessel, M. M., E. Bowersox, and W. Jester (1960) Bacteria in electronically cooked foods. *J. Am. Diet. Assoc.* **37**:230.
Dumansky, Y. D., and V. F. Rudichenko (1976) Dependence of the functional activity of liver mitochondria on super-high frequency radiation. *Gig. Sanit.* **4**:16.
Dutta, S. K., W. H. Nelson, C. F. Blackman, and D. J. Brusick (1979a) Lack of microbial genetic response to 2.45-GHz CW and 8.5–9.6-GHz pulsed microwaves. *J. Microwave Power* **14**:275.
Dutta, S. K., M. A. Hossain, H. S. Ho, and C. F. Blackman (1979b) Effects of 8.6 GHz pulsed electromagnetic radiation on an *Escherichia coli* repair deficient mutant. In: *Electromagnetic Fields in Biological Systems,* S. S. Stuchly (ed.). IMPI, Edmonton, Canada, pp. 76–95.
Dutta, S. K., W. H. Nelson, C. F. Blackman, and D. J. Brusick (1980) Cellular effects in microbial tester strains caused by exposure to microwaves or elevated temperatures. *J. Environ. Pathol. Toxicol.* **3**:195.

Elder, J. A., and J. S. Ali (1975) The effect of microwaves (2450 MHz) on isolated rat liver mitochondria. *Ann. N.Y. Acad. Sci.* **247**:251.

Elder, J. A., J. S. Ali, M. D. Long, and G. E. Anderson (1976) A coaxial air line microwave exposure system. 1. Respiratory activities of mitochondria irradiated at 2–4 GHz. In: *Biological Effects of Electromagnetic Waves,* Vol. I, C. C. Johnson and M. L. Shore (eds.). HEW Publ. (FDA) 77–8010, pp. 352–365.

Epstein, N., and H. Cook (1951) The effects of microwaves on the Rous N 1 fowl sarcoma virus, *Br. J. Cancer* **5**:244.

Evans, H. J. (1967) Actions of radiations on chromosomes. In: *Scientific Basis of Medicine.* Annual Reviews, Palo Alto, Calif., pp. 321–339.

Fabian, F. W., and H. T. Graham (1933) Influence of high-frequency displacement currents on bacteria. *J. Infect. Dis.* **55**:76.

Faitel'berg-Blank, V. R., and G. Sivorinovs'kiy (1972) The effect of ultrasound and superhigh frequency (3 cm wavelength) electromagnetic field on liver and kidney mitochondrial oxidative phosphorylation. *Fiziol. Zh. Akad. Nauk UKR* SRS **18**:808.

Fleming, H. (1944) Effect of high frequency fields on microorganisms. *Electrical Eng.* **63**:18.

Frank-Kamenetskii, D. A. (1961) Plasma effects in semiconductors and biological effect of radiowaves. *Dokl. Akad. Sci. USSR* **136**:476. English translation in *Sov. Phys. Dokl.* **6**:91.

Friend, A. W., Jr., E. D. Finch, and H. P. Schwan (1975) Low frequency (1 Hz–10 MHz) electric field-induced changes in the shape and motility of amoebas. *Science* **187**:357.

Frings, H. (1952) Factors determining the effects of radio-frequency electromagnetic fields on insects and materials they infest. *J. Econ. Entomol.* **45**:396.

Fröhlich, H. (1975) The extraordinary dielectric properties of biological materials and the action of enzymes. *Proc. Natl. Acad. Sci. USA.* **72**:4211.

Gilles, E. (1944) Lethal effects of ultrashort waves on micro-organisms. *C. R. Soc. Biol.* **123**:546.

Goldblith, S. A., and D. I. Wang (1967) Effect of microwaves on *Escherichia coli* and *Bacillus subtilis*. *Appl. Microbiol.* **15**:1371.

Grant, E. (1978) Determination of bound water in biologic materials from dielectric measurements. In: *The Physical Basis of Electromagnetic Interactions with Biological Systems,* L. S. Taylor and A. Y. Cheung (eds.). HEW Publ. (FDA) 78–8055, pp. 113–119.

Green, D. R., Jr., F. S. Rosenbaum, and W. F. Pickard (1977) Biological effects of microwaves on the pupae of Tenebrio molitor. In: *Biological Effects and Measurement of Radiofrequency/Microwaves,* D. G. Hazard (ed.). HEW Publ. (FDA) 77–8026, pp. 253–262.

Grundler, W., and F. Keilmann (1980) Frequency fine-tuning studies of microwave influenced yeast growth. Presented at the *International Symposium on Electromagnetic Waves and Biology,* Jouy-en-Josas, France.

Grundler, W., F. Keilmann, and H. Fröhlich (1977) Resonant growth rate response of yeast cells irradiated by weak microwaves. *Phys. Lett.* **62A**:463.

Guy, A. W. (1977) A method for exposing cell cultures to EM fields under conditions of controlled temperature and field strength. *Radio Sci.* **12**(6S):87.

Hamnerius, Y., H. Olofsson, A. Rasmuson, and B. Rasmuson (1979) A negative test for mutagenic action of microwave radiation in Drosophila melanogaster. *Mutat. Res.* **68**:217.

Hamrick, P. E. (1973) Thermal denaturation of DNA exposed to 2450 MHz CW microwave radiation. *Radiat. Res.* **56**:400.

Hamrick, P. E., and B. T. Butler (1973) Exposure of bacteria to 2450 MHz microwave radiation. *J. Microwave Power* **8**:227.

Harrison, G. H., J. E. Robinson, D. McCulloch, and A. Y. Cheung (1980) Comparison of

hyperthermal cellular survival in the presence or absence of 2.45 GHz microwave radiation. Presented at the *International Symposium on Electromagnetic Waves and Biology*, Jouy-en-Josas, France.
Heller, J. H. (1970) Cellular effects of microwave radiation. In: *Biological Effects and Health Implications of Microwave Radiation*, S. F. Cleary (ed.). HEW PHS, BRH/DBE 70-2, p. 116.
Heller, J. H., and G. H. Mickey (1961) Non-thermal effects of radiofrequency in biological systems. In: *Digest of the 1961 International Conference on Medical Electronics*, New York City, p. 152.
Heller, J. H., and A. A. Teixeira-Pinto (1959) A new physical method of creating chromosomal aberrations. *Nature (London)* **183**:905.
Henderson, H. M., K. Hergenroeder, and S. S. Stuchly (1975) Effect of 2450 MHz microwave radiation on horseradish peroxidase. *J. Microwave Power* **10**:27.
Hershberger, W. D. (1978) Microwave transmission through normal and tumor cells. *IEEE Trans. Microwave Theory Tech.* **MTT-26**:618.
Hill, D. W., M. J. Hagmann, A. Riazi, O. P. Gandhi, L. M. Partlow, and L. J. Stensaas (1978) Effect of millimeter waves on bacteria and viruses. *Proc. Biol. Eff. E.M. Waves.* XIX Gen. Assembly. Int. Union Radio Sci., Helsinki (Abst.).
Hirose, T., I. Abe, M. Kohno, T. Suziki, K. Oshima, and T. Okakura (1975) The use of microwave heating to control insects in cigarette manufacture. *J. Microwave Power* **10**:181.
Huang, A. T., M. E. Engle, J. A. Elder, J. B. Kinn, and T. R. Ward (1977) The effect of microwave radiation (2450 MHz) on the morphology and chromosomes of lymphocytes. *Radio Sci.* **12**:173.
Illinger, K. (1976) The attenuation function for biological fluids at millimeter and far-infrared wavelengths. In: *Biological Effects of Electromagnetic Waves*, Vol. II, C. C. Johnson and M. L. Shore (eds). HEW Publ. (FDA) 77-8011, pp. 169–183.
Illinger, K. (1978) Millimeter wave and far-infrared absorption in biological systems. In: *The Physical Basis of Electromagnetic Interaction with Biological Systems*, L. S. Taylor and A. T. Cheung (eds.). HEW Publ. (FDA) 78-8055, pp. 43–64.
Imig, C. J., and G. W. Searle (1962) Review of Work Conducted at State University of Iowa on Organisms exposed to 2450 mc cw Microwave Irradiation. Griffiss AFB, Rome Air Development Center, Rome, N.Y.
Ingram, M. (1969) Clinical and laboratory observations useful in estimating degree of radiation injury. In: *A Study of Early Radiation-Induced Biological Changes as Indicators of Radiation Injury*. FASEB, Bethesda.
Ismailov, E. S. (1966) Effect of microwaves on *Opalina ranarum*. *Vestn. Leningr. Univ. Ser. Biol. Geogr. Geol.* **2**:147.
Ismailov, E. S. (1977) Infrared spectra of erythrocyte ghosts in the region of the amide I and amide II bands on microwave irradiation. *Biophysics* **21**:960 (translation of *Biofizika* **21**:940, 1976).
Jacobs, S. E., M. J. Thornley, and P. Maurice (1950) The survival of bacteria in high-frequency electric fields. *Proc. Soc. Appl. Bacteriol.* **2**:161.
Janes, D. E., W. M. Leach, W. A. Mills, R. E. Moore, and M. L. Shore (1969) Effect of 2450 MHz microwaves on protein synthesis and on chromosomes in Chinese hamsters. *Non-Ioniz. Radiat.* **1**:125.
Janiak, M., and S. Szmigielski (1977) Injury of cell membranes in normal and SV40-virus transformed fibroblasts exposed in vitro to microwave (2,450 MHz) or water-bath hyperthermia (43 deg C). In: *Abstracts of the 1977 International Symposium on the Biological Effects of Electromagnetic Waves*, Airlie, Va.
Jaski, T., and C. Süsskind (1961) Electromagnetic radiation as a tool in the life sciences. *Science* **133**:443.

Kadoum, A. M., H. J. Ball, and S. O. Nelson (1967a) Morphological abnormalities resulting from radiofrequency treatment of larvae of Tenebrio molitor. *Ann. Entomol. Soc. Am.* **60:**889.

Kadoum, A. M., H. J. Ball, and L. E. Stetson (1967b) Metabolism in the yellow mealworm, Tenebrio molitor (Coleoptera tenbrionidae), following exposures to radiofrequency electric fields. *Ann. Entomol. Soc. Am.* **60:**1195.

Kadoum, A. M., S. O. Nelson, and L. E. Stetson (1967c) Mortality and internal heating in radiofrequency-treated larvae of Tenebrio molitor. *Ann. Entomol. Soc. Am.* **60:**885.

Kalant, H. (1959) Physiologic hazards of microwave radiation, survey of published literature. *Can. Med. Assoc. J.* **81:**575.

Kamat, G. P., and J. W. Laskey (1970) Enzyme inactivation in vitro with 2450 MHz microwaves. In: *Radiation Bio-effects Summary Report, January–December 1970.* HEW, PHS, BRH Publ. BRH/DBE 70-7 (December), p. 26.

Keilmann, F. (1978) Nonthermal microwave resonances in living cells. In: *Coherence in Spectroscopy and Modern Physics,* F. T. Arecchi, R. Bonifacio, and M. O. Scully (eds.). NATO Advanced Study Institute Series, Ser. B, Vol. 37, Plenum Press, New York, pp. 347–360.

Kerova, N. I. (1964) The effect of super-high frequencies of an electromagnetic field on the activity of polynucleases and content of nucleic acid. In: *Biological Effects of Ultrasound and Super-High-Ultra-High Frequency Electromagnetic Oscillations,* A. A. Gorodetskiy (ed.). Kiev, p. 108 (Libr. Cong. ATD pp. 65–68, Washington, D.C.).

Key, M., and K. N. Charyulu (1976) The thermal, non-thermal and therapeutic effects of 2450 MHz radiation on mammalian cells. *24th Annual Meeting of the Radiation Research Society,* San Francisco (Abst.).

Kolodub, F. A., and G. I. Yevtushenko (1972) Biochemical aspects of the biological effect of a low-frequency pulsed electromagnetic field. *Gig. Tr. Prof. Zabol.* **6:**13 (JPRS 56583, 1972).

Kulin, E. T., and E. I. Morozov (1964) The effect of decimeter radio-emission on the phagocytic functions of unicellular organisms. *Dokl. Akad. Nauk SSSR* **8:**329.

Kulin, E. T., and E. I. Morozov (1965) Some features of the effect of electromagnetic fields of the SHF range on the phagocytic function of paramecia. *Vestn. Akad. Navuk B SSR Ser. Biyal. Navuk* **4:**91.

Leach, W. M. (1976) On the induction of chromosomal aberrations by 2450 MHz microwave radiation. *J. Cell Biol.* **70**(S):387A (Abst.).

Lechowich, R. V., L. R. Beuchat, K. I. Fox, and F. H. Webster (1969) Procedure for evaluating the effects of 2450 megahertz microwaves upon *Streptococcus faecalis* and *Saccharomyces cerevisiae. Appl. Microbiol.* **17:**106.

Leonard, A., and G. DeKnudt (1967) Relation between the X-ray dose and the rate of chromosome rearrangements in spermatogonia of mice. *Radiat. Res.* **32:**35.

Lindauer, G. A., L. M. Liu, G. W. Skewes, and F. J. Rosenbaum (1974) Further experiments seeking evidence of nonthermal biological effects of microwave radiation. *IEEE Trans. Microwave Theory Tech.* **MTT-22:**790.

Lindegren, D. (1972) The temperature influence on the spontaneous mutation rate. *Hereditas* **70:**165.

Liu, L. M., and S. F. Cleary (1977) Effects of microwave radiation on erythrocyte membranes. In: *Abstracts of the 1977 International Symposium on the Biological Effects of Electromagnetic Waves,* Airlie, Va. (Abst.).

Liu, L. M., F. J. Rosenbaum, and W. F. Pickard (1975) The relation of teratogenesis in Tenebrio molitor to the incidence of low-level microwaves. *IEEE Trans. Microwave Theory Tech.* **MTT-23:**929.

Luczak, M., S. Szmigielski, M. Janiak, M. Kolus, and E. deClerq (1976) Effect of microwaves on virus multiplication in mammalian cells. *J. Microwave Power* **11:**173.

Lystov, V. N., and D. A. Frank-Kamenetskii (1965) Effect of centimeter radiowaves on vegetative cells, spores, and transforming DNA. *Biofizika* **10**:105 (English translation in *Biophysics* **10**:114).
McLees, B. D., and E. D. Finch (1971) The effects of radiofrequency radiation on regenerating hepatic tissue. In: *Proc. DOD Electromagnetic Radiation Research Workshop*, Bur. Med. Surg., Washington, D.C., p. 175.
McLees, B. D., E. D. Finch, and M. L. Albright (1972) An examination of regenerating hepatic tissue subjected to radiofrequency irradiation. *J. Appl. Physiol.* **32**:78.
McRee, D. I., G. K. Livingston, and G. MacNichols (1978) Incidence of sister chromatid exchange in bone marrow cells of the mouse following microwave exposure. In: *Symposium on Electromagnetic Fields in Biological Systems*, IEEE/IMPI, Ottawa, Canada, pp. 15–16 (abstract).
Madson, R. A., J. T. Cordaro, R. L. Killer, and G. E. Voelker (1970) Effects of Microwaves on Bacteria in Frozen Foods. USAF School of Aerospace Medicine Rep. SAM-TR-70-87.
Manikowska, E., J. M. Luciani, B. Servantie, P. Czerski, J. Obrenovitch, and A. Stahl (1979) Effects of 9.4 GHz microwave exposure on meiosis in mice. *Experientia* **35**:388.
Marha, K., J. Musil, and H. Tuha (1968) *Electromagnetic Fields and the Living Environment*. State Health Publishing House, Prague (Transl. SBN 911302-13-7, San Francisco Press, 1971).
Marmor, J. B., N. Hahn, and G. M. Hahn (1977) Tumor cure and cell survival after localized radiofrequency heating. *Cancer Res.* **37**:879.
Meisel, N. (1973) Microwave applications to food processing and food systems in Europe. *J. Microwave Power* **8**:143.
Mendecki, J., E. Friedenthal, and C. Botstein (1976) Effects of microwave-induced local hyperthermia on mammary adenocarcinoma in C_3H mice. *Cancer Res.* **36**:2113.
Michaelson, S. M. (1970) Discussion following the paper "Effects of 2450 MHz microwave radiation on cultivated kangaroo rat cells". In: *Biological Effects and Health Implications of Microwave Radiation*, S. F. Cleary (ed.). HEW Publ. BRH/DBE 70-2, p. 133.
Michaelson, S. M. (1978) Biologic and pathophysiologic effects of exposure to microwaves. In: *Microwave Bioeffects and Radiation Safety*, M. A. Stuchly (ed.). IMPI, Edmonton, Canada, pp. 55–94.
Mickey, G. H. (1963) Electromagnetism and its effect on the organism. *N.Y. State J. Med.* **63**:1935.
Miro, L., R. Loubiere, and A. Pfister (1974) Effects of microwaves on the cell metabolism of the reticulo-endothelial system. In: *Biological Effects and Health Hazards of Microwave Radiation*, P. Czerski, K. Ostrowski, M. L. Shore, C. Silverman, M. J. Suess, and B. Waldeskog (eds.). Polish Medical Publishers, Warsaw, pp. 89–97.
Mittler, S. (1976) Failure of 2- and 10-meter radio waves to induce genetic damage in Drosophila melanogaster. *Environ. Res.* **11**:326.
Mittler, S. (1977) Failure of chronic exposure to nonthermal FM radiowaves to mutate Drosophila. *J. Hered.* **68**:257.
Moore, H. A., R. Raymond, M. Fox, and A. G. Galsky (1979) Low-intensity microwave radiation and the virulence of *Agrobacterium tumefaciens* strain B_6. *Appl. Environ. Microbiol.* **37**:127.
Moressi, W. J. (1964) Mortality patterns of mouse sarcoma 180 cells resulting from direct heating and chronic microwave irradiation. *Exp. Cell Res.* **33**:240.
Nicols, W. W. (1966) Studies on the role of viruses in somatic mutation. *Hereditas* **55**:1.
Nyrop, J. E. (1946) A specific effect of high-frequency electric currents on biological objects. *Nature (London)* **157**:51.
Olsen, C. M. (1965) Microwaves inhibit bread mold. *Food Eng.* **37**:51.

Olsen, C. M., C. L. Drake, and S. L. Bunch (1966) Some biological effects of microwave energy. *J. Microwave Power* **1**:45.

Olsen, R. G. (1977) Insect teratogenesis in a standing wave irradiation system. *Radio Sci.* **12**(S):199.

Overgaard, K., and J. Overgaard (1972) Investigations on the possibility of a thermic tumor therapy. II. Action of combined heat–roentgen treatment on a transplanted mouse mammary carcinoma. *Eur. J. Cancer* **8**:573.

Pay, T. L., E. C. Beyer, and C. F. Reichelderfer (1972) Microwave effects on reproductive capacity and genetic transmission in Drosophila melanogaster. *J. Microwave Power* **7**:75.

Pederson, P. D., Jr., and A. W. Blomquist (1967) Microwave Applications. Tech. Rep. AFTAL-TR-67-196. Air Force Armament Lab., Eglin AFB, Fla.

Pratt, C. B., and C. Sheard (1935) The effects of intravenous injection into rabbits of strains of streptococci which have been exposed to the high-frequency field. *Protoplasma* **23**:24.

Presman, A. S. (1965) The effect of microwaves on living organisms and biological structures. *Usp. Fiz. Nauk* **86**:263.

Presman, A. S., and S. M. Rappeport (1965) Effect of microwaves on the excitable system of paramecia. *Byull. Eksp. Biol. Med.* **4**:48.

Presman, A. S., Y. I. Kamenskiy, and N. A. Levitina (1961) Biological effect of microwaves. *Usp. Sovrem. Biol.* **51**:84.

Prince, J. E., L. H. Mori, J. W. Frazer, and J. C. Mitchell (1972) Cytologic aspect of RF radiation in the monkey. *Aerosp. Med.* **43**:759.

Prohofsky, E. W., and K. C. Lu (1979) Resonant melting of the double helix and a possible strand separation and propulsion mechanism for enzymes. *Biophys. J.* **25**:183A.

Robe, K. (1966) Improved flavor of pasteurized products (cooked with microwave radiation). *Food Process. Mark.* **27**:84.

Saito, M., and H. P. Schwan (1961) The time constants of pearl-chain formation. In: *Biological Effects of Microwave Radiation*, Vol. 1, M. F. Peyton (ed.). Plenum Press, New York, p. 85.

Savage, J. R. K. (1971) Use and abuse of chromosomal aberrations as an indicator of genetic damage. *Int. J. Environ. Stud.* **1**:233.

Sawicki, W., and K. Ostrowski (1968) Non-thermal effect of microwave radiation *in vitro* on peritoneal mast cells of the rat. *Am. J. Phys. Med.* **47**:225.

Schwan, H. P. (1968) Radiation biology, medical applications and radiation hazards. In: *Microwave Power Engineering*, Vol. 2, E. C. Okress (ed.). Academic Press, New York, p. 213.

Schwan, H. P., and G. M. Piersol (1954) The absorption of electromagnetic energy in body tissues, a review and critical analysis. Part I. Biophysical aspects. *Am. J. Phys. Med.* **33**:371.

Searle, G. W., R. W. Dahlen, C. J. Imig, C. C. Wunder, J. D. Thomson, J. A. Thomas, and W. J. Moressi (1961) Effect of 2450 mc microwaves in dogs, rats and larvae of the common fruit fly. In: *Biological Effects of Microwave Radiation*, Vol. 1, M. F. Peyton (ed.). Plenum Press, New York, p. 187.

Sharp, J. C., and C. J. Paperiello (1971) The effects of microwave exposure on thymidine-H^3 uptake in albino rats. *Radiat. Res.* **45**:434.

Sheridan, J. P., B. P. Gaber, F. Cavatorta, and P. E. Schoen (1979) Molecular level effects of microwaves on natural and model membranes: A Raman spectroscopic investigation. Presented at the joint meeting of USNC/URSI and the Bioelectromagnetics Society, Seattle (Abst.).

Smolyanskaya, A. Z., and R. L. Vilenskaya (1973) Effects of millimeter-band electromagnetic radiation on the functional activity of certain genetic elements of bacterial cells. *Usp. Fiz. Nauk* **110**:571.

Stodolnik-Baranska, W. (1974) The effects of microwaves on human lymphocyte cultures. In: *Biological Effects and Health Hazards of Microwave Radiation,* P. Czerski, K. Ostrowski, M. L. Shore, C. Silverman, M. J. Suess, and B. Waldeskog (eds.). Polish Medical Publishers, Warsaw, p. 189.

Straub, K. D., and P. Carver (1975) Effects of electromagnetic fields on microsomal ATPase and mitochondrial oxidative phosphorylation. *Ann. N.Y. Acad. Sci.* **247**:292.

Suzuki, T., and K. Oshima (1973) Applications of microwave power to the food industry in Japan. *J. Microwave Power* **8**:149.

Syngayevskaya, V. A. (1970) Metabolic changes. In: *Influence of Microwave Radiation on the Organism of Man and Animals,* I. R. Petrov (ed.). Meditsina Press, Leningrad, p. 48 (NASA TT F-708).

Szmigielski, M., M. Luczak, M. Bielec, M. Janiak, M. Kobus, W. E. Stewart II, and E. deClerq (1976) Effect of microwaves combined with interferon and/or interferon inducers (poly I–poly C) on development of sarcoma 180 in mice. *J. Microwave Power* **11**:174.

Takashima, S. (1966) Studies on the effect of radio frequency waves on biological macromolecules. *IEEE Trans. Biomed. Eng.* **BME-13**: 28.

Teixeira-Pinto, A. A., L. L. Nejelski, J. L. Cutler, and J. H. Heller (1960) The behavior of unicellular organisms in an electromagnetic field. *Exp. Cell Res.* **20**:548.

Tell, R. A. (1972) Microwave absorption characteristics of *Drosophila melanogaster*. In: *Twinbrook Research Laboratory Annual Report 1971,* EPA, Washington, D.C., p. 155.

Tyazhelov, V. V., S. I. Alekseyev, and P. A. Grigor'ev (1979) Change in the conductivity of phospholipid membranes modified by alamethicin on exposure to a high frequency electromagnetic field. *Biophysics* **23**:750 (translation of *Biofizika* **23**:732, 1978).

Valtonen, E. J. (1966) The effects of microwave radiation on the cellular elements in the peritoneal fluid and peripheral blood of the rat. *Acta Rheumatol. Scand.* **12**:129.

Valtonen, E. (1967) Observations on the fine structure of giant mast cells produced by microwave radiation of the peritoneal fluid. *Z. Zellforsch. Mikrosk. Anat.* **80**:322.

Van Ummersen, C. A., and F. C. Cogan (1970) Effects of microwave radiation on lens epithelial cells (summary). In: *Biological Effects and Health Implications of Microwave Radiation,* S. F. Cleary (ed.). HEW, PHS, BRH/DBE 70-2, p. 122.

Varma, M. M., and E. A. Traboulay, Jr. (1975) Biological effects of microwave radiation on the testes of Swiss mice. *Experientia* **31**:301.

Varma, M. M., and E. A. Traboulay, Jr. (1976) Evaluation of dominant lethal test and DNA studies in measuring mutagenicity caused by non-ionizing radiation. In: *Biological Effects of Electromagnetic Waves,* Vol. I, C. C. Johnson and M. L. Shore (eds.). HEW Publ. (FDA) 77-8010, pp. 386–396.

Varma, M. M., and E. A. Traboulay, Jr. (1977) Comparison of native and microwave irradiated DNA. *Experientia* **33**:1649.

Varma, M. M., E. L. Dage, and S. R. Joshi (1976) Mutagenicity induced by nonionizing radiation in Swiss male mice. In: *Biological Effects of Electromagnetic Waves,* Vol. I, C. C. Johnson and M. L. Shore (eds.). HEW Publ. (FDA) 77-8010, pp. 397–405.

Wald, N., A. C. Upton, V. T. Jenkins, and W. H. Borges (1964) Radiation-induced mouse leukemia: Consistent occurrence of an extra and a marker chromosome. *Science* **143**:810.

Ward, T. R., J. W. Allis, and J. A. Elder (1975) Measure of enzymatic activity coincident with 2450 MHz microwave exposure. *J. Microwave Power* **10**:315.

Webb, S. J. (1975) Genetic continuity and metabolic regulation as seen by the effects of various microwave and black light frequencies on these phenomena. *Ann. N.Y. Acad. Sci.* **247**:327.

Webb, S. J., and A. D. Booth (1969) Absorption of microwaves by microorganisms. *Nature (London)* **222**:1199.

Webb, S. J., and D. D. Dodds (1968) Inhibition of bacterial cell growth by 136 gc microwaves. *Nature (London)* **218**:374.

Whitney, W. K., S. O. Nelson, and H. H. Walkden (1961) Effects of high frequency electric fields on certain species of stored-grain insects. U.S. Dep. Agric. Mark. Res. Rep. No. 453, p. 52.

Wiktor-Jedrzejczak, W., A. Ahmed, P. Czerski, W. M. Leach, and K. W. Sell (1976) Microwaves (2450 MHz) stimulate maturation of B lymphoid cells in spleens of exposed mice. *Proc. 1976 Annu. Meet. IURS,* Amherst (Abst.).

Wildervanck, A., K. G. Wakim, J. F. Herrick, and F. H. Krusen (1959) Certain experimental observations on a pulsed diathermy machine. *Arch. Phys. Med.* **40**:45.

Yao, K. T. S. (1976) Cytogenetic consequences of microwave incubation of mammalian cells in culture. *Genetics* **83**(suppl.):584A.

Yao, K. T. S. (1978) Microwave radiation-induced chromosomal aberrations in corneal epithelium of Chinese hamsters. *J. Hered.* **69**:409.

Yao, K. T. S., and M. M. Jiles (1970) Effects of 2450 MHz microwave radiation on cultivated kangaroo rat cells. In: *Biological Effects and Health Implications of Microwave Radiation,* S. F. Cleary (ed.). HEW, PHS, BRH/DBE 70-2, p. 123.

Yerushalmi, A. (1975) Cure of a solid tumor by simultaneous administration of microwaves and X-ray irradiation. *Radiat. Res.* **64**:602.

Zalyubovskaya, N. P. (1973) Reactions of living organisms to exposure to millimeter-band electromagnetic waves. *Usp. Fiz. Nauk* **110**:574.

Zufarov, K. A., and V. B. Shnaivais (1970) Response of white mice liver cell mitochondria from electromagnetic field irradiation. *Tsitologiya* **12**:146.

8

Reproduction, Development, and Growth

8.1. REPRODUCTION

Reproductive efficiency concerns the capacity of the dam or sire to effect a conception and bear and rear offspring. Changes in this capacity might be due to alterations in behavior, physiology, or morphology.

Pay *et al.* (1978) exposed *Drosophila* to 2450 MHz at SARs from 400 to 800 W/kg. The reproductive efficiency, in this case the production of eggs, was significantly reduced in both heated and microwave-irradiated females as compared to the shams. However, there appeared to be no significant difference in the production of eggs in females exposed to microwaves and those exposed to heat alone.

In 28-week-old hens that had been irradiated on day 1 of age for 4.5 sec at a power of 800 W in a multimodal cavity (est. SAR 2770 W/kg), there appeared to be no differences in the production of eggs during the 100 days of laying between the control group and the group irradiated previously with microwaves on day 1 of age (Davidson *et al.*, 1976). The authors also stated that an exposure of 2500 W/kg for 9 sec at a frequency of 2450 MHz is a lethal dose, and that 42% of the day-old chicks that received 2810 W/kg for 6 sec at this frequency died. Those animals that survived were unconscious for a period of up to 5 min. Approximately the same sublethal SAR was absorbed by the day-old chicks used in the examination for latent reproductive effects (2770 W/kg for 4.5 sec), but there were no deaths that could be directly attributed to the microwave exposure. From these experiments, it is concluded that the massive doses of this experimental regimen produced no latent alterations of reproductive efficiency.

Some studies on the effects of microwave exposure on reproductive organs of mice and rats (Table 8-1) have been summarized by Leach (1980).

Rugh *et al.* (1975) examined the differences in the average lethal absorbed dose of microwaves (2450 MHz) during the estrous cycle of CF1 mice (29–31 g). There was a prior 20-min acclimatization to the waveguide exposure chamber, and environmental conditions were 23.5°C,

TABLE 8-1
Summary of Animal Studies on Effects of Microwave Exposure on Reproductive Organs[a]

Animal	Exposure power density (mW/cm²)	Radiation frequency (GHz)	Effect	Reference
Mouse	10 (2 hr daily for 5 or more months)	3.0	Testicular changes	Bereznitskaya and Kazbekov (1973)[b]
	50 (30–40 min)	1.7	Altered spermatogenesis	Varma and Traboulay (1975)[b]
	10 (100 min)	9.27 (pulsed)	Testicular degeneration	Prausnitz and Süsskind (1962)[b]
	100 (4.5 min 5 days/week for 59 weeks)	2.45	Testicular damage	Haidt and McTighe (1973)
	6.5 (total of 230 hr over 2-month period)			
	400 (5 min)	~10(?) (3-cm waves)	Testicular lesions, lesions of Graafian follicles, change in sexual cycle in females	Gorodetskaya (1964)[b]
	0.344 (30 min) 20–50 times prior to mating	~10(?) (3-cm waves) (pulsed)	No deviations from normal values for duration of pregnancy, number of offspring, or development of offspring of irradiated mothers	Povzhitkov et al. (1961)[b]
Rat	250 (5–15 min)	24.0	Testicular damage	Gunn et al. (1961)
	80 (10–80 min)	2.45	Testicular damage	Muraca et al. (1977)
	0.1, 1.3 (4 hr daily for 62–80 days)	2.98 (pulsed)	Change in sexual cycle in females	Letowski (1967), Letowski et al. (1971)

[a] Modified from Leach (1980).
[b] Studies having data on irradiated animals' ability to sire offspring.

50% relative humidity, and an air flow of 38 liters/min (0.38 km/hr). There was a significant lowering of the average lethal absorbed dose (expressed in cal/g) of the females that were in estrus, compared to those that were in diestrus ($p < 0.01$). The forward power was 8.24 W. It would thus appear that changes during the reproductive cycle could affect the radiosensitivity to microwaves.

Exposure to 3000 MHz, 8 mW/cm^2 did not affect mating of mice or rats (Miro et al., 1965). Pituitary gonadotropic function was preserved in female mice exposed to 3000 MHz, 10 mW/cm^2, twice daily for 5 months (Bereznitskaya, 1968).

Among offspring of irradiated animals, increased stillbirths were detected in two studies (Bereznitskaya and Kazbekov, 1973; Gorodetskaya, 1964); no effects on progeny were observed in two other studies (Prausnitz and Süsskind, 1962; Povzhitkov et al., 1961). Although some data suggest the importance of multiple exposures (Bereznitskaya and Kazbekov, 1973; Letowski, 1967; Letowski et al., 1971), two such studies showed no deleterious effects among offspring (Prausnitz ard Süsskind, 1962; Povzhitkov et al., 1961), even though testicular damage had been reported in one of these studies (Prausnitz and Süsskind, 1962). In summary, it appears that the efficiency of the reproductive system of the female is not easily altered. Only extremely high power densities can produce any discernible changes in reproductive patterns.

The effect of microwaves on the testes has been studied fairly extensively (Ely et al., 1957, 1964; Gorodetskaya, 1963; Imig et al., 1948; de Seguin and Castelain, 1947). Exposure of the scrotal area at high power densities (> 50 mW/cm^2) results in varying degrees of testicular damage such as edema, enlargement of the testes, atrophy, fibrosis, and coagulation necrosis of seminiferous tubules in rats and rabbits, exposed to 2450, 3000, and 10,000 MHz.

Muraca et al. (1977) exposed the testes of rats to 2450-MHz microwaves (est. SAR to the testis = 60 W/kg). Intratesticular temperatures of 36, 38, 40, and 42°C were produced. The duration of each exposure at a power density of 80 mW/cm^2 varied from 10 to 73 minutes. The animals were exposed once or repeatedly on five consecutive days. Five days after the treatment, the animals were sacrificed. There appeared to be no significant change in the number of animals that had abnormal testicular tissue. After a single exposure of 10 min during which the intratesticular temperature was allowed to reach 42°C, there was a threefold increase in the number of animals that had some abnormal changes. In the multiple exposures, even where the temperature reached only 36°C for 60 min, all the testes had some changes in the spermatogenic epithelium. When intratesticular temperatures were allowed to reach 40°C for repeated short periods (10 to 27 min, five times), severe degeneration in the spermatic tubules was seen in all the testes. The testes of rats that were subjected to heating by water-bath immersion were less affected by similar intratesticular temperatures maintained for similar durations. This difference, however, may be a consequence of different heating rates or thermal gradients produced by the two heating modalities.

Fahim *et al.* (1975) conducted an experiment comparing the contraceptive capability of microwaves to other heating modalities. Male Sprague–Dawley rats (Holtzman strain) were exposed to 2450-MHz microwaves (from a diathermy unit of maximum output of 100 W) after pentobarbital anesthesia. The applicator of the diathermy unit was 3 inches from the testes of the rat and provided near-field exposures, which do not allow a good estimate of the associated SAR. By varying the power output of the unit and also the exposure time from 1 to 15 min, the authors developed four subgroups of animals: those where the testicular temperature reached 65 or 45°C for 15 min, and those where the testicular temperature reached 39°C for 1 or 5 min. The rats were allowed to mate with normal females beginning 24 hr after treatment, and every 5 days thereafter until pregnancy was observed. "The endpoint for fertility was the amount of time required for every surviving male in the treatment group to impregnate a female." Later the gonads were weighed, and histological examinations were made of the testes and secondary sex organs. Raising the temperature of the testes to 45°C for 15 min caused complete infertility in the males for a period of 10 months. When the testes were examined histologically, there was no observable spermatogenesis. When the temperature was raised to 39°C, 70% of the males remained normal in their breeding capability, while the remaining 30% recovered their fertility so that they were able to impregnate females within 2 weeks. Histological sections indicated normal spermatogenesis. There appeared to be no differences in the weights of testes or of secondary sex organs, even in the group (45°C, 15 min) that was sterile 10 months after the microwave exposure. This experiment demonstrates that a minimum temperature of 45°C, produced by microwave exposure, must be attained in rat testes in order to produce a permanent sterility. Temperatures that ranged to 39°C, somewhat above the colonic temperature, but induced for only a short period (5 min), were not effective and produced only temporary, if any infertility. Along with the permanent sterility induced by the high temperatures (minimum of 45°C), there was damage to the tubules themselves and a lack of spermatogenesis.

In a study attempting to demonstrate alteration in functional fertility and mutagenesis conducted by Berman *et al.* (1980), male rats were exposed to 2450 MHz in an anechoic chamber: (1) at a power density of

5 mW/cm^2, 4 hr/day, daily from day 6 of gestation through 90 days of age; (2) at a power density of 10 mW/cm^2, 5 hr/day for 5 days, beginning on day 90; and (3) to 28 mW/cm^2, 4 hr/day, 5 days/week, for 4 weeks, beginning on day 90. The rats were bred to untreated female rats shortly after the end of the treatment period. No mutagenic effect was demonstrable. In the first experiment, the SAR varied with the growth of the animals from approximately 4.5 W/kg in neonates to approximately 0.9 W/kg at 90 days of age. SARs are estimated to be 2 W/kg at a power density of 10 mW/cm^2, and 5.5 W/kg at 28 mW/cm^2. Testicular temperatures taken in rats exposed for up to 90 min to 28 mW/cm^2 showed an increase from a preexposure level of 34°C to almost 38°C after exposure. Simultaneous colonic temperatures were approximately 3°C higher than testicular temperatures during the entire period. Sham-irradiated animals had testcular temperatures ranging from almost 32°C to approximately 35°C. The exposure to 28 mW/cm^2 during the 90 min produced a testicular temperature equivalent to normal colonic temperature.

The chronic exposure to 5 mW/cm^2 from day 6 of gestation through 90 days of age appeared to have no effect on the reproductive efficiency of the male rats when bred to normal females. Also, exposure to a power density of 10 mW/cm^2 (SAR ~ 2 W/kg) at 90 days of age for a period of 5 days had no effect on the reproductive efficiency of the males. Only exposure to 28 mW/cm^2 for approximately 4 weeks (est. SAR 5.5 W/kg) caused any alteration in reproductive function. Only 50% of the females that were available to the males for breeding became pregnant during the week immediately following the exposure period. The breeding returned to normal beginning at the 3rd week after irradiation. The animals bred normally thereafter. No examination was made of the testes of the animals that were exposed to 28 mW/cm^2. The temperatures reached in the testes at the high power density (28 mW/cm^2) were similar to those reported by Fahim *et al.* (1975) where histological changes were seen.

Gunn *et al.* (1961) described the effect of 24-GHz energy on interstitial cell morphology and function in rats. They exposed rats once for 5 min at a power density of 250 mW/cm^2, causing a temperature rise to 41°C in the testes. Scrotal burns, edema, and spermatic tubular degeneration, but no interstitial cell pathology were noted. Zinc uptake by the dorsolateral prostate was decreased. This suggested decreased prostate function because of decreased testosterone secretion.

Ely *et al.* (1957, 1964), using 2880 MHz, tried to determine the lowest power density that would produce minimal testicular changes in the most sensitive animal in a group of dogs. As part of these studies, they irradiated the testes of anesthetized dogs. Testicular temperature was measured about 1 cm from that surface nearest the microwave source, which was the location of greatest temperature development.

Testicular temperatures were found to equalize throughout the organ with relative rapidity. For the testis, an initial temperature of 35.6°C was used, as this is the maximum in normal humans. The threshold temperature of 37°C induced by 5 mW/cm^2 was the lowest damaging temperature found in this study. It should be noted that this is based on a single animal, and may be spurious. Not enough controls were used nor was the temperature increment noted. There may have been a normal incidence of histological damage in these animals. The field intensity required (5 mW/cm^2) to maintain a threshold temperature was chosen from the most sensitive of the 35 dogs exposed. It is of considerable significance that this is about the same figure that would result if computation were based on a 1.4°C temperature rise rather than a recorded temperature of 37°C. It should be noted, however, that, in general, mean power densities greater than 23 ± 15 mW/cm^2 were required to maintain testicular temperatures of 36°C or above or an increase of 1.4°C over the preexposure temperature. The authors point out that the damage observed at such low power levels is slight, almost certainly fully recoverable, and the response of the testes to heating from a radar source is similar to that from other sources of heat. The same effect, which is reversible, can also be caused by a hot bath or constrictive clothing and should therefore not be considered hazardous. It is questionable, therefore, whether such effects should be legitimately considered as a basis for appraisal of hazard from microwave exposure (Kalant, 1959).

Whole-body exposure of dogs to 24,000 MHz (Deichmann *et al.*, 1963) or guinea pigs to 3000 MHz (Follis, 1946) did not affect reproduction.

Saunders and Kowalczuk (1981b) exposed the posterior halves of the bodies of anesthetized male C3H mice in a waveguide for 30 min to 2.45-GHz microwaves and the effects on the testes were compared to those produced by direct heating. Damage measured 6 days after exposure ranged in severity from depletion of the spermatocytes to extensive necrosis of the germinal epithelium. The observed effects are consistent with the hypothesis that heat damage is the primary effect of microwave exposure. Temperature-sensitive probes implanted in the testes revealed a threshold effect for depletion of the spermatocytes of approximately 39°C and an LD_{50}^6 (50% cell death after 6 days) of about 41°C after microwave exposure or direct heating. The corresponding effective threshold effect and LD_{50}^6 expressed in terms of absorbed microwave power were 20 and 30 W/kg. It is probable that a conscious animal is better able to regulate testicular temperature and hence adjust to higher dose-rates. An "effective" dose-rate to the testis in excess of about 20 W/kg, approximately $2\frac{1}{2}$ times the basal metabolic rate, maintained for periods of 30 min, damages the temperature-sensitive cells—the spermatocytes—in the anesthetized mouse. The higher the dose-rate, the more severe is the depletion. The LD_{50}^6 occurred around 30 W/kg at a temperature of approximately 41°C. This is about 4°C higher than normal body temperature but approximately 7°C higher than testicular temperature in the conscious animal. In a previous study by Saunders and Kowalczuk (1981a), the effects of far-field radiation on mouse testes were quantitatively examined. No effects were seen, although exposures ranged from 1000 W/m^2 for 5 min to 100 W/m^2 for 260 min. Exposure of the mice to 500 W/m^2 for 45 min raised colonic temperature as high as 42.5°C but had no discernible effect on the testis. The dose-rate in this example was 33 W/kg. However, the mice were not anesthetized and were able to regulate their body and testicular temperatures normally by, for example, increasing blood flow through the tail and ears by moving the testes farther into the scrotal sac. Higher exposures are clearly required in conscious mice to raise testicular temperature to a damaging level. Thus, the threshold value of 20 W/kg and an LD_{50}^6 of 30 W/kg for acute exposure in the anesthetized animal are probably pessimistic values for the conscious animal. Using these data, it can be estimated that dose-rates in man in excess of 20 W/kg would only be produced by exposure to power densities greatly in excess of 100 W/m^2 (10 mW/cm^2) (Saunders and Kowalczuk, 1981b).

Reports of human sterility from exposure to microwaves are questionable. Barron and Baraff (1958) and Barron et al. (1955) found no evidence of fertility changes in their human surveys. Reports of altered fertility in man even with unusually large exposures to microwaves are not available (Rosenthal and Beering, 1968).

There are reports that chronic "low-level" exposure can result in impairment of spermatogenesis and reproductive function without measurable testicular temperature increase (Bereznitskaya and Kazbekov, 1973; Dumansky et al., 1972).

There is general agreement that high power density exposure can affect the testes and ovaries. These responses can be related to the heating of the organs. The sensitivity of the testes to heat is well known (van Demark and Free, 1973). Comparable heating of rat scrota with 2450-MHz CW microwaves or by immersion in water to temperatures of 36, 38, 40, and 42°C resulted in comparable damage at each temperature (Muraca et al., 1977).

There is a vast literature on the effects of temperature increases on fertility. High environmental temperatures, when sustained, can produce infertility in male rats. Pucak et al. (1977) described deaths in a large rat production colony where temperatures in the room accidentally reached 31.6°C for 2 days and as high as 37.7°C in individual cages. Under these conditions, approximately 3000 of 14,000 Sprague–Dawley rats died from heat prostration. When examined 18 days after the incident, 25% of the surviving males had bilateral atrophy of the testicles, which were approximately half the size of normal. Histological examination showed atrophy of the spermatic tubules and failure of spermatogenesis. The proportion of affected testes ranged from 50 to 75%. Five weeks after the incident, those animals with small testes were still sterile. In comparison to the temperatures seen in this study, raising the testicular temperature to 42°C by microwave exposure appears to be an extreme thermal burden.

Effects in humans (Marha *et al.*, 1968 ; Marha, 1970) include: decreased spermatogenesis, altered sex ratio of births, changes in menstrual patterns, retarded fetal development, congenital effects in the newborn, and decreased lactation in nursing mothers. They also report an increased incidence of miscarriages in women working with microwaves. Because of these reports, adolescent and pregnant women are not permitted to work with HF, VHF, or UHF equipment in Czechoslovakia. According to these authors, the above-mentioned effects occur at thermal microwave exposure intensities (greater than 10 mW/cm^2).

It appears highly unlikely that serious or permanent damage to human testes will occur except from inordinately high exposure levels. Damage to the testes from microwaves is considered to be completely reversible. Although temporary sterility and damage to seminiferous tubules may occur at high power densities, the condition does not appear to be of a permanent nature and will ultimately correct itself.

8.2. EMBRYONIC DEVELOPMENT

There are reports suggesting that particular combinations of exposure frequency, duration, and power density produce effects on embryonic development and postnatal growth. Alterations in development have been reported in insects (Carpenter and Livstone, 1971; Lindauer *et al.*, 1974; Liu *et al.*, 1975), chick embryos (Van Ummersen, 1961, 1963), and rodents (Bereznitskaya, 1968, 1972; Bereznitskaya and Rysina, 1974; Chernovetz *et al.*, 1975, 1977, 1979a,b; Berman *et al.*, 1978; Rugh *et al.*, 1974, 1975, 1976; Rugh and McManaway, 1976, 1977).

Van Ummersen (1961, 1963) investigated the effects of microwave energy on chick embryo development. Embryos at the 48-hr stage of development were exposed to 2450 MHz CW through the intact shell. Exposure to 400 mW/cm^2 for 1 to $1\frac{1}{2}$ min, 280 mW/cm^2 for 7 to $8\frac{1}{2}$ min, 200 mW/cm^2 for 13 to 14 min, or 20 to 40 mW/cm^2 for 280 to 300 min caused significant temperature elevations (ΔT up to 19°C) in the yolk.

Estimates of the SAR for these power densities are 140, 98, 70, and 7 to 14 W/kg, respectively. The embryos were then studied at the 96-hr stage of development. Of 183 embryos so treated, 16 continued to develop normally, 48 died, and 119 developed abnormally. In general, the abnormalities appeared to be the result of inhibition of growth and/or differentiation, so that many embryos were only as large as 72-hr rather than 96-hr embryos. In many cases, further differentiation of the brain, eye, wing buds, and heart had been inhibited. Development of hind limbs, tail, and allantois was suppressed. The temperature of the yolk at a position immediately beneath the embryo was recorded at all three power densities, and was found to increase with exposure at a rate proportional to power density. In all cases, a yolk temperature of approximately 59°C proved to be lethal. The conclusion reached was that microwave exposure appears to inhibit cellular differentiation in the developing chick embryo. In structures that have already begun to differentiate, cellular proliferation continues, but no further degree of differentiation occurs. Structures that have not yet begun to differentiate fail to do so subsequent to irradiation, and their development is therefore suppressed. Since all embryos in which effects were produced reached a temperature of 55°C, the results of these studies suggest that the deleterious effects observed are due to heating. Since protein denaturation takes place in the neighborhood of 45°C, anything that elevates the temperature to this level could start degeneration of cell structures. The high power densities that were used in this study would be sufficient to cause protein denaturation on a thermal basis.

Osborne (1958, 1959) found that at no stage of development was the chick embryo affected by prolonged 200-MHz CW exposure. In these experiments, the temperature rise within the egg was never more than 1°C.

Krueger et al. (1975) irradiated poultry at 260, 915, and 2435 MHz for 4 weeks at several power densities and observed decreased egg production but no effect on fertility, hatches, or sex ratios. Also, no macroscopic abnormalities were noted in newly hatched chicks or in dead embryos. These experiments, however, were fraught with difficulties, including death and infertility in controls, small sample size, inadequate temperature controls, and a loss and change of power. It is thus difficult to obtain meaningful results from this work.

Quail embryos exposed to 30 mW/cm^2 (14 mW/g), 2450 MHz CW for 4 hr on one or each of the first 5 days of incubation, did not develop gross deformities or changes in hatchability that could be correlated with exposure (McRee et al., 1975). Microwave-induced temperature within the eggs varied from 34°C to 37°C, which is the normal incubation temperature. The only statistically significant finding was decreased hemoglobin associated with exposure on day 2 but it was elevated when exposures were on day 5. Day 2 produced decreases in white blood count, and in percentage of lymphocytes and neutrophils.

In further investigations of exposures on day 2 of the incubation period, Hamrick and McRee (1975) found no significant effects following exposure to 2.45-GHz energy at 14 mW/g. The temperature of the eggs was not elevated beyond that normally associated with incubation. Although no effects were noted, there were large temperature differences across the grid between different eggs as well as temperature gradients in individual eggs.

In another study, Japanese quail embryos were exposed during the first 12 days of development to 2.45-GHz microwaves at an incident power density of 5 mW/cm^2 and SAR of 4.03 mW/g. Environmental temperature was 35.5°C (McRee and Hamrick, 1977). No gross deformities were observed in the exposed quail when sacrificed and examined at 24 to 36 hr after hatch. No significant changes in the total body weight or weight of the heart, liver, gizzard, adrenals, or pancreas were found in the treated birds. Hematological parameters were also measured in this study. The results showed a statistically significant increase in hemoglobin and a statistically significant decrease in monocytes in birds exposed to microwaves. No statistically significant changes in hematocrit, red blood cells, total white blood cells, lymphocytes, neutrophils, basophils, or eosinophils were detected. The authors hypothesized that the decreased monocyte count might indicate a change in immune responsiveness and thus the latest in this series of studies (Hamrick and McRee, 1975) assessed the development of immunological competence. Quail eggs were exposed throughout the first 12 days of development to 2.45-GHz microwaves at 5 mW/cm^2. The eggs during exposure were between 37.5 and 38°C. The animals were observed from hatch to 5 weeks of age. The mean of body mass as assessed at hatch and weekly thereafter was numerically but not statistically lower in exposed than in control animals. Organ masses (spleen and bursa of Fabricius) did not differ. No difference was observed in mortality. Both sexes developed normally and showed normal immune potential. Regrettably these studies were analyzed using multiple comparison t tests even though the data are time dependent. The authors did demonstrate, however, the importance ambient temperature can play in experiments where microwaves are the agent under investigation. They included the results of an experiment where the Japanese quail eggs were in an environment at a temperature only slightly higher ($+1.5$°C) than in the main experiment (35.5°C). The authors began their study using the higher ambient temperature (37°C), which is the temperature at which quail eggs are conventionally incubated. This ambient temperature, however, with the addition of an SAR of 4 W/kg, was sufficient to cause a death rate of 93% of the fertilized eggs. The eggs that were irradiated at the same SAR, but at an ambient temperature 1.5°C lower (35.5°C), had a death rate of only 42%. The results of this apparently slight (1.5°C) increase in incubation temperature during microwave exposure show that for the quail egg, the temperature at which the egg is maintained during exposure is critical.

Rugh et al. (1974) reported abnormalities in CF-1 mouse fetuses exposed in an environmentally controlled waveguide at days 7 to 13 of gestation to 12.6 to 33.5 J/g, 2450-MHz CW microwaves for 5 min, equivalent to 123 mW/cm^2 incident power. The approximate SARs for these exposures ranged from 85 to 112 W/kg, which are exceedingly high energy inputs. Hemorrhages, resorptions, exencephaly, stunting, and fetal death were observed. The number of abnormalities (specific malformations and resorptions) increased in relation to the microwave dose. Differential effects at different gestation days suggest thermal sensitivity of embryos. The actual data were reported graphically with each point representing the percentage of abnormal fetuses of a single litter. The more common statistics, i.e., the percentage of litters at a given power or dose rate that contained abnormalities or the percentage of abnormalities per implantation, were not reported. The primary anatomical abnormality was exencephaly. The percentage of fetuses in a litter showing the exencephaly appeared to increase as microwave dose increased.

In another study reported by Rugh et al. (1975), temperature, relative humidity, and air flow were closely regulated. The temperature humidity index (THI) was monitored and maintained during the exposures at a level of 71.6. They concluded that the average lethal dose of radiation decreased as the THI increased. They also found that diestrous females had an average lethal dose of approximately 48 J/g as compared with averages of approximately 44.5 J/g for estrous females. The authors concluded that the female mouse is more susceptible to microwave radiation during estrus.

Rugh and McManaway (1976) reported studies on CF-1 mice exposed to 2450-MHz microwaves for 4 min at dose rates of 78.8 to 136.2 mW/g. The majority of the observed abnormalities resulted from exposures on day 8 or 10 of gestation. In a later study in which the average dose rate was 107.4 mW/g, Rugh and McManaway (1977) observed that 68% of the animals exposed on day 8 were either resorbed, dead, or abnormal as compared with 38% of the animals exposed on day 10, and with 20% of the animals exposed on day 3 or 4. The authors suggested two main peaks of teratogenic susceptibility: the first on day 4, which corresponds to the time of implantation of the embryo in the uterine horn, and the second on day 8, which corresponds to the beginning of organogenesis. It is important to note that 100 mW/g for 4 min is the convulsive threshold for this strain of mouse. Rugh and McManaway (1976) and Rugh et al. (1976) also demonstrated that lowering the dam's body temperature with pentobarbital anesthesia could prevent the teratogenic effects of thermal loading with microwaves.

Lin et al. (1979) studied the effect of repeated exposure of C3H mice to 48 MHz. The animals were exposed to 0.5 mW/cm^2 (63.25 V/m) in a TEM exposure chamber for 1 hr/day, 5 days/week, beginning on the 4th to 7th days *postpartum,* for 10 weeks. The formed elements in the blood were not affected by the exposure. The means of body mass of the irradiated and control animals were comparable. No significant differences in lesion onset, incidence, prevalence, extent, or type were observed when repeatedly RF-exposed animals were compared with sham control groups. During the period of the study, no cataracts were noted. Fertility differences among irradiated and control animals were not found. Body growth patterns did not differ among sham- and RF-exposed animals.

Employing a multimodal cavity at 2450 MHz, Chernovetz et al. (1975) irradiated pregnant C3H/HeJ mice with a single "intense" dose of 38 mW/g (estimated incident energy 160 mW/cm) for 10 min (22.8 J/g) on gestation day 11, 12, 13, or 14. This exposure resulted in a 2.2°C temperature increase and 10% maternal lethality. The exposure during late organogenesis or early fetal stage caused no change in fetal mortality or morbidity when compared to shams. This factorially designed study involved microwaves alone as well as in combination with cortisone acetate, a known teratogen. The cortisone was given in 5-mg i.p. injections 37 ± 8 min before irradiation or sham-irradiation was initiated. A sham-irradiated group of mice, and a group receiving only the cortisone served as controls. Microwave exposure alone did not increase or alter the incidence of malformations. There was some indication that tail abnormalities were associated with the microwave as well as with the cortisone treatments but small increases in frequency of this defect were not reliable. The highest incidence of abnormality was associated with the combined microwave and cortisone treatment on day 14 of gestation.

A second study in this series involved exposures of mice to 2450-MHz microwaves for 10 min on gestation day 14. Four groups of mice were respectively given a sham or microwave exposure, cortisone, or a combination of microwaves and cortisone. The animals were allowed to come to term. The results indicated that cortisone treatment reduced the survival rate but that microwaves had no effect. The survival rate of pups whose dams had been given the combined treatment was reliably higher than that of pups from dams that received cortisone only. There was also some indication that the microwave exposure alleviated the amount of fetal insult attributable to cortisone.

Another study assessed the functional competence of the prenatally exposed animals. After weaning, the animals were challenged by a reversal-learning task in a modified Lashly III water maze. There was no statistical evidence of functional deficits resulting from microwave exposure.

Bereznitskaya (1968, 1972) exposed mice to 300 MHz, 10 mW/cm^2, which resulted in increased fetal wastage. No definite abnormalities or inborn genetic defects were found (Bereznitskaya and Rysina, 1974).

Neonatal mice exposed to 10.5, 19.27, or 26.6 MHz pulsed in a magnetic field of 55 A/m and an electric field of 8000 V/m 40 min/day for 5 days did not show any evidence of alteration in growth or development (Stavinoha et al., 1975).

Berman et al. (1978) exposed CD-1 mice to 2450-MHz microwaves for 100 min daily throughout gestation (day 1 through day 18), at 3.4 mW/cm^2 (2 mW/g), 13.6 mW/cm^2 (8.1 mW/g), or 28 mW/cm^2 (22.2 mW/g). The temperature and humidity in the anechoic chamber were maintained at 20.2 ± 0.5°C and 50% humidity. The authors reported that the treatments resulted in no thermal increment. The mean mass of live fetuses per litter was significantly decreased in the animals exposed at 28 mW/cm^2. The occurrence of cranioschisis (brain herniation) in the animals exposed to microwaves was not different from controls at any one power density but when summed across groups a significantly higher number of fetuses with cranioschisis occurred in the irradiated groups. The lack of brain-herniated litters in the sham-irradiated groups makes the data difficult to interpret with confidence since the spontaneous rate of brain hernias in the CD-1 mouse is approximately 0.2% of all fetuses (Perraud, 1976). As there were approximately 3500 live fetuses in the 336 sham-irradiated litters, one might expect a spontaneous incidence of seven brain hernias in the sham-irradiated litters, but the incidence was zero. Therefore, the seven affected microwave-irradiated litters may well be the result of unequal distribution of the spontaneous incidence instead of the result of (2 to 22 mW/kg) microwave exposure.

Nelson et al. (1979) exposed C3H mice at 148 MHz for 1 hr daily from day 2 through day 19 of gestation in a rectangular coaxial exposure system at 0.5 mW/cm^2 corresponding to an SAR of 0.013 mW/g. The experiment was conducted as three separate replications. In each of the experiments, some of the dams were allowed to come to term and the fetuses were assessed for weight at birth and again at 60 days of age while in others the uterus was extirpated on day 19 of gestation. No differences in percentage of resorbed, stillborn, or abnormal fetuses were observed in any of the three experiments.

The embryofetal toxicity and teratogenicity of 2.45-GHz CW microwaves at different intensities were investigated in the CD-1 mouse by Nawrot et al. (1981). Mice were exposed on days 1 to 15 of gestation to an incident power density of 5 mW/cm² (SAR 6.7 mW/g) and on either days 1 to 6 or 6 to 15 of gestation to 21 mW/cm² (SAR 28.14 mW/g) or to 30 mW/cm² (SAR 40.2 mW/g) for 8 hr daily. Exposure on days 1 to 6 or 6 to 15 of gestation to a power density of 21 or 30 mW/cm² caused an increase in colonic temperature of exposed dams of 1 and 2.3°C, respectively. To distinguish between "thermal" and "nonthermal" effects of 21 or 30 mW/cm², groups of mice were also exposed to elevated ambient temperature to raise their body temperature to the level of those animals exposed to microwaves. Ambient temperatures of 30 and 31°C increased the deep colonic temperature to that obtained with the 21 and 30 mW/cm² microwave exposure, respectively. The temperature-exposed mice were handled in exactly the same manner as the microwave-exposed mice. A significant reduction in maternal weight gain, during treatment on days 1 to 6 or 6 to 15 of gestation, was observed in females of all handled groups. Handling plus exposure to elevated ambient temperature (30 or 31°C) during days 6 to 15 of gestation increased this reduction in maternal weight gain. A significant decrease in implantation sites per litter and reduction in fetal weight were noted in the group exposed to 30 mW/cm² during days 1 to 6 of gestation. Exposure of mice to 30 mW/cm² (days 6 to 15 of gestation) resulted in a slight but significant increase in the percentage of malformed fetuses, predominantly with cleft palate, when compared to all other groups.

In an interesting study, Preskorn *et al.* (1978) reported retarded tumor growth and greater longevity in CFW mice following fetal irradiation by 2450 MHz at 35 ± 3 mW/g for 20 min on days 11, 12, 13, and 14 of gestation. The mice were implanted with a homogenate of a lymphoreticular cell sarcoma on day 16 postpartum. Microwave treatments did not alter the incidence of tumor but the tumors developed at a slower rate in the fetally irradiated animals.

Budd *et al.* (1970) investigated the sensitivity of the fetal rat's hematological system following *in utero* microwave irradiation. Pregnant Sprague–Dawley rats were exposed one at a time for $8\frac{1}{2}$ min to whole-body 2450-MHz CW microwaves, 100 mW/cm², at day 15 of gestation. Under these conditions, the rectal temperature of the pregnant rats increased 4.2°C above that of the controls. Hematological factors were measured in the pregnant rats at 4 hr, 24 hr, and 5 days postirradiation (shortly before the fetuses were removed). Body and spleen weights, and hematological changes were measured in the fetal rats at day 20 of gestation. No significant differences were found between control and microwave-exposed pregnant rats in body weight, total leukocyte count, erythrocyte count, hematocrit, or hemoglobin value. Microwave-irradiated fetuses had significantly lower spleen weights ($P < 0.05$), total leukocyte counts ($P < 0.01$), and somewhat lower hemoglobin values ($P < 0.10$) than controls. No appreciable differences were observed between microwave-irradiated fetuses and their controls in body weight, ^{59}Fe uptake in blood, or fetal resorption.

Laskey et al. (1970) exposed pregnant rats to 2450-MHz CW microwaves, 100 mW/cm^2, for 8 to 13 min on days 2, 5 (preimplantation stage), 8 (organogenesis stage), or 15 (fetal stage). These exposures produced group mean rectal temperatures ranging from 41.4 to 42.8°C (sham = 38.0°C). No changes occurred in the day 5 embryos, but there was an increased number of resorbed fetuses in the day 8 exposure and a decrease in weight of live fetuses exposed on day 8 or day 15. No obvious abnormalities were seen in any of the litters when examined on day 19 of gestation.

Dietzel and colleagues (Dietzel and Kern, 1970; Dietzel et al., 1972; Dietzel, 1975) exposed pregnant rats with a 27.12-MHz diathermy unit at power settings of 55, 70, and 100 W for 5, 10, and 10 min, respectively, which was sufficient to raise the animals' colonic temperatures to 39, 40.5, and 42°C. The rats were exposed once between days 1 and 16 of gestation. The fetuses were examined near term. The peak incidence of anomalies was found to occur on gestation days 13 to 14, when 16% of the fetuses were abnormal. This fetal wastage, as in the studies by Rugh et al. (1974, 1975), is clearly associated with a general body temperature increase in the dam.

Offspring of Sprague–Dawley rats exposed to 2450 MHz, 10 mW/cm^2 (est. SAR 2.2 W/kg), 5 hr daily on days 14 through 20 of gestation showed a relative decrease in body weight on postnatal day 3 (Shore et al., 1977). At parturition there were no differences in litter size. Body mass did not differ 1 or 2 weeks after birth. The authors noted that environmental temperature was not controlled. Temperature for the sham-exposed rats averaged 22.8 ± 0.2°C compared to 25.5 ± 0.7°C for the experimental chamber. Rats were grouped by E- or H-field orientation during exposures, and only the 3-day-old rats exposed parallel to the E field had significantly lower body and brain weights. This preferential decrement is difficult to explain on the basis of either age or orientation during exposure. It is most likely there is no significant difference in SAR in rats due to orientation at this frequency (Gage et al., 1979).

Smialowicz et al. (1979) exposed rats to 2450 MHz daily for 4 hr/day at a power density of 4 mW/cm^2 in utero from day 6 of gestation through 40 days of age. The SARs were determined by twin-well calorimetry for several ages of the animals. Pregnant dams weighing 300 to 350 g had a mean SAR of 0.7 W/kg; animals that were 1 to 5 days of age and weighed 6 to 10 g absorbed approximately 4.7 W/kg. There was no significant difference between the mean body weights of the males (female offspring were not used in this experiment) in the 12 sham-irradiated litters when compared to the mean body weights of the males in the 12 microwave-irradiated litters.

In studies of effects of *in utero* exposure of Long–Evans rats to 2450 MHz CW, Michaelson *et al.* (1976, 1978) found no adverse effects on the dam or offspring when gestation length or litter size was examined. The dams were exposed at 10 or 40 mW/cm^2 (est. SAR 2.5 or 10 W/kg) for 1 hr on day 9 (organogenesis) or day 16 (fetal stage) of gestation. Exposure to 40 mW/cm^2 caused an increase in colonic temperature of approximately 1 to 2°C over the sham-exposed animals. The exposure to 10 mW/cm^2 on day 9 or 16 of gestation caused a significant increase (~ 0.5 to 1°C) in the temperature of dams on day 16 of gestation. In general, there were no apparent differences in growth rate, development, or brain weight in pups from irradiated or nonexposed dams through the nursing period to weaning. Oxygen consumption in cold-stressed ratlets from the 40 mW/cm^2 exposed dams was increased (ca. 75 ml O$_2$/min per kg) relative to controls and 10 mW/cm^2 exposures (ca. 50 and 43 ml O$_2$/min per kg, respectively). There was no apparent difference in oxygen consumption at neutral temperature. Enhanced maturation as indicated by adrenocortical response was suggested.

Johnson *et al.* (1978) exposed pregnant rats for 20 hr daily for 19 days to 918 MHz at 5 mW/cm^2 (2.5 W/kg). This study is especially interesting, because it was conducted at a frequency close to resonance of the experimental subject (rats) and it is the only reported study conducted with continuous exposure. The eight microwave- and eight sham-irradiated pregnant dams were maintained in a waveguide exposure apparatus at 22°C, 45% relative humidity, and *ad lib* access to rat chow and water. The exposure was begun on the first day of pregnancy, the day on which the copulatory plug was first seen. The dams remained in the exposure waveguide or sham condition until gestation day 20. At 4 days of age, the litters were culled to four males and four females per litter, and then observed through 91 days of age. There appeared to be no differences in the litter means for the number of pups born, or number dead during the first day after birth. There were no pups in any of these litters (which included microwave-irradiated, sham-irradiated, and cage controls) reported to have any visible physical defects. Body weights at birth, at 28 days of age, and at 91 days of age did not reveal any significant alterations due to microwave exposure. There appeared to be a significant shift to earlier eye-opening in the exposed animals and this earlier maturation was approximately 1 day. However, eye-opening observations were made only twice daily, and the timing of birth had at least an 8-hr error, and thus these cumulative sources of experimental error diminish confidence in the result.

Jensh *et al.* (1978a) examined the effects of protracted prenatal exposure of Wistar-derived rats to 2450-MHz microwaves for 8 hr daily throughout gestation. The mean exposure time was 115 hr to incident energy at 20 mW/cm^2. No statistically significant differences were observed between control and exposed animals for maternal mass, embryonic and fetal resorption rate, abnormality rate, and term fetal and placental masses. These authors also reported similar experiments in which 915-MHz microwaves were employed (Jensh et al., 1977, 1978b). They exposed Wistar rats at 10 mW/cm^2 for 8 hr daily throughout gestation for an average of 110 hr of exposure. Postexposure colonic temperatures of dams showed no increase over baseline colonic temperatures. No differences were observed in embryonic or fetal death, abnormalities, fetal mass, litter size, placental mass, fetal sex ratio, maternal mass, or maternal gain of mass.

In another study (Jensh and Ludlow, 1980), gravid Wistar rats were exposed 8 hr daily throughout pregnancy to 915-MHz microwaves at 10 mW/cm^2. The average exposure time was 109 hr. In this study, dams were allowed to deliver their offspring. Within 3 days after birth, the pups were given three tests for reflexes. After the pups were weaned, a series of performance tests were given. The postweaning tests began on postpartum day 60 and were completed by day 90. No detrimental effects were observed concerning performance in a water T-maze, avoidance behavior, open-field behavior, forelimb hanging, or performance in a 24-hr activity wheel. Jensh et al. (1979) also reported no observable teratological effects in rats exposed throughout gestation to 6000 MHz, 35 mW/cm^2. The authors of the three studies state that the irradiation was "nonthermal," but no doses or dose rates were given for any of the exposure conditions.

To summarize studies of the rat: most of the significant results are based on exposures of dams to highly intense radiation, which is frequently fatal for the dam. Increases in resorption rate and decreases of fetal mass are the most common reported "defects."

Chernovetz et al. (1977) exposed Holtzman-derived, Sprague–Dawley rats to 2450-MHz microwaves in a multimode cavity at a dose rate of 31 ± 3 mW/g for 20 min. The microwave treatment was matched to infrared treatment on the basis of duration and averaged increment of colonic temperature ($\Delta T = 3.4°C$). The animals were acutely exposed once on day 10, 11, 12, 13, 14, 15, or 16 of gestation.

An increased number of fetal resorptions but no specific fetal abnormalities occurred in dams exposed to microwaves. Fetal mass was smaller than that of controls among dams subjected to either microwaves or infrared. Fetal brains of microwave-exposed animals contained less norepinephrine. Dopamine content of the fetal brain, although reduced in microwave-exposed animals, was not significantly different from that in control and infrared-irradiated animals.

Microwave-exposed dams differed from infrared-irradiated dams only in exhibiting a greater number of resorptions. Both microwave- and infrared-exposed dams differed from controls in exhibiting more resorptions; their fetuses were also smaller. No specific anatomical abnormalities were observed, although the dose of microwave energy was at the LD_{23} level for the dam. The authors speculated that the probability of teratogenic insult from the microwave exposure of the rat is smaller than the dam's probability of mortality. No quantitative data of the gross teratologic consequences of this microwave exposure were presented in the paper. But comments were made in the text by the authors regarding the lack of any structural abnormalities. The number of resorptions was significantly higher ($\sim$ sixfold) in the microwave- than in the sham-exposed fetuses, especially in the dams that had been exposed on day 11 of gestation. Fetal weights were also altered by the irradiation regimen with a small but statistically significant decrease in fetal mass. The alterations seen in the fetuses, in this case decreased fetal weights and death (in the form of resorptions), reflect the thermally induced teratological potential of microwave exposure in the rat. It is important to remember that the fetal alterations were found from microwave exposure regimens where colonic temperatures rose above 40°C.

In another study on rats, Chernovetz et al. (1979a) employed dose rates of 28 and 14 mW/g for 20 min and reported no specific abnormalities or increase of resorptions from exposure of fetuses to 2450-MHz microwaves in a multimode cavity on day 8, 10, 13, or 14 of gestation. No lethality resulted from the treatment although the posttreatment temperature of the dams receiving 28 mW/g reached 42°C. A third study employed elevated dose rates of 31 and 17 mW/g for 20 min on gestation days 8, 10, 12, or 14 resulting in average posttreatment temperatures of 43 and 41°C with a lethality rate of 21% for the dams exposed to the higher level of microwaves (Chernovetz et al., 1979b). Both resorptions and abnormalities were increased at 31 mW/g. Exencephaly was the most frequently observed abnormality. Fetal body mass was smaller at 31 mW/g and fetal brain mass was affected by both the treatment and the day of gestation on which exposure occurred. Regression analysis revealed that both peak temperature and dose rate were related positively to the occurrence of resorptions and abnormalities. The regression of fetal brain mass on fetal body mass revealed a tendency for animals exposed to 31 mW/g to be macrocephalic while the 17 mW/g exposed animals tended to be microcephalic. The three studies taken together would appear to support the authors' earlier speculation that in the laboratory rat the teratogenic threshold for thermal levels of microwaves is near the mortality threshold for the exposed dam. In addition, the results of the three studies clearly parallel the heat stress literature in the observation of a narrow thermal window in which fetal damage will occur in the rat.

Berman et al. (1978) exposed Sprague–Dawley rats to 2.45 GHz at a power density of 0 or 28 mW/cm^2 for 100 min daily from days 6 to 15 after breeding. Additional animals were exposed to 40 mW/cm^2. They concluded that 2.45-GHz microwaves do not produce a strong teratogenic effect in the rat unless the dam is thermally stressed.

Berman et al. (1981) were not able to elicit any fetotoxic or teratological responses (body weight; numbers alive and dead; external, visceral, or skeletal morphology) in fetal rats irradiated daily (100 min/day) during gestation, even with the use of a large number of litters. The dams were exposed to 2450-MHz radiation at power densities of 0 or 28 mW/cm^2 (4.2 W/kg). These conditions produced a mean colonic temperature of 40.3°C by the end of the 100-min exposure.

A series of experiments was conducted on rats to assess the teratological effects of 27 MHz because of the large-scale utilization of this frequency in industry such as RF heat sealers (Lary et al., 1979, 1980; Conover et al., 1980; Lacy et al., 1980a,b). At various days of gestation, the investigators used energy levels sufficient to cause and sustain high body temperatures (up to 43°C, 20 to 40 min). These experiments showed that day 9 was the most sensitive day of pregnancy.

A variety of malformations, including decreased body weight, were found. Thermal (maternal) threshold was 41.5°C. Gross microscopic teratogenic effects were equivalent when maternal temperature was the result of microwaves or hot-water immersion. The threshold was approximately 12 mW/g for 30 min.

Conover et al. (1978) reported on single, 20- and 30-min exposures of fetal rats on day 10, 12, or 14 of gestation to 27.12 MHz at SAR, of 17 to 35 mW/g. Preliminary results suggested that fetal wastage occurred after exposure on day 10 or 14 of gestation. Grossly observable malformations occurred in animals exposed on day 10 for 30 min while visceral abnormalities occurred after exposure on day 10 or 14. Fetal mass and fetal crown–rump length were smaller in the fetuses exposed to microwaves. The same investigators (Lary et al., 1979) reported on eight groups of 16 to 28 gravid rats exposed to 27.12 MHz. The facility for exposure was an RF near-field synthesizer operating in the dominant magnetic field mode at a field strength of 55 A/m. The dams were exposed on gestation day 2, 4, 6, 8, 10, 12, 14, or 16 for 20–40 min at an average dose rate of 125 mW/g until their colonic temperature reached 43.0°C. Eight groups were sham-irradiated for 30 min and one group of 29 rats served as cage controls. Rats irradiated on days 8–16 (organogenesis) had a significant increase in gross malformations and a significant decrease in fetal weight and fetal crown–rump length.

Rats were exposed to 2450 MHz on day 13 of gestation to varying power densities and durations (Sharp and Paperiello, 1971). The fetuses were removed on day 19 of gestation and weighed. The authors noted that if 13-day-old fetuses were exposed to 10 mW/cm^2 for 10 min and body weight measured on day 19 of gestation, there was an increase of approximately 10% in the weight of the exposed fetuses as compared to the nonexposed controls. Exposure to 33 mW/cm^2 for 10 min resulted in a median increase in live fetal weights but also an increase in weight variability and an increase in the number of resorptions.

Wise et al. (1949) showed that exposure to 2450 MHz at power densities in excess of 100 mW/cm^2, sufficient to cause injury to soft tissues in rats, may produce shortening and deformity of bones, or partial or complete epiphyseal destruction. However, at power densities less than 100 mW/cm^2, no appreciable effect on bone growth was noted.

An investigation by Granberry and Janes (1963) did not reveal any effect of microwave diathermy on bone growth. One knee joint from each of seven (4–5 month old) puppies was exposed to 2450-MHz microwaves, approximately 200 mW/cm^2, for two 1-hr periods/day (3-hr intervals) for a total of 100 hr over 9 weeks. The animals were sacrificed and bones from exposed and unexposed legs examined roentgenographically and histologically. No changes in growth were found.

Boak et al. (1932) administered "shortwave" radiation (10 MHz) to rabbits from day 29 of life through several matings and pregnancies. The total exposure time ranged between 30 and 75 hr, during which the temperatures of the animals were raised to 41 to 42°C. There was no interference with mating, fertilization, or development of the young *in utero*. Litter sizes were not significantly different from those of control animals.

Deichmann et al. (1963) exposed two female (21 month old) beagles to 24,000 MHz (pulsed) at a power level estimated to be 24 mW/cm^2 for a period of 20 months. One dog was exposed for 400 min/day, 5 days/week for a total of 2631 hr and the other for $16\frac{1}{2}$ hr/day, 4 days/week for a total of 3970 hr. The dogs were bred during the experiment and delivered a total of three litters. The first dog had five pups (one stillborn) after 1500 hr exposure; the second had one litter (five pups, two stillborn) after 200 hr exposure, and another litter (four pups, one stillborn) after 1950 hr exposure. The bitches were not exposed during the week before and 3 weeks after parturition. All offspring developed normally.

Shively (1970) studied the effect of exposure to microwave energy on puppies. Newborn dogs were selected for study since their retina and cerebellum are immature at birth and the sensitivity of these organs to damage by exposure to ionizing radiation had been previously demonstrated (Shively et al., 1967). Two- or three-day-old dogs were positioned facing a 2450-MHz microwave source and exposed for varying periods of time from 3 to 24 min at 100 or 300 mW/cm^2. Complete necropsy was performed 1–70 days after exposure. Subcellular changes were not detected in the retinas studied by electron microscopy. Under the conditions used in this pilot experiment, morphological changes attributable to microwave exposure were not found.

Kaplan (1981) reported a study of the postnatal effects of *in utero* exposure to up to 3.4 W/kg of 2.45-MHz microwaves in squirrel monkeys. The authors observed an increase in neonatal deaths. However, a more intensive examination, by replication, was not able to demonstrate any change in death rate, and not able to confirm the earlier report (Kaplan, 1981).

Conclusion

In a review, O'Connor (1980) noted that with respect to basic design, procedure, and variables assessed, the teratogenic studies reported to date have been more diverse than decisive. Wide variation in exposure parameters makes it difficult to compare the results; additional difficulty is generated because many of the reports do not contain information on critical variables such as the manner in which the day of gestation was timed. The day on which the animal is sperm or sperm-plug positive can be timed as day 0, although a more common procedure is to consider this day 1. The manner in which control animals were treated is often not given. Many kinds of controls have been employed including passive cage controls, sham-exposed controls, heat (infrared irradiated) controls, and historic controls. In some reports, statistical or probability statements have been substituted for data from control animals. Multiple control procedures in single experiments have not been used extensively.

Many of the investigators who have reported defects have employed acute, intense irradiation, which obviously placed a thermal burden on the exposed subject. Some studies attempt to control for heat by including controls heated by means of infrared. Of importance in this regard are the comparisons with the literature on heat stress.

Many of the teratogenic studies of RF exposure have been performed without a sufficient number of animals, and others lack sophisticated design and thus do not allow for observation of low-probability events. One could argue that any increase in the incidence of fetal damage, regardless of how low, should be considered as a possible biologically significant event even if it is not statistically reliable. While few adequate and rigorous designs have been employed, more critical to the assessment of demonstrated teratogenic potential of microwaves is the fact that the statistical analyses are usually not given in enough detail to permit evaluation (O'Connor, 1980).

If attention is focused not on procedural questions but only on similarities in the results of the studies, several trends are apparent. The most common result from fetal exposure to microwaves would appear to be a nonspecific response, that of reduced or retarded gain of body mass. Without further study, it is impossible to know if this decrease is maintained after birth and when, if ever, the exposed stunted fetuses catch up. It is important to note that this general suppression of body mass is the only effect that appears to be common across the range of species that have been studied.

Another more general deleterious response seen in the mammal is increased rate of fetal resorption. The increase may be indicative of malformed fetuses, but the resorbed nature of the fetal material precludes a more fine-grained analysis and thus identification of which, if any, specific structure was damaged. The increased rate of resorption and the range of exposures within which it occurs are remarkably similar to the effects of heat stress. Particularly in the rat, the resorption rate appears to increase within a rather narrow thermal window, the other side of which is thermal death. The majority of defects have been observed following high-level, acute exposures with obvious thermal components (O'Connor, 1980).

It does appear that abnormalities in small animal fetuses can be produced with microwaves in conjunction, however, with systemic hyperthermia of 2.5–5°C above the normal temperature for the species for some time period during specific critical developmental stages. From a survey of the lilterature, it appears that it is the temperature rise in the fetus, irrespective of the manner in which it is produced, that causes damage. It is important to realize that in all species there is a constantly evolving pattern of maturation during gestation and in the rat this continues during the first 3 weeks of postnatal life. In interpreting teratological effects of microwaves, as with any agent it is important to realize that many fetal defects such as hemorrhage, resorption, stillbirth, and exencephaly occur spontaneously in mice (Chernovetz et al., 1975).

In man, infections such as rubella, influenza, and smallpox, occurring during early pregancy, are known to cause abortions and fetal malformations (Wilson, 1959; Gruenwald, 1947). In general, it appears that any infection giving rise to fever in the early stages of pregnancy in man or animals, is capable of producing fetal malformation or abortion. It is well known that induction of fever can lead to the early termination of pregnancy (Cameron, 1943). There are numerous reports of abnormalities resulting from the induction of systemic hyperthermia of 2.5–5°C above the normal temperature for the species for 1 hr or longer during specific critical developmental stages of the fetus by exposure of the pregnant animals to elevated temperatures and humidity in environmental chambers. Fetal resorption, growth retardation, microphthalmia, and malformations affecting the central nervous system, musculoskeletal system, and other organs, have been observed in mammalian species, e.g., the guinea pig (Edwards, 1967, 1969) and the rat (Edwards, 1968; Garrison, 1940; Hsu, 1948). In experiments on rats, hyperthermia of 4 to 4.5°C for 40 to 60 min during specific developmental stages produces increased fetal resorptions, retardation of growth, microphthalmia, anencephaly, and defects of tails, limbs, toes, palate, and body, depending upon the gestational stage at which the hyperthermia occurred (Edwards, 1968). These results indicate that the occurrence of fetal malformations in mammals in early pregnancy is probably related not as much to the viral or bacterial toxemia, but to the fever–hyperthermia occurring at a particular critical stage of organogenesis. The threshold appears to be an elevation of 2.5–5.0°C above the normal temperature of the species, sustained for 1 hr or more.

As noted by Martson and Voronina (1976) from the standpoint of public health, one must consider the difficulty of extrapolating data from experimental teratology to the human fetus. Such an extrapolation becomes feasible only after detailed analysis of the fine mechanisms of teratogenesis. Also of great importance is the need for appropriate scaling factors to permit extrapolation of experimental data obtained on small animals, to the human. The concepts of scaling are discussed in another chapter.

The reports on effects of microwave exposure on early development have been reviewed by Baranski and Czerski (1976) who concluded that no serious effects are to be expected at power densities below 10 mW/cm^2 under usual exposure conditions. They further note that defects, when observed, are the result of hyperthermia. There are numerous reports of abnormalities from the induction of systemic hyperthermia of 2.5–5°C above the normal temperature for the species, by exposure of the pregnant animal to elevated temperatures at specific critical developmental stages of the fetus (Edwards, 1968, 1969). It would thus appear that in the reports of microwave-induced developmental abnormalities, it is the temperature rise in the fetus, irrespective of the manner in which it was produced, that caused the damage.

RF/MW energies are weak teratogens that must be applied at high SARs ($> 15 \text{ W/kg}$) approaching lethal levels for the mother in experimental animal studies. High maternal body temperatures are known to be associated with birth defects. There appears to be a threshold for the induction of experimental birth defects when a maternal colonic temperature of 41 to 42°C is reached. Any agent capable of producing elevated internal temperatures in this range is a potential teratogen.

Studies involving prenatal exposures have not shown effects on growth and development. Temperature in the testes of greater than 45°C caused by any modality can cause permanent sterility; from 37 to 42°C, mature sperm may be killed with a temporary loss of spermatogenic epithelium. Changes in reproductive efficiency have not been directly associated with RF/MW exposure.

REFERENCES

Baranski, S., and P. Czerski (1976) *Biological Effects of Microwaves*. Dowden, Hutchinson & Ross, Stroudsburg, Pa.

Barron, C. I., and A. A. Baraff (1958) Medical considerations of exposure to microwaves (radar). *J. Am. Med. Assoc.* **168**:1194.

Barron, C. I., A. A. Love, and A. A. Baraff (1955) Physical evaluation of personnel exposed to microwave emanations. *J. Aviat. Med.* **26**:442.

Bereznitskaya, A. N. (1968) The effect of 10-centimeter and ultrashort waves on the reproductive function of female mice. *Gig. Tr. Prof. Zabol.* **9**:33.

Bereznitskaya, A. N. (1972) Research on the reproductive function in female mice under the impact of low-intensity radio waves of different ranges. In: *Industrial Health and Biological Effects of Radio Frequency Electromagnetic Waves*. Material of the Fourth All-Union Symposium, Moscow.

Bereznitskaya, A. N., and I. M. Kazbekov (1973) Studies on the reproduction and testicular microstructure of mice exposed to microwaves. In: *Biological Effects of Radiofrequency Electromagnetic Fields*, Z. V. Gordon (ed.). No. 4, Moscow, pp. 221–229 (JPRS 63321, 1974).

Bereznitskaya, A. N., and T. Z. Rysina (1974) Embryotropic effects of microwaves. In: *Biological Effects of Radiofrequency Electromagnetic Fields*, Z. V. Gordon (ed.). JPRS 63321, pp. 168–174.

Berman, E., J. B. Kinn, and H. B. Carter (1978) Observations of mouse fetuses after irradiation with 2.45 GHz microwaves. *Health Phys.* **35**:791.

Berman, E., H. B. Carter, and D. House (1980) Tests of mutagenesis and reproduction in male rats exposed to 2450 MHz (CW) microwaves. *Bioelectromagnetics* **1**:65.

Berman, E., H. B. Carter, and D. House (1981) Observations of rat fetuses after irradiation with 2450 MHz (CW) microwaves. *J. Microwave Power* **16**:9.

Boak, R. A., C. M. Carpenter, and S. L. Warren (1932) Studies on the physiological effects of fever temperatures. II. The effect of repeated short wave (30 meter) fevers on growth and fertility of rabbits. *J. Exp. Med.* **56**:725.

Budd, R. A., J. Laskey, and C. Kelly (1970) Hematological response of fetal rats following 2450 MHz microwave irradiation. In: *Radiation Bio-effects Summary Report, January–December 1970*, D. M. Hodge (ed.). HEW, PHS, BRH Publ. BRH/DBE 70-7 (December), p. 161.

Cameron, J. A. (1943) Termination of early pregnancy by artificial fever. *Proc. Soc. Exp. Biol. Med.* **52**:76.

Carpenter, R. L., and E. M. Livstone (1971) Evidence for nonthermal effects of microwave radiation: Abnormal development of irradiated insect pupae. *IEEE Trans. Microwave Theory Tech.* **MTT-19**: 173.

Chernovetz, M. E., D. R. Justesen, N. W. King, and J. E. Wagner (1975) Tetratology, survival, and reversal learning after fetal irradiation of mice by 2450 MHz microwave energy. *J. Microwave Power* **10**:391.

Chernovetz, M. E., D. R. Justesen, and A. F. Oke (1977) A teratologic study of the rat: Microwave and infrared radiations compared. *Radio Sci.* **12**(6S):191.

Chernovetz, M. E., D. R. Justesen, and D. M. Levinson (1979a) Acceleration and deceleration of fetal growth of rats by 2450 MHz microwave radiation. In: *Electromagnetic Fields in Biological Systems*, S. Stuchly (ed.). IMPI, Edmonton, Canada, pp. 175-193.
Chernovetz, M. E., D. Reeves, and D. R. Justesen (1979b) Teratology in rats exposed to 2450 MHz microwaves at intense and intermediate dose rates. Presented at the *Biolectromagnetics Symposium*, Seattle.
Conover, D., J. M. Lary, and E. Foley (1978) Induction of teratogenic effects in rats by 27.12 MHz RF radiation. Presented at the *1978 Symposium on Electromagnetic Fields in Biological Systems*, Ottawa, Canada.
Conover, D. L., J. M. Lary, and P. L. Hanser (1980) Thermal threshold for teratogenic response in rats irradiated at 27.12 MHz. *Bioelectromagnetics* **1**:204.
Davidson, J. A., B. A. Kondra, and M. A. K. Hamid (1976) Effects of microwave radiation on eggs, embryos and chickens. *Can. J. Anim. Sci.* **56**:709.
Deichmann, W. B., M. Keplinger, and E. Bernal (1963) Effects on dogs of chronic exposure to microwave radiation. *J. Occup. Med.* **5**:418.
de Seguin, L., and G. Castelian (1947) Action of ultrahigh frequency radiation (wavelength 21 cm) on temperature of small laboratory animals. *C. R. Acad. Sci.* **224**:1662.
Dietzel, F. (1975) Effects of non-ionizing electro-magnetic radiation on the development and intrauterine implantation of the rat. *Ann. N. Y. Acad. Sci.* **247**:367.
Dietzel, F., and W. Kern (1970) Abortion following ultra-shortwave hyperthermia animal experiments. *Arch. Gynaekol.* **209**:445.
Dietzel, F., W. Kern, and R. Steckenmesser (1972) Deformity and intrauterine death after short-wave therapy in early pregnancy in experimental animals. *Muench. Med. Wochenschr.* **114**:228.
Dumansky, Y. D., A. M. Serdyuk, C. I. Litvinova, L. A. Tomashevskaya, and V. M. Popovich (1972) Experimental research on the biological effects of 12-centimeter low-intensity waves. In: *Health in Inhabited Localities*. Ed. II, Kiev, p. 29.
Edwards, M. J. (1967) Congenital defects in guinea pigs following induced hyperthermia during gestation. *Arch. Pathol.* **84**:42.
Edwards, M. J. (1968) Congenital malformations in the rat following induced hyperthermia during gestation. *Teratology* **1**:173.
Edwards, M. J. (1969) Congenital defects in guinea pigs: Fetal resorptions, abortions, and malformations following induced hyperthermia during early gestation. *Teratology* **2**:313.
Ely, T. S., D. E. Goldman, J. Hearon, R. B. Williams, and H. M. Carpenter (1957) Heating characteristics of laboratory animals exposed to ten-centimeter microwaves. U.S. Nav. Med. Res. Inst. (Res. Rep. Proj. NM 001-056.13.02). *IEEE Trans. Biomed. Eng.* **BME-11**: 123 (1964).
Fahim, M. N., Z. Fahim, R. Der, D. G. Hal, and J. Harman (1975) Heat in male contraception (hot water 60°C, infrared, microwave and ultrasound). *Contraception* **11**(5):549.
Follis, R. H., Jr. (1946) Studies on the biological effect of high frequency radio waves (radar). *Am. J. Physiol.* **147**:281.
Gage, M. I., E. Berman, and J. B. Kinn (1979) Videotape observation of rats and mice during an exposure to 2450 MHz microwave radiation. *Radio Sci.* **14**(6S):227.
Garrison, L. H. (1940) The effect of fever on the development of the rat incisor. *J. Dent. Res.* **19**:215.
Gorodetskaya, S. F. (1963) The effect of centimeter radio waves on mouse fertility. *Fiziol. Zh. (Kiev)* **9**:394.
Gorodetskaya, S. F. (1964) The influence of SHF electromagnetic fields on fertility, peripheral blood picture, conditioned reflexes, and morphology of internal organs of

white mice. In: *Biological Action of Ultrasound and SHF-UHF Electromagnetic Oscillations,* A. A. Gorodetskii (ed.). Nauk Dumka, Kiev, p. 80.

Granberry, W. M., and J. M. Janes (1963) The lack of effect of microwave diathermy on bone of the growing dog. *J. Bone J. Surg.* **45A:**773.

Gruenwald, P. (1947) Mechanisms of abnormal development. *Arch. Pathol.* **44:**398.

Gunn, S. A., T. C. Gould, and W. A. D. Anderson (1961) The effect of microwave radiation on morphology and function of rat testis. *Lab. Invest.* **10:**301.

Haidt, S. J., and A. H. McTighe (1973) The effect of chronic, low-level microwave radiation on the testicles of mice. In: *1973 IEEE-G-MTT International Microwave Symposium,* S. W. Maley (ed.) pp. 324–325.

Hamrick, P. E., and D. I. McRee (1975) Exposure of the Japanese quail embryo to 2.45 GHz microwave radiation during the second day of development. *J. Microwave Power* **10:**211.

Hsu, C. (1948) Influence of temperature on development of rat embryos. *Anat. Rec.* **100:**79.

Imig, C. J., J. D. Thomson, and H. M. Hines (1948) Testicular degeneration as a result of microwave irradiation. *Proc. Soc. Exp. Biol. Med.* **69:**382.

Jensh, R. P., and J. Ludlow (1980) Behavioral teratology: Application in low dose chronic microwave irradiation studies. In: *Advances in the Study of Birth Defects,* Vol. 4, T. V. N. Persand (ed.). MTP Press, Lancaster, U.K., pp. 135–162.

Jensh, R. P., J. Ludlow, L. Weinburg, W. H. Vogel, T. Rudder, and R. L. Brent (1977) Teratogenic effects on rat offspring of non-thermal chronic prenatal microwave irradiation. *Teratology* **15**(2):14A.

Jensh, R. P., J. Ludlow, L. Weinburg, W. H. Vogel, T. Rudder, and R. L. Brent (1978a) Studies concerning the post natal effects of protracted low dose prenatal 915 MHz microwave radiation. *Teratology* **17:**21A.

Jensh, R. P., J. Ludlow, L. Weinburg, W. H. Vogel, T. Rudder, and R. L. Brent (1978b) Studies concerning the protracted prenatal exposure to a non-thermal level of 2450 MHz microwave radiation in the pregnant rat. *Teratology* **17:**48A.

Jensh, R. P., W. H. Vogel, J. Ludlow, and T. McHugh (1979) Studies concerning the effects of low dosage prenatal 6000 MHz microwave radiation on growth and development in the rat. *Teratology* **19**(2):32A.

Johnson, R. B., S. Mizumori, and R. H. Lovely (1978) Adult behavioral deficits in rats exposed prenatally to 918-MHz microwaves. In: *Developmental Toxicology of Energy-Related Pollutants,* D. D. Mahlum, M. R. Sikov, P. L. Hackett, and F. D. Andrew (eds.). Department of Energy Symposium Series 47, pp. 281–299.

Kalant, H. (1959) Physiologic hazards of microwave radiation, survey of published literature. *Can. Med. Assoc. J.* **81:**575.

Kaplan, J. N. (1981) Study of the lethal effects of microwaves in the developing squirrel monkey. Final report for Contract No. 68-02-3210, U.S. Environmental Protection Agency.

Krueger, W. F., A. J. Giarola, J. W. Bradley, and A. Shrekenhamer (1975) Effects of electromagnetic fields on fecundity in the chicken. *Ann. N.Y. Acad. Sci.* **247:**323.

Lacy, K. K., J. M. Desesso, and J. M. Lary (1980a) A comparison of the teratogenic effects of radiofrequency radiation and hyperthermia: Gross evaluation. *Teratology* **21:**51A.

Lacy, K. K., J. M. Dessesso, T. W. Sadler, and J. M. Lary (1980b) A comparison of the teratogenic effects of radiofrequency radiation and hyperthermia: Light microscopic evaluation. *Teratology* **21:**52A.

Lary, J. M., D. L. Conover, E. D. Foley, and P. L. Hanser (1979) Teratogenicity of 27.12 MHz radiofrequency radiation in rats. *Teratology* **19:**36A.

Lary, J. M., D. L. Conover, E. D. Foley, and P. L. Hanser (1980) Teratogenicity of 27.12 MHz radiofrequency radiation in rats. *Bioelectromagnetics* **1:**402.

Laskey, J., D. Dawes, and M. Howes (1970) Progress report on 2450 MHz irradiation of pregnant rats and the effect on the fetus. In: *Radiation Bio-effects Summary Report, January–December 1970*, D. M. Hodge (ed.). HEW, PHS, BRH Publ. BRH/DBE 70-7 (December), pp. 167–173.

Leach, W. M. (1980) Genetic, growth, and reproductive effects of microwave radiation. *Bull. N.Y. Acad. Med.* **56**:249.

Letowski, A. (1967) Badania doswiadzalne nad wplywem aparatury radarowej na ustroj szczurow ze szczegolnym narzadow plciowych zenskich. *Ginekol. Pol. Supl.* **7**:51.

Letowski, A., T. Bartoszewicz, and A. Lankienicki (1971) Proba oceny metoda cytohormonalna i histochemiczna estrogenow u szczurzyc ciczarnych napromienianych microfalami. *Lek. Wojsk.* **47**:551.

Lin, J. C., J. C. Nelson, and M. E. Ekstrom (1979) Effects of repeated exposure to 148 MHz radiowaves on growth and hematology of mice. *Radio Sci.* **14**:173.

Lindauer, G. A., L. M. Liu, G. W. Skewes, and F. J. Rosenbaum (1974) Further experiments seeking evidence of nonthermal biological effects of microwave radiation. *IEEE Trans. Microwave Theory Tech.* **MTT-22**:790.

Liu, L. M., F. J. Rosenbaum, and W. F. Pickard (1975) The relation of teratogenesis in *Tenebrio molitor* to the incidence of low level microwaves. *IEEE Trans. Microwave Theory Tech.* **MTT-23**:929.

McRee, D. I., and P. E. Hamrick (1977) Exposure of Japanese quail embryos to 2.45 GHz microwave radiation during development. *Radiat. Res.* **71**:355.

McRee, D. I., P. E. Hamrick, J. E. Zinkl, P. Thaxton, and C. R. Parkhurst (1975) Some effects of exposure of the Japanese quail embryo to 2.45 GHz microwave radiation. *Ann. N.Y. Acad. Sci.* **247**:377.

Marha, K. (1970) Maximum admissible values of HF and UHF electromagnetic radiation at work places in Czechoslovakia. In: *Biological Effects and Health Implications of Microwave Radiation*, S. F. Cleary (ed.). Symposium Proceedings, HEW Publ. BRH/DBE 70-2, p. 188.

Marha, K., J. Musil, and H. Tuha (1968) *Electromagnetic Fields and the Living Environment*. State Health Publishing House, Prague (Transl. SBN 911302-13-7, San Francisco Press, 1971).

Martson, L. V., and V. M. Voronina (1976) Experimental study of the effect of a series of phosphoroorganic pesticides (Dipterex and Imidan) on embryogenesis. *Environ. Health Perspect.* **13**:121.

Michaelson, S. M., R. Guillet, M. A. Catallo, J. Small, G. Inamine, and F. W. Heggeness (1976) Influence of 2450 MHz microwaves on rats exposed in utero. *J. Microwave Power* **11**:165.

Michaelson, S. M., R. Guillet, and F. W. Heggeness (1978) The influence of microwave exposure on functional maturation of the rat. In: *Developmental Toxicology of Energy-Related Pollutants*, D. D. Mahlum, M. R. Sikov, P. L. Hackett, and F. D. Andrew (eds.). Department of Energy Symposium Series 47, pp. 300–316.

Miro, L., R. Loubiere, and A. Pfister (1965) Studies of visceral lesions observed in mice and rats exposed to UHF waves: A particular study of the effects of these waves on the reproduction of these animals. *Rev. Med. Aeronaut. (Paris)* **4**:37.

Muraca, G. J., Jr., E. S. Ferri, and F. L. Buchta (1977) A study of the effects of microwave irradiation of the rat testes. II. In: *Biological Effects of Electromagnetic Waves*, Vol. 1, C. C. Johnson and M. L. Shore (eds.). HEW Publ. (FDA) 77-8010, pp. 484–494.

Nawrot, P. S., D. I. McRee, and R. E. Staples (1981) Effects of 2.45 GHz CW microwave radiation on embryofetal development in mice. *Teratology* **24**:303.

Nelson, J. C., J. C. Lin, and M. E. Ekstrom (1979) Teratogenic effects of RF radiation on mice. Presented at *Bioelectromagnetics Symposium*, Seattle.

O'Connor, M. E. (1980) Mammalian teratogenesis and radiofrequency fields. *Proc. IEEE* **68:**56.
Osborne, C. (1958) Studies on the biological effects of 200 mc. In: *Proceedings of the Second Annual Tri-Service Conference on Biological Effects of Microwave Energy,* E. G. Pattishall and F. W. Banghart (eds.). University of Virginia, Charlottesville, p. 196.
Osborne, C. (1959) Studies on the biological effects of 200 mc. In: *Investigators' Conference on Biological Effects of Electronic Radiating Equipments.* Rome Air Development Center, Air Research and Development Command, Rome, N.Y., ASTIA Document No. AD 214 693, p. 20.
Pay, P. L., A. F. Anderson, and G. L. Jessup, Jr. (1978) A comparative study of the effects of microwave radiation and conventional heating on the reproductive capacity of *Drosophila melanogaster. Radiat. Res.* **76:**271.
Perraud, J. (1976) Levels of spontaneous malformations in the CD rat and CD-1 mouse. *Lab. Anim. Sci.* **26:**293.
Povzhitkov, A. A., N. V. Tyagin, and A. M. Grebieshetchnikova (1961) Vlijanie sverchvysokotchastronogo impulsnogo elektromagnitnogo polja na zatchatie i tetchenie bieremennosti u belych myshei. *Byull. Eksp. Biol. Med.* **5:**103.
Prausnitz, S., and C. Süsskind (1962) Effects of chronic microwave irradiation on mice. *IRE Trans. Bio-Med. Electron.* **9:**104.
Preskorn, S. H., W. P. Edwards; and D. R. Justesen (1978) Retarded tumor growth and greater longevity in mice after irradiation by 2450 MHz microwaves. *J. Surg. Oncol.* **10:**438.
Pucak, G. J., C. S. Lee, and A. S. Zaino (1977) Effects of prolonged high temperature on testicular development and fertility in the male rat. *Lab. Anim. Sci.* **27:**76.
Rosenthal, D. S. and S. C. Beering (1968) Hypogonadism after microwave radiation, *J. Am. Med. Assoc.* **205:**345.
Rugh, R., and M. McManaway (1976) Anesthesia as an effective agent against the production of congenital anomalies in mouse fetuses exposed to electromagnetic radiation. *J. Exp. Zool.* **197:**363.
Rugh, R., and M. McManaway (1977) Mouse fetal sensitivity to microwave radiation. *Congenital Anomalies (Senten Ijo)* **17:**39.
Rugh, R., E. I. Ginns, H. S. Ho, and W. M. Leach (1974) Are microwaves teratogenic? In: *Biological Effects and Health Hazards of Microwave Radiation,* P. Czerski, K. Ostrowski, M. L. Shore, C. Silverman, M. J. Suess, and B. Waldeskog (eds.). Polish Medical Publishers, Warsaw, pp. 98–107.
Rugh, R., E. I. Ginns, H. S. Ho, and W. M. Leach (1975) Responses of the mouse to microwave radiation during estrous cycle and pregancy. *Radiat. Res.* **62:**225.
Rugh, R., H. Ho, and M. McManaway (1976) The relation of dose rate of microwave radiation to the time of death and total absorbed dose in the mouse. *J. Microwave Power* **11:**279.
Saunders, R. D., and C. I. Kowalczuk (1981a) The effect of acute far-field exposure at 2.45 GHz on the mouse testes. *Int. J. Radiat. Biol.* **39:**587.
Saunders, R. D., and C. I. Kowalczuk (1981b) Effects of 2.45 GHz microwave radiation and heat on mouse spermatogenic epithelium. *Int. J. Radiat. Biol.* **40:**623.
Sharp, J. S., and C. J. Paperiello (1971) The effects of microwave exposure on thymidine-H^3 uptake in albino rats. *Radiat. Res.* **45:**434.
Shively, J. N. (1970) A pilot study of effects of microwave exposure on ontogenesis. In: *Radiation Bio-effects Summary Report, January–December 1970,* D. M. Hodge (ed.). HEW, PHS, BRH Publ. BRH/DBE 70-7 (December), p. 201.
Shively, J. N., R. D. Phemister, and G. P. Epling (1967) Alterations in the fine structure of the mature retina of dogs irradiated as neonates. *Exp. Eye Res.* **6:**278.
Shore, M. L., R. P. Felten, and A. Lamanna (1977) The effect of repetitive prenatal

low-level microwave exposure on development in the rat. In: *Biological Effects and Measurement of Radiofrequency/Microwaves,* D. G. Hazzard (ed.). HEW Publ. (FDA) 77-8026, pp. 280–289.

Smialowicz, R. J., J. B. Kinn, and J. A. Elder (1979) Prenatal exposure of rats to 2450-MHz CW microwave radiation: Effects on lymphocytes. *Radio Sci.* **14**(6S):147.

Stavinoha, W. B., A. Modak, M. A. Medina, and A. E. Gass (1975) Growth and development of neonatal mice exposed to high-frequency electromagnetic fields. Report SAM-TR-75-51, School of Aerospace Medicine, Brooks AFB, Texas.

van Demark, W. R., and J. R. Free (1973) Temperature effects. In: *The Testis,* Vol. III, A. D. Johnson, W. R. Gomes, and M. L. van Demark (eds.). Academic Press, New York, pp. 233–312.

Van Ummersen, C. A. (1961) The effect of 2450 mc radiation on the development of the chick embryo. In: *Biological Effects of Microwave Radiation,* Vol. 1, M. F. Peyton (ed.). Plenum Press, New York, p. 201.

Van Ummersen, C. A. (1963) An Experimental Study of Development Abnormalities Induced in the Chick Embryo by Exposure to Radio Frequency Waves. Ph.D. dissertation, Tufts University, Medford, Mass.

Varma, M. M., and E. A. Traboulay, Jr. (1975) Biological effects of microwave radiation on the testes of Swiss mice. *Experientia* **31**:301.

Wilson, G. J. (1959) Experimental studies on congenital malformations. *J. Chronic Dis.* **10**:111.

Wise, C. W., B. Castleman, and A. L. Watkins (1949) Effect of diathermy on bone growth in the albino rat. *J. Bone Joint Surg.* **31A**:487.

9

Thermoregulation

9.1. PHYSIOLOGIC REGULATION

If biological perturbations as a result of exposure to electromagnetic energies should occur, they could be manifested by general "stress" responses characterized by functional changes in regulatory systems of the body. The main integrators of these regulatory systems appear to be the brain and central nervous system (CNS). The CNS and the hypothalamus in particular mediate the classical biological responses to factors that may impose a strain on the homeostatic mechanisms of the body.

Physiological integration results from cooperating processes at work within an individual. Regulation and therefore integration typically deals with cooperation among two or more different processes. For example, heart rate and other circulatory functions are modified in response to messages from specific muscles, viscera, or glands. In those tissues, augmented blood flow increases the supplies of oxygen and other substances at active local sites. Messages are transmitted at various kinds of junctions and chemical receptors (Adolph, 1979).

Physiologic regulation represented by neuroendocrine function, neurochemical activity, thermoregulation, and immune responses are exquisitely "tuned" interrelated systems that constitute sensitive indicators of body responses to environmental insults. Pituitary hormones and neurotransmitters are intimately linked to the functions of the CNS. There are reports that exposure to electromagnetic fields may affect neuroendocrine, neurochemical activities and behavior. Little, however, has been learned of the underlying mechanisms that bring about these effects. It is quite possible that many of the reported observations, especially those related to behavioral responses, are manifestations of perception or detection of the field rather than a direct coupling of the energy into the responding body function. Study of the integration and correlation of many body functions relative to the homeostatic or homeokinetic status of the exposed subject is thus required.

Regulation requires activation of processes and limitation (usually by feedback) of the processes and their speeds. Every regulation involves integration among actions. Thus, regulation of body heat depends on shifts of heat production and heat elimination. One can conclude that integration of body heat depends on detailed regulations, oscillations, blood flows, and so on. There is no boundary or distinction between regulation and integration (Adolph, 1979).

Reactions of mammals to stimuli are mainly achieved by neural and endocrine mechanisms. Separation of neural and endocrine control, in the present state of the art, is impossible. Since neural response is one of the primary controllers over body function in protection of mammals against adverse conditions, the importance and significance of neuroendocrine and neurotransmitter perturbations are evident.

Thermoregulation serves as an example of relations by which several integrating functions yield a complex result. Thus, body content of heat is equilibrated by approach to equality of two overall processes, gain and loss. Integration exists in that these two counteractions respond to disturbances and they restore a normative result. Heat production and heat loss are both locally and integrally controlled in a complex manner and many sensory and central factors are intricately interrelated. Thus, multiple sensations from the skin, hypothalamus, spinal cord, abdominal cavity, and respiratory passages have been shown to converge in the CNS.

For the body as a whole, each response to temperature sensations appears to recognize a threshold. This threshold can be conveniently imagined to contribute to a so-called set point. The set point, however, is not fixed under all conditions (Adolph, 1979). In addition to the physiological responses of heat production and vasoconstriction, other actions that the individual takes may be regarded as behavioral.

Fever represents a form of heat integration. Pyrogen that escapes from a parasitic organism gives rise to outputs of norepinephrine and prostaglandin E. These hormones influence hypothalamic neurons to command extra heat production and at the same time to diminish heat loss. Thus, fever can be illustrative of aroused integrative function (Adolph, 1979).

To maintain homeostasis, a mammal possesses two control mechanisms that react to changes in internal and external environments (stimuli or stress). These two control mechanisms are the neural and endocrine systems. Separation of endocrine from neural control is impossible as neural signals are integrated at the hypothalamus to react to deviations in the internal or external environments. Hypothalamic–hypophysial–adrenocortical (HHA), hypothalamic–hypophysial–thyroidal (HHT), and hypothalamic–hypophysial–somatotropic (HHS) are three endocrine systems that participate in the "stress" response. Generally, they operate through a negative feedback mechanism.

Adrenergic neurons in the hypothalamus stimulate thyrotropin-releasing hormone (TRH) acting on the anterior pituitary to increase thyrotropin (TSH), entering the general circulation to stimulate thyroid secretion of triiodothyronine (T_3) and thyroxine (T_4). T_3 and T_4 then act by negative feedback control on hypophysial TSH secretion.

There is evidence that suppression of central adrenergic tone is responsible for a reduction of growth hormone (GH) release. A specific growth-hormone-inhibiting factor (GIF) is present in the hypothalamus. GIF inhibits the release of GH and counteracts the effects of growth-hormone-releasing factor (GRF) from the hypothalamus. GRF acts on the anterior pituitary to release GH into the general circulation. GH acts on target tissue to increase the glucose level (by decreased utilization) and nonesterified fatty acid levels (by mobilization) and to decrease the amino acid pool for protein synthesis. It is these substrates, especially glucose, that provide a feedback control on the hypothalamus for GH release. GH also acts directly by a short-loop negative feedback control on the hypothalamus and anterior pituitary. Physical stimuli, emotions, or any interference with the body's ability to maintain homeostasis (heat, cold, infections, toxins, lack of oxygen, injury) can result in the liberation of corticotropin-releasing factor (CRF), which in turn stimulates the release of adrenocorticotropic hormone (ACTH) from the anterior pituitary (hypophysis). ACTH then stimulates the secretion by the adrenal cortex of glucocorticoids, which are hormones related to the immune response.

The pathophysiologic picture of "stress" has been characterized as the "general adaptation syndrome," which develops in three stages, the alarm reaction, the stage of resistance, and the stage of exhaustion (Selye, 1950). The classic triad of the alarm reaction (adrenocortical stimulation, thymicolymphatic hypotrophy, and gastrointestinal ulcer) denotes the stereotyped response of the body to any demand that severely taxes the regulatory processes. The triad of the alarm reaction also points out the involvement of the HHA system and autonomic control. Only recently has the secretory pattern of adenohypophysial hormones (other than ACTH) been found to be involved in the nonspecific stress responses. It is now well established that in rats, acute stress inhibits GH secretion and stimulates ACTH and prolactin release. In general, stress-induced hormonal changes are not related to the nature, but rather to the intensity and duration of the stressing agent.

Standard laboratory stressors can easily be found in the experimental procedures that are used in biomedical studies. Such commonplace procedures as handling, novelty of experimental environment and procedures, extreme environmental temperatures, forced muscular exercise, immobilization, transportation, noise, electrical shock, ether anesthesia, and so on can act as stressors under certain conditions. Great care must thus be exercised to ensure that the changes in hormone levels are the response to the specific stressor in question (i.e., electric or electromagnetic fields) rather than to some extraneous factors.

There is a dissociation of the modes of pituitary–adrenal activation for the stress response and the rhythmicity at the level of the hypothalamic CRF neurons. The transient nature of shifts in circadian periodicity emphasizes the importance of homeothermic adaptive mechanisms in the mammal.

One of the major functions of thyroid hormones is their effect on basal and resting metabolic rate. Pituitary secretion of TSH has been shown to respond in a specific, metabolic pattern to extreme environmental temperature, and appears to respond in a nonspecific manner to other stressful stimuli. TSH secretion is under the control of the CNS, as are the secretions of the other adenohypophysial hormones.

The release of TSH by the anterior pituitary is regulated by an interaction between hypothalamic TRH, which stimulates TSH release, and the calorigenic ("metabolically active") thyroid hormones T_4 and T_3, which suppress it.

In addition to mediating somatic growth of the organism, GH is an important component of the endocrine control of circulating metabolites. Like the other adenohypophysial hormones, GH under the control of the CNS is mediated through the hypothalamic inhibiting hormone, somatostatin, and a hypothalamic releasing factor. As noted earlier, changes in GH secretion during stress are considered to be a nonspecific response to a stimulus. Unlike TSH or ACTH, the GH stress response is somewhat species dependent, with a decrease in rodents, and an increase in dogs and primates including the human.

The CNS provides an interface between afferent nervous pathways from sensor and efferent nervous pathways to effectors. It is also the structure in which the sensor-to-effector pathways are integrated so that an animal can respond in a systematic way to complex patterns of signals from sensors. In this way the existence of the organism as a whole is sustained in the context of its external environment, while its constituent cells are maintained in their immediate milieu (Bligh, 1979).

It is well established that intraneuronal communication in the brain is achieved by releasing specific chemical mediators and that the neuroexcitability is partly a function of synaptic transmission. Altered neurotransmitter function has been demonstrated in a variety of behavioral as well as neurological abnormalities.

Neuroendocrine function and neurotransmitter activity react to alterations in internal or external environments to maintain homeostasis. Changes in hormone levels can result in modification of energy utilization, carbohydrate, fat, and protein metabolism, immune competence, and electrolyte balance. They can also modify perception, neural function, behavior, and mentality. Neuroendocrine functions are the controllers that maintain homeostasis of man and animals in relation to diverse stimuli. The importance of these neuroendocrine factors is that they are slower and more persistent controllers of body functions than the quickly reactive neural mechanisms.

9.2. THERMOREGULATION

According to the Glossary Committee of the International Union of Physiological Science (Bligh and Johnson, 1973), the following definitions have been accepted "to improve precision of meaning and uniformity in the usage of technical terms in thermal physiology":

> TEMPERATURE REGULATION: The maintenance of the temperature or temperatures of a body within a restricted range under conditions involving variable internal and/or external heat loads. Biologically, the existence of some degree of body temperature regulation by autonomic or behavioral means. Antonym: TEMPERATURE CONFORMITY.
>
> TEMPERATURE REGULATION, BEHAVIORAL: The regulation of body temperature by complex patterns of responses of the skeletal musculature to heat and cold which modify the rates of heat production and/or heat loss (e.g., by exercise, change in body conformation, and in the thermal insulation of bedding and (in man) of clothing, and by the selection of an environment which reduces thermal stress).

Thermoregulation, which is part of the complex control system involving circulation, metabolism, respiration, as well as neural structures, can be reasonably divided into two components: a physiological component made up of heat production and heat loss mechanisms, and a behavioral component that has sensory, motivational, and response aspects (Lipton *et al.*, 1970). Physiological thermoregulation controls body temperature within narrow limits although its power to counteract thermal stress is relatively small. Behavioral thermoregulation, on the other hand, exerts a less precise control but is very powerful in defending against great temperature extremes through the initiation and maintenance of various voluntary actions (Benzinger *et al.*, 1963). While in the normal life of homeotherms both components interact to assure a viable thermal level, the great power and modifiability of the behavioral component are of particular interest for theoretical and practical reasons. Ivanov (1975) has examined the significance of specific heat-sensitive structures such as neurons, interoceptors, and cutaneous thermoreceptors, in heat regulation. He concludes that temperature signals from cutaneous thermoreceptors reach the somatosensory region of the cerebral cortex. The main processing of thermal signals from cutaneous thermoreceptors reaches the somatosensory region of the cerebral cortex. The main processing of thermal signals and generation of a controlling signal for the effector part of thermoregulation takes place in the hypothalamus.

There is no aspect of an organism's behavior that is not to some extent controlled by environmental stimuli. As noted by Stolwijk (1977), "Body temperatures are probably sensed by a number of temperature-sensitive neural structures. Animal studies have shown that temperature-sensitive neurons exist in the skin. Local thermal stimulation of these regions in animals produces physiological responses of greater thermal magnitude than the stimulus."

"The heat exchange between the human body and the environment can be described by the general heat balance equation:

$$S = M - W - E \pm R \pm C$$

in which S = rate of heat storage; M = rate of metabolic heat production (proportional to rate of oxygen consumption); W = mechanical work done on the environment; E = evaporative heat loss rate (via respiration or sweating); R = heat gain or loss through radiation; C = heat gain or loss through convection. All terms are expressed in watts per square meter body surface area (W/m^2). Imbalance of the internal heat production term (M) and the remaining terms, causes heat to be stored in or lost from the body, with resultant changes in body temperature. For a 75 kg man, a heat storage rate of 100 W for 1 hr will cause a rise in mean body temperature of 1.33°C. Well-trained individuals can sustain a metabolic production at the rate of 1,000 W for up to 0.5 hr, so that substantial heat dissipation mechanisms are required to protect against excessive hyperthermia during heavy exercise. During hard work or in fever, central temperatures may rise to 40–41°C for short periods."

Nonhibernating mammals maintain an internal body temperature within a few degrees centigrade in spite of the wide (ca. 100°C) variation of environmental temperature. Numerous physiologic responses that contribute to thermal equilibrium include vasomotor, respiratory, and metabolic adjustments, as well as sweating, shivering, and piloerection. Behavioral responses of the animal also contribute to thermal balance (Carlisle, 1970).

Temperature information is derived from two sets of receptors: one set located peripherally (cutaneous receptors) and the other centrally (hypothalamic temperature-sensitive neurons) (Nakayama et al., 1963). Temperature regulation can best be understood as a dual-control system involving central cutaneous modulation of a hypothalamic controller. The nature of the control system will not be dealt with here, and the reader is referred to the excellent reviews by Hardy (1961), Bligh (1966), Hammel (1968), and Corbit (1970) for more information.

An animal with a body temperature of about 38°C is faced with a clear regulatory problem when a flow of heat is committed to the environment by the body–ambient temperature difference. The rate of change of internal temperature is determined by the balance or imbalance between rates of heat production and heat loss. The behavioral regulation of body temperature can be very accurate under some conditions. Weiss and Laties (1960, 1961) and Laties and Weiss (1959, 1960), in an elegant series of experiments, have shown that behavior is a markedly sensitive mechanism in the regulation of body temperature.

An avoidance response has been used successfully with lizards; this work demonstrated that the behavioral avoidance of thermal extremes was a joint function of hypothalamic and peripheral temperatures (Hammel et al., 1967). A natural response of rats, when heat-stressed, is to groom saliva into the ventral body surface, thereby increasing evaporative heat loss (Hainsworth, 1967). Behavioral and physiologic responses are wired in parallel; if the physiologic response is an activation of heat-loss mechanisms, then the behavioral response will be in the same direction. If physiologic responsiveness is impaired (or strained), then behavioral responses increase in order to compensate for this heat stress (Lipton, 1968).

Thermal motivation arises in situations of thermal stress. On the warm side, it is the uncomfortable feeling of excessive warmth and the desire for temperature reduction; on the cold side, it involves the unpleasant feeling of being too cold and the desire for temperature increase. The biological significance of thermal motivation is that, by acting in such a way as to minimize thermal discomfort and maximize thermal comfort, the organism tends to escape from situations of thermal stress and to locate itself in a physiologically neutral thermal environment, thereby solving the problem of physiological temperature regulation (Corbit, 1973).

The problem of thermal motivation can help us to refine our understanding of the neural basis of motivation, because it provides a context in which the important general theoretical issues can be brought into unusually sharp focus. This is so because the input variables or stimuli for thermally motivated behavior are simply various body temperatures, and existing technology makes it not only possible but also easy to measure and control these temperatures with whatever degree of precision is required. The ease with which precise specification of the input variables can be achieved has enabled workers from several disciplines to take a quantitative approach in their studies of the input–output characteristics of the system. Consequently, there is now a set of relatively clear statements for the laws relating temperatures on the input side to measures of neural activity, autonomic thermoregulatory reactions, behavior of the whole animal, and subjective experience on the output side (Corbit, 1973).

Weiss and Laties (1961), who introduced the methods of operant conditioning to the study of thermal motivation, identified skin temperature as one stimulus for thermoregulatory behavior, and Satinoff (1964) showed that thermoregulatory behavior is influenced by locally produced changes in hypothalamic temperature, as well as by changes in peripheral temperature. Thus, thermal motivation depends on central (hypothalamic) as well as on peripheral (cutaneous) temperature stimuli.

This suggests that the driving forces for the behavioral and autonomic thermoregulatory responses are generated by similar neural mechanisms. Raising hypothalamic temperature above its neutral value gives rise to an aversive motivational state (Corbit, 1973).

Thermal experience varies along two main dimensions: one, sensory (warm–cold) and the other, affective (pleasant–unpleasant). The intensity of warm or cold sensations increases with increasing deviation of skin temperature above or below the neutral value of about 33°C (Stevens and Stevens, 1960; Gagge and Stevens, 1968). The intensity of the unpleasant feeling of thermal discomfort increases with increasing deviation of skin temperature away from 33°C (Winslow *et al.*, 1937; Hardy, 1953–1954) and with increasing deviation of internal body temperature from its normal value of about 37°C (Chatonnet and Cabanac, 1965; Cabanac, 1969, 1971). It is apparent that knowledge of behavioral thermoregulation is essential if one is to evaluate experimental data from microwave bioeffects studies.

Extensive investigations into microwave bioeffects during the last quarter century indicate that, for frequencies between 200 and 24,500 MHz, exposure to a power density of 100 mW/cm^2 or greater than 4 mW/g for several minutes or hours can result in physiological manifestations of a thermal nature in laboratory animals. Such effects may or may not be characterized by a measurable temperature rise, which is a function of the thermal regulatory processes and active adaptation of the animal. The end result is either reversible or irreversible change, depending on the conditions of the exposure and the physiological state of the animal. At lower power densities, evidence of pathological change or physiological alteration is nonexistent or equivocal. A great deal of discussion, nevertheless, has concerned the relative importance of thermal or nonthermal effects of RF/MW radiation.

The results of some *in vitro* studies have been considered as evidence of nonthermal effects of RF radiation. Although some investigators and reviewers still question the interpretation of these so-called nonthermal effects (Michaelson, 1970, 1974a; Milroy and Michaelson, 1971; Saito and Schwan, 1961; Sher et al., 1970), several support *nonthermal* interactions between tissues and electric and magnetic fields (Kholodov, 1966; Gordon, 1955; Marha et al., 1968; Petrov, 1970; Presman, 1968).

Temperature increase during exposure to microwaves depends on: (1) the specific area of the body exposed and the efficiency of heat elimination; (2) intensity or field strength; (3) duration of exposure; (4) specific frequency or wavelength; and (5) thickness of skin and subcutaneous tissue. These variables determine the percentage of radiant energy absorbed by various tissues of the body (Schwan and Piersol, 1954, 1955).

In partial-body exposure under normal conditions, the body acts as a cooling reservoir, which stabilizes the temperature of the exposed part. The stabilization is due to an equilibrium established between the energy absorbed by the exposed part of the body and the amount of heat carried away from it. This heat transport is due to increased blood flow to cooler parts of the body, maintained at normal temperature by heat-regulating mechanisms such as heat loss due to evaporation, radiation, and convection. If the amount of absorbed energy exceeds the optimal amount of heat energy that can be handled by the mechanisms of temperature regulation, the excess energy will cause continuous temperature rise with time. Hyperthermia and, under some circumstances, local tissue destruction can result.

Elucidation of the biological effects of microwave exposure requires an understanding of the physiology of thermal regulation and a careful review and critical analysis of the available literature. Such review requires the appreciation and differentiation of the established effects and mechanisms from speculative and unsubstantiated reports. Although most of the experimental data support the concept that the effects of microwave exposure are primarily, if not only, a response to hyperthermia or altered thermal gradients in the body, there are large areas of confusion, uncertainty, and actual misinformation.

Certain organs and organ systems are reported to be affected by MW/RF exposure, in terms of functional disturbance, structural alterations, or both. Some reactions to MW/RF exposure may lead to measurable biological effects that remain within the range of normal (physiological) compensation, and thus an effect is not necessarily a hazard. Some reactions, on the other hand, may lead to potential or actual health hazards.

In this context, Czerski and Szmigielski (1974) have noted:

1. All detectable changes in function and structure, above the molecular level, may be termed biological effects.

2. The immediate effect at the site of a primary interaction may induce further changes (secondary or indirect effects).
3. Measurable biological effects that remain within the range of normal compensation are not necessarily hazardous; some effects may improve the efficiency of certain physiological processes and are used for therapeutic purposes.
4. Biological effects that may be detrimental to the efficiency of a living system should be considered hazardous.

Most of the biological reactions elicited by microwave exposure can be attributed to thermal energy conversion, almost exclusively as enthalpic energy (heating) phenomena. This, however, does not provide a predictive model of the biological consequences of nonuniform absorption of energy in animals and humans. The nonuniform, largely unpredictable distribution of energy absorption may give rise to temperature increases and rates of heating that can result in unique biological effects. It should be noted, however, that under ordinary circumstances the body experiences numerous thermal gradients and nonhomogeneities. Furthermore, induced temperature gradients in deep body organs may act as a stimulus to alter normal function both in the heated organ and in other organs of the system. The nonuniform characteristics of microwave absorption, with differing rates of temperature rise in different tissues, results in heating patterns that cannot be replicated with radiant, convected, or conducted heat. Indirect effects can be thus be mediated in organs removed from the site of the primary interaction. It should also be pointed out that temperature rises from diverse etiologies may induce chromosomal alterations, mutagenesis, virus activation and inactivation, as well as behavioral and immunological reactions.

Irradiation of biological systems with MW/RF energy leads to temperature elevation when the rate of energy absorption exceeds the rate of energy dissipation. Whether the resultant temperature elevation is diffuse or confined to specific anatomical sites depends on:

1. The electromagnetic field characteristics and distributions within the body
2. The passive and active thermoregulatory mechanisms available to the particular biological entity

The passive thermoregulatory mechanisms available consist of heat radiation, conduction, convection, and evaporative cooling. In furbearing animals and clothed humans, heat loss by radiation and evaporative cooling is poor. The efficiency of heat convection between a body and its immediate environment is a function of the environmental conditions.

Active thermoregulatory mechanisms make use of passive heat transfer mechanisms by employing internal circulating fluids (such as blood) to transfer heat from internal regions to external regions where passive heat radiation and convection are more effective. In some fur-bearing animals, an efficient mechanism is the movement of internally warmed blood to the lungs; heat in the lungs is then transferred to the inspired air by convection and is then expired into the environment. Another mechanism (especially in the human) is cutaneous vasodilation, resulting in the transfer of internal heat to the skin, where it can be radiated and convected into the surrounding environment. Sweating from the skin of humans and the paws and snout of fur-bearing animals provides a means of heat transfer; evaporation of the fluid permits rapid heat loss into the environment.

While respiratory and cutaneous heat transfer is well documented (Bligh, 1973), no information is available on any alteration of vascular perfusion patterns of internal organs in response to local temperature changes. As a result, the possibility of local internal "hot spots" exists if

1. The rate of energy absorption is relatively high compared to the vascular heat transfer capacity of the local region (e.g., lens of the eye, necrotic center of tumor)
2. The rate of energy absorption is relatively uniform throughout the region, but the vascular perfusion patterns are such that confluence or pooling occurs (i.e., venous system in the splanchnic region and above the spinal cord)

9.3. THE PHYSIOLOGY OF THERMOREGULATION

As a class, biological organisms are capable of existing over a wide range of temperatures. Certain plants and microorganisms grow and reproduce at temperatures well below freezing, while others thrive at temperatures approaching that of boiling water. Mammals and birds, the warm-blooded animals or *homeotherms,* are capable of existing only in a relatively restricted range of body temperatures around 38°C. Irving (1966) noted that "In all climates and everywhere on the earth, mammals maintain a body temperature of about 38°C. It looks as if evolution has settled this temperature as an optimum for the mammalian class."

The ability of homeotherms to maintain a relatively constant body temperature confers many advantages. First, consistency of the regulatory processes is assured, as most physiological processes involve chemical reactions that, in turn, proceed at rates dependent on temperature. If body temperature varied, as in cold-blooded or *poikilothermic* animals, the various biochemical and physiological processes would vary with body temperature and hence sometimes be ineffective. Second, constant body temperature enables homeotherms to function efficiently over a wide range of ambient temperatures, an advantage over the poikilotherms. There are also disadvantages. First, although suitably protected (humans can exist at ambient temperatures from $-70°C$ to $100°C$), the inner core temperature cannot change by more than about $4°C$ without impairment of physical and mental capabilities. In mammals, the CNS ceases to function at 44 to $45°C$ and the heart stops beating at $48°C$. A rise in temperature of $5°C$ causes a two- to threefold increase in pulse rate, oxygen consumption, and so on. Second, maintaining a fixed body temperature requires a relatively high metabolic rate; the homeotherms must pay for their advantages in the currency of food intake.

Man is generally considered the best homeothermic regulator, with a regulation to a body temperature of $36.9 \pm 1°C$. Other species exhibit similar, but usually less stable regulation, while some are capable of different levels of regulation. The hibernators, for example, can depress their regulated temperature by as much as $35°C$, or just a few degrees above ambient temperature. This depression produces a dormant state, which is reversed by rewarming to homeothermic regulatory activity.

In relation to the time involved for evolution of the species, man has only recently learned to protect himself against cold, using clothing and suitable housing. This means that humans are essentially tropical animals and are not cold adapted, as they must artificially maintain their immediate ambient temperatures at suitably high levels to exist. Human thermal regulation, as well as that of many animals, is then actually geared to the opposite problem, that of protecting the body against overheating (Hardy, 1961, 1967). As the absorption of external electromagnetic energy causes heating, it is this regulatory capability that is of interest in the discussion of thermal regulation in this chapter.

Normally the body maintains temperature equilibrium by regulating metabolism (M), loss or gain from body heat stores (S), evaporation (E), and radiation, convection, and conduction (H) according to

$$M + S = H + E \tag{9.1}$$

M is always positive. The body may use heat from its stores, in which case S is positive, or store heat, in which case S is negative. When heat is lost through radiation, convection, and conduction, H is positive. Heat may also be added to the body by these mechanisms; if their aggregate is a gain rather than a loss, H becomes negative. E is always positive. These sign conventions then mean that in the above equation, M and S are regarded as heat sources, and H and E as heat sinks. The normal physiological significance of these quantities is discussed in physiology texts (Bullard, 1971).

For a resting human at 30°C, the metabolic rate is 60 to 90 kcal/h, or 70 to 100 W. Muscular work can increase this metabolic rate. For short (5 to 10 min) activity periods, well-trained athletes may support a metabolic rate of approximately 2000 W (Astrand and Rodahl, 1970). This then means that, as a source of heat, the human body produces from 70 to 2000 W, depending on ambient temperature, physiological factors, and activity.

If the body absorbs external electromagnetic radiation in amounts adequate to affect thermal regulation, then an additional external radiation converted to heat (R) must be added to the source side of (9.1):

$$M + S + R = H + E \qquad (9.2)$$

The relation of external absorbed radiant energy to the customary physiological parameters and its role in affecting thermal regulation are the subjects of the material of this chapter. The effects of heating can be subdivided into those acting at (1) the cellular level, (2) the organ level, and (3) the total self-regulatory mechanisms. In dealing with the whole organism, the effects at these three levels are interrelated and occur simultaneously.

Successful strategies or mechanisms to maintain body temperatures in a narrow and desirable range in a complex and varying thermal environment are termed thermoregulatory. Although such strategies or mechanisms are found in great variety, they fall into two main categories: voluntary and behavioral adjustments, and involuntary physiological adjustments (Stolwijk, 1977).

The limits of effectiveness of involuntary physiological thermoregulation are rather narrow and we must rely on behavioral methods of thermoregulation over most of the range of environmental temperatures to which we are often exposed. Changes in body temperatures bring about not only autonomic drives but also behavioral drives.

The duration of the tissue temperature elevation is important in determining the extent of the biological reaction. The rate of the rise of temperature also plays a role in determining the extent of the biological response. This is due in part to the fact that out of the total period of heat application, only that limited portion will be biologically operative during which an effective temperature level is attained in the tissues. Thus, a modality that will rapidly raise the temperature to biologically effective levels will produce a more pronounced effect than a modality that raises the tissue temperature more slowly, provided both modalities are applied over the same period of time (Lehmann, 1971).

In all mammals, the metabolic rate is lowest at a temperature lower than the regulated body temperature. This is the normal temperature, which is actually defined by the minimum on the metabolic rate curve. When ambient temperature falls below the normal temperature, the regulatory mechanisms respond by increasing the metabolic rate. The rate of the metabolic process increases with slowly rising temperature, at first exponentially, becoming maximal at an optimal temperature, then decreasing more and more quickly until, at a certain temperature, metabolism ceases completely and death ensues. Although the general shape of these "metabolic rate–temperature" curves is the same for all living systems, tissue or cells, and even whole organisms devoid of a temperature regulatory mechanism, they differ very much with regard to the temperature for maximal activity and that at which death occurs. These latter characteristics vary as a rule, more with species differences than with differences between various tissues of the same animal. Even such differences, however, can be of practical importance [e.g., the optimal temperature for the human testis is considerably lower than for most human tissues (Fischer and Solomon, 1965)].

Associated with the changes in tissue metabolism are changes in enzyme reactions. These may be speeded up by moderate tissue temperature elevation and may be gradually abolished at higher temperatures. This may be explained by the fact that the rate of the chemical reaction is increased by temperature elevation while the protein component of the enzyme system is destroyed at higher temperatures. As a result of the temperature elevation, proteins may be denatured and the resulting products, such as polypeptides and histaminelike substances, in turn may become biologically effective. Also, the rate of filtration and of diffusion across biological membranes is increased because of greater permeability with a resulting escape of plasma proteins.

All animals have an optimal environmental temperature range within which they can most successfully carry on their activities. Whenever the environmental temperature deviates from this optimum range, the organism becomes handicapped. At extremes of temperature, life is not possible. The temperature range at which organisms remain active is somewhat less than that at which life is possible. The optimum temperature range varies from one species to another, and that which would be fatal for one organism may be well within the optimum range for another. These differences undoubtedly arise by adaptation. However, rapid change of environmental temperature might be fatal to an organism, while gradual changes might not (Gilstrap et al., 1964).

Although animals vary in their endurance to extreme heat, it is known that proteins coagulate and become denatured and enzymes are inactivated at a temperature of about 50°C. This inactivation frequently starts at about 40°C and proceeds more rapidly as the temperature rises. If the thermal destruction of protein and enzymes goes beyond a certain point, it cannot be alleviated by lowering the temperature. Lethal heat stress of an organism depends not only on the temperature but also on the duration during which this stress is applied; this is substantiated by enzyme inactivation also being dependent on these two factors (Gilstrap et al., 1964).

The activity–temperature relation for living systems is complicated by the fact that such systems usually exhibit considerable hysteresis; i.e., the rate of function is dependent not only on the present conditions, of which the temperature is one, but also on the past history of the systems. Thus, the activity–temperature curve depends to a certain extent on the speed of the temperature changes, and especially on whether a given temperature is reached from a lower or higher temperature. If the rate of temperature change is rapid, it may also act as a stimulus and cause, like any other adequate stimulus, a typical response of the system (muscle, nerve). On the other hand, the behavior of living systems can be affected by adaptive changes caused by a prolonged exposure to relatively high temperatures, but well inside the activity range of the system. Thus, some systems become considerably warm adapted (Fischer and Solomon, 1965).

Thermally, the body is considered to be an inner core at the constant regulated temperature and an outer shell of variable temperature. In humans, roughly two-thirds of the body is at the core temperature while one-third is at the shell temperature. The core temperature (T_r) is usually easily defined and measured as the rectal or some other internal temperature, while the shell temperature (T_s) can be expressed only as the weighted mean of several skin temperature measurements. This is done with a radiometer or by attaching thermal detectors to the skin at several locations. The weighting factors are (Newburgh, 1949)

Head	0.07
Arms	0.14
Hands	0.05
Feet	0.07
Legs	0.13
Thighs	0.19
Trunk	0.35
	1.00

The temperature of the body (T_b) is then considered to be

$$T_b = 0.67T_r + 0.33T_s \qquad (9.3)$$

The heat content of the body can be computed from T_b as follows:

In thermal terms, the body is mostly water, but also contains biological material of lower specific heat. The average specific heat of the body is approximately 0.83 kcal/kg, so the heat content for a body weight of W kilograms is

$$\text{body heat content} = 0.83 T_b W \text{ kcal} \qquad (9.4)$$

Most recent publications concerned with nonionizing radiation effects use the SI units now standard for scientific work. The SI unit of energy is the joule (1 cal = 4.186 J). Thus equation (9.4) should be multiplied by 4186 to yield body heat content in joules.

Physiologically, changes in body heat content are of greater interest than total heat content in assessing the effects of absorbed microwave energy. In addition, it is convenient to speak in terms of power, as the magnitudes of most electromagnetic insults to which the body is exposed are so expressed. Using the conversion of 1 cal = 1/860 W-hr, equation (9.4) can be rewritten as

$$\frac{\text{Change in body heat content per hour}}{} = \frac{0.965(T_{b2} - T_{b1})W}{\text{time in hours}} = \text{watts} \qquad (9.5)$$

where T_{b2} and T_{b1} are the body temperatures in degrees Celsius at the end and start of the time period in question, and W is the body weight in kilograms.

The concept of a "constant" body temperature applies only to the core. Even assuming theoretically perfect temperature regulation, the core temperature itself is not uniform, because the temperature of each organ in the core depends on the relative level of its metabolism and on the temperature and volume of its blood supply. Because the mean shell temperature is lower than the mean core temperature, the shell supports a thermal gradient from the core down to the skin. One of the main factors in the thermal regulation of mammals is the capacity to alter the temperature gradient in the shell and to change, to a certain extent, the ratio of shell volume to core volume. The gradient exists because the body loses heat from its surface by conduction, convection, radiation, and evaporation [factors H and E of equation (9.1)], since under ordinary conditions ambient temperature is below body temperature. The heat loss or gain of any body increases with the difference between the temperature of its surface and that of the surrounding environment. Any increase in this differential increases the heat loss or gain at a rate much higher than that corresponding to the change in temperature alone (Fischer and Solomon, 1965).

The core of the mammalian body will remain at a constant temperature (heat balance) when the heat generated by the metabolism of the body is equal to the heat lost from its surface. Since the latter depends on the difference between surface and environmental temperature, under the condition of heat balance, the skin surface temperature has a well-defined value for a given heat production by the body and for a given environmental temperature. If the environmental temperature suddenly increases, the difference between the latter and the skin decreases, the heat loss decreases considerably, and other heat sources balance losses to heat sinks. When the environmental temperature remains constant, but body heat increases, heat balance is disrupted and can be restored only when the skin temperature has increased enough to produce a differential to the environmental temperature that permits an increased heat loss, equaling the increased heat production. The necessary skin temperature changes are caused by circulatory changes.

Although the magnitude of the temperature difference between core and skin is regulated according to the requirements for heat balance, the slope of the temperature gradient in the shell and the width of the shell depend on two main factors: where the heat is mainly liberated—in the deeper parts of the trunk, or in muscle activity in the limbs; and the character of heat transport from the core to the skin. The latter occurs partly by physical conduction, depending on the heat conductivity of the various tissues, and partly by the more important heat convection inside the body by the circulating blood. Circulation can be regarded as a cooling system for the core and as a heating system for the shell. The higher the environmental temperature, the lower is the gradient slope and the higher the blood flow through the skin. Clothing or covering only a part of the body will diminish the local gradients because the heat loss from the covered area is determined mainly by the surface temperature of the clothing or the cover. The slower the heat conduction through the covering (depending on its thickness and how poor the heat conductivity of the material), the higher will be the skin temperature and skin blood flow (Fischer and Solomon, 1965).

In all mammals, cardiovascular, hormonal, and nervous control are involved in temperature regulation, which are the regulatory mechanisms that enable the mammal to maintain a fairly constant body temperature despite considerable variation in environmental temperatures (Fischer and Solomon, 1965). In the control and regulation of the function of the organism as a whole, the vascular system plays an important role, not only by controlling the nutritional state of the tissues (supply of oxygen and fuel, removal of waste products including CO_2), but also as the means of transport of heat and the various hormones for hormonal control. The nervous and endocrine systems are the other main control mechanisms. The direct temperature effect upon blood vessels is vasomotor: a dilatation with increase, and a constriction with decrease in temperature. This mechanism plays an important, but not exclusive role in the effect of temperature upon the blood flow through an organ.

All the partial mechanisms of heat regulation are integrated by hormonal and nervous control as well as by a direct temperature effect of the blood supplying the "highest" center of integration of the nervous temperature regulation, located in the anterior part of the hypothalamus. The hypothalamic center can be influenced experimentally by direct heating. The threshold for direct heat activation is an increase in temperature of 0.5 to 0.6°C (Fischer and Solomon, 1965).

Mammals, as homeothermic animals, maintain an almost constant body temperature. The variation from species to species is not great, being only a few degrees at most. However, mammals have developed means by which they can compensate for or regulate these temperature changes. These compensations can be either physiological, as in the case of the human, or partly anatomical, as in the case of fur-covered animals.

The physiological basis of the temperature-regulating mechanism is generally the same for all homeotherms. Usually overheating is prevented by evaporation of water or sweating. Not all animals are able to do this, and therefore some animals accomplish evaporation of water by panting, which consists of the evaporation of water from the tongue and upper respiratory tract (Gilstrap *et al.*, 1964).

For humans, when the ambient temperature exceeds 31°C, air convection and thermal radiation are inadequate to supply the required cooling, and the evaporation of water, produced by sweating, is the only cooling mechanism available. In addition, when the ambient temperature exceeds 34°C, radiation and convection cease to cool and begin to warm the body. This accounts for the rapid rise of evaporative cooling necessary to maintain cooling at temperatures above 31°C to 34°C. At these elevated temperatures, the body sends as much blood as possible to the skin to become cooled. In addition, physical activity involving work output increases the metabolic rate which, to maintain regulation, is generally compensated for by sweating. Sweating is a particularly effective cooling mechanism: working humans can maintain a sweat rate of approximately 2 litres/hr for 5 hr or more, which is a cooling power of approximately 1400 W/hr (Bullard, 1971).

In the ambient temperature range of approximately 25 to 33°C, blood flow, as controlled by vasomotor mechanisms, is usually adequate to achieve regulation without cooling by sweating or heating, by increased metabolic activity. At ambient temperatures below about 25°C, radiation and convection cause increasing heat loss. Regulation is then maintained by increased metabolic activity and stored heat. The increased metabolic activity may be maintained by voluntary physical activity, or by involuntary physical activity, such as shivering.

The net result of the summed chemical and physical reactions to temperature stress is the regulation of core temperature despite varying thermal gradients between body and environment. Impulses from temperature receptors ascend via lateral spinothalamic tracts and the thalamus to the hypothalamus, from which various autonomic reflex responses are activated. The various heating and cooling mechanisms are then activated to achieve regulation. In the human, as well as some other species, the aggregate temperature control mechanisms are dynamic; approaching the sensitivity of an engineered system (Gilstrap et al., 1964).

The mechanisms of heat regulation are activated in two ways: by thermal receptors in the skin, and by direct stimulation of the hypothalamus by changes in blood temperature. Thermal receptors are distributed in a definite pattern in the skin; some may be encapsulated, but many are free nerve endings. Much sensory summation occurs so that the threshold for stimulation decreases as the size of the area stimulated increases. The density of temperature receptors of the skin varies for different surface areas of the body and also from subject to subject. Results of temperature differentiation studies over the human body indicate that the following degrees of difference can be registered: eyelids, 0.05°C; lips, 0.10°C; outside surface of arm, 0.25°C; palm of hand, 0.5°C (Gilstrap et al., 1964).

Under normal conditions, the main vascular reactions to heat application are elicited from the temperature receptors of the skin by segmental reflexes; but reflexes involving larger parts of the spinal cord, when the full mechanism of heat regulation acts, are elicited by reflex mechanisms involving the medullary and, especially, the hypothalamic vasomotor centers. The spreading of vascular dilatation elicited by local heat application into deeper tissues and remote skin areas (consensual reaction) is due to true spinal reflexes elicited by the thermoreceptors of the skin (Fischer and Solomon, 1965).

There are some indications that the local vascular response of the skin depends not only upon its temperature, but also can be altered by the speed and the direction of temperature changes. Vasodilatation of the skin, elicited by local heating of the heat-regulating area in the hypothalamus, is brought about mainly by stimulation in that area of inhibitory neurons acting upon the lower vasoconstrictor centers in the medulla and spinal cord, which dimininishes their vasoconstrictor tone and results in vasodilatation (Fischer and Solomon, 1965).

When heat is applied to certain areas of the body, the vascular beds increase and blood flows through them at highly increased speeds, while in other areas only minor decreases in vascular beds and in blood flow occur, resulting in considerable shifts of blood from one region of the body to others and an increase in circulating blood volume. In the human, this type of shift, in which blood from an organ is released for use where it is needed, occurs mainly in the lungs, liver, and the extensive subpapillary plexuses of the skin (Fischer and Solomon, 1965).

An increase in temperature leads to an increase in capillary permeability as well as increased capillary hydrostatic pressure and dilation, which increases capillary surface area. If the heat-induced permeability increase is great enough, plasma protein can escape into the interstitial space, resulting in an increased local fluid retention.

Ambient temperature changes also result in shifts in the volumes of fluid compartments. Hemodilution, the plasma dilution evidenced by a decrease in blood solids, plasma protein concentration, and hemoglobin concentration, is one such shift resulting from increased ambient temperature. Hemodilution is generally less than 5%. If the ambient temperature is adequate to induce sweating, hemodilution occurs only during the first 30 min of exposure before sweating occurs. As might be expected, copious perspiration results in *hemoconcentration.* It has been further shown that with prolonged heat exposure, there occurs a secondary increase in red cell volume. How much the increased red cell volume represents an increased mobilization of cells from hemopoietic tissue or a mobilization of blood reserves has not been established. If hyperpyrexia is great enough to produce shock, marked decrease in blood volume occurs, as in any type of shock (Adolph, 1947).

For prolonged exposure to heat, fluid shifts play a major role in "heat acclimatization." As defined by Bass and Henschel (1956), "heat acclimatization" is a dramatic increase in ability to do work. This improvement is associated with disappearance of subjective discomfort and reduction of physical strain during work. The physiological adaptations are (1) reduction in cardiovascular strain, (2) improved maintenance of body temperature, and (3) increased secretion of a more dilute sweat. Acclimatization results in an expansion of extracellular fluid and plasma volume.

Adolph (1947) observed that a consistent sign of lethality for different mammalian species is a rectal temperature in the range of 41.7–43.4°C. Deep body temperature above 42°C leads rapidly to irreversibly damage and irrecoverable hyperthermia.

Local temperature may profoundly affect the flow resistance of the various skin vessels. Local application of heat causes increased blood flow due to arteriolar and capillary dilatation. The rate of filtration and of diffusion across biological membranes is also increased. There may be a greater capillary membrane permeability with a resulting escape of plasma proteins. Vigorous heating may result in cellular responses associated with an inflammatory reaction, ranging in degree from mild to severe. Tissue metabolism is initially increased, as a result of the temperature elevation; if temperatures are elevated extensively and maintained for a prolonged period of time, tissue metabolism may be decreased (Lehmann, 1971).

A consensual response is usually observed in areas distant from the site of local tissue temperature elevation. This action is always less pronounced than the local response to heat application, and its magnitude is dependent on the size of the area heated. If the skin is heated, the vessels of the musculature beneath show no increase in diameter or may even show a vasoconstriction. If the skin of the abdominal wall is heated, it has been observed that a blanching of the gastric mucosa occurs. Relaxation of the smooth musculature of the gastrointestinal tract (decrease in peristalsis) during superficial heat application, has also been observed (Fischer and Solomon, 1965).

Clinically, it has been noted that heating of the superficial tissues produces marked relaxation of the striated skeletal muscles, and even protective muscle spasms may result. It is conceivable that the reaction is reflex in nature and is triggered by the effect on the temperature receptors in the skin. It is also conceivable that this effect may have a strong psychological component (Lehmann, 1971).

Reactions occurring distant from the site of tissue temperature elevation are reflex in nature. Some of them may be produced by an elevation of the core temperature of the body, which in turn produces those reactions that are commonly a part of the mechanism regulating the body temperature.

Jahns (1976) demonstrated the presence of midbrain raphe (MRP) neurons responding to scrotal skin temperature with positive thermal coefficients. Since many of the thermosensitive neurons in other parts of the brain respond to peripheral temperature and the majority of such neurons have the same type of thermal coefficients to both local and peripheral temperatures (Bligh, 1973; Boulant and Hardy, 1974), it is highly probable that some MRP neurons have dual thermosensitivities to both local and peripheral temperatures (Hori and Harada, 1976).

An organism's physiological response to heat is determined by the level, duration, and rate of rise of temperature elevation of the pertinent tissues. All tissues exhibit threshold responses: below a certain temperature no reactions are observed, while above these thresholds any minor change in tissue temperature may produce a major change in physiological response.

The duration and rate of rise are interdependent quantities. For temperature elevations that are noninjurious, duration of elevation determines the extent of reaction. The minimum effective duration of exposure is approximately 3 to 5 min, whereas complete reactions are obtained after exposure of approximately 30 min. The rate of rise to an elevated temperature is important in two respects. First, for a given period of time, the rate of rise effectively determines the duration of exposure to the elevated temperature involved. Second, all biological systems respond to changes in a manner similar to mathematical integration altered by compensating and adaptive mechanisms. These factors mean that a modality that raises temperature rapidly will have a more pronounced effect than one that effects a slower rise, provided that both are applied over the same period of time (Lehmann, 1971).

The "relative heating" or relative amount of energy converted into heat at any given point throughout the tissues, determines the pattern of the tissue temperature distribution. The temperature distribution is also modified by the tissue thermal conductivity if heating extends over a period of time long enough for heat flow to occur. The final temperature distribution in live tissues is then modified by physiological factors, such as the temperature distribution in the tissues prior to the application of heat and blood flow changes. Any temperature elevation produced by application of heat is superimposed upon the existing physiological temperature distribution. As heat is applied, the local blood flow may increase in response to the tissue temperature elevation. This may result in cooling, because blood temperature is usually lower than that of the heated tissue. The temperature distribution may be modified in this fashion (Lehmann, 1971).

The stabilization of temperature after an initial rise can be ascribed to an adjustment of the local circulation, with vasodilatation, and to the eventual equilibrium of heat loss and heat gain. The time taken for equilibrium to occur depends upon the area exposed (Boyle *et al.*, 1950, 1952).

9.4. ADAPTATION

There are data suggesting an adaptive or physiological adjustment to the thermal effects of microwave exposure. Kalyada (1973), in the book *The Problem of Adaptation in Labor Hygiene,* has stressed the adaptation of the body to "radiowave" exposure. She noted that extremely modest attention is being devoted to research on adaptive possibilities of the body to RF irradiation, and yet experimental research in animals has demonstrated the possibility for adaptation of the body to superhigh-frequency fields of rather high thermogenic intensity (Subbota and Svetlova, 1972).

Kalyada quotes Petrov (1970) as saying the function of the hypophysial–adrenal axis is the earliest and most generally nonspecific adaptive reaction in response to various stimuli, including microwaves. Apparently, such reactions can be interpreted as the first phase of development of adaptive changes.

Czerski (1975), in describing his studies on lymphocytes, noted that after a period of response, the animals become adapted to the microwaves. The phenomenon of physiological adaptation or diminished responsiveness, as a result of repeated exposure to microwaves, has also been reported by Michaelson *et al.* (1967), Michaelson (1974b), Phillips *et al.* (1975), Gordon (1966), Baranski and Czerski (1976), and Petrov (1970).

9.5. THERMAL STRESS

Physiologically, thermal stresses to which homeothermic animals are subjected may be classified in terms of whether or not the thermoregulatory system can cope with the heat involved. If the system cannot cope and regulation fails, adverse symptoms appear. If the system can cope and continues to regulate, the organism may or may not exhibit behavioral maneuvers in response to the imposed stress. The symptoms of exceeding heat tolerance limits are physiologically and clinically well documented. The effects of thermal stresses within tolerance limits are less well understood.

Locally produced heat dissipates rapidly throughout the body without causing high local tissue temperatures (Stolwijk, 1975). The body has a great tolerance for additional endogenous heat (Hastings and Harmison, 1969). In order to define limits on tolerance of added endogenous heat from an internal source, using blood as a coolant, electrically energized heaters were surgically implanted in the descending thoracic aorta of miniature swine and power levels of 0 to 60 W ($0-4.7$ W/cm^2 flux, $0-1.1$ W/kg body wt) applied for periods up to and exceeding 12 months (Gillis and Walkup, 1969). High ambient temperature ($>27-30°C$) or pyrexic states produced severe hyperthermia at the higher power levels, necessitating discontinuance of power to prevent death. Otherwise, no alteration of physiological function was observed. Whole-body exposure of dogs to 2880-MHz pulsed (360 pps, 2 to 3 μsec

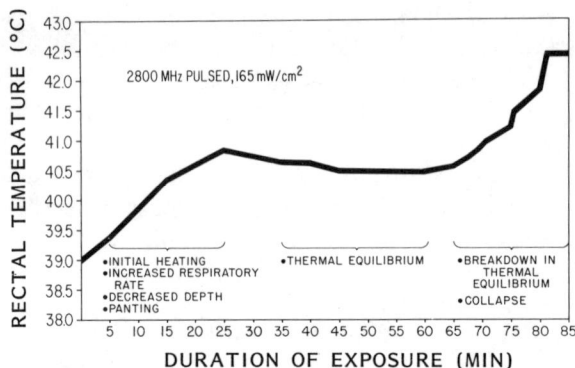

FIGURE 9-1. Response of dogs exposed to microwaves.

pulse width) microwave fields at an average power density of $1\,\text{kW/m}^2$ (SAR = 3.7 W/kg) for 6 hr or $1.65\,\text{kW/m}^2$ (SAR = 6.1 W/kg) for 2 to 3 hr produces a characteristic triphasic change in internal body temperature (Fig. 9-1): (1) an initial increase in core temperature, (2) a plateau phase at the hyperthermic level, and (3) thermoregulatory failure. Presumably, specific heat loss mechanisms (e.g., panting) mobilized by these exposures are able to counterbalance partially the thermalizing energy absorbed by the animal, but only temporarily. The strain placed upon the thermoregulatory system ultimately exhausts the heat loss capabilities of the dog and death ensues due to hyperpyrexia unless the animal is removed from the field (Michaelson, 1974, 1983; Michaelson *et al.*, 1961).

The environmental temperature at which the exposure occurs is also very important. Thus, dogs can tolerate exposures at SARs of 3.7 and 6.1 W/kg when T = 11°C and exposures at 3.7 W/kg when T = 22°C without becoming hyperthermic. However, at T = 40.5°C, dangerous hyperthermia can occur within 20 min at SAR = 6.1 (a value roughly twice the resting metabolic heat production of the dog) (Fig. 9-2).

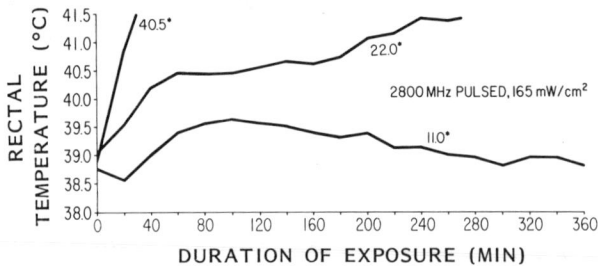

FIGURE 9-2. Response of dogs exposed to microwaves at various environmental temperatures.

Hydration during microwave exposure permits an extended tolerance at high SARs, presumably through an increased capacity for respiratory evaporative heat loss (panting). One notable finding was the development of tolerance to RF exposure at SAR = 6.1 W/kg as the number of such exposures increased; e.g., it took 60 min on the first day, but 220 min on the 34th day, for dogs to generate a rise in rectal temperature of 1.5°C. This phenomenon resembles acclimatization to hot environments as described by Goldman (1983).

In short-term experiments in which respiratory frequency, respiratory evaporative heat loss, and certain body temperatures were measured in dogs, it was confirmed that no significant thermoregulatory responses could be elicited in 25-kg dogs subjected to additional endogenous heat loads of 0.6–0.7 W/kg in a neutral or warm environment (Rawson, 1969). In 50- to 60-kg sheep, a 0.5–0.6 W/kg heat input was immediately followed by a significant increase in panting in the absence of a rise in temperature of skin or brain thermoreceptors. This was interpreted as evidence of the operation of unknown deep body temperature receptors. These studies by Rawson (1969) indicate that an additional heat load of up to 0.6 W/kg in dogs in neutral or slightly warm environments is easily dissipated in the conscious animal by increased respiratory heat loss. Unshorn sheep, in a 38°C environment, underwent a body temperature increase that leveled off at about 0.5°C higher than basal level. Also, in short-term sheep experiments, it was clearly demonstrated that the respiratory mechanism could be overdriven to cool the cerebral circulation and decrease the hypothalamic temperature—a phenomenon probably dependent upon unknown deep body thermoreceptors.

Studies by Norman et al. (1969) have shown that the temperature regulation mechanisms of dogs adjust to dissipate additional endogenous heat loads of up to 0.8 W/kg (corresponding to a heat flux of 1 W/cm^2 and a maximum blood temperature rise of 4°C). The additional endogenous heat was tolerated without apparent ill effects for periods of up to 13 months. Serial hematological, endocrine, hepatic, and renal function tests were within normal limits.

The question quite often asked is whether individuals with cardiac problems can tolerate increased body heat. An interesting paper in this respect is that of Sancetta et al. (1958), who reported on a study in which 16 patients, 8 with and 8 without left ventricular failure, were subjected for 2 hr to an ambient temperature of 98°F. "Neither group of subjects showed any significant change in minute ventilation, oxygen consumption, arteriovenous oxygen difference, and cardiac output. Both groups showed significant decreases in brachial and pulmonary artery pressure, systemic and total pulmonary resistances, and left ventricular work." The authors "speculated that the short-term exposure to a warm, dry environment under circumstances which produce the above changes is not deleterious, but may actually be beneficial to certain patients with left ventricular failure."

9.6. RESPONSE TO ABSORBED RF ENERGY

The amount of incident electromagnetic energy absorbed by an exposed body depends on the frequency, geometry, and polarization of the incident electromagnetic field, the orientation of the body with respect to the field, and body geometry and dielectric properties.

The basic physical principle of conservation of energy demands that all the electromagnetic energy absorbed by any physical body must be converted into another form of energy or be reradiated. Because animals are mostly water, they are poor electromagnetic reradiators, and almost all the electromagnetic energy they absorb is converted into heat.

Animal and human modeling data for electromagnetic absorption have been obtained (Beischer and Reno, 1974; Allen, 1975; Guy, 1975). Under physically "ideal" conditions, an exposed body may absorb up to 50% of the aggregate incident microwave energy; the remainder is either reflected or scattered. It is this absorbed energy that is available for conversion into heat in body tissue, and hence must be considered as an externally applied heat load.

The responses evoked by externally applied heat loads depend on their area of application and their magnitude. For humans, the application may be local and unintentional, such as is the case for most accidental exposures; local and intentional such as for therapeutic uses; or whole-body. These three application categories will be discussed in the following. The aggregate effect of a thermal insult depends on its magnitude relative to the ongoing activity of the thermoregulatory system or its various physiological mechanisms. For instance, for whole-body exposure at 10 mW/cm^2, an average human of frontal area approximately 3000 to 5000 cm^2 would absorb a maximum of 15 to 25 W, which is of the order of one-third the minimum metabolic rate.

Schwan (1958) noted that the human body's heat turnover, determined at a caloric uptake of about 2000 kcal/day, corresponds to an energy flux of about 0.05 W/cm^2 body surface. Local applications of comparable energy flux values can be taken care of by the body's heat regulation mechanism without noticeable general or local rise in body temperature. Based on the assumption of an effective depth of penetration of between 2 and 5 cm (2450 MHz) and if values for the heat capacity of tissue similar to those of water are introduced, a tissue volume of 5-cm depth should heat up with a speed of about $0.2°C/\text{min}$, if supplied with an energy of 0.1 W/cm^2.

The basal metabolic rate (BMR) of 1800–2000 cal/day may be increased threefold under conditions of sustained heavy work. Higher metabolic rates can be sustained for shorter periods of time, i.e., the average metabolic rate for a long-distance runner competing for an hour is about 10 times the BMR. Typical values for incident radiation in bright sunlight at the earth's surface is about 600 cal/m^2 per hr (Leden et al., 1947). About half of this is absorbed in the skin. A human with typically a 1.9-m^2 surface area would thus absorb energy at a rate of about 8000 cal/day through the skin (with appropriate allowance for reradiation) when standing unclothed in bright sunlight. Such an individual would thereby absorb 4 times as much energy as his BMR.

The thermal and physiological properties of the body tissues successively exposed to an external electromagnetic energy insult are also vital in determining the character of the final thermal stress. For instance, fatty tissue has a considerably lower heat conductance than muscular tissue. As a consequence, the subcutaneous fat layer tends to establish a temperature barrier between inside and outside of the human body. If heat is developed predominantly in the skin or the fat itself, the resulting temperature rise in these tissues will establish heat conduction to the outside even though the internal body temperature does not rise much (Schwan, 1958).

Depth of penetration in the muscular tissues is only a rough guide as to the eventual temperature distribution, except during the linear transient period. After heat conductance starts to effectively contribute to the final temperature distribution, "effective" depth of penetration may often be larger than "primary" depth of penetration. Hence, once heat has been successfully delivered beyond the subcutaneous fat layer, blood flow and heat conductance will help to establish a deep-reaching, but still localized, temperature elevation.

It has been shown that in heating due to microwave exposure, muscle blood flow increases, but the muscle temperature increase affects muscle blood flow much less than a comparable skin temperature increase affects skin blood flow (Fischer and Solomon, 1965). An increase in blood flow that is closely related to the increase in tissue temperature has been measured during microwave exposure. Investigations by Lehmann (1971) suggest that during microwave application, the resulting blood flow changes are most marked in the skin and subcutaneous tissues. The blood apparently has a lower temperature than the heated tissues and thus acts as a cooling agent, selectively decreasing the temperature in the superficial tissues, therefore providing for a relatively better depth heating. Heated tissues cool more slowly with the blood flow occluded than when it is intact, thus illustrating the role of blood flow in cooling.

Gersten et al. (1949) determined the effect of various power densities and different periods of exposure to microwave diathermy (2450 MHz) on the peripheral circulation and tissue temperature in the exposed limb of human volunteers. The duration of exposure varied from 1 to 30 min. Significant increases in blood flow and in temperature of the tissues were produced in the exposed extremities. Changes in body temperature, heart rate, and blood flow in the unexposed extremities were insignificant. The average temperature rise in muscle was significantly greater than that of the subcutaneous tissues, while the average subcutaneous temperature increase was greater than that of the skin. After 20 min of exposure, the blood flow continued to increase and reached a maximum after 30 min of exposure, at which time the average total increase was 65%, After 30 min of heating, the decline in tissue temperature from the peak attained at 20 min was directly proportional to the increased blood flow during the same period.

The physiological effects observed to result from shortwave (27 MHz) diathermy applications are also due to heating (Kottke *et al.*, 1949). Changes in blood flow due to 27-MHz exposure have been investigated (Wise *et al.*, 1949). Abramson *et al.* (1957, 1960) found, in human volunteers, that associated with the increase in circulation was a definite increase in local oxygen uptake with the maximal rise being more than twice the control level. The response was observed to extend into the postexposure period for an average of approximately one-half hour. At a higher exposure, vasospasm and decrease in blood flow were observed. When kidney and blood flow function were tested, either no change in the "majority of the subjects" (Lehmann, 1971) or a decrease was observed (Kottke *et al.*, 1949). The sodium clearance in skin and muscle was greatly increased during exposure (Millard, 1961).

Silverman and Pendleton (1968) compared the effect of CW and pulsed 27-MHz exposure on peripheral circulation by exposing volunteers for 20 min. A significant increase in circulation was found with each modality but no significant difference in the effect of pulsed versus continuous output was seen. No threshold reactions were observed that might be attributed to the high pulse peak power.

9.7. ACUTE LETHALITY

The duration of irradiation by RF/MW of various frequencies and intensities sufficiently to kill an animal (immediately or within a few days after exposure) has been studied (Michaelson *et al.*, 1967; Deichmann *et al.*, 1959a,b,c; Mirutenko, 1964a; Tyagin, 1957; Lobanova, 1960; Addington *et al.*, 1961; Fukalova, 1964; Solov'ev, 1963; Schrot and Hawkins, 1974).

Deichmann et al. (1959c) investigated the thermal stress effects of exposure to an interrupted microwave field (simulating the continuous 360° sweeping action of a radar scanner). Using rats subjected to a constantly rotating microwave frequency of 24,000 MHz, 300 mW/cm^2, they found that the ratio of exposure time to nonexposure time in the field, as the scanner completed its full circle was critical to the length of total safe exposure. When compared with continuous exposure (0.30 W/cm^2), which killed a rat in 15 min, intermittent whole-body exposure to 50% of this energy per unit of time over a period of 31 min (generator—1 min on, 1 min off) killed in 16 min of actual exposure time, while 17% of the above microwave energy (1 min on, 5 min off) killed in 34 min of actual exposure time. These results suggest the animals had a chance to dissipate some of the absorbed heat during the nonexposure intervals.

Prausnitz and Süsskind (1962) and Süsskind (1958) have reported similar findings with mice exposed to 10,000 MHz, but note that when the mice are removed from the microwave field, the slight latency period before body temperature decreases indicates their inability to dissipate heat if the exposure–nonexposure cycle is too rapid. This would result in a situation similar to almost-continuous exposure.

Exposure of rats and mice to 24,000 MHz indicates that there is an inverse relationship between power density and exposure duration for lethality from total-body exposure. For the following power densities (W/cm^2), the minimum lethal exposure periods were as follows: 0.15—rats 35 min, mice 5 min; 0.08—rats 56 min, mice 13 min; 0.05—rats 80 min, mice 35 min; 0.03—rats 135 min, mice 140 min. Within the limits of these experiments, the survival time was directly related to body weight (Deichmann, 1966; Deichmann et al., 1959a,b, 1964; Deichmann and Stephens, 1961).

Tolerance to microwave exposure decreases as the ambient temperature increases (Michaelson et al., 1959; Michaelson, 1974a,b). Rats subjected to 24,000 MHz, 250 mW/cm^2, showed a twofold increase in survival time when the environmental temperature was reduced from 35°C to 15°C. Increased air circulation also resulted in a prolongation of survival time (Deichmann et al., 1959a).

In mice exposed to 10,000 MHz, the median survival (LD$_{50}$) could be obtained by exposure to 0.100 W/cm^2 for 12 min; to 0.270 W/cm^2 for 3.75 min (Prausnitz and Süsskind, 1962). Whole-body exposure to microwaves caused a rise in the body temperature of the animal; death could be correlated with the maximum body temperature reached, so that 50% of the mice died if their body temperature reached 44.1°C, or 6.7°C above normal. (Treatment with chlorpromazine, which lowers body temperature by several degrees, permitted correspondingly larger temperature rises.) All deaths were found to occur within 24 hr of irradiation. In another study, the LD_{50} for mice was reported to be $5 \, mW/cm^2$ (10,000 MHz) for 188 min or $8.6 \, mW/cm^2$ for 33 min of exposure. At 10,000 MHz, $400 \, mW/cm^2$, rats died in 13–14 min (Mirutenko, 1964a,b). For irradiation at $200 \, mW/cm^2$, survival time was 25–30 min (Hyde and Friedman, 1968).

When anesthetized dogs were exposed to 2450 MHz CW at a calculated power density of $0.8 \, W/cm^2$ localized to the head, damage threshold (42.5°C) for the skin of the scalp was approached but not exceeded (Imig and Searle, 1962; Searle et al., 1961). The survival time ranged from 180 to 390 min (mean = 311 min). Heart rate increased steadily throughout the exposure period. The diastolic pressure was significantly higher than the initial level at the half and three-quarter marks, then fell. The systolic pressure did not change significantly until the terminal quarter of the period. No marked change occurred in the cerebrospinal fluid pressure throughout. The fatal termination appeared to be one of circulatory collapse. The rapid pulse and the falling pulse pressure could have been the result of peripheral vasodilation set in motion to maintain normal limits of body temperature. Panting, which was seen almost from the beginning of the exposures, was inadequate to control the body temperature increase.

At 3000 MHz, $100 \, mW/cm^2$, 100% lethality occurred in rabbits after 103 min and in rats after 25 min of exposure (Tyagin, 1957; Lobanova, 1960). Lethality in rats occurred after 15 min at 2450 MHz, $70 \, mW/cm^2$ (Richardson, 1958).

Samaras et al. (1971) exposed male rats weighing 275 to 325 g to approximately $100 \, mW/cm^2$ microwaves at 2450 MHz for as long as 3 hr while maintaining normal body temperature by means of external convection. Animals exposed with no cooling air flowing through the chamber died within 17 ± 2 min with colonic temperatures reaching 45 to 47°C at the time of death. None of the animals exposed with cooled air flowing showed visible distress during or immediately after irradiation, and their colonic temperatures remained stable at about 38°C. No lesions or other signs of stress were noted during the 30-day postirradiation observation period nor at necropsy following that time. Specimens of lung, ovary, eye, brain, liver, kidney, thyroid, and adrenal gland were normal on microscopic examination.

Exposure to 400 MHz resulted in death in rabbits after 30–40 min at $50 \, mW/cm^2$ (Boyle et al., 1950) and in rats after 30 min at 100–$200 \, mW/cm^2$ (Lubin et al., 1960). At 200 MHz CW, one dog died after 31 min at $200 \, mW/cm^2$; in guinea pigs, death occurred after exposure to 432, 500, or $680 \, mW/cm^2$ for 28, 40, or 18 min, respectively (Addington et al., 1959).

An approximate median lethal dose for dogs was obtained with

15 min exposure to 200 MHz CW, 330 mW/cm^2, with perpendicular orientation (Addington *et al.*, 1961). Markedly lower rates of lethality were produced with slightly longer durations of exposure at 220 and 194 mW/cm^2, and no deaths resulted from exposures of 0.5 to 1.0 hr at power densities of 165 mW/cm^2 and less (all at perpendicular polarization). All of the dogs that died had colonic temperature increases of 4.0°C or more. Because of the small number of animals used, the data have little statistical significance; they do, however, give some idea of the range of lethality for 200 MHz.

Rats died after 100 min exposure to 2000 V/m of 69.7 MHz or 5000 V/m of 14.88 MHz; 5 min exposure to 5000 V/m of 69.7 MHz was lethal (Fukalova, 1964). The LD$_{50}$ for mice exposed to 500 Hz was 650,000 V/m for 90 min; for 50 Hz, the LD$_{50}$ was 650,000 V/m for 270 min (Solov'ev, 1963).

Schrot and Hawkins (1974), in a series of experiments, confirmed the earlier theoretical study by Hoeft (1965), which indicated that at a given power density, small animals die sooner than larger ones.

It is well recognized that lethality is a function of higher power density–exposure duration relationships. In a report by Polson *et al.* (1974), lethality for rats exposed to different frequencies (0.95–7.44 GHz) was studied. They noted that for the most lethal frequency, the lethal energy constant was 36.643 mW-sec/cm^2 or 10.2 mW-hr/cm^2. This is a factor of 10 or greater than the ANSI (1973) radiation protection guide of 1 mW-hr/cm^2. This, of course, has to be related to the small body size of the rat in contrast to larger animals. Thus, for the human, this factor of 10 could be increased considerably. In addition, by comparing energy density and exposure duration. Polson *et al.* (1974) determined a function designated as "tissue power dissipation" or the ability of the organism to dissipate the absorbed energy. On this basis, the minimum "tissue power dissipation" value (at the most lethal frequency) was 78 mW/cm^2. Here again, when one considers scaling factors for differences in body size, for the human the "tissue power dissipation" value would be considerably greater than for the rat.

Review of these reports reveals that lethality depends on a number of conditions of irradiation, on the dimensions of the animal, and on the combined conditions. For a given intensity, a shorter exposure will kill the animal when the temperatures of the body and the environment are higher, and when the dimensions of the animal are small.

That death of animals from exposure to an exceedingly high power density of certain microwave frequencies can occur, is incontrovertible. Body temperature rather than power density is, however, the determining factor as to when death will occur. This generalization, however, has to be placed in its proper context. It is known that if body temperature is raised by more than 5 to 10°C, macromolecular denaturation occurs and irreversible effects result. There are no substantiated reports of human deaths from exposure to microwave-generating equipment under normal conditions of operation or even at levels in excess of prevailing standards.

9.8. RESPONSE TO LOCAL EXPOSURE TO MW/RF ENERGIES

Some consideration has been given in animal experiments and man to the temperature rise in various organs and tissues as functions of incident energy wavelength, thickness of the subcutaneous fatty layer, rate of blood circulation, and other factors. The increase in temperature of tissues during local exposure is linear for short periods (1–3 min) and proportional to the magnitude of the microwave energy absorbed. With exposures in excess of 3 min, the extent of the thermal effect and distribution of heat in tissues is determined by heat-regulating mechanisms (Mirutenko, 1962, 1964b). Worden *et al.* (1948) reported that the thermal effect depends on exposure duration and that deep-lying muscles are heated to a greater extent only during the first 20 min of exposure. When the thigh region is exposed to microwaves, there is a greater temperature rise in the muscles than in the skin and subcutaneous fatty layer (Cook, 1952; Herrick and Krusen, 1953; Krusen *et al.*, 1947; Rae *et al.*, 1949). The distribution of temperatures among the various tissues depends on the rate of blood circulation. Thus, rapid heating of all tissues was observed in rabbit thighs during microwave exposure when the local blood supply was occluded. When the paws of rabbits were exposed to 2450 MHz, the temperature rise in the deep tissues of the leg could vary substantially with repeated local exposures. While the temperature in the thigh muscles rose 4°C after the first 10-min exposure at 120–150 mW/cm^2, the rise was only about 2°C after the sixth or seventh treatment, suggesting that adaptive reactions had come int play. Adaptive reactions were also noted on the opposite unexposed leg after daily conditioning exposures to microwaves. After denervation of the rear extremity, the temperature rise in the thigh muscles remained the same regardless of the number of exposures (Semenov, 1965).

Engle *et al.* (1960), Gersten *et al.* (1949), and Rae *et al.* (1949) exposed the hindlegs of dogs and the forearms of human volunteers and found that increments in temperature of muscle were slightly higher than those of subcutaneous fat. Lehmann *et al.* (1962a,b) noted that consideration of the thickness of the subcutaneous tissues involved may explain apparent differences in results of various investigations. Examination of the hindleg of a dog reveals that the subcutaneous layer is usually only a few millimeters thick, and in many cases contains little fat.

Similarly, the human forearm has a comparatively thin layer of subcutaneous fat in most cases. Thus, one explanation for the greater increments in temperature of muscle than of fat in some studies might be that, under the particular conditions of the experiments, relatively small amounts of energy were absorbed in the thin layer of subcutaneous fat.

9.9. COMPARISON OF EXPOSURE TO MICROWAVES AND INFRARED

According to some investigators (Gordon, 1960; Gordon and Lobanova, 1960; Tyagin, 1957), hyperthermia develops much more efficiently with microwaves than with infrared exposure. With 2450 MHz, 50 mW/cm^2, 30 min exposure of the spinal region in rabbits, a 1–1.5°C rectal temperature rise was observed, while 350 mW/cm^2 was necessary to produce the same effect with infrared.

Several studies, notably those of Lehmann et al. (1964, 1965, 1966), have compared the heating patterns and temperature distributions resulting from 2450- and 915-MHz microwave exposure to those resulting from infrared exposure, using volunteers. The highest temperature distributions with infrared application were obtained in the most superficial tissues, while the highest temperatures from microwave application were obtained close to the subcutaneous fat–muscle interface. Microwave application produced somewhat higher temperatures in all cases in the deep tissues. A marked difference was found between temperature distributions produced by the two microwave frequencies prior to the blood flow changes resulting from temperature increases in the tissues. The 915-MHz exposure produced a greater increase in the temperature of the deeper musculature. This difference was much less pronounced after blood flow changed, about 10 min after the start of the exposure, since the increased flow cooled the skin and subcutaneous tissues specifically. Thus, after blood flow increased, the difference in the deep-heating properties between the two frequencies diminished.

Lehmann et al. (1964) suggested that there are no major modifying factors in live tissues beyond the blood flow change and the physiological initial temperature distribution, which may alter the temperature distribution obtained during microwave exposure.

9.10. THERAPEUTIC APPLICATION OF RF/MW ENERGIES (DIATHERMY)

Diathermy is the therapeutic induction of heat in the tissue beneath skin and subcutaneous fat. The temperature elevation results in increased metabolic activity and in the dilation of blood vessels, causing increased blood flow. The increased blood flow increases the oxygen supply to the treated areas and accelerates the removal of carbon dioxide and metabolic products. In addition, microscopic thrombi may be unclogged or removed when constricted vessels are opened.

Diathermy has proven particularly useful in the treatment of arthritic and rheumatic diseases. The clinical aspects of diathermy are beyond the scope of this book; the texts by Krusen *et al.* (1971) and Lehmann (1982) are recommended as sources of more complete information for the interested reader.

There are three diathermy modalities currently in use: ultrasonic, shortwave, and microwave. All are similar in that an applicator is placed over the area to be treated and incident power density and exposure time are adjusted to achieve the effect considered necessary. They differ, however, in the mechanism of heating involved. In ultrasonic diathermy, an applicator comprising a piezoelectric transducer focuses a beam of high-frequency acoustic energy, which penetrates into deeper tissue layers. Shortwave and microwave diathermy are similar in that they both involve application of electromagnetic energy. However, as their frequencies are different, usually 13.56 MHz for shortwave diathermy and 2450 MHz for microwave diathermy, their depths of penetration and hence methods of application differ. Shortwave diathermy relies more on induced fields, while microwave diathermy relies more on a focused beam of electromagnetic energy to achieve the final desired conversion into heat. The present discussion will be limited to microwave diathermy.

Most microwave diathermy units consist of a microwave generator feeding an applicator through a length of waveguide or coaxial cable. The generator usually has controls for varying the applied power level and the duration of exposure. The applicator is simply a microwave antenna designed for transferring a maximum amount of energy to a body in contact with its surface.

The exposure factors utilized in microwave diathermy include:

- Dose rate: The total power, or energy applied per unit time, in watts.
- Energy flux: The power density, or dose rate per unit body surface, in watts per square centimeter of body surface.
- Dose: The total energy applied in watt-seconds, or joules. It is equal to the energy flux times the surface area exposed times the exposure duration.
- Specific absorption rate (SAR): The rate at which microwave energy is imparted to a material per unit mass of the material. The

SAR is obtained from the relationship:

$$\mathrm{SAR} = \frac{4.19 \times 10^3 cT}{t}$$

where c is the specific heat of the material (kcal/kg per °C), T is the temperature rise in the material (°C), t is the time of energy deposition in the material (seconds), and SAR is the specific absorption rate (W/kg).

The total heat developed in the body, due to microwave exposure, is determined by the total energy uptake.

In diathermy treatment, while total applied dosage increases somewhat with the area exposed treatment, it rarely exceeds 1000 W-min. The energy flux is generally kept beneath 1 W/cm^2, and the dose rate seldom exceeds 100 W. Time of treatment varies from 3 to 30 min According to Schwan (1958), the above figures cannot be exceeded significantly without danger of overheating and burning. On the other hand, these figures cannot be lowered by much more than about a factor of 10, without reducing heat development to an insignificant amount. It is difficult to estimate more accurately the lowest flux level that can bring about significant effects. Aside from energy flux, quantities such as depth of penetration, configuration of tissues, and physiological factors (e.g., dilatation of blood vessels) determine temperature rise.

Several studies have yielded experimental results defining those physical properties of the tissues that determine microwave energy propagation and absorption, and hence are useful in diathermy (Cook, 1951; England, 1950; Herrick *et al.*, 1950; Schwan, 1957, 1958, 1960; Schwan and Carstensen, 1953). Determination has also been made of the patterns of relative heating and temperature distributions produced in specimens by exposure to 2450 and 900 MHz (Lehmann *et al.*, 1962a,b). It has been documented that heating of the superficial tissues produces relatively few mild physiological and therapeutic reactions. On the other hand, certain beneficial biological and therapeutic effects can be obtained readily by heating the deep tissues directly (Lehmann, 1971).

Lehmann *et al.* (1965) have shown that in order to produce vigorous physiological and therapeutic reactions to heat, it is necessary to elevate temperatures close to tolerance levels in those tissues where the desired effect is to be obtained. It is important that the peak value of the distribution is in the tissues to be treated, in order to avoid destructive effects from exceeding the tolerable temperature elsewhere. The assumption that microwaves may heat muscle selectively is based on muscle having a high coefficient of absorption because of its high water content (Schwan, 1958). The studies by Lehmann *et al.* (1982a,b) indicate that microwave energy produced by commercially available 2450-MHz diathermy equipment and applied by a commonly used applicator, results in a distribution of temperature with the highest level in subcutaneous fat, if this layer is of a thickness of approximately 1 cm or more. It appears, based on studies conducted by Lehmann *et al.* (1978), that 238 W/kg would result in a temperature of 42–43°C over the course of a 15 to 30-min treatment.

Of considerable interest is the possibility of using microwaves to induce local or whole-body hyperthermia in the treatment of cancer.

9.11. SUMMARY

The conversion of any form of physical energy into heat is determined by the physical properties of the absorbing matter. Heat development may occur at either localized sites (specific heating) or involve more or less uniformly the total medium (volume heating). A closer examination of the mode of energy transfer into heat shows that molecular friction is responsible for the generation of heat. Hence, heat is developed at the boundaries that separate the molecule responsible for heat production from its environment. It is difficult to describe mechanisms that do not include some energy transfer into heat (Schwan, 1958).

The membranes that surround tissue cells have no influence on the electrical properties of tissues at ultrahigh frequencies. This means that electromagnetic waves and fields proceed without being affected by the cell membranes. Hence, the cell interior and exterior are exposed equally to the electric field and warmed to nearly the same extent, since their electrical characteristics are quite similar (Schwan, 1957). As a consequence, electromagnetic waves and fields cause "volume" heating, not only on a macroscopic, but also on a microscopic level. This volume heating is completely due to the movement of ions of the tissue electrolytes with the electrical field (Schwan, 1958).

Thermal responses are the most thoroughly investigated and documented effects of exposure to microwaves. The absorbed energy is transformed into increased kinetic energy of the absorbing molecules, thereby producing a general heating of the tissue. The heating results from both ionic conduction and vibration of the dipole molecules of water and proteins. The temperature rise is a function of the thermoregulatory capacity of the body in relation to the thermal properties of the tissues and neurocirculatory mechanisms.

Frequencies greater than 3000 MHz approach those in which surface heating predominates. Since the skin contains most of the body's nerve endings or sensory elements, heating of this layer is perceived immediately.

Schwan (1958) has described the sequence of events following exposure of tissues to microwaves:

1. Primary process—the radiant or electric energy, in its interaction with the molecules of the various tissues, is ultimately "absorbed." That is, it is transformed from radiant or electric energy into heat. The details of this transformation are determined by the electrical properties of the biological substances. Hence, a determination of these properties is needed to understand the primary processes.
2. Following the primary process of heat development, heat conduction will occur from sites of higher to sites of lower temperature. Heat development and heat conduction together determine ultimately the temperature rise that occurs at any specific location.
3. Temperature rise will have physiological consequences. Metabolic activity is increased, since ion transfer processes are accelerated at higher temperatures. With sufficient temperature increase, blood flow often increases due to dilatation of blood vessels. Vasodilatation in turn further supports increased metabolic activity.

The human body is well adapted to withstand surface heating. The basal metabolic rate (BMR) may rise in individuals engaged in certain activities. Although such increased rate cannot be sustained indefinitely, it does indicate there is a large heat tolerance reserve in healthy individuals so that even allowing for diminution of this reserve in certain individuals, there is still a reserve for extra heat loading.

In the final analysis, research on metabolic rate and heat development in the human for various work loads, suggests that an added heat input, comparable to the BMR, is easily tolerated. In fact, the human body is often exposed to considerably higher loads without ill effects.

An excessive increase in body temperature produces damage indistinguishable from hyperthermia of other origin. When the thermoregulatory capability of the body or portion of the body exposed is exceeded, tissue damage can result. Such injury occurs at absorbed power levels far above the metabolic output of the body. Intermittent exposure can be better tolerated for longer periods than constant exposure at comparable power levels, owing to processes of heat dissipation. Heat produced is diffused from the irradiated portions of the body by the vascular system and conduction.

REFERENCES

Abramson, D. I., A. J. Harris, P. Beaconsfield, and J. M. Schroeder (1957) Changes in peripheral blood flow produced by short-wave diathermy. *Arch. Phys. Med.* **38:**369.

Abramson, D. I., Y. Bell, H. Rejal, S. Tuck, C. Burnett, and C. J. Fleischer (1960) Changes in blood flow, oxygen uptake, and tissue temperatures produced by therapeutic physical agents. II. Effect of short wave diathermy. *Am. J. Phys. Med.* **39:**87.

Addington, C. H., C. Osborn, G. Swartz, F. P. Fischer, and Y. T. Sarkees (1959) Thermal effects of 200 megacycles (CW) irradiation as related to shape, location, and orientation in the field. In: *Proceedings of the Third Annual Tri-Service Conference on Biological Effects of Microwave Radiating Equipments,* C. Süsskind (ed.). University of California, Berkeley, pp. 10–14.

Addington, C. H., C. Osborn, G. Swartz, F. P. Fischer, R. A. Neubauer, and Y. T. Sarkees (1961) Biological effects of microwave energy at 200 Mc. In: *Biological Effects of Microwave Radiation,* Vol. 1, M. F. Peyton (ed.). Plenum Press, New York, p. 177.

Adolph, E. F. (1947) Tolerance to heat and dehydration in several species of mammals. *Am. J. Physiol.* **151:**564.

Adolph, E. F. (1979) Look at physiological integration. *Am. J. Physiol.* **6:**R255.

Allen, S. J. (1975) Measurements of power absorption by human phantoms immersed in radiofrequency fields. *Ann. N.Y. Acad. Sci.* **247:**494.

American National Standards Institute (1973) Techniques and Instrumentation for the Measurement of Potentially Hazardous Electromagnetic Radiation at Microwave Frequencies. ANSI Publ. C95.3-1973, NY.

Astrand, P.-O., and K. Rodahl (1970) Temperature regulation. *Textbook of Work Physiology.* McGraw-Hill, New York, pp. 491–536.

Baranski, S., and P. Czerski (1976) *Biological Effects of Microwaves.* Dowden, Hutchinson & Ross, Stroudsburg, Penn.

Bass, D. E., and A. Henschel (1956) Responses of body fluid compartments to heat and cold. *Physiol. Rev.* **36:**128.

Beischer, D. E., and V. R. Reno (1974) Microwave reflection and diffraction by man. In: *Biological Effects and Health Hazards of Microwave Radiation,* P. Czerski, K. Ostrowski, M. L. Shore, C. Silverman, M. J. Suess, and B. Waldeskog (eds.). Polish Medical Publishers, Warsaw, pp. 254–259.

Benzinger, T. H., C. Kitzinger, and A. W. Pratt (1963) The human thermostat. In: *Temperature—Its Measurement and Control in Science and Industry,* Vol. 3, J. D. Hardy (ed.). Reinhold, New York, p. 637.

Bligh, J. (1966) The thermosensitivity of the hypothalamus and thermoregulation in mammals. *Biol. Rev.* **41:**317.

Bligh, J. (1973) *Temperature Regulation in Mammals and Other Vertebrates.* North-Holland, Amsterdam.

Bligh, J. (1979) The central neurology of mammalian thermoregulation. *Neuroscience* **4:**1213.

Bligh, J., and K. G. Johnson (1973) Glossary of terms for thermal physiology. *J. Appl. Physiol.* **35:**941.

Boulant, J. A., and J. D. Hardy (1974) The effect of spinal and skin temperatures on the firing rate and thermosensitivity of preoptic neurones. *J. Physiol. (London)* **240:**639.

Boyle, A. C., H. F. Cook, and T. J. Buchanan (1950) The effects of micro-waves; a preliminary investigation. *Br. J. Phys. Med.* **13**:2.
Boyle, A. C., H. F. Cook, and D. L. Woolf (1952) Further investigations into effects of microwaves. *Ann. Phys. Med.* **1**:3.
Bullard, R. W. (1971) Temperature regulation. In: *Physiology,* 3rd edition, E. E. Selkurt (ed.). Little, Brown, Boston, p. 651.
Cabanac, M. (1969) Plaisir ou deplaisir de la sensation thermique et homeothermie. *Physiol. Behav.* **4**:359.
Cabanac, M. (1971) Physiological role of pleasure. *Science* **173**:1103.
Carlisle, H. J. (1970) Thermal reinforcement and temperature regulation. In: *Animal Psychophysics, the Design and Conduct of Sensory Experiments,* W. C. Stebbins (ed.). Appleton-Century-Crofts, New York, pp. 211–229.
Chatonnet, J., and M. Cabanac (1965) The perception of thermal comfort. *Int. J. Biometeorol.* **9**:183.
Cook, H. F. (1951) The dielectric behavior of some types of human tissues at microwave frequencies. *Br. J. Appl. Phys.* **2**:295.
Cook, H. F. (1952) A physical investigation of the heat production in human tissues when exposed to microwaves. *Br. J. Appl. Phys.* **3**:245.
Corbit, J. D. (1970) Behavioral regulation of body temperature. In: *Physiological and Behavioral Temperature Regulation,* J. Hardy, A. P. Gagge, and J. A. J. Stolwijk (eds.). Thomas, Springfield, Ill., pp. 777–830.
Corbit, J. D. (1973) Thermal motivation. *Neurosci. Res. Program Bull.* **11**(4):317.
Czerski, P. (1975) Microwave effects on the blood-forming system with particular reference to the lymphocyte. *Ann. N.Y. Acad. Sci.* **247**:232.
Czerski, P., and S. Szmigielski (1974) Microwave bioeffects, current status and concepts. In: *Proc. 5th European Microwave Conference,* Hamburg, pp. 348–354.
Deichmann, W. B. (1966) Biological effects of microwave radiation of 24,000 megacycles. *Arch. Toxicol.* **22**:24.
Deichmann, W. B., and F. H. Stephens, Jr. (1961) Microwave radiation of 10 mW/cm^2 and factors that influence biological effects at various power densities. *Ind. Med. Surg.* **30**:221.
Deichmann, W. B., M. Keplinger, and E. Bernal (1959a) Relation of interrupted pulsed microwaves to biological hazards. In: *Proceedings of the Third Annual Tri-Service Conference on Biological Effects of Microwave Radiating Equipments,* C. Süsskind (ed.). University of California, Berkeley, p. 77.
Deichmann, W. B., E. Bernal, and M. Keplinger (1959b) Effects of environmental temperature and air volume exchange on survival of rats exposed to microwave radiation of 24,000 megacycles. *Ind. Med. Surg.* **28**:535.
Deichmann, W. B., F. H. Stephens, M. Keplinger, and K. F. Lampe (1959c) Acute effects of microwave radiation on experimental animals (24,000 Mc). *J. Occup. Med.* **1**:369.
Deichmann, W. B., J. Miale, and K. Landeen (1964) Effect of microwave radiation on the hemopoietic system of the rat. *Toxicol. Appl. Pharmacol.* **6**:71.
England, T. S. (1950) Dielectric properties of human body for wave-length in 1–10 cm range. *Nature (London)* **166**:480.
Engle, J. P., J. F. Herrick, K. G. Wakim, J. H. Grindlay, and F. H. Krusen (1950) The effects of microwaves on bone and bone marrow and on adjacent tissues. *Arch. Phys. Med.* **31**:453.
Fischer, E., and S. Solomon (1965) Physiological responses to heat and cold. In: *Therapeutic Heat and Cold,* S. Licht (ed.). E. Licht, New Haven, Conn., p. 126.
Fukalova, P. P. (1964) The effect of short and ultrashort waves on body temperature and survival of experimental animals. In: *The Biological Effect of Radio-frequency*

Electromagnetic Fields. Institute of Work Hygiene and Occupational Diseases, AMN, SSR, Issue 2, Moscow, pp. 78–79.

Gagge, A. P., and J. C. Stevens (1968) Thermal sensitivity and comfort. In: *The Skin Senses*, D. R. Kenshalo (ed.). Thomas, Springfield, Ill., p. 345.

Gersten, J. W., K. G. Wakim, J. F. Herrick, and F. H. Krusen (1949) Effect of microwave diathermy on the peripheral circulation and on tissue temperature in man. *Arch. Phys. Med.* **30:**7.

Gillis, M. F., and P. C. Walkup (1969) Studies on the effects of added endogenous heat and on heat exchanger designs. In: *Proc. Artificial Heart Program Conference*, R. J. Hegeli (ed.). HEW, NIH, Washington, D.C., pp. 883–892.

Gilstrap, L. O., Jr., J. S. McNeil, L. P. Greenberg, and R. B. Spodak (1964) *A Compilation of Biological Laws, Effects and Phenomena, with Associated Physical Analogs.* Wright-Patterson AFB, Ohio.

Goldman, R. F. (1983) Acclimation to heat and suggestion, by inference, for microwave radiation. In: *Microwaves and Thermoregulation*, E. R. Adair (ed.). Academic Press, New York.

Gordon, Z. V. (1955) Occupational health aspects of radio-frequency electromagnetic radiation. In: *Ergonomics and Physical Environmental Factors.* Occupational Safety and Health Series, No. 21, International Labour Office, Geneva, p. 159.

Gordon, Z. V. (1960) The problem of the biological action of UHF. *Tr. Nii Gig. Tr. Prof. USSR* **1:**5.

Gordon, Z. V. (1966) Biological Effect of Microwaves in Occupational Hygiene. Izd. Med., Leningrad (TT 70-50087, NASA TT F-633, 1970).

Gordon, Z. V., and Y. A. Lobanoya (1960) The temperature reaction of animals under the influence of SHF-UHF. *Tr. Nii Gig. Tr. Prof. USSR* **1:**59.

Guy, A. W. (1975) Engineering considerations and measurements. In: *AGARD Lecture Series No. 78 on Radiation Hazards.* AGARD Document LS-78, pp. 9-1–9-36.

Hainsworth, F. R. (1967) Saliva spreading, activity, and body temperature regulation in the rat. *Am. J. Physiol.* **212:**1288.

Hammel, H. T. (1968) Regulation of internal body temperature. *Ann. Rev. Physiol.* **30:**641.

Hammel, H. T., F. T. Caldwell, Jr., and R. M. Abrams (1967) Regulation of body temperature in the blue-tongued lizard. *Science* **156:**1260.

Hardy, J. D. (1953–1954) Control of heat loss and heat production in physiologic temperature regulation. *Harvey Lect.* p. 242.

Hardy, J. D. (1961) Physiology of temperature regulation. *Physiol. Rev.* **41:**521.

Hardy, J. D. (1967) Central and peripheral factors in physiological temperature regulation. In: *Les concepts de Claude Bernard sur le Milieu Interieur.* Masson, Paris, p. 247.

Hastings, F. W., and L. T. Harmison (1969) *Artificial Heart Program Conference*, R. J. Hegyeli (ed.). HEW, NIH, Washington, D.C.

Herrick, J. F., and F. H. Krusen (1953) Certain physiologic and pathologic effects of microwaves. *Electrical Eng.* **72:**239.

Herrick, J. F., D. G. Jelatis, and G. H. Lee (1950) Dielectric properties of tissues important in microwave diathermy. *Fed. Proc.* **9:**60.

Hoeft, L. O. (1965) Microwave heating, a study of the critical exposure variables for man and experimental animals. *Aerosp. Med.* **36:**621.

Hori, T., and Y. Harada (1976) Responses of midbrain raphe neurons to local temperature. *Pfluegers Arch.* **364:**205.

Hyde, A. S., and J. J. Friedman (1968) Some effects of acute and chronic microwave irradiation of mice. In: *Thermal Problems in Aerospace Medicine*, J. D. Hardy (ed.). Unwin, Ltd., Old Woking, Surrey, pp. 163–175.

Imig, C. J., and G. W. Searle (1962) Studies on Organisms Exposed to 2450 Mc-CW

Microwave Irradiation. RADC-TDR-62-358, Contract AF 41 (657)113, Griffiths AFB, New York.
Irving, I. (1966) Adaptations to cold. *Sci. Am.* **214**:94.
Ivanov, K. P. (1975) Temperature signalization and its processing in an organism. In: *Mechanisms of Information Processing in Sensory Systems.* Izdatel'stvo Nauka, Leningrad, p. 7.
Jahns, R. (1976) Difference projections of cutaneous thermal inputs to single units of the midbrain raphe nuclei. *Brain Res.* **101**:355.
Kalyada, T. V. (1973) Adaptive reactions of the human body in response to radiowave irradiation. In: *The Problem of Adaptation in Labor Hygiene,* Y. I. Lynblina and N. A. Minkina (eds.). Moscow, p. 89.
Kholodov, Y. A. (1966) *The Effect of Electromagnetic and Magnetic Fields on the Central Nervous System.* Nauka, Moscow, p. 283 (NASA TT-F-465).
Kottke, F., D. Koza, W. Kubicek, and M. Olson (1949) Deep circulatory response to short wave diathermy and microwave diathermy in man. *Arch. Phys. Med.* **30**:431.
Krusen, F. H., J. F. Herrick, U. Leden, and K. G. Wakim (1947) Microkymatotherapy: Preliminary report of experimental studies of the heating effect of microwaves (radar) in living tissues. *Proc. Mayo Clin.* **22**:209.
Krusen, F. H., F. J. Kottke, and P. M. Ellwood (eds.) (1971) *Handbook of Physical Medicine and Rehabilitation.* Saunders, Philadelphia.
Laties, V. G., and B. Weiss (1959) Thyroid state and working for heat in the cold. *Am. J. Physiol.* **197**:1028.
Laties, V. G., and B. Weiss (1980) Behavior in the cold after acclimation. *Science* **131**:1891.
Leden, U. M., J. F. Herrick, K. G. Wakim, and F. H. Krusen (1947) Preliminary studies on the heating and circulating effects of microwaves (radar). *Br. J. Phys. Med.* **10**:177.
Lehmann, J. F. (1971) Diathermy. In: *Handbook of Physical Medicine and Rehabilitation,* F. H. Krusen, F. J. Kottke, and P. M. Ellwood (eds.). Saunders, Philadelphia, p. 273.
Lehmann, J. F. (ed.). (1982) *Therapeutic Heat and Cold.* Williams and Wilkins, Baltimore.
Lehmann, J. F., A. W. Guy, V. C. Johnston, G. D. Brunner, and J. W. Bell (1962a) Comparison of relative heating patterns produced in tissues by exposure to microwave energy at frequencies of 2450 and 900 meagcycles. *Arch. Phys. Med.* **43**:69.
Lehmann, J. F., J. A. McMillan, G. D. Brunner, and V. C. Johnston (1962b) Heating patterns produced in specimens by microwaves of the frequency of 2456 megacycles when applied with the "A", "B", and "C" directors. *Arch. Phys. Med.* **43**:538.
Lehmann, J. F., G. D. Brunner, J. A. McMillan, D. R. Silverman, and V. C. Johnston (1964) Modification of heating patterns produced by microwaves at the frequencies of 2456 and 900 Mc by physiologic factors in the human. *Arch. Phys. Med. Rehabil.* **45**:555.
Lehmann, J. F., V. C. Johnston, J. A. McMillan, D. R. Silverman, G. D. Brunner, and L. A. Rathbun (1965) Comparison of deep heating by microwaves at frequencies of 2456 and 900 megacycles. *Arch. Phys. Med.* **46**:307.
Lehmann, J. F., D. R. Silverman, B. A. Baum, N. L. Kirk, and V. C. Johnston (1966) Temperature distributions in the human thigh, produced by infrared, hot pack and microwave application. *Arch. Phys. Med. Rehabil.* **47**:291.
Lehmann, J. F., A. W. Guy, J. B. Stonebridge, and B. J. de Lateur (1978) Evaluation of a therapeutic direct contact 915 MHz microwave applicator for effective deep tissue heating in humans. *IEEE Trans. Microwave Theory Tech.* **MTT-26**: 556.
Lipton, J. M. (1968) Effects of preoptic lesions on heat-escape responding colonic temperature in the rat. *Physiol. Behav.* **3**:165.
Lipton, J. M., D. D. Avery, and D. R. Marotto (1970) Determinants of behavioral thermoregulation against heat: Thermal intensity and skin temperature levels. *Physiol. Behav.* **5**:1083.

Lobanova, Y. A. (1960) Survival and development of animals at various intensities and duration of SHF action. *Tr. Nii Gig. Tr. Prof. AMN SSSR* **1**:61.

Lubin, M., G. W. Curtis, H. R. Dudley, L. E. Bird, P. F. Daley, D. G. Cogan, and J. Fricker (1960) Effects of ultrahigh frequency radiation on animals. *AMA Arch. Ind. Health* **21**:555.

Marha, K., J. Musil, and H. Tuha (1968) *Electromagnetic Fields and the Living Environment*. State Health Publishing House, Prague (Transl. SBN 911302-13-7, San Francisco Press, 1971).

Michaelson, S. M. (1970) Biological effects of microwave exposure. In: *Biological Effects and Health Implications of Microwave Radiation*, S. F. Cleary (ed.). Symposium Proceedings, HEW Publ. BRH/DBE 70-2, p. 35.

Michaelson, S. M. (1974a) Effects of exposure to microwaves: Problems and perspectives. *Environ. Health Perspect.* **8**:133.

Michaelson, S. M. (1974b) Thermal effects of single and repeated exposures to microwaves—A review. In: *Biological Effects and Health Hazards of Microwave Radiation*, P. Czerski, K. Ostrowski, M. L. Shore, C. Silverman, M. J. Suess, and B. Waldeskog (eds.). Polish Medical Publishers, Warsaw, p. 1.

Michaelson, S. M. (1983) Thermoregulation in intense microwave fields. In: *Microwave and Thermoregulation*, E. R. Adair (ed.). Academic Press, New York, pp. 283–295.

Michaelson, S. M., J. Howland, R. A. E. Thomson, and H. Mermagen (1959) Comparison of responses to 2800 Mc and 200 Mc microwaves or increased environmental temperature. In: *Proceedings of the Third Annual Tri-Service Conference on Biological Effects of Microwave Radiating Equipments*, C. Süsskind (ed.). University of California, Berkeley.

Michaelson, S. M., R. A. E. Thomson, and J. W. Howland (1961) Physiologic aspects of microwave irradiation of mammals. *Am. I. Physiol.* **201**:351.

Michaelson, S. M., R. A. E. Thomson, and J. W. Howland (1967) *Biologic Effects of Microwave Exposure*. Tech. Rep. RADC-TR-67-461, Griffiths AFB, Rome Air Development Center, Rome, N.Y.

Millard, J. B. (1961) Effect of high-frequency currents and infra-red rays on the circulation of the lower limb in man. *Ann. Phys. Med.* **6**:45.

Milroy, W. C., and S. M. Michaelson (1971) Biological effects of microwave radiation. *Health Phys.* **20**:567.

Mirutenko, V. I. (1962) Investigating local thermal effect of electromagnetic (3 cm) waves on animals. *Fiziol. Zh. Akad. Nauk UKR SSR* **8**:382.

Mirutenko, V. I. (1964a) The thermal effects of a SHF electromagnetic field on animals, and some problems of SHF-field dosimetry. In: *The Biological Action of Ultrasound and Super High Frequency Electromagnetic Vibrations*. Nauk Dumka Akad. Nauk UKR SSR Inst. Fiziol., Kiev, p. 62.

Mirutenko, V. I. (1964b) Effect of blood circulation on the distribution of heat, and the magnitude of the thermal effect during action of a SHF–UHF electromagnetic field on animals. *Fiziol. Zh. Akad. Nauk UKR SSR* **10**:641.

Nakayama, T., H. T. Hammel, J. D. Hardy, and J. S. Eisenman (1983) Thermal stimulation of electrical activity of single units of the preoptic region. *Am. J. Physiol.* **204**:1122.

Newburgh, L. H. (1949) *Physiology of Heat Regulation and the Science of Clothing*. Saunders, Philadelphia.

Norman, J., C. Pegg, G. Sandberg, R. Lee, and F. Huffman (1969) Effects of intracorporeal heat and radiation on dogs. In: *Proc. Artificial Heart Program Conference*, R. J. Hegyeli (ed.). HEW, NIH, Washington, D.C., pp. 901–912.

Petrov, I. R. (ed.) (1970) *Influence of Microwave Radiation on the Organism of Man and Animals*. Meditsina Press, Leningrad (NASA TT F-708, 1971).

Phillips, R. D., E. L. Hunt, R. D. Castro, and N. W. King (1975) Thermoregulatory, metabolic and cardiovascular response of rats to microwaves. *J. Appl. Physiol.* **38**:630.

Polson, P., D. C. L. Jones, A. Karp, and J. S. Krebs (1974) Mortality in Rats Exposed to CW Microwave Radiation at 0.95, 2.45, 4.54, and 7.44 GHz. Final Technical Report, Stanford Research Institute, Menlo Park, Calif.

Prausnitz, S., and C. Süsskind (1959) Temperature regulation in laboratory animals irradiated with 3-cm microwaves. In: *Proceedings of the Third Annual Tri-Service Conference on Biological Effects of Microwave Radiating Equipments*, C. Süsskind (ed.). University of California, Berkeley, p. 33.

Prausnitz, S., and C. Süsskind (1962) Effects of chronic microwave irradiation on mice. *IRE Trans. Bio-Med. Electron.* **BME-9**:104.

Presman, A. S. (1968) *Electromagnetic Fields and Life*, Izd-vo Nauka, Moscow (Transl. Plenum Press, 1970).

Rae, J. W., Jr., J. F. Herrick, K. G. Wakim, and F. H. Krusen (1949) A comparative study of temperatures produced by microwave and short wave diathermy. *Arch. Phys. Med.* **30**:199.

Rawson, R. (1969) Studies of the effects of additional endogenous heat. In: *Proc. Artificial Heart Program Conference*, R. J. Hegyeli (ed.). HEW, NIH, Washington, D.C., pp. 893–912.

Richardson, A. V. (1958) Review of the work conducted at the St. Louis University School of Medicine. In: *Proceedings of the Second Annual Tri-Service Conference on Biological Effects of Microwave Energy*, E. G. Pattishall and F. W. Banghart (eds.). University of Virginia, Charlottesville, pp. 169–174.

Saito, M., and H. P. Schwan (1961) The time constants of pearl-chain formation. In: *Biological Effects of Microwave Radiation*, Vol. I. M. F. Peyton (ed.). Plenum Press, New York, p. 85.

Samaras, G. M., L. R. Muroff, and G. E. Anderson (1971) Prolongation of life during high-intensity microwave exposures. *IEEE Trans. Microwave Theory Tech.* **MTT-19**:245.

Sancetta, S. M., J. Kramer, and E. Husni (1958) The effects of "dry" heat on the circulation of man. I. General hemodynamics. *Am. Heart J.* **56**:212.

Satinoff, E. (1964) Behavioral thermoregulation in response to local cooling of the rat brain. *Am. J. Physiol.* **206**:1389.

Schrot, J., and T. D. Hawkins (1974) Lethal effects of 3000 MHz radiation on the rat. *Radiat. Res.* **59**:504.

Schwan, H. P. (1957) Electrical properties of tissues and cell suspension. *Adv. Biol. Med. Phys.* **5**:147.

Schwan, H. P. (1958) Biophysics of diathermy. In: *Therapeutic Heat*, S. H. Licht (ed.). E. Licht, New Haven, Conn., pp. 55–115.

Schwan, H. P. (1960) Characteristics of absorption and energy transfer of microwaves and ultrasound in tissue. In: *Medical Physics*, Vol. 3, O. Glasser (ed.). Year Book Medical, Chicago, p. 1.

Schwan, H. P., and E. Carstensen (1953) Application of electric and acoustic impedance measuring techniques to problems in diathermy. *Am. Inst. Electrical Eng. Trans.* **72**:106.

Schwan, H. P., and G. M. Piersol (1954) The absorption of electromagnetic energy in body tissues, a review and critical analysis. Part I. Biophysical aspects. *Am. J. Phys. Med.* **33**:371.

Schwan, H. P., and G. M. Piersol (1955) The absorption of electromagnetic energy in body tissues, a review and critical analysis. Part II. Physiological and clinical aspects. *Am. J. Phys. Med.* **34**:425.

Searle, G. W., R. W. Dahlen, C. J. Imig, C. C. Wunder, J. D. Thomson, J. A. Thomas, and W. J. Moressi (1961) Effects of 2450 Mc microwaves in dogs, rats and larvae of the common fruit fly. In: *Biological Effects of Microwave Radiation,* Vol. I, M. F. Peyton (ed.). Plenum Press, New York, p. 187.

Selye, H. (1950) *Stress.* Acta, Inc., Montreal.

Semenov, A. I. (1965) The effect of UHF on the temperature or rabbit femoral tissues. *Byull. Eksp. Biol. Med.* **60:**64.

Sher, L. D., E. Kresch, and H. P. Schwan (1970) On the possibility of nonthermal biological effects of pulsed electromagnetic radiation. *Biophys. J.* **10:**970.

Silverman, D. R., and L. Pendleton (1968) A comparison of the effects of continuous and pulsed short-wave diathermy on peripheral circulation. *Arch. Phys. Med.* **4:**429.

Solov'ev, N. A. (1963) Responses of the entire living organism to an electromagnetic field. *Tr. Vses. Nauchno Issled. Inst. Med. Instrum. Oborudovaniya* **3:**120.

Stevens, J. C., and S. S. Stevens (1980) Warmth and cold: Dynamics of sensory intensity. *J. Exp. Psychol.* **60:**183.

Stolwijk, J. A. J. (1975) Physiological response to whole body and regional hyperthermia. In: *Proceedings of the International Symposium on Cancer Therapy by Hyperthermia and Radiation.* Washington, D.C., pp. 28–30.

Stolwijk, J. A. J. (1977) Responses to the thermal environment. *Fed. Proc.* **36:**1655.

Subbota, A. G., and Z. B. Svetlova (1972) *Labor Hygiene and the Biological Action of Radio-Frequency Electromagnetic Waves.* Moscow, p. 13.

Süsskind, C. (1958) *Biological Effects of Microwave Radiations.* Ann. Sci. Rep., Univ. California, Inst. Eng. Res., Ser. 60(205), RADC-TR-298.

Tyagin, N. V. (1957) Study of the thermal effect of SHF–UHF electromagnetic fields on various animals using the thermometric method. *Tr. Voen. Med. Akad. Kirov* **73:**9.

Weiss, B., and V. G. Laties (1960) Magnitude of reinforcement as a variable in thermoregulatory behavior. *J. Comp. Physiol. Psychol.* **53:**603.

Weiss, B., and V. G. Laties (1961) Behavioral thermoregulation. *Science* **133:**1338.

Winslow, C. E. A., L. P. Herrington, and A. P. Gagge (1937) Relationship between atmospheric conditions, physiological reactions and sensations of pleasantness. *Am. J. Hyg.* **26:**103.

Wise, C. W., B. Castlemen, and A. L. Watkins (1949) Effects of diathermy on bone growth in the albino rat. *J. Bone Joint Surg.* **31A:**487.

Worden, R. E., J. F. Herrick, K. G. Wakim, and F. H. Krusen (1948) The heating effects of microwaves with and without ischemia. *Arch. Phys. Med.* **29:**751.

10

Neural Effects of Microwave/Radiofrequency Energies

There has been a concerted effort to assess the sensitivity of the central nervous system (CNS) to "low levels' of microwave energy. To date there is no convincing evidence of the existence of "low-intensity" microwave effects on the human CNS. Animal studies suggest that the mechanisms that are the basis for reported effects, involve microwave-induced nonuniform temperature distributions and/or thermal gradients (Cleary, 1977).

10.1. ANATOMY AND PHYSIOLOGY OF THE NERVOUS SYSTEM

The nervous system, in many cases inextricably related to the endocrine organs (neuroendocrine system), is one of the most essential integrators of the organism as a whole, playing an important role in the vital processes of highly developed animals. In conjunction with the endocrine system, the nervous system adapts and regulates the internal environment (milieu intérieur) of the organism in relation to the requirements of the external environment to maintain homeostasis within physiological limits.

Since any disturbance in the usual functions of the nervous system could result in changes in other body systems, it is important to determine and understand the influence of RF or microwaves on the nervous system, in order to distinguish the responses of various organs and organ systems as a direct effect or indirectly mediated through the nervous system.

The nervous system is usually divided, for convenience, into the CNS, which includes the brain and spinal cord; the peripheral nervous system (PNS) (peripheral nerves); and the autonomic nervous system (ANS). The brain has three main parts: (1) the brain stem or medulla is an extension of the spinal cord responsible for unconscious and involuntary control of important reflex actions such as heart rate and breathing; the medulla also relays nerve impulses to other parts of the brain; (2) the cerebellum is the center of coordination and balance; (3) the cerebrum is the center of voluntary actions, consciousness, and sensation. The brain lies within and nearly fills the cranial cavity; it is continuous with the spinal cord, which lies within the vertebral canal. The brain and spinal cord are protected by the nonneural meninges: the outer tough dura mater, the fragile arachnoid, and the delicate, highly vascular pia mater. The subarachnoid space is filled with the cerebrospinal fluid (CSF), which protects the brain and spinal cord.

Craniospinal nerves include 12 pairs of cranial nerves that originate at the level of the brain, and 31 pairs of segmentally arranged spinal nerves from the spinal cord. Branches of the craniospinal nerves reach all parts of the body and consist of hundreds of nerve fibers, which may be motor, sensory, or have an autonomic function. Each nerve fiber is a peripherally extended part of an individual nerve cell, the body of which lies either in the CNS or within a ganglion (an aggregation of nerve cell bodies lying outside the CNS). The ANS is a description of the fibers that innervate smooth muscle, myocardium, and the glands of the body.

Nervous tissue consists of two types of cells, neurons (or nerve cells) and supporting elements called neuroglia (or glial cells). In the PNS, the nerve fibers are contained in bundles called nerves. The capacity of the nervous system to recover or regenerate after disease or injury is different in its peripheral and central portions. If a peripheral nerve is divided, new fibers may grow out from the central stump only if the two cut surfaces are approximated. On the other hand, in the CNS only abortive attempts at recovery are observed and new fibers are never formed.

Next to the blood vascular system, the nervous system is the most widely distributed system in the body, bringing back to the CNS by means of afferent (or sensory) peripheral nerve fibers impulses from receptors located in all parts of the body, both external and internal. By means of efferent (or motor) nerve fibers, the CNS is in communication with all effector organs in the body, both somatic and visceral, whether striated muscle to move limbs, cardiac muscle to augment the beat of the heart or to inhibit the flow of gastric secretion. The CNS is, then, the mediator or the integrator, into which information concerning the circumambient environment, the surface of the body, and all the internal environment is constantly being funneled by the sensory nerves. This information may be stored in the memory or it may be acted upon by sending appropriate impulses out over the motor nerves. A very large part of this constant activity takes place at levels below consciousness.

It is the responsibility of the ANS to maintain body homeostasis. Mobilization of the resources of the body to meet an emergency, such as a sudden change in its external environment (e.g., severe temperature change, severe hemorrhage, combat, or attack), is achieved by stimulation of the sympathetic division of the ANS with resultant secretion of epinephrine. This sympathetico-adrenal activity is demonstrated maximally in an animal by cardiac acceleration, sweating, pilomotor activity, deep respiration, and gastrointestinal inhibition. The parasympathetic division of the ANS, on the other hand, is primarily concerned with the protection, conservation, and restoration of the body resources. In most individual viscera the two divisions of the ANS tend to have antagonistic actions as in the heart where the sympathetic accelerates and the parasympathetic slows the beat, or in the gut where the actions are reversed, the parasympathetic augmenting and the sympathetic inhibiting peristalsis.

In order to grasp the significance of some of the reports of the CNS response to RF/MW exposure, an understanding of reflexes (involuntary action from a nerve stimulation) is necessary. Reflexes may be divided into two groups. Both spinal and brain-stem reflexes belong to the group of inborn, stereotyped invariable reflexes that are peculiar to the species. The number of these is very great. The cardiovascular reflexes, the reflexes of respiration and digestion, the reflexes of metabolism and elimination, the postural and locomotor reflexes, and even that body of more complex reactions sometimes referred to as instinct, all belong to this group, many of which have been studied (Ekel, 1974). Reflexes of this kind were designated as unconditioned reflexes by Pavlov (1927).

The second group of reflexes includes all those reflexes that are gained by the individual in the course of its existence. These are conditional responses, so called because they depend on many conditions for their formation and maintenance. They are also known as individual or acquired reflexes and are in many instances at least the same as those nervous reactions long known as associations. Conditional responses may be acquired either naturally or artificially, i.e., experimentally. When food is placed in the mouth of a dog, saliva is secreted. This is known as an inborn reflex. As a dog develops, he acquires a response that causes him to secrete saliva if he is hungry, when he sees food with which he is familiar, or smells food. This is a natural conditional response. If, when a dog is fed, a certain sound is made, and this combination of sound and food is frequently repeated, there comes a time when the sound alone will cause the secretion of saliva. This is an artificial conditional response. There is no fundamental difference between these two kinds of conditional responses.

According to Pavlov, the formation and maintenance of conditional responses are dependent upon the cerebral cortex, as complete removal not only abolishes all such reactions but makes the acquisition of additional responses impossible. The removal of localized areas causes less severe effects. After a period of disturbance, preexisting conditional responses may return.

The *integrative action* of the nervous system was particularly emphasized by Pavlov. If any one of the bodily organs and systems is affected by a noxious agent, the effect is most likely to show expression in the activity of the affected system and in the nervous system, but at the same time may not show at all in other bodily systems and organs (Ekel, 1974).

In addition to this integrative nature of the nervous system, it is probably the most vulnerable of all the bodily systems to adverse agents (e.g., it is the first system to die when the oxygen supply is stopped). The cerebral cortex is the part of the brain that is most vulnerable. This *vulnerability* of the nervous system, and of the cerebral cortex in particular, may also explain the fact that a very low level of intoxication may not show effects in other bodily systems or organs, but may show effects in the activity of the nervous system, and of the cerebral cortex in particular [i.e., in conditional reflex activity (CR)]. Thus, CR methods are used to investigate directly the functional state of the cerebral cortex, the organ most likely to be affected due to its *integrative nature* and *high vulnerability*. Usually the conditioned reflexes (CR) are categorized into two classes: (1) classical CR (known also as respondent behavior), and (2) instrumental CR (known also as operant behavior). Another important reflex is the orienting reflex (OR), which is a very specific unconditioned reflex. According to Pavlov, the unconditioned stimulus for it is "novelty" (any change in the usual environment of the animal); the reaction is a directing of the sense organs toward the source of the new stimulus (turning head, and so on) and it involves an inhibition of the ongoing conditioned activity. It is now generally recognized that there are four classes of component in the OR: (1) motor (turning the head and the body so as to set the appropriate sense organs to receive the stimulus), (2) vegetative (vasomotor reflexes of a very complex nature and galvanic skin reflex), (3) sensory (an increase in sensitivity of the receptors), (4) central (inhibition of the ongoing conditioned activity and changes in EEG).

The interesting property of the CR is that to evoke it, the stimulus need not be very strong; it is sufficient that it be novel. In fact, there are experimental data showing that stimuli within the threshold range of intensity evoke a more pronounced OR than stimuli just above this range (Ekel, 1974).

In order to get some appreciation for the literature on neural effects, definition of some commonly used words is necessary.

- *Anorexia*: Loss of appetite.
- *Asthenia*: Weakness or general debility, with no reference as to cause. A very general term.

- *Conditioned reflex* (*reflex*: the sum total of any particular involuntary activity—may be voluntary at some point in its development or evolution): A reflex that does not occur naturally in the animal, but may be gradually developed by training and through frequent repetition of a stimulus.
- *Dermographia* (*dermatographia*): A condition of the skin whereby tracings on the skin surface with a pointed object result in elevated reddish wheals that persist. Seen in disorders of adrenal function. The Soviets use a provocative test with histamine infusion and time the appearance and quality of the response. It is considered a sign of vascular instability due to altered neurohumoral function in the autonomic centers of the brain.
- *Functional*: Of, or pertaining to a function. Affecting the operations of a part, but not the structure necessarily. Physiologists study living things as functional entities. Physicians use the term in two senses: one in the absolute physiological meaning with the connotation that measurable physical parameters exist to measure functions of a living thing; the other is a very broad use, i.e., a functional disorder, meaning that no measurable alteration of structure causes the "functional" symptoms presented. It is used as opposed to organic ailment, denoting that a measurable physical alteration in structure or physical makeup has occurred to explain the symptoms as presented. Subjective complaints such as headache, fatigue, nervousness are termed "functional" in the absence of demonstrable correlative pathology.
- *Hidrosis*: Moisture, sweat.
- *Hyperhidrosis*: A lot of moisture, a lot of sweat! Soviets use galvanic skin response measurements as one of their physiological parameters of body function (autonomic nervous system).
- *Myocardial dystrophic changes*: Dystrophy means a specific change in the capabilities and structure of muscle, and is degenerative, i.e., muscular dystrophy. To the Soviets this phrase means a disorder of neural regulation to the heart with an alteration of function (usually condition abnormalities) that is entirely reversible, and of which the patient may have no awareness. In the Soviet context there is no change in the cardiac muscle itself, its intrinsic properties, or its internal conduction mechanism; only in its neural regulation. The several changes described have no significance for Western cardiologists. They are listed as normal variations when encountered, unless there is demonstrable correlative pathology.
- *Neurasthenia*: Used to denote nervous prostration; in the West, a descriptive term, without pathological reference, meaning nervous

exhaustion characterized by fatigability. It is usually due to a long and excessive expenditure of energy, and is marked by fatigue, lack of drive, vague pains, often in the back, loss of memory, insomnia, constipation. To the Soviets, regardless of origin, it means a specific disease entity as it is used. It is the neme given to a list of broad non-specific "functional" symptoms, that, taken together mean there exists a disorder of the nervous system of a *functional* nature.
- *Reflexogenic*: Producing or increasing a reflex action. Used to denote an area of the brain also (reflexogenic area of the cortex).
- *Vagotonia* (*vagos,* wandering; *tonos,* tension): Hyperexcitability of the vagus nerve. A condition of dominance of the vagus nerve in general body functioning. It is marked by vasomotor instability (dilatation of cutaneous blood vessels, constriction of visceral blood vessels), constipation, sweating, viscid salivation, pupillary constriction, involuntary motor spasms and pain, slowing of the heart, and so on.
- *Vegetative*: Concerned with growth and nutrition. Functioning involuntarily or unconsciously. Vegetative nervous system is another way of saying autonomic nervous system (meaning parasympathetic and sympathetic).

10.2. FUNDAMENTALS OF ELECTROMAGNETIC ENERGY–NEURAL TISSUE INTERACTION

The normal brain of the mammal is electrically polarized. Two forms of a steady potential are evident: a "resting" potential present in the absence of stimuli, and a second potential that is apparently due to incoming sensory volleys. The importance of these potentials is emphasized by the DC shifts associated with external and locally applied stimulation.

An extensive discussion of the possible mechanisms of electromagnetic energy–neural tissue interaction is not possible in this book. For in-depth discussion of such mechanisms, the reader is referred to reviews by Schwan (1957, 1971, 1977), Adey (1977), and Adey and Bawin (1977). As noted by Schwan (1977), "The electrical properties of biological membranes, capacitance and conductance, linear and nonlinear have been the subject of extensive investigations for more than half a century." Membrane capacitance values are available for many cell types from bulk measurements and with electrode systems impaled into the cells and directly measuring across the membrane. Based on such measurement, the capacitance is of the order of $1\ \mu\text{F/cm}^2$ with a range extending from 0.6 to 1.3 μF/cm^2 and an accuracy of about 20 or 30% in most cases. This capacitance appears to be frequency independent for the range from about 1 kHz to 100 MHz.

The membrane capacitance is polarized by an applied external field with cytoplasmic and extracellular tissue fluids serving as access impedance elements in series with the membrane capacitance. Thus, the invoked membrane potential is given by the applied field sampled over the cell dimensions. Larger cells receive a given membrane potential from an external field more effectively than smaller ones. Available data indicate membrane conductance values of the order of 10 mmho/cm^2 but varying over a wide range depending on numerous circumstances.

Membrane capacitance and conductance are linear, i.e., do not change if the applied external field evokes membrane potentials that are small in comparison with the resting potential of about 70 mV. However, if the membrane becomes depolarized, the membrane conductance increases dramatically at least in nerve and muscle cells to values of the order of 100 times those observed in the resting state.

On the basis of his own work and a comprehensive review of the literature, Schwan (1977) concludes that microwave fields cannot be coupled effectively into membranes. Current density values must be well above 1 mA/cm^2 to be potentially harmful. From Ohm's law the corresponding field strength in tissue would then have to be close to 0.1 V/cm. Adey and Bawin (1977), on the other hand, do consider brain interactions with weak electromagnetic fields by "cooperative" mechanisms. Although individual tissue components (electrolytes, membranes, or biopolymers) are not sensitive to an electric field, complex biological systems at higher levels of biological organization may be sensitive to low electric fields. No cooperative principles have, however, been established.

The neuronal structure of the CNS of experimental animals can be altered by acute, high-level exposures (> 4 W/kg). The changes, which include swelling axons and decreased dendritic spines, are qualitatively similar but quantitatively different and almost always reversible. Several investigators nevertheless state that the CNS is the most sensitive of all body systems to microwaves at intensities below "thermal" thresholds. According to some of these authors (Gordon, 1964; Presman, 1968), the reaction of the nervous system to microwaves is due to the spontaneous effect of the energy on skin receptors or brain cells. Receptor cells react to external stimuli while brain cells react to specific coded signals transmitted by receptor cells. The response is dependent on wavelength. Direct effects on the brain are intensified with increase in wavelength. Reactions attributed to skin receptor stimulation increase as the wavelength is decreased. When the reactions are due to a combination of peripheral and CNS stimulation, it is impossible to correlate the degree of reaction with wavelength.

Presman (1968) suggests that resonant absorption at superhigh frequencies (gigahertz range) could cause transitions of molecules, especially protein molecules, to excited states. Also, he discusses changes in the Na^+-K^+ gradient across cell membranes, owing to different effects of microwaves on degrees of hydration of these ions, as well as changes in cell permeability by the disruption of protein hydration at the cell membrane. It must be emphasized that all this is purely speculative, and no supporting experimental data are available (Petrov, 1970). On the other hand, Presman (1968) has also stated that the changes in functions of the nervous system produced by microwaves are not specific.

The resting membrane potential of animal muscle and nerve cells is generally in the range of -70 to -110 mV; animal cells cultured *in vitro* may show values as low as -10 to -30 mV; and protozoan cells have been shown to display potentials in the range of -30 to -100 mV. Due to their selective permeability, electrical double layers are formed at biological membranes, which cause differences of potential across the membranes. Therefore, the membranes are placed within electrical fields that are conditioned by electrical double layers. The amplitude of these fields is considerable. It amounts to 10^5 V/cm with a potential difference of 100 mV and a thickness of membrane of 100 Å. Very high fields would thus be required to cause a direct effect on nervous tissue (Schwan, 1971).

Microwave fields are only capable of applying a potential to a biological membrane that is many orders of magnitude smaller than the resting potential and, for this reason, should be unable to excite or change normal patterns (Schwan, 1957, 1971, 1977). Using a theoretical approach, based on biophysical principles and electromagnetic field theory, wave propagation and absorption in tissues, Schwan (1971) calculated that nerve cell membranes cannot be excited at field strengths below thermal levels of frequencies greater than 100 MHz, above which membranes are short-circuited. The electric field strength that exists in a nerve membrane is about 500 kV/cm. The field strengths applied by a microwave field to the human body are infinitely smaller, and hence cannot evoke stimulation (Schwan, 1971).

The possibility that microwaves may interact with the CNS by some mechanism other than heating has been suggested by several investigators (Petrov, 1970; Kholodov, 1966; Marha *et al.*, 1968; Novitskii *et al.*, 1971; Gordon, 1960, 1970a; Presman, 1968; Tolgskaya and Gordon, 1973; Baranski and Czerski, 1976). These reports come chiefly from the Soviet and Eastern European literature. These investigators stress that the CNS must be considered as being moderately or highly sensitive to radiation injuries. Their conceptual basis for this view is largely centered about Pavlovian conditional response methods and the principle of "nervism", which may be interpreted to mean that the CNS exerts a controlling influence over all primary reactions in the organism. Nonnervous reactions are considered as only of secondary importance because of the basic controlling role of the CNS in the whole organism. It should be pointed out, however, that although the nervism principle of Secenov and Pavlov does constitute one of the most important theoretical bases for Soviet medicine in general, specific studies are related to the discipline within which a given effect is studied, i.e., electroencephalography, biochemistry, cardiovascular pathophysiology (Z. V. Gordon, personal communication).

The reported nonthermal effects are based on a definition of thermal as being those effects associated with a measurable local or whole-organism temperature rise from an equilibrated baseline (Petrov, 1970; Gordon, 1960). Most Western investigators use the term *thermal* in a somewhat more refined sense, taking into account the fact that an organism can be affected thermally without a demonstrable temperature rise. In fact, when the temperature rises, it means that the functional reserves of the organism for maintaining homeostasis have been exceeded in some manner, and thermal regulation has been instituted.

Temperature input signals arise in many body structures among which the following have been identified experimentally: (1) preoptic–anterior hypothalamus, (2) posterior hypothalamus, (3) midbrain, medulla, motor cortex, and thalamus, (4) spinal cord, (5) skin, (6) respiratory tract, and (7) viscera. All these except the motor cortex and thalamus have been shown to evoke behavioral and/or physiological responses to changes in local temperature (Hardy, 1973).

Changes may be produced by means of stimulation or variation of the excitability of the peripheral and central parts of the nervous system. Since biological objects are electrically heterogeneous and microwave-range electromagnetic fields (EMF) have a known selective thermal effect on various tissues and organs, a difference between a microwave effect and a neutral heat effect is not necessarily due to an unknown extrathermal factor, but might well be a function of an uneven distribution of heat in the organism that could exert its own peculiar effect.

According to Presman (1968), intensities below $10\,mW/cm^2$ may be considered nonthermal for pulsed and CW microwaves of biologically effective frequencies in either whole-body or local irradiation. With intensities of $10\,mW/cm^2$ or less, conversion of microwave to thermal energy does not exceed the heat loss from $1\,cm^2$ of body surface under normal environmental conditions.

Evidence of microscopic changes in the structure of neurons due to microwave energy absorption is inconclusive. It is quite evident that changes observed are due to heating effects. There are some reports, however, that these same effects have been observed with low-power-density energy (Tolgskaya and Gordon, 1973). It is questionable whether these responses, if they do in fact occur as reported, are unrelated to heating effects, and their clinical significance to the human, if any, is not known. A few investigators have refused to accept the possibility of nonthermal neural stimulation, and explain these effects entirely as due to local heating.

McAfee (1961, 1963) has noted that an EMF can be reinforced in the region of peripheral nervous tissue causing a temperature rise, even while nearby muscle and skin show no measurable temperature effect. When peripheral nerves are heated above a minimum level, they may trigger spontaneously and produce the neurophysiological and behavioral changes that have been reported. The interaction between the PNS and the CNS could also account for reported cardiovascular effects. Pinneo *et al.* (1962) postulated that many so-called "nonthermal" effects may actually be direct thermal actions on certain neural structures. They examined the thermal stimulation of peripheral nerves exposed to 3000- and 10,000-MHz microwave and infrared energies. Their experiments showed that all three sources of energy produced the same effects on the CNS. They suggested that experiments purporting to show nonthermal effects should be examined with the possibility in mind that a thermally induced neurophysiological response may have occurred.

McAfee (1961, 1963) believes that the neural effects of microwave stimulation are due solely to the thermal effects of the energy and that these effects arise from stimulation of afferent pathways of the PNS structures. The studies by McAfee and associates suggest that the presumed nonthermal effects of microwaves on the CNS are a result of thermal stimulation of PNS structures. Studies claiming CNS effects of microwaves should include controls for possible PNS effects. These studies provide an explanation for behavioral effects in terms of responses evoked by microwave-induced heating of afferent nerve fibers, and also demonstrate errors that can be encountered when comparing responses obtained by irradiation of different regions of the animals. Such experiments and conclusions deserve careful consideration when physiological changes in animals exposed to microwaves are attributed to specific or nonthermal effects of microwave exposure.

10.3. IN VITRO STUDIES

Wachtel *et al.* (1975) and Seaman and Wachtel (1978) exposed *Aplysia* ganglia in a stripline to 1.5- and 2.45-GHz, CW and pulse-modulated microwaves. Changes in the firing rate of *Aplysia* neurons were reported with effective absorbed power ≤45 mW/cm^2. In a majority of cases, the firing rate of pacemaker cells increases with an increase in temperature, and decreases with a decrease in temperature. In a minority of cases (13%) for the pacemaker cells, the microwave irradiation reversed the normal change in firing rate, i.e., the rate decreased or stopped with a microwave-induced increase in temperature. The authors were able to detect slow and rapid components. The slow component, occurring in 30 to 60 sec, was correlated with the slow temperature change due to exposure. The rapid component, occurring within 1 sec, appeared to correlate with the presence of the microwave field. The rapid component was always found to be a decrease in firing rate in the presence of the field and was not produced by convective heating. Similar but more variable effects were found for the bursting cells. The threshold for the slow component was about 7 W/kg, but in one case the rapid component was found at an SAR as low as 1 W/kg. In all cases where effects were found, the firing rates returned to normal when the exposure was terminated, and the temperature returned to normal. According to the authors, the effects were in large part attributable to slight ganglionic warming; however, in some cases, effects were induced by microwave exposure that could not be reproduced by thermal means. Although they observed a decrease in the firing rate that could be produced by simply heating the preparation (2–3°C), they also noted that heating the preparation sometimes produced a change in firing rate opposite to that produced by microwaves, i.e., an increase in firing rate. These results suggested to the authors that the observed changes in firing rate are not produced solely by heating effects of microwaves. The authors hypothesized that at a dose rate of about 1 W/kg, conversion of 0.1% of the microwave energy into a polarizing current density across the cell membrane would be sufficient to affect the firing rate of pacemaker neurons. Yamaura and Chichibu (1967) found results similar to those of Wachtel using ganglia of crayfish and prawn exposed at 11 GHz. The regular firing rate of the ganglia decreased rapidly during microwave exposure, rebounded to a higher than normal rate when the exposure was terminated, and returned to normal. Temperature controls showed only an increased firing rate as the temperature was increased. The authors stated that the SAR was about 199 W/kg but did not describe the method of measurement.

Arber (1976) found a hyperpolarization of the resting potential of giant neurons of the mollusk *Helix pomatia* during exposure to 2.45-GHz CW microwaves. In this experiment, the ganglion was isolated and mounted in a stripline. The cell potential was measured, as in Wachtel's experiment, by inserting microelectrodes into the neuron. Exposure to microwaves with an SAR of about 15 W/kg for an hour produced a 5 to

10% increase in resting potential, followed by a stabilization or slight additional increase by an hour postexposure. This result is presumably caused by a change in the sodium–potassium balance in the cell. When Arber treated the cells with ouabain (postexposure), which inhibits Na^+,K^+-ATPase, he found that part of the hyperpolarization could be accounted for by the action of this enzyme under the influence of the microwaves. The remainder was attributed to changes in passive ion transport. The existence of microwave-induced alterations in the firing pattern of *Aplysia* ganglia at the intensities employed in this study has been considered as evidence of field rectification by neuronal membranes although no mechanism for such an effect is indicated (Baranski and Czerski, 1976).

It should be noted in this context that *Aplysia* pacemaker cells are sensitive to small changes in temperature and the firing rate may double with a 2°C increase in temperature. The firing rate of these pacemaker cells is controlled by pump currents as well as passive ion leakage currents each having opposite temperature dependence (Carpenter, 1967; Willis *et al.*, 1974). The apparent rectification may be an artifact resulting from the asymmetric nature of the cell membrane (Cole, 1968) or by rectification that would occur in the electrode itself.

Pickard *et al.* (1980) have presented results in which single cells from the plant *Nitella flexilis* exhibited a large voltage step-increase when exposed to pulses of 0.1 to 5 MHz (250-msec pulse duration, 6.3-sec pulse interval). These authors also found a fast and a slow component, the slow component correlating with a temperature rise in the sample. The authors suggest that the fast component is produced by the rectification of the oscillating electric field by the cell membrane. The fast component disappears into noise at about 667 V/m and may be a high-field effect.

In summary, the available literature on cellular and subcellular effects of microwaves does not yet definitely establish whether effects unrelated to heating the medium do exist. Several investigators report effects, but a majority do not find the effects unrelated to temperature variations. In some cases, results conflict. In other cases, the effects found are somewhat equivocal. Heating effects may not be clearly eliminated, or, as in the case of neuronal firing rate, the change in the rate may occur only in a minority of cases (Seaman and Wachtel, 1978).

Portela *et al.* (1975) studied the effect of 2.88-GHz pulsed microwaves on passive and dynamic electrical properties and on cell water parameters in frog muscle. They concluded that 120 min exposure at $10\,mW/cm^2$ did not produce permanent effects on electrical and cell water parameters.

Several investigators have shown that RF/MW energies do not affect simple nerve preparations if the temperature is carefully controlled. In studies by Chou (1975), exposure of vagus nerves and superior cervical ganglia at absorbed power densities of 0.3 to 1500 W/kg CW and 0.03 to 220 kW/kg peak pulsed fields induced no significant changes in compound action potentials. Conduction characteristics of the neurons were independent of electrical field polarization. Observations on the contractile tension of rat diaphragm muscles subjected to 0.3 to 1500 W/kg CW fields or 0.3 to 220 kW/kg peak intensities for pulse-modulated fields could not be dissociated from thermal mechanisms. Thus, it is believed that these fields would have little, if any, effects on peripheral nerves unless there is field-induced heating.

Using 2450 MHz, Taylor and Ashleman (1974) showed that nerve impulses were significantly attenuated when transmitted through the spinal cord of the cat exposed to microwaves. These effects, however, were reproduced by convective heating. The fact that the time course over which the detected effects occurred following microwave exposure differed from that due to other modalities of heating was attributed to differences in the time course of temperature elevations. It was stated that if the tissues were appropriately cooled during microwave exposure, the effects on the spinal cord were ameliorated or reversed. Exposure of hypothermic spinal cords changed the activity to the normal state, indicating that a given level of microwave energy acts on the spinal cord by elevating the tissue temperature. The authors concluded that these findings, together with those previously obtained with evoked thalamic potentials and isolated peripheral nerves, support the view that microwave effects on nervous system mechanisms are thermal in nature.

Bawin et al. (1975) and Bawin and Adey (1976, 1977) have reported calcium efflux from chick brains exposed *in vitro* to 147-MHz electromagnetic fields, amplitude modulated at 9, 11, 16, and 20 Hz at 1 to 2 mW/cm^2. Unmodulated fields and fields modulated at 0.5 and 3 Hz did not induce any significant changes in $^{45}Ca^{2+}$ efflux, as contrasted with progressive increases in efflux from brains exposed to fields modulated at 6, 9, 11, and 16 Hz. The effects gradually decreased as the pulse-modulation frequency was increased above 20 Hz. The authors note that no effect on Ca^{2+} efflux was produced by unmodulated fields and a pulse repetition rate-dependent maximum rate of efflux was detected at 11 and 16 Hz indicating that Ca^{2+} movement was critically related to specific slow components of the field.

Bawin et al. (1978) also investigated the effects on Ca^{2+} efflux from chick brains exposed *in vitro* to 450-MHz microwaves, amplitude modulated at 16 Hz, at intensities of 0.5, 0.1, 1, and 5 mW/cm^2. They found that 20 min exposure to 0.1 or 1 mW/cm^2 but not 0.5 or 5 mW/cm^2 (16-Hz modulation) resulted in a significant (9 to 10%) increase in calcium released relative to controls. ELF fields also indicated the frequency sensitivity of the brain tissue, but the net effect on calcium was a significant decrease in release rather than the increase seen at 147 and 450 MHz (Bawin and Adey, 1977). The authors suggested that the increase and decrease in calcium in the above experiments could reflect the binding properties of calcium and that different frequencies might react with different binding sites. Blackman et al. (1979) replicated the 147-MHz studies of Bawin et al. (1975), which had demonstrated a modulation "frequency window" at an SAR estimated to be < 0.002 W/kg. In this case, the increased release of calcium by a 16-Hz amplitude-modulated carrier frequency was effective only at specific power densities rather than over a continuum above the threshold.

Bawin et al. (1975) and Bawin and Adey (1976, 1977) suggest that electromagnetic fields may induce conformational changes of the neuronal membrane resulting in displacement of the surface-bound cations. On the basis of physicochemical principles, it is difficult to see how the authors were able to measure Ca^{2+} efflux in bulk tissue such as cerebral hemispheres. In these studies, similar external fields for both ELF and microwaves were used. The results suggest that it is not necessarily the internal field but the similar electrostatic interaction of the field with the sample that may be responsible for the observed effects. In addition, it is quite possible some induced current could have been injected into the brain tissue. Nevertheless, Blackman et al. (1979, 1980) were able to replicate these studies. They did indicate, however, the sensitive nature of the test, which is influenced by temperature deviations and sample size or number of tubes tested at any one time. Their data also showed considerable drift in control samples, which apparently was not taken into consideration.

Calcium plays a central role in neural excitation, regulating neurotransmitter secretion, hormone molecule binding at membrane receptor sites, and prostaglandin metabolism. To explain the interaction of electromagnetic fields with the CNS based on the observation of Ca^{2+} efflux from the brain, Grodsky (1975) presented an electrochemical model of the "greater membrane" concept, comprising the neuronal phospholipid sheet and the constituents of the intercellular spaces in brain tissue as a paradigm for the explanation of the interaction of electromagnetic fields consisting of gradients below those needed for direct intervention of action potentials at synaptic sites within the CNS. The essence of the model is a nonlinear feedback structure between the dipole sheet and the calcium-specific properties of the glycoproteins in the interstitial environment.

Several attempts have been made to model such highly cooperative effects. Some of these, however, concern only the frequency range of about 100 GHz where water loses its damping properties (Fröhlich, 1977). The possibility of highly cooperative phenomena that are field induced and take place in a "greater membrane" is interesting. Available dielectric data could well be supportive of such a concept, but also permit different interpretations (Schwan, 1977). In the few cases where cooperative effects of electric fields have been demonstrated, field levels greater than 10 kV/cm are required (Schwarz, 1962).

Some of the experiments by Bawin et al. (1975) and Bawin and Adey (1977) also explored the importance of bicarbonate ions on calcium efflux as well as the probable pool of calcium affected by electromagnetic energy. Contradictory evidence on the effects of electromagnetic fields on calcium efflux has been reported (Albert et al., 1980a; Shelton and Merritt, 1979, 1980). The calcium efflux work has been extensively critiqued by Myers and Ross (1981).

Albert et al. (1980a) investigated the effects of sinusoidally modulated 147-MHz fields on isolated chick quarter brains and cerebral cortical slices. The tissues were prepared and treated somewhat differently than did Bawin et al. (1975, 1978), Bawin and Adey (1977), and Blackman et al. (1979, 1980) to increase the survivability of the brain tissue and to facilitate exchange of metabolites. The calcium-labeled tissues were then exposed for 30 min to 147-MHz electromagnetic fields sinusoidally modulated at 16 Hz, 0.75 or 2 mW/cm². The amount of calcium released from quarter brains after irradiation at 0.75 mW/cm² was not significantly different in experimental tissues than in controls. However, there appeared to be a 10% decrease in calcium efflux from quarter brains after irradiation with 2 mW/cm². These data do not confirm previous studies on calcium efflux, although the 10% decrease at 2 mW/cm² mimics the effect observed by Bawin and Adey (1977) after exposure to ELF fields.

Shelton and Merritt (1979) failed to observe significant differences in calcium efflux between control and exposed rat brain tissues. They exposed $^{45}Ca^{2+}$-labeled rat cerebral tissue *in vivo* for 20 min to far-field pulsed 1-GHz microwave irradiation at 0.5, 1.0, 2.0, and 15 mW/cm², modulated at 16 Hz. Shelton and Merritt (1980) also reported that neither 1- nor 2.45-GHz, 16-Hz modulated microwave irradiation at 1 or 10 mW/cm² (est. SAR 0.07 to 0.7 W/kg) induced calcium release from rat brain labeled *in vivo* with ^{45}Ca but irradiated *in vitro* for 20 min. It should be noted that the latter authors used pulsed and not sinusoidal modulation. Bawin et al. (1975) did not find any effect of 147-MHz modulated fields on the skeletal muscle. On the other hand, Albert et al. (1980b), using similar exposure parameters, found an increase of calcium efflux from rat pancreatic tissue after 1 to 2 hr of irradiation. However, this increase in calcium efflux was not accompanied by a change in pancreatic protein secretion, thus raising questions about the biological significance of such findings.

10.4. EFFECTS IN EXPERIMENTAL ANIMALS

In one of the earliest studies on neurological effects of microwaves, focal coagulation necrosis was found in brains of rabbits exposed to 2450-MHz microwaves (Oldendorf, 1949). The first report on the effect of microwave energy on conditional response activity of experimental animals was made by Gordon et al. (1955). In subsequent years, the study of the "nonthermal" effects of microwaves gradually occupied the central role in electrophysiological studies in the Soviet Union (Novitskii et al., 1971).

Yakovleva et al. (1968) reported that single and repeated exposures of rats to microwaves, 5 to 15 mW/cm^2, weakened the "excitation process" and decreased the "functional mobility" of cells in the cerebral cortex. Edematous changes were most often noted throughout the cortex. The greatest number of altered cells was noted with repeated exposures at 15 mW/cm^2.

In a study with audiogenic seizure-susceptible mice and rats, Kitsovskaya (1960, 1968a) found that the seizure response to noise was transiently suppressed after exposure to 3000-MHz pulsed microwaves at an average power density of 10 mW/cm^2. Changes in olfactory threshold in humans following occupational exposures have been reported (Lobanova and Gordon, 1960; Fukalova, 1964; Goncharova et al., 1966).

Tolgskaya et al. (1960) studied the effects of pulsed and CW 3000- and 10,000-MHz microwaves at various intensities on rats. More pronounced morphological changes in the CNS were found following 3000 MHz than 10,000 MHz at 1 to 10 mW/cm^2. Pulsed waves were more effective than CW—an observation also made by Marha (1963). Additional studies comparing pulsed and CW microwaves can be found in the monograph by Tolgskaya and Gordon (1973). They noted that microwave-induced CNS alterations are functional in nature and are reversible; disappearing at the same time the conditional reflex activity of the animals is being restored upon cessation of exposure to microwaves. Using audiogenic-susceptible rats, Stverak et al. (1974) found reduced sensitivity to seizures following exposure to 2850 MHz pulsed for 10-μsec repetition frequency, 769.2 Hz, at an average power density of 30 mW/cm^2, 4 hr/day for 10 weeks.

Some investigators suggest that microwave energy absorption may affect hypothalamic and midbrain function and also affect cerebral, cortical, and reticular system function (Thompson and Bourgeois, 1965;

Yermakov, 1969). According to Gvozdikova et al. (1964), the greatest cortical sensitivity occurs in the meter range, less in the decimeter, and least in the centimeter microwave band.

In studies reported by Dumansky and Shandala (1974) and Bilokrinitsky and Dumansky (1974), untoward effects were noted in the CNS, cardiovascular system, and endocrine system of rabbits and rats following systematic long-term (8 h/day for 4 months) exposure to SHF (12 cm CW or 3 cm pulsed) at 5–20 μW/cm^2 power densities. These authors also reported that the various enzymes involved in aerobic and anaerobic metabolism differ in the degree of activity, both in the cells of the cortex and the subcortical formations, as well as in the epithelial cells of the vascular plexuses in the brain ventricles and its meninges. The reliability of those reports is questioned as will be discussed later.

10.4.1. Electroencephalographic Changes

Several investigators have reported that microwave exposure produces alterations in the electroencephalogram (EEG) (Baldwin et al., 1960; Gvozdikova et al., 1964; Kholodov, 1963, 1964, 1966; Livanov et al., 1960; Baranski and Edelwejn, 1967; Bawin et al., 1973; Servantie et al., 1975).

Baldwin et al. (1960) exposed the heads of rhesus monkeys to 225 to 400 MHz CW in a resonant cavity and noted a progressively generalized slowing and some increase in amplitude of EEG patterns accompanied by signs of agitation, drowsiness, akinesia, and nystagmus, as well as autonomic sensory and motor abnormalities. There were signs of diencephalic and mesencephalic disturbances, alternation of arousal and drowsiness, together with confirming EEG signs. The response depended on orientation of the head in the field and reflections from the surrounding enclosure.

EEG tracings in rabbits exposed to 3000 MHz (pulsed), 5 mW/cm^2, showed a slight desynchronization from the motor region; at 20 mW/cm^2, variations in the amplitude were observed; 300 MHz had a greater effect than 3000 MHz (Chizenkova, 1967, 1969). Pulsed microwaves produced a greater effect than CW microwaves. Baranski and Edelwejn (1967, 1975) reported that rabbits exposed to 10,000 MHz (pulsed), 4 mW/cm^2 (single exposure), showed no changes in EEG tracings, but exposure to 3000 MHz, 7 mW/cm^2, 3 hr/day for 60 days produced functional and morphological changes. Serdiuk (1969) reported changes in the EEG and conditional responses in rats and rabbits exposed to 50 MHz, 0.5 to 6 V/m, 10–12 hr/day for 180 days. Changes in conditional reflexes were also reported in rats exposed to 70 MHz, 150 V/m, 60 min/day for 4 months (Lobanova and Goncharova, 1971).

Bawin et al. (1973) reported that electromagnetic energy at 147 MHz, amplitude modulated at brain wave frequencies (8 and 16 Hz), influenced spontaneous and conditioned EEG patterns in cats at 1 mW/cm^2. These amplitude-modulated 147-MHz fields induced changes only when the amplitude modulation frequency approached that of physiological bioelectric function rhythms; no effects were seen at modulation frequencies below 8 Hz or above 16 Hz.

Takashima et al. (1979) exposed male rabbits to 1- to 10-Hz fields amplitude modulated at 14 to 16 Hz or 60 Hz for 2 to 3 hr (single exposure) or 4 to 6 weeks (chronic exposure). The field strengths ranged from 60 to 500 V/m. There was no temperature rise in exposed animals. EEG recordings under sodium pentabarbital anesthesia after acute exposures at 60 to 500 V/m or chronic exposures up to 70 V/m showed no differences between control and experimental animals. However, chronic irradiation at higher field strengths showed abnormal patterns. These consisted of bursts of high-amplitude spindles at 90 V/m as well as suppression of activity at 500 V/m. All brain activity returned to normal a few hours after irradiation. The results in this study appear to be free of electrode artifacts, because all recordings were made in the absence of fields. The effects of anesthesia are not clear and the natural fluctuations of the brain activity also complicate interpretation of the results. Although the occurrence of high-amplitude spindles in irradiated animals in this study is similar to that described by Bawin et al. (1973), it is difficult to compare the two results, because in the latter study chronically implanted electrodes may have interfered with the imposed fields. Takashima et al. (1979) confirmed the existence of artifacts when electrodes were implanted during irradiation.

It appears that the electrical activity of the brain, measured by means of the EEG, may be influenced by a wide variety of exposure regimes. Early experimentation in this area has been reviewed by Kholodov (1966). Long-term, repeated exposures of dogs, cats, rabbits, rats, frogs, and mice at power densities between 2 and 5 mW/cm^2 were reported to lead to alterations, such as the desynchronization of basal rhythms and later a flattening in EEG tracings (Baranski and Edelwejn, 1968; Bychkov and Dronov, 1974; Bychkov et al., 1974; Gillard et al., 1976). However, these earlier-reported effects are questionable since experiments were carried out using EEG electrodes or wires that significantly perturbed the field.

A review of the publications on EEG effects requires an awareness of certain deficiencies in methodology and interpretation. The EEG is difficult to quantify due to its time-varying waveform. The use of metallic electrodes either implanted in the brain or attached to the scalp also makes many of the reports on EEG or evoked responses (ER) questionable. Johnson and Guy (1972) pointed out that such metallic electrodes grossly perturb the field and produce greatly enhanced absorption of energy in the vicinity of the electrodes. Such enhancement produces artifacts in the biological material under investigation (Tyazhelov et al., 1977).

10.4.2. Biochemical Changes

10.4.2.1. In Vitro Studies

The functional properties of the microtubule assembly system extracted from brain cells of rabbits were studied after exposure to 3.1 GHz by Paulsson et al. (1977). The binding of a drug, colchicine, to the microtubule precursor protein, tubulin, was measured after exposure to pulsed microwaves for 15 min at average dose rates of 112 and 243 W/kg (pulse repetition frequency, 200 MHz; pulse duration, 1.4 μsec). Colchicine normally blocks the formation of microtubules, thus halting cell division. The normal assembly of microtubules from tubulin exposed for 10 min to pulsed microwaves (as above) at 430 W/kg was also studied. No noticeable effect on either process was found. The data indicate that a change of about 15% in the colchicine binding and about 10% in the microtubule assembly measurement would have been noted. Paulsson et al. also studied the migration of proteins within the axonal membrane of the rabbit vagus nerve. In this case, the samples were exposed for 24 hr at an SAR of 10 to 100 W/kg (est.) using a pulse repetition rate of 100 Hz and pulse duration of 1.4 μsec. The distribution of tritium-labeled protein in the axonal membrane was found to be the same in exposed and control samples. A difference of more than 20% would have been required for detection in this experiment.

10.4.2.2. Cholinesterase

Because of the reports of possible interaction of RF/MW energies and neural tissues, considerable research on cholinesterase has developed especially among Soviet investigators in an attempt to elucidate a possible mechanism of action of these energies. Cholinesterase is an enzyme contained in numerous tissues that catalyzes the hydrolysis of acetylcholine, which is liberated from the preganglionic and postganglionic endings of parasympathetic fibers and from the preganglionic fibers of sympathetic nerves. The functional state of the nervous system is determined to a considerable extent by its level of acetylcholine, as the chemical mediator in the transmission of impulses in CNS synapses. It is readily apparent that alteration in normal nerve transmission could be reflected by changes in cholinesterase levels in the body. Acetylcholine is liberated at the nerve endings upon reduction in the number of calcium ions. This phenomenon is associated with the activating property of calcium with respect to adenosine triphosphatase, the enzyme that splits ATP with release of the energy needed for conduction of the nerve impulse. The importance of serum cholinesterase in this context is, however, questionable. Although Soviet investigators report changes in blood cholinesterase, there is no correlation between blood cholinesterase and neural activity and one has to question the reliability of cholinesterase determinations.

Nikogosyan (1960, 1964) obtained data suggesting a parasympathetic effect in rabbits elicited by exposure to 3000 MHz at 40 mW/cm^2, 30 min/session, 65 sessions over $2\frac{1}{2}$ months; 10 mW/cm^2 for 90 min/session, 120 sessions over 5 months; 1 mW/cm^2 for 90 min/session, 185 sessions over 8 months. Measurements were made of cholinesterase activity in blood and tissue, liver, cerebrum, brain stem, and heart. In the 10 and 40 mW/cm^2 groups, there were significant reductions in cholinesterase activity. The level returned to normal 5–6 weeks after the study ended. The most pronounced changes were within 14 days of the initiation of the experiment. There was no change in cholinesterase activity in rabbits exposed to 1 mW/cm^2. In rabbits exposed at 5 mW/cm^2, a 13–29% decrease in cholinesterase activity in the cortex, cerebellum, brain stem, and medulla oblongata was observed. Stavinoha et al. (1970) reported that acetylcholine levels in the brains of rats that had been rapidly killed by microwave irradiation were significantly higher than previously reported. Presumably, the rapid inactivation of acetylcholinesterase was responsible for this difference.

Chronic exposure of rats to 3000 MHz also caused a decrease in the activity of cholinesterase in the CNS. Its effect in the cerebral hemispheres varied depending on the functional state of the CNS. In audiogenic-susceptible rats, the decrease in cholinesterase activity was more pronounced than in conventional rats (Kitsovskaya, 1968a).

Kitsovskaya (1968a,b) also reported disturbance of cholinergic processes in rats under the influence of microwaves. These changes are expressed as a reduced activity of cholinesterase in the cerebral hemispheres and brain stem, an increase of acetylcholine in the cerebral hemispheres, a decrease of SH groups in the brain stem, and an increase of Na$^+$ and a decrease of K$^+$ ions in the cerebral hemispheres and brain stem.

At lower frequencies (VHF), Mishchenko (1968) also noted a decrease in the amount of acetylcholine in the rat brain. Acetylcholinesterase activity was lower in the brain tissues of irradiated animals at both "thermogenic" and "nonthermogenic" intensities.

Similar decrease in cholinesterase activity has been reported by other investigators (Tomashevskaya and Makarenko, 1967). Baranski (1972) found inconsistent changes in cholinesterase activity in rabbit and guinea pig brains following 3 months of exposure, 1 hr/day with pulsed fields of 2.45 GHz, 25 mW/cm^2. He also found a decrease in cholinesterase activity in the brains of guinea pigs after a single 3-hr exposure to 3.5 mW/cm^2. An increase in incident power density to 25 mW/cm^2 caused a further decrease in activity. Pulsed exposures were found to have a greater effect than CW exposures of the same average power density, suggesting that these effects are due to peak fields.

Because of the implications of altered cholinesterase levels in the body, it is important to consider some of the problems in measurement of this enzyme. These have been reviewed by Cornish (1971). It has been suggested that measurement of plasma or red cell cholinesterase is an indirect way of attempting to assess cholinesterase activity in the various parts of the nervous system. A variety of methods have been described for the determination of cholinesterase activity in tissues. Whatever the method utilized for the determination of cholinesterase activity, there are a number of general sources of error common to most procedures. For example, a dietary effect on cholinesterase activity has been reported (Casterline and Williams, 1969). In rats on a low calcium intake (25% of normal) for 30 days, serum and liver cholinesterase values were elevated by 16 to 89% while animals on a high calcium or magnesium intake had liver and brain cholinesterase levels from 17 to 52% above comparable control groups on similar dietary regimens. Thus, interpretation of reports of cholinesterase changes requires considerable circumspection.

10.4.2.3. Trace Metals

Changes in zinc concentration have been reported to be related to temperature and MW/RF exposure (Gunn et al., 1961; Rupp et al., 1975). Whereas zinc content was increased significantly in the cerebral cortex and liver of 19-MHz-irradiated rats (Stavinoha et al., 1976), testicular zinc uptake was decreased in rats following a 5-min exposure to 24.5 GHz, 250 mW/cm^2 (Gunn et al., 1961). Rupp et al. (1975) also reported a significant loss of zinc from whole-liver homogenates of rats with a core temperature increase to 45°C. Alteration in zinc content has previously been associated with deficiency diseases, in thermal environments, or in surgical trauma (Stavinoha et al., 1976).

In rats exposed whole body to 1600-MHz microwaves at 80 mW/cm^2 (SAR 48 W/kg) for 10 min, iron levels were increased in the hypothalamus, corpus striatum, midbrain, hippocampus, cerebellum, medulla, and cortex of the brain (Chamness et al., 1976). Manganese was increased in the cortex and medulla, and copper was increased in the cortex; calcium, zinc, sodium, and potassium were unchanged. These changes were probably a result of hyperthermia, since the irradiated animals showed a colonic temperature increase of 4.5°C and most alterations were also observed in rats subjected to a hot environment. The biological or physiological significance of these changes is not apparent.

10.4.2.4. Brain Chemistry

Specific brain loci containing various neurotransmitters are known to affect the inhibitory or excitatory states of the brain. The relative firing rates of these neuronal systems are reflected in the turnover of their neurotransmitters. Since microwaves have been reported to stimulate or depress CNS activity, several studies on the effects of microwaves on CNS neurotransmitters have been performed.

In a report by Snyder (1970), rats were exposed to 3000 MHz CW, 10 mW/cm^2 (2 mW/g) and 40 mW/cm^2 (8 mW/g). He observed that 1 hr of exposure at 40 mW/cm^2 resulted in a significant increase of 5-hydroxyindoleacetic acid (5-HIAA) and 5-hydroxytryptamine (5-HT; serotonin) in discrete nuclei of the brain. After 7 days exposure for 8 hr/day, there was a marked slowing of 5-HIAA and 5-HT turnover in the brain. This suggested to the author that microwave exposure decreases the firing rate of 5-HT neurons in the brain. Since these neurons are known to participate in the regulation of sleep and wakefulness as well as body temperature, these findings have been related to certain of the behavioral effects purportedly produced by microwave exposure. In rats exposed to 10 mW/cm^2, there was a 1–2°C increase in colonic temperature over that of controls and the exposed rats showed signs of moderate heat stress. It is well known that there is a relationship between body temperature increase and release of catecholamines in rabbits and of 5-HT in cats (Veninga, 1971), and thus the effect is most likely thermally mediated.

Snyder (1970) also tested the effects of nonmicrowave heating on rats whose body temperature was raised equivalent to that observed after 10 mW/cm^2 irradiation. He found no difference in the turnover rate of norepinephrine or 5-HT or steady-state levels of 5-HIAA between heated and control animals. He concluded that chronic microwave exposure was distinctly different in producing effects on levels of 5-HT and 5-HIAA on rat brains than conventional heating when repeated daily over 7 days.

Zeman et al. (1973) investigated the effects of acute and chronic exposure of rats to 2860 MHz pulsed (average power 300 W) on rat brain γ-aminobutyric acid (GABA). Chronic exposures were conducted at 10 mW/cm^2 (est. SAR 2 W/kg) and lasted 4 to 8 hr/day, 4 to 6 weeks.

Acute exposures were conducted at 40 to 80 mW/cm^2 (est. SAR 8 to 16 W/kg) for either 5 or 20 min. No significant change in body temperature was noted during chronic exposures at 10 mW/cm^2, while colonic temperature increased by 3°C after acute exposures at 40 to 80 mW/cm^2. There was no significant difference in whole-brain GABA levels between control and exposed animals in acute or chronic experiments. These results would have been more meaningful if they had been conducted on discrete areas of the brain rich in GABA rather than whole brains.

Merritt *et al.* (1975) reported decreased norepinephrine, dopamine, and 5-HT in discrete areas of rat brains after whole-body exposure to 1.6-GHz microwaves at 80 mW/cm^2 (est. SAR 24 W/kg) for 10 min. These exposures raised colonic temperatures by 3.7°C. Hypothalamic epinephrine decreased significantly in microwave-irradiated and hyperthermal controls, but 5-HT levels decreased in hippocampus of irradiated but not hyperthermal control rats. There were no differences in the 5-HT levels in hypothalamus and striatum between hyperthermal controls and microwave-irradiated animals. Merritt *et al.* (1975) concluded that, in general, hyperthermia rather than a direct microwave effect is responsible for the changes in neurotransmitters.

In a separate study, Merritt *et al.* (1977) observed a decrease in rat hypothalamic norepinephrine and dopamine after a 10-min whole-body exposure to 1.6-GHz microwaves at 20 mW/cm^2 (est. SAR 6.0 W/kg) but not at 10 mW/cm^2. The former power density was associated with increased temperature, while the latter was not. Hypothalamic 5-HT was unaffected by microwaves even at power densities of 80 mW/cm^2.

In rats exposed to 48 MHz at a "nonthermogenic intensity," Mishchenko (1969) found the amount of lactic and pyruvic acid in brain tissue increased, and the amount of glycogen decreased. These changes depended on field intensity and duration of exposure.

Stavinoha *et al.* (1976) exposed rats to 19-MHz energy with a magnetic field of 55 A/m and an electric field of 8000 V/m in a "near field synthesizer." After one exposure of rats for 40 min, the average rise in colonic temperature was approximately 1°C. No lethality was observed in either irradiated or thermally exposed animals. No remarkable changes were seen in the levels of acetylcholine or catecholamines in the rats after RF or thermal exposure. No changes were seen in cyclic AMP but there were some irradiation-related changes in high-energy phosphates. Significant changes were seen, however, in the concentrations of several cations in the brain after exposure. Most notably, the concentration of zinc in the cerebral cortex increased from 0.28 μmole/mg to 0.53 μmole/mg after irradiation.

Schmidt *et al.* (1971) employed microwave irradiation as a means of tissue fixation of cyclic AMP in brain areas. Using rats exposed to

2450 MHz at a power density high enough to cause death within 3–5 sec of irradiation, the authors found that amounts of cyclic AMP were highest in the cerebellum and brain stem, intermediate in the hypothalamus and midbrain, and lowest in the hippocampus and cortex. Decapitation increased the concentration of cyclic AMP in all brain areas, although the increase in the cerebellum was three to four times greater than that in other areas.

Microwave irradiation appears to rapidly arrest enzymatic activity in the brain, permitting easy dissection of the brain into its component parts. In some experiments, it was found that 10 sec of microwave exposure increased the temperature of the brain to 55°C and that after 20 sec of exposure (70°C) adenyl cyclase and phosphodiesterase were no longer active. The authors concluded that this method of killing the animal appears to offer the advantages of minimum stress before death, rapid tissue fixation, and easy dissection of the brain into its component parts.

10.4.3. Histopathology

Some investigators have reported that severe damage to the brain occurs when electromagnetic energy of a variety of frequencies at high power density (> 40 mW/cm^2), producing frank heating, is employed. These changes consist of hemorrhages, edema, and vacuolation of neurons after 40 min exposure to 3000- or 10,000-MHz pulsed or CW microwaves of 40 to 100 mW/cm^2 power density. At 20 mW/cm^2, similar but less severe effects were observed. More marked changes were produced at 3000 MHz than 10,000 MHz of equal power density (Gordon, 1970b; Tolgskaya and Gordon, 1973).

Cellular changes in the nervous system of small animals following microwave exposure at 10 mW/cm^2 have been reported (Tolgskaya, 1959; Tolgskaya and Gordon, 1964, 1973). Degeneration of neurons in the cerebral cortex and tissue changes in the kidney and myocardium of rabbits have been produced by exposure to 200 MHz. Head exposure of rabbits to 2450 MHz resulted in focal lesions in the cerebral cortex; whole-body exposures of rats to 1430 MHz produced lesions of the brain (Oldendorf, 1949; de Seguin and Castelain, 1947; Tolgskaya and Gordon, 1960).

Exposure of cats for 1 hr to 10,000 MHz, 400 mW/cm^2, resulted in injury to cerebral and spinal cord nerve cells; changes occurred in the Nissl bodies and other components of nerve cells (Bilokrinitsky, 1966). On the other hand, rabbits exposed to 10,000 MHz (pulsed), 4 mW/cm^2, showed no evidence of morphological damage to the brain, but exposure to 3000 MHz did produce such changes (Baranski and Edelwejn, 1967).

Tolgskaya et al. (1960) investigated the influence of pulsed and CW 3000 and 10,000-MHz microwaves on the morphology of nervous tissue in rats and rabbits. With exposure to 3000 MHz (110 and 40 mW/cm^2), symptoms of overheating were observed, often leading to death. Vascular disorders such as edema and hemorrhages in the brain and internal organs were predominant. In repeated, but less prolonged exposure, vascular disorders and degenerative changes in internal organs and the nervous system were less severe. With repeated exposures, the animals were better able to withstand successive exposures; they continued to gain weight, body temperature after irradiation quickly recovered, and overheating was not evident.

At high field intensities, when death is a result of hyperthermia, the vascular changes are those of hyperemia, hemorrhage, and acute dystrophic manifestations (Baranski et al., 1963; Dolina, 1961; Minecki and Bilski, 1961). At lower field intensities, the changes are of a more general dystrophic character, and proliferation of the glia and vascular changes are not as prominent.

Baranski (1972) exposed guinea pigs and rabbits to CW and pulsed 3000-MHz microwaves at power densities of 3.5 and 5 mW/cm^2, 3 hr daily for 3 months (chronic exposure), and at power densities of 3.5 and 25 mW/cm^2 (est. SAR 0.4–2.9 W/kg) in single 3-hr exposures. Morphological and histochemical investigations were carried out; acetylcholinesterase, cytochrome oxidase, and succinic acid dehydrogenase activities were determined. The results indicated that chronic repeated exposure to microwaves, at power densities that do not cause a temperature rise, may lead to the appearance of morphological lesions indicative of metabolic disturbances in myelin sheaths and glial cells, as expressed by the appearance of peculiar metachromatic spherical bodies in the white matter of the brain and cerebellum. A proliferative reaction of glial cells was also described. In contrast, Austin and Horvath (1954) did not observe similar changes in the brains of rats that became convulsive and hyperthermic (brain temperatures 43.5°C) in a single exposure to 2450 MHz. These authors observed only mild pyknosis and hyperemia in some areas of the brain.

Albert and DeSantis (1975) reported morphological changes in the brains of Chinese hamsters following exposure to 2450-MHz CW microwaves at power densities of 25 and 50 mW/cm^2. Exposure durations varied from 30 min to 14 hr/day for 22 days. Both light and electron microscopic examination revealed alterations in the hypothalamus and subthalamic structures of exposed animals whereas other regions of the brain appeared unaltered. It should be noted that SARs as high as 4 W/kg per incident mW/cm^2 could occur under these conditions. Peak SARs could reach 40 to 200 W/kg in selected brain regions. The effects detected in this investigation are typical of the response of neurons to heat.

Albert and DeSantis (1975, 1977) did not observe hemorrhage, gliosis, or focal necrosis in Chinese hamsters exposed to 2450 MHz CW at 50 mW/cm^2 (est. SAR 17.5 W/kg) for 30 to 120 min, but they did observe swollen neurons with frothy cytoplasm in the hypothalamic and thalamic regions of the brain. Such observations were not seen in the cerebellum, pons, or spinal cord. Histological changes in the brains of rats have also been reported at low (< 10 mW/cm^2) power densities of 3000-MHz microwaves after multiple 30-min exposures. All of the above changes were reversible after 3 to 4 weeks.

In subsequent studies at 1760 and 2450 MHz, 10 and 20 mW/cm^2, Albert (1977a, 1978a,b) described similar cytoplasmic vacuolation of neurons, irregular swelling of axons, and decrease in dendritic spines of cortical neurons. The axonal swelling and spine changes were seen only in chronic exposures, whereas neuronal changes were observed in acute exposure. In all studies, no signs of permanent degenerative changes were seen, and reversibility was noted 2 hr after exposure (Albert, 1977b, 1978a,b). The author concluded that while it is possible the higher exposure levels (25 and 50 mW/cm^2) could result in thermal effects, it is unlikely that 10 mW/cm^2 would result in significant heating of the whole brain, but the possibility of "hot spots" was not ruled out. Exposures of rats at 10 mW/cm^2 to 2450 and 2800 MHz resulted in average hypothalamic temperature increases of 0.4°C, or less.

In general, there is agreement that qualitatively the morphological effects on the CNS are similar at 10 and 50 mW/cm^2 power densities, but quantitatively they are greater at higher power densities. There is also agreement that these power densities can raise the body temperature. Soviet investigators consider small increases in temperature as physiological and therefore nonthermal. Further, Soviet scientists continue to find similar morphological changes even at 1 mW/cm^2 after chronic exposure, and they do not consider morphological alterations at 1 mW/cm^2 to be of thermogenic origin. Tolgskaya and Gordon (1973), Baranski (1972), and Baranski and Edelwejn (1968) further state that morphological effects are more marked after pulsed wave or chronic exposure than after CW or acute exposure. Most Eastern European studies claim full recovery in animals 1 to 3 weeks after exposure to less than 10 mW/cm^2. Albert and DeSantis (1975) found continued presence of neuronal cytopathology in animals 2 weeks after exposure. Perhaps a longer recovery period in the latter study would have shown complete reversibility.

Switzer and Mitchell (1977) described myelin figures in dendrites of rat brains exposed to 2450 MHz CW over a 110-hr period (av. SAR 2.3 W/kg) and allowed to recover for 6 weeks. The authors did not observe any gliosis, perivascular edema, or synaptic pathology, although the exposed rats exhibited marked disruption of discriminative performance during exposure.

Albert et al. (1980c) reported permanent loss of cerebellar Purkinje cells in rat pups after exposure of pregnant dams to 100- and 2450-MHz energies. There was a reversible decrease in cerebellar Purkinje cells in newborn rat pups exposed to 2450-MHz microwave irradiation.

The occurrence of platelet aggregation in some cerebral vessels of a few experimental animals was first described by Albert (1978a,b) in Chinese hamsters exposed to 2450 MHz, 10 mW/cm^2. McKee et al. (1980) reported pyknotic neurons in the hypothalamus, cerebral cortex, and hippocampus, and platelet aggregation with occlusion of some vessels in Chinese hamsters irradiated with 1700-MHz CW microwaves at 10 and 25 mW/cm^2 (est. SAR 5 and 12.5 W/kg) for 30 to 120 min. Albert (1978a) did not see platelet aggregation in rats or monkeys, which raises the question of possible species specificity.

10.4.4. Influence of Drugs

Microwave exposure has been reported to alter effects of drugs that influence CNS function. Edelwejn (1968) reported altered EEG tracings and decreased tolerance to Cardiasol (a CNS stimulant) in individuals occupationally exposed to microwaves. He also found that administration of Phenactil (a depressant of cortical activity) to rabbits followed by exposure to pulsed 3000-MHz microwaves at 20 mW/cm^2 (est. SAR 3.0 W/kg) for 20 min resulted in EEG desynchronization, suggesting a stimulatory effect of microwaves on the reticular formation of the brain. Under the same exposure conditions, Edelwejn (1968) demonstrated that Cardiasol administration required half the amount of drug to obtain the same EEG reaction as in control animals without previous microwave irradiation, suggesting that microwaves enhance CNS stimulation. Chronic exposure of rabbits to 3000-MHz pulsed microwaves at 7 mW/cm^2 (est. SAR 1.0 W/kg) for 3 hr/day for a total of 70 to 80 hr resulted in convulsions after injection of the same dose of Cardiasol (3 mg/kg) as in controls, thus indicating that tolerance to Cardiasol was decidedly lower in chronically exposed animals than in controls. Chronic exposure also resulted in EEG desynchronization with high recording potentials. In this study, thermal effects of microwaves were considered unlikely, and it was suggested that microwaves may exert a stimulating effect on specific areas of the CNS.

Servantie et al. (1974) investigated the effect of microwave exposure on Pentetrazol (a convulsant drug) administered to CD1 mice subjected to 3000-MHz pulsed microwaves (maximum peak power 600 kW) a few minutes a day for 8, 15, 20, 27, and 36 days. At the end of the exposure, 50 mg/kg of Penetrazol was administered intraperitoneally. Microwave exposure affected the time for convulsion onset and mortality rate. There was no difference between controls and experimentals receiving 8 days of exposure. After 15 days of irradiation, microwaves delayed the appearance of convulsions and rendered animals less susceptible to the epileptic action of Pentetrazol. However, after 27 to 36 days of exposure, the effect was reversed. The results suggest a biphasic response of mice over 36 days. Microwaves also decreased the incidence of mortality in drug-injected animals if the animals were irradiated more than 8 days.

Servantie et al. (1974) also investigated the effect of curarelike drugs on *in vivo* and *in vitro* preparations of the rat sciatic nerve. They found that irradiated rats were less susceptible to paralyzing drugs. Similar findings were noted in isolated rat sciatic preparations. Additionally, sciatic nerves isolated from irradiated rats were paralyzed to a lesser extent and recovered sooner than those from control rats. These results suggest that the effect of microwaves is more likely at the neuromuscular junction (synapse) and less likely due to secondary effects on the metabolism or binding of the drugs.

Goldstein and Sisko (1974) investigated the effects of pentobarbital and 9.3-GHz CW microwaves at a power density of 0.7–2.8 mW/cm^2 (est. SAR 0.1–0.4 W/kg) on the behavior and EEG patterns of rabbits. They reported no difference in EEG patterns between control (pentobarbital-injected) and pentobarbital plus microwave (0.7 mW/cm^2) irradiation during the first 5 min. However, after a latent period, cycles of intense arousal and sedation occurred in experimental animals but not in controls. Similar, but more pronounced, effects were seen with 2 mW/cm^2 (est. SAR 0.2 W/kg).

Thomas et al. (1979) reported that acute low-level (av. 1 mW/cm^2) pulsed microwaves (2450 MHz) (est. SAR 0.2 W/kg) potentiate the tranquilizing effects of chlordiazepoxide in rats.

It appears that mice, rats, and rabbits subjected to various regimens of microwave exposure can show an increased susceptibility to convulsant drugs (Baranski and Edelwejn, 1968; Servantie et al., 1974, 1975). According to Baranski and Czerski (1976), detailed analyses of EEG data and results of pharmacological studies indicate that the reticular formation of the midbrain is the structure in which exposure to MW/RF may induce effects.

The mechanism of altered susceptibility to drugs (particularly convulsant drugs acting on the nervous system) after repeated microwave exposures is unclear. On the other hand, as the action of many drugs is well understood, the phenomenon may serve to clarify mechanisms of the action of MW/RF energies on the nervous system (Czerski, 1975).

10.5. EFFECTS ON THE BLOOD–BRAIN BARRIER

In the past few years, there have been contradictory reports concerning the effects of microwave exposure on the permeability of the blood–brain barrier (BBB). Some of these studies suggest direct microwave effects in experimental animals resulting in increased BBB permeability (Frey et al., 1975; Oscar and Hawkins, 1977; Albert and DeSantis, 1977; Albert, 1979). Others indicate that increased permeability might be mediated by hyperthermia induced by microwave energy absorption (Sutton and Carroll, 1979; Merritt et al., 1978; Lin and Lin, 1980), while still others (Preston et al., 1979; Preston and Prefontaine, 1980; Williams et al., 1984a,b,c,d) report negative findings. Some of these discrepancies may be attributed to differences in techniques employed to assess changes of permeability. These include gross examination of brain slices, single-passage isotope tracers, fluorometric measurements, and electron microscopic tracers. All of these techniques have some inherent shortcomings, either in quantitation or in sensitivity. Therefore, one must consider the limitations of techniques applied as well as physical parameters of microwave exposure before arriving at conclusions regarding effects of microwaves on the BBB.

The BBB is not a discrete anatomical entity as the name implies, but designates a functional interposition between the blood and the cerebrospinal fluid (CSF). The concept of a BBB has existed ever since it was shown that certain intravenously injected dyes stained all tissues except those of the CNS. Substances that do not easily enter the CSF are excluded from neural tissue. Thus, it appears that a barrier exists both in regard to free passage from the blood of the choroid plexus and from the blood supplying the tissues of the brain and spinal cord. While differences in the concentration of a large number of substances between blood plasma and CSF can be demonstrated, the idea of a barrier between blood and brain has met with considerable controversy. The extracellular space revealed by electron microscopy of the brain is in accord with the volume distribution of poorly penetrating substances such as sucrose or inulin. Thus, the contention has developed that the so-called BBB is not due to some physical impediment to outflow from capillaries, but a reflection of a small extracellular fluid phase.

The BBB system has been used to investigate effects on the CNS of various types of physiological activity and stress (Brightman et al., 1970) such as cold, heat, photic stimulation, pressure, ionizing radiation (Nair and Roth, 1964), seizures (Clawson et al., 1966), drugs (Lorenzo et al., 1972), and sensory input. Bondy and Purdy (1974) have shown increased penetration of tyrosine into brain areas receiving reduced sensory input. Sabbot and Costin (1974) have shown increased uptake of $^{45}Ca^{2+}$ in brain tissue as a result of cold stress. Concussions have been studied experimentally by the creation of pressure pulses induced by sudden introduction of a small volume of fluid extradurally through a parietal trephine hole (Rinder and Olsson, 1968). Low-magnitude pressure pulses gave abnormal penetration of protein tracer within the walls of the blood vessels.

Sutton et al. (1973) used 2450 MHz to produce selective hyperthermia of the brain in rats. They then studied the integrity of the BBB with horseradish peroxidase (HRP), a protein tracer that can be detected quantitatively. The rat brains were heated to 40, 42, and 45°C. Barrier integrity was disrupted after heating for more than 45 min at 40°C. Animals with brains heated to 45°C survived for only 8 to 15 min. The most common site of vascular leakage was the white matter adjacent to the granular cell layer of the cerebellum. The authors concluded that to prevent BBB disruption, brain temperatures must not exceed 40°C in the absence of body-core hypothermia.

Frey et al. (1975) reported an increase in permeability of the rat BBB after microwave exposure. They reported that 30 min exposure of rats to 1.2-GHz CW microwaves with an average power density of 2.4 mW/cm^2 (est. SAR 1.0 W/kg) resulted in a statistically significant increase of fluorescein in brain slices of exposed animals over controls. Most of the fluorescein appeared to be concentrated in the vicinity of the lateral and third ventricles. Some dye was detected in the metencephalon. The authors also reported similar alterations in BBB permeability among rats irradiated with pulsed microwaves (modulated at 2.1 mW/cm^2 peak and 0.2 mW/cm^2 average power density with an SAR estimated at 0.8 W/kg). This report suggested that pulsed microwave irradiation was more effective in altering BBB permeability than CW irradiation. The possibility of artifacts cannot be ruled out in this study.

Merritt et al. (1978) were unable to replicate the fluorescein studies of Frey et al. (1975). They exposed rats to 1.2-GHz CW and pulsed microwaves for 30 min at power densities from 2 to 75 mW/cm^2 and found no BBB alteration unless there had been an increase of 4°C in the brain. Increased brain permeation of fluorescein–albumin (molecular weight 60,000) was produced in rats heated to 40°C by either hot air or microwaves. They concluded that hypothermia per se and not microwave irradiation is an essential determinant of increased permeability. Using sodium fluorescein and Evans blue as indicator molecules, Lin and Lin (1980) also found no change in BBB permeation after a single 20-min exposure of the head at 0.5 to 1000 mW/cm^2 (est. SAR 0.04 to 80 W/kg) at 2450 MHz pulsed.

Albert (1977a) used HRP as a tracer and reported regions of leakage in the microvasculature of the brains of Chinese hamsters exposed to

2450 MHz at 10 mW/cm² for 2 to 8 hr. In control animals, an extravascular reaction product was found only in brain regions normally lacking a BBB. In a later paper, Albert (1977b) reported that continuation of his earlier studies indicated that a partial restoration of BBB impermeability may have occurred within 1 hr after exposure ceased, and that restoration was virtually complete within 2 hr. Albert believes that these changes may be clinically subacute and probably cause no lasting ill effects. It is important nevertheless to note that such leakage of the microvasculature of the brain occurs irregularly; it was observed in approximately 50% of exposed animals and in 20% of control animals studied by Albert (1977a,b).

Albert (1977a,b, 1979) and Albert and Kerns (1981), using electron microscopic tracer methodology, followed the movement of HRP (M_r 40,000) in rat and Chinese hamster brains after exposure to 2450 MHz CW, 10 mW/cm² (est. SAR 0.9 to 2.0 W/kg), in the far field. The authors reported focal areas of increased permeability in brains of 35% of irradiated animals versus 10% of controls. Areas with increased permeability were seen with greater frequency in the thalamus, hypothalamus, medulla, and cerebellum than in cortex and hippocampus. Using the same species and parameters of exposure as above, Albert (1979) and Albert and Kerns (1981) showed that within 2 to 4 hr post-irradiation, there was no evidence of increased BBB permeability, thus demonstrating complete reversibility of the initial effect. It was also shown that the increased BBB permeability appeared to be due to stepped-up pinocytotic transport of the tracer rather than opening of the endothelial tight junctions (Albert and Kerns, 1981).

Isotope tracers were used by Oscar and Hawkins (1977) in rats exposed to 1.3-GHz CW and pulsed microwaves for 20 min. Using the dual indicator technique of Oldendorf (1970), they found that after CW exposure at 1 mW/cm² (est. SAR 0.4 W/kg) there was a significantly greater uptake of mannitol (M_r 182) and inulin (M_r 5000), but not of dextran (M_r 60,000), in exposed animals. Similar, but greater, uptake of these compounds was observed after pulsed irradiation (av. power 0.3 mW/cm², est. SAR 0.1 W/kg) than after CW irradiation. Uptake of mannitol by the brain was quite dependent on power density, pulse width, and number of pulses per second. This suggested that microwave exposure induces a temporary change in the permeability of small inert polar molecules across the BBB of rats. Increase in permeability was observed for mannitol and inulin but not for dextran, both immediately and 4 hr after exposure, but not 24 hr after exposure. D-Mannitol is small and easily passes with slight BBB alterations; inulin, which is similar in molecular weight to many unbound dyes that are used for tracers, and dextran, with a molecular weight of 60,000 to 75,000, would be similar in weight to dye–protein complexes. It is important to note that even in this study, the most sensitive indicator (mannitol) was no different in exposed animals relative to controls between 4 and 24 hr after exposure. The authors suggest that BBB alteration is a function of peak power density, pulse width, and number of pulses per second. For a given average power density, one can get a higher permeability change by raising the peak power and lowering the number of pulses per second than by raising the pulses per second and lowering the peak power. In this study dextran, which is similar in molecular weight to protein, did not penetrate the barrier, but inulin, which is similar in molecular weight to many dyes used as tracers, did. This suggests that in earlier microwave studies, which used dyes as tracers, penetration of unbound dye rather than penetration of dye complexes was being observed. The authors consider the possibility of local heating due to "hot spots" since the greatest BBB alteration occurs in the cerebellum and medulla or close to the neck region of rats. Attempts to duplicate the findings of Oscar and Hawkins (1977) have yielded equivocal results (Chang *et al.*, 1978) or have resulted in failure (Preston *et al.*, 1978, 1979; Preston and Prefontaine, 1980; Spackman and Riley, 1978; Williams *et al.*, 1984a,b,c,d).

Merritt *et al.* (1978) also used the Oldendorf technique and reported no significant change in uptake of mannitol or inulin in rats exposed to microwaves under conditions similar to those used by Oscar and Hawkins (1977).

In the studies by Oscar and Hawkins (1977), a quantitative radioactive isotope technique was used. The technique, developed by Oldendorf (1970, 1971), permits quantitative measurement of the relative amount of test substance entering a particular region of the brain in reference to a highly diffusible substance such as tritiated water. This method allows measurement of the penetration of a variety of test substances as a function of any of several variables such as microwave characteristics, brain region, time after exposure, molecular weight of test substance, and so on. While this technique does not allow the detailed localization of tracers and display of the BBB alteration site that staining and observation with an electron microscope might, it should permit limited mapping of tracer penetration. This technique also lends itself well to simple statistical interpretation as to whether a certain insult produces a BBB permeability change (Oscar, 1980).

Sutton and Carroll (1979) observed increased rat brain permeability to HRP when brain temperatures were elevated to 40 to 45°C for a few minutes by intense microwave (2450 MHz CW) heating. A significant observation was that BBB integrity and survival times at 45°C cerebral temperature could be prolonged if the colonic temperature was maintained at 30°C. They hypothesized that perfusion of the vessels with cool blood had a protective effect. This study suggested that severe hyperthermia induced by microwave irradiation results in increased permeability of tracer proteins in the brains of rats.

Preston et al. (1979) also used the Oldendorf technique. Rats were exposed to 2450 MHz CW for 30 min at 0.1 to 30 mW/cm^2 (est. SAR 0.02 to 6 W/kg); no change in the brain uptake of mannitol was found. They also speculated that the changes reported by Oscar and Hawkins (1977) may have been due to change in blood flow. Later, Oscar et al. (1980) and Oscar (1981) measured the blood flow in several brain regions during microwave exposure to 15 mW/cm^2 average power at 2800 MHz pulsed for 5 to 60 min and found increased local blood flow. They then suggested previously reported BBB permeability changes (Oscar and Hawkins, 1977) to be of smaller magnitude than originally indicated. In fact, Oscar and his associates (Gruneau et al., 1982) reported that in unanesthetized rats exposed to 2.8 GHz CW 10–40 mW/cm^2 or pulsed at 1–15 mW/cm^2 for 30 min, there was no evidence of BBB alteration using [^{14}C]sucrose as a tracer.

Preston and Prefontaine (1980) had described studies at 2450 MHz CW in both the near and far field using [^{14}C]sucrose as a tracer. The far-field exposure took place in an anechoic chamber at 1 or 10 mW/cm^2 (est. SAR 0.2 and 2.0 W/kg) for 30 min. In a second study, a microwave applicator was placed on the rat's head for a near-field exposure. The exposure consisted of a single 25-min exposure at SARs of 0.08 to 1.6 W/kg. In the second study, the microwave exposure took place after the tracer was injected into the animal so that they were looking at BBB function during irradiation. No permeability changes were found in either study.

Oscar (1980; Oscar et al., 1981) performed experiments to examine local cerebral blood flow, using the *in vivo* [^{14}C]iodoantipyrine technique with brain homogenization and liquid scintillation counting. All experiments employed conscious rats during microwave exposure and blood flow measurement. The experiments demonstrated that microwaves increased local cerebral blood flow in rats. The first brain region affected, after only 5 min of exposure, was the inferior colliculus. By 60 min of exposure, the blood flow in all 17 brain regions sampled increased a minimum of 39% with many increasing well over 100%. The largest blood flow increases were in the pineal, pituitary, temporal cortex, inferior colliculus, and lateral and medial geniculate.

Oscar (1980) believes that the blood flow increases at short exposure times are due to increases in metabolic activity through excitation or activation of brain tissue receptors. The larger blood flow increases at longer exposure times are due to gross alteration of brain function owing to stress. This stress may be from excessive sensory stimulation, heat, pressure, and so on. As brain functional activity, cerebral temperature, blood volume, metabolism, BBB permeability, and blood flow are coupled, Oscar (1980) believes that the increased blood flow and pressure causes the small BBB permeability changes. He believes microwaves could alter the uptake of low-molecular-weight saccharides in the BBB of rats. The greater permeability, however, occurred for low- but not high-molecular-weight saccharides. The permeability returned to normal after 24 hr and was of greatest magnitude in the medulla, cerebellum, and hypothalamus. The absolute level of permeability could not be quantified because in the next set of experiments it was discovered that microwaves alter the local cerebral blood flow of rats, and all techniques capable of measuring small differences in permeability uptake rely on constant blood flow during the experiment.

It is known that microwave exposure causes nonuniform distribution of energy inside a body due to the body's geometry and electrical properties. These nonuniform temperature rises or "hot spots" are created at tissue interfaces, geometrical focusing points, and loci of electric and magnetic resonance.

Such effects in rats cannot be assumed to occur in the human. The induced temperature rise is a function of the incident microwave parameters, geometry of the irradiated object, and electrical properties of the object. As the electrical properties are frequency dependent, one cannot duplicate the temperature distribution in man by simply frequency scaling the exposure given to a rat.

It is possible that the increase in brain uptake index (BUI) noted by Oscar and Hawkins (1977) occurs because of the reduced uptake of tritiated water, rather than because of the increased uptake of mannitol and inulin. Dextran, which is similar in molecular weight to protein, did not penetrate the barrier; but inulin, which is similar in molecular weight to many dyes used as tracers, did. This suggests that in earlier microwave studies that used dyes as tracers, a penetration of unbound dye was being observed rather than a penetration of dye–protein complexes (Oscar, 1980).

The reports by Oscar (1980) and Oscar and Hawkins (1977) do not address the question of whether the microwave exposure interacts directly to alter the BBB system or whether the microwave exposure causes an indirect effect. The data also do not address the question of whether BBB alterations are due to lesions or increases in micropinocytotic vesicle transfer (Reese and Karnovsky, 1967; Olsson and Reese, 1969; Rene et al., 1973).

It is important to realize that the methods used to investigate BBB permeability are still controversial. Permeability changes in cerebral blood vessels occur under various conditions, including those that produce heat necrosis (Rodzilsky and Olszewsky, 1957). Most techniques used to measure BBB permeability, in fact, measure the net influence of several variables on brain uptake, and do not differentiate among the effects of changes in the vascular space, alterations of blood flow, and variations in membrane permeability (Oscar and Hawkins, 1977).

The selection of techniques to quantitatively measure the effects of microwaves on BBB permeability is controversial. The dual indicator techniques of Oldendorf (1970, 1971, 1974) or Crone (1963, 1965) use either highly diffusible or relatively nondiffusible internal standards and rely on constant circulatory flux during the experiment. A dual compartment technique to measure cerebrovascular permeability has been developed by Rapoport *et al.* (1978), and accounts for changes in the brain–blood flow. This technique has the sensitivity to measure low-permeability substances, but may not have the ability to detect subtle changes in that permeability. Most previous studies reporting BBB permeability changes due to microwave exposure used protein-bound markers and observation with optical, fluorescent, or electron microscopy. Oscar and Hawkins (1977) reported quantitative measurement of microwave-induced BBB permeability increases using the Oldendorf technique with tritiated water as the internal standard. Water does not freely equilibrate in the brain and as cerebral blood flow increases, water's diffusion is lowered (Raichle *et al.*, 1974, 1976). Since the Oldendorf technique measures the ratio of a test substance to the internal standard as blood flow increases and causes the brain tissue level of water to decrease, the reported ratios of BBB permeability may be overly high. The small BBB permeability increases that have been reported in microscopy studies may be a secondary effect caused by thermally induced alterations of blood flow (Williams *et al.*, 1984a,b,c,d,e).

In the final analysis, it should be recognized that in the reported studies on BBB alteration or alteration in cerebral blood flow as a result of microwave exposure, the response is transient (less than 24 hr). It was hoped that such alteration could actually be beneficial by enhancing the permeability of therapeutic agents and the use of certain chemotherapeutic agents in the treatment of cancers of the brain and leukemia in children. Currently no information conclusively shows RF affects the BBB at SARs below 2 W/kg (Ward *et al.*, 1982; Williamson *et al.*, 1984).

10.6. OBSERVATIONS IN THE HUMAN

Soviet and other East European investigators have contributed most of the studies on the human effects of exposure to microwaves; the greatest emphasis is on effects produced at less than "thermogenic" power flux densities ($< 10\,\text{mW/cm}^2$) in occupational exposures. According to these authors, the responses of an organism to microwave exposure are directly or indirectly referable to the CNS (Gordon, 1958, 1966; Petrov, 1970; Presman, 1968).

A number of human effects referable to CNS sensitivity have been described, i.e., fatigability, headache, sleepiness, irritability, loss of appetite, and memory difficulties. Psychic changes that include unstable mood, hypochondriasis, and anxiety have been observed. According to some reports, persons working in microwave fields of various intensities often complain of a heavy feeling in their head, headaches, fatigue, drowsiness in the daytime, irritability, poor memory, and a pain in the heart, usually of the aching, stabbing type. In addition, bright red, diffuse, persistent dermographia, hyperhidrosis, unstable arterial pressure, and angiopathy of the retina have been described. Autonomic vascular instability is reflected in changes in the electrocardiogram (bradycardia, disturbance in intraventricular conduction). The above-mentioned signs and symptoms are often expressed in certain neurological syndromes: asthenia, and particularly autonomic vascular dysfunctions (D'Yachenko, 1970a,b; Muratov and Turaeva, 1972; Rogussky *et al.*, 1970; Sadchikova and Nikonova, 1971; Tyagin, 1971). Most of these signs and symptoms are reversible, and pathological damage to neural structures is insignificant. Most of the reports are based on subjective rather than objective findings. It should be noted that individuals suffering from a variety of chronic diseases may exhibit the same dysfunctions of the central nervous and cardiovascular systems as those attributed to microwave exposure.

The observed effects from exposure to electromagnetic radiation have been organized into categories by wavelength, organ system, or clinical syndrome. Many of the reports in the human can be classified into categories such as: (1) neurasthenic syndrome, (2) autonomic vagotonic dystonia, and (3) diencephalic syndrome (Dodge and Kassel, 1966). Drogichina *et al.* (1966) report all three classes of symptoms in personnel subjected to microwave fields of "a few mW/cm^2." The basic symptomatology and neuropathology underlying all of these syndromes are reportedly due to a functional disturbance often in the CNS caused by purportedly "nonthermal" mechanisms. These effects do not appear in relation to observed rise in body temperature, and are reported to occur at levels far below those required to produce a temperature rise. Such syndromes are completely reversible in most cases, with little or no time lost from work (Osipov, 1965). In contrast, other authors emphasize the resultant time lost from work, and the necessary hospitalization (Gordon, 1966; Letavet and Gordon, 1960). One author reported that physical activity in both organized and unorganized forms modifies the incidence of functional cardiovascular disorders in radar operators, but he does stress "environmental factors and job immobility" as contributing to the incidence (D'Yachenko, 1970b).

Clinical observations of humans exposed to microwave fields have suggested that motor effects may be accompanied by sleep disturbances, a lower resistance to fatigue, increased irritability, and memory concentration deficits (Edelwejn and Haduch, 1962; Kevork'yan, 1948; Sadchikova, 1962; Sadchikova and Orlova, 1958; Sercl et al., 1961). Kevork'yan (1948) reported that workers exposed to "moderate"-intensity microwave fields are prone to a syndrome including sleep disturbances, memory changes, and rapid fatigue under work requiring mental concentration. Sadchikova and Orlova (1958) also found general debility, listlessness, and increased irritability in individuals chronically exposed to "low to moderate"-intensity microwave fields in an industrial environment. They classified the people according to exposure: (1) periodic to $3-4\,mW/cm^2$, (2) periodic to less than $1\,mW/cm^2$, and (3) constant to less than $0.1\,mW/cm^2$. In group 1, a vagotonic reaction was observed with symptoms of bradycardia, and prolongation of intraauricular and intraventricular conduction. In those exposed continuously (group 3), an asthenic syndrome with irritability was reported. The control group apparently was not composed of matched workers, but consisted of a group of college students between the ages of 25 and 40.

Alteration of olfactory thresholds was reported in occupationally exposed individuals in fields between 30 MHz and 300 GHz (Fukalova, 1964; Goncharova et al., 1966; Gordon, 1958; Karamyshev, 1966; Lobanova and Gordon, 1960). Some reduction in the excitability of the olfactory and optical analyzers has been reported in workers. Increase in olfactory threshold and curtailment of chronaxie have also been reported. Lobanova and Gordon (1960) found lower olfactory sensitivities among 358 workers exposed to microwaves than among members of a control group. Among experimental subjects exposed continuously to power densities of up to $1\,mW/cm^2$, the lowest sensitivity was in those exposed less than 1 year or more than 6 years; among subjects exposed periodically to power densities up to several mW/cm^2, the sensitivity decreased with increasing exposure time.

In a study of the functional condition of the vestibular and visual analyzers in people subjected to lengthy exposure to "low-intensity" microwaves, Nikogosyan (1971) found that the threshold of stimulation had risen. When Grinbarg (1959) applied 50-MHz energy through electrodes, the threshold for pain was raised. Sheyvekhman (1949), using electrodes to apply 50-MHz energy for 5 min to the head of humans, found auditory threshold changes in the exposed individuals.

EEG examination has revealed various cortical alterations. The most pronounced changes were observed in persons with severe symptoms from the action of centimeter waves. According to Ginzburg and Sadchikova (1964), the character of the changes (generalized paroxysmal activity) indicates "functional damage at the mesodiencephalic level." Kolesnik and Malyshev (1967) reported that accidental exposure of the head and upper trunk of a man to 10,000 MHz, 10 mW/cm^2, for 15 min resulted in asthenia, and on the EEG he showed lowered voltage, a rapid beta rhythm, and a slow theta rhythm.

The results of long-term neurological observation of 500 persons exposed to electromagnetic fields were evaluated by Klimkova-Deutschova (1974). The most frequent subjective symptoms were: headache, fatigue, and sleep disturbances. Less frequent were cases of anxiety, hyperexcitability, and vegetative disorders. The objective symptomatology was characterized by labyrinthine deviations and disturbances of pyramidal and extrapyramidal motor systems. The incidence of neurosis was significantly higher than in controls. Experimental physiological and EEG methods showed mostly reduced vigilance and pathological records independent of the intensity of the field. "The disturbances in metabolic, EEG, and clinical symptoms suggest an impairment of the regulative mechanism in the mesodiencephalic region."

On the basis of extensive material dealing with "electrophysiological research conducted on different subjects with electrographic and excitometric methods *in vitro* and *in vivo* and neuropharmacological loads", Bychkov (1972) concluded that "the evolution of the integral effect of low-intensity microwaves on the central nervous system has three stages: (1) An initial effect on the cortex, manifested in a moderate deactivation, which may be considered an initial adaptive reaction; (2) an adaptive-reaction stage related to non-specific adaptive compensatory mechanisms of the reticular formation of the brain stem and hypothalamus; (3) a stage of pathological reactions caused by suppression of the compensatory mechanisms and dysfunction of the brain."

With regard to the question of the so-called "neurasthenic responses," reported by Soviet authors, Cohen and White (1972) presented an extensive review of neurocirculatory asthenia as a clinical syndrome that has implications in assessing the reported effects of "low-level" microwaves. The authors relate that onset of the syndrome in predisposed individuals is usually precipitated or made worse by emotion-provoking circumstances, medical illness, unaccustomed or hard muscular labor (particularly if involuntary), pregnancy, and in various situations in military service. Exact etiological relationships are unknown.

More sophisticated studies are needed to learn if the prevalence of such disorders associated with occupational exposure to microwaves as described by Soviet investigators is greater than in the general population. Since most of the complaints are subjective, every means should be taken to avoid a bias or prejudgment on the part of the examiner and the subject. The examiner should not be aware of the occupation of the subject, and the subject should not be influenced to respond a certain way.

10.7. THE SOVIET APPROACH TO BIOLOGY AND MEDICINE

In order to understand the apparent inconsistencies in the Western and Eastern European literature, consideration of the differences in approach to biology and medicine is appropriate in a discussion of neural effects. Soviet and American interest in the biological effects of electromagnetic fields has increased since 1950. Although some Soviet investigators recognize the thermal nature of the biological effects of microwaves, there are numerous reports suggesting that microwave exposure at field intensities that do not produce an appreciable thermal effect may produce functional changes in the nervous and cardiovascular systems. The effects on the nervous system include changes in "excitation and inhibition relationships of the cerebral cortex." Cardiovascular changes such as arterial hypotension, bradycardia, sinus arrhythmia, lengthening of the conduction time in the heart, reduction of the amplitude of the spikes of the ECG, are noted and referable to CNS effects.

Presman (1965, 1968) believes that the stress stimulus from microwaves comes not only from the thermal receptors of the skin, but also from other sensory skin receptors. Under comparable conditions, microwave irradiation causes a more intense flow of afferent impulses and a more intense stimulation of hypothalamic–hypophyseal activity than does thermal irradiation. The apparent adaptation to repeated microwave exposures is also referable to stimulation of skin receptors.

Soviet investigators suggest that chronic irradiation of animals with low-intensity microwaves ($< 15 \text{ mW/cm}^2$) may induce functional changes in the nervous and cardiovascular systems without a rise in tissue temperature. The changes are observed with chronic or single exposures.

The majority of Soviet investigators concerned with the biological effects of microwaves are of the opinion that this energy directly affects neural structures and that these structures, especially the CNS, are the most sensitive to microwaves. CNS effects have been reported as a result of exposure to both "nonthermal" and "thermal" intensities of pulsed and CW MW/RF fields.

Osipov (1965) noted that while microwaves may have a biological, and especially a neural effect at field intensities that do not produce measurable temperature rises, it is experimentally impossible to demonstrate a specific, e.g., nonthermal microwave effect by comparing the alleged effect with a thermoequivalent control. He reasons that since biological objects are electrically heterogeneous and since microwave-range electromagnetic fields have a known selective thermal effect on various tissues and organs, a difference between a microwave effect and a neutral heat effect is not necessarily due to an unknown extrathermal factor, but might well be a function of an uneven distribution of heat in the organism which could exert its own peculiar effect. He feels that the reported "nonthermal" microwave effects may well be "microthermal" effects in the absence of conclusive experimental evidence to the contrary.

Presman (1968), on the other hand, is more inclined to believe that if a microwave EMF does not result in any perceptible temperature shifts in an organism, any change in its behavior, function, or structure can be attributed to the nonthermal mechanism of the EMF, even if it is experimentally impossible to demonstrate that thermogenic and nonthermogenic EMF intensities each give rise to different reactions. In short, Presman feels that there is ample evidence of the nonthermal effects of microwave-range EMFs by virtue of an absolute temperature criterion, whereas Osipov feels that while nonthermal effects are entirely possible, they have not as yet been as well substantiated physiologically as have thermal effects.

Soviet investigators have a great interest in conditional response phenomena. Because of their interest in electrosleep, extrasensory perception, thought transmission, and other neural phenomena related to thought control, the interest and dogma that arose from Pavlov's work and subsequent theories of thought and behavior are quite apparent. This central theme has remained at the root of Soviet medicine. The Soviets actively seek a direct or indirect CNS mechanism for all pathological processes and physiological functions, as well as for behavior, thought, memory, and judgment. When one reads their scientific, and most particularly their medical and biological literature, this theme is omnipresent. To understand Soviet reports, one must read them in the context in which they are written, whether one accepts the precepts behind the writing or not. The Soviet investigators do not think of the CNS as merely an integrative component of bodily function and response, but as *the* iniating, monitoring, and controlling functionary over all life processes. This explains to some degree why Soviet investigators accept many things and events as important while others do not ascribe any clinical or functional significance to them.

It is readily apparent that Soviet investigators base much of their conceptual approach on Pavlovian conditional response techniques and interpretation. The framework of Pavlovian "nervism" as a philosophy means that not only are all motor responses influenced, integrated, and mediated by the CNS, but *all* bodily functions as well. This includes such seemingly remote physiological activities as cellular response to injury, hematopoiesis, and specific organ responses to local metabolic demands. In this context, all responses of an organism to a physical agent are CNS responses, either directly or indirectly.

Without diminishing the importance of the CNS as an integrating and initiating functional unit mechanism, Western physiologists and neurophysiologists do not ascribe such profound functional abilities and controlling processes, or at least do not emphasize them as much as do the Soviets. This is especially true in the utilization of conditional response studies as a means of evaluating these functional abilities. In terms of acceptance of Soviet reports, Western investigators are skeptical because of the limited statistical analyses presented, lack of controls, and the intrinsic difficulties of objectively analyzing the results.

Soviet experimental design philosophy appears to differ from our own. It is sometimes difficult to interpret their experiments due to this, and also due to differences in style of reporting and difficulty in translation. In evaluating what "cortical inhibition" means, for example, one is struck by the parallel situation created by a warm external environment. This is known to cause less encephalographic activity at the cortical and reticular activating system levels, with the end result of somnolence. By its volume heating characteristics, microwaves under some conditions could be expected to produce similar responses, and indeed may be the mechanism in some reported experiments. This is inhibition as the Soviets describe it, and it can be explained very reasonably on thermal grounds, without invoking an unproven "nonthermal" effect mechanism. Nevertheless, at prevailing protection guides, heating to produce such effects would not occur.

Pazderova (1968), in a review of the microwave literature, noted that much of the Soviet work was unacceptable, since it presented little data and could not be statistically analyzed. She also related that the Soviet work was based mostly on subjective rather than objective findings, and that "dosimetry" in most cases was poor, and not comparable from worker to worker.

In a recent review, Pazderova-Vejlupkova (1981) reiterated her criticism of the Soviet reports, noting "Our findings are at variance to many of those reported in the earlier Soviet and Polish literature." Apparently "working conditions involving exposure levels over the past 10 years have improved drastically. It is not surprising, therefore, that observed frequencies of field-related maladies are very low at the present time."

REFERENCES

Adey, W. R. (1977) Anatomy and biophysics of brain cells in weak ELF fields. In: *Biologic Effects of Electric and Magnetic Fields Associated with Proposed Project Seafarer.* National Academy of Sciences, Washington, D.C., pp. 389–399.

Adey, W. R., and S. M. Bawin (eds.) (1977) *Brain Interactions with Weak Electric and Magnetic Fields. Neurosci. Res. Program Bull.* **15**.

Albert, E. N. (1977a) Light and electron microscopic observations on the blood brain barrier after microwave irradiation. In: *Biological Effects and Measurement of Radiofrequency/Microwaves*, D. G. Hazzard (ed.). HEW Publ. (FDA) 77-8026, pp. 294–309.

Albert, E. N. (1977b) Reversibility of the blood brain barrier. *URSI/USNC Int. Symp. Biol. Eff. Electromagnetic Waves*, Airlie, Va. (abstract).

Albert, E. N. (1978a) Ultrastructural pathology associated with microwave induced blood–brain barrier permeability. In: *URSI International Symposium on Biological Effects of Electromagnetic Waves*, Helsinki, p. 58.

Albert, E. N. (1978b) Ultrastructural pathology associated with microwave induced alterations in blood–brain barrier permeability. In: *Proc. Biol. Eff. E.M. Waves.* XIX Gen. Assembly. Int. Union Radio Sci., Helsinki, p. 58.

Albert, E. N. (1979) Reversibility of microwave induced blood–brain barrier permeability. *Radio Sci.* **14**: 323.

Albert, E. N., and M. DeSantis (1975) Do microwaves alter nervous system-structure? *Ann. N.Y. Acad. Sci.* **247**: 87.

Albert, E. N., and M. E. DeSantis (1977) Histological observations on central nervous system. In: *Biological Effects of Electromagnetic Waves*, Vol. I, C. C. Johnson and M. L. Shore (eds.). HEW Publ. (FDA) 77-8010, pp. 299–310.

Albert, E. N., and J. Kerns (1981) Reversible microwave effects on the blood–brain barrier. *Brain Res.* **230**: 153.

Albert, E. N., F. J. Slaby, K. Patunraj, and D. Balzano (1980a) 147 MHz RF irradiation does not increase calcium release from chick brains. *Bioelectromagnetics* **1**: 212A.

Albert, E. N., C. F. Blackman, and F. Slaby (1980b) Calcium dependent secretory protein release and calcium efflux after VHF electromagnetic radiation of rat pancreatic tissue. In: *Proc. URSI Symposium on Electromagnetic Waves and Biology*, A. J. Berteaud (ed.). Paris, pp. 330–336.

Albert, E. N., M. F. Sherif, N. J. Papadopoulos, F. J. Slaby, and J. Monahan (1980a) Effect of 100 MHz and 2.45 GHz on rat cerebellar Purkinje cells. *Bioelectromagnetics* **1**:206A.

Arber, S. L. (1976) Effect of microwaves on resting potential of giant neurons of mollusk *Helix pomatia. Elektron. Obrab. Mater.* **6**:78.

Austin, G. N., and S. M. Horvath (1954) Production of convulsions in rats by high frequency electrical currents. *Am. J. Phys. Med.* **3**:141.

Baldwin, M. S., S. A. Bach, and S. A. Lewis (1960) Effects of radio frequency energy on primate cerebral activity. *Neurology* **10**:178.

Baranski, S. (1972) Histological and histochemical effects of microwave irradiation on the central nervous system of rabbits and guinea pigs. *Am. J. Phys. Med.* **51**:182.

Baranski, S., and P. Czerski (1976) *Biological Effects of Microwaves.* Dowden, Hutchinson & Ross, Stroudsburg, Pa.

Baranski, S., and Z. Edelwejn (1967) Electroencephalographic and morphological investigations on the influence of microwaves on the central nervous system. *Acta Physiol. Pol.* **18**:423.

Baranski, S., and Z. Edelwejn (1968) Studies on the combined effects of microwaves and some drugs on bioelectric activity of rabbit CNS. *Acta Physiol. Pol.* **19**:37.

Baranski, S., and Z. Edelwejn (1975) Experimental morphologic and electroencephalographic studies of microwave effects on the nervous system. *Ann. N.Y. Acad. Sci.* **247**:109.

Baranski, S., L. Czekalinski, P. Czerski, and S. Haduch (1963) Experimental research on fatal effect of micrometric wave electromagnetic radiation. *Rev. Med. Aeronaut. (Paris)* **2**:108.

Bawin, S. M., and W. R. Adey (1976) Sensitivity of calcium binding in cerebral tissue to weak environmental electric fields oscillating at low frequency. *Proc. Natl. Acad. Sci. USA* **73**:1999.

Bawin, S. M., and W. R. Adey (1977) Calcium binding in cerebral tissues. In: *Biological Effects and Measurement of Radiofrequency/Microwaves*, D. G. Hazzard (ed.) HEW Publ. (FDA) 77-8026, PP. 305–313.

Bawin, S. M., R. J. Gavalas-Medici, and W. R. Adey (1973) Effects of modulated very high frequency fields on specific brain rhythms in cats. *Brain Res.* **58**:365.

Bawin, S. M., L. K. Kaczmarek, and W. R. Adey (1975) Effects of modulated VHF fields on the central nervous system. *Ann. N.Y. Acad. Sci.* **247**:74.

Bawin, S. M., A. R. Sheppard, and W. R. Adey (1978) Possible mechanisms of weak electromagnetic field coupling in brain tissue. *Bioelectrochem. Bioenerg.* **5**:67.

Bilokrinitsky, V. S. (1966) Changes in the tigroid substance of neurons under the effect of radio waves. *Fiziol. Zh. (Kiev)* **12**:70.

Bilokrinitsky, V. S., and Y. D. Dumansky (1974) Histochemical characteristics of brain enzymes with exposure to a low intensity SHF field. Presented at the 2nd Industrial and Environmental Neurology Congress, Prague.

Blackman, C. F., J. A. Elder, C. M. Weil, S. G. Benane, D. C. Eichinger, and D. E. House (1979) Induction of calcium ion efflux from brain tissue by radiofrequency radiation: Effects of modulation frequency and field strength. *Radio Sci.* **14**: 93.

Blackman, C. F., S. G. Benane, J. A. Edler, D. E. House, J. A. Lampe, and J. M. Faulk (1980) Induction of calcium-ion efflux from brain tissue by radiofrequency radiation: Effect of sample number and modulation frequency on the power-density window. *Bioelectromagnetics* **1**:35.

Bondy, S. C., and J. L. Purdy (1974) Selective regulation of the blood–brain barrier by sensory input. *Brain Res.* **76**:542.

Brightman, M. W., I. Klatzo, Y. Olsson, and T. S. Reese (1970) The blood–brain barrier to protein under normal and pathological conditions. *J. Neurol. Sci.* **10**:215.

Bychkov, M. S. (1972) Neurophysiological characterization of the action mechanism of super-high frequency electromagnetic waves. In: *Industrial Health and Biological Effects of Radio-Frequency Electromagnetic Waves*. Materials of the Fourth All-Union Symposium, Moscow, p. 46.

Bychkov, M. S., and I. S. Dronov (1974) Electroencephalographic data on the effects of very weak microwaves at the level of the midbrain reticular formation–hypothalamus–cerebellar cortex level. (Translation in NTIS Rep. JPRS 63321.)

Bychkov, M. S., V. Markov, and V. Rychkov (1974) Electroencephalographic changes under the influence of low intensity chronic microwave irradiation. (Translation in NTIS Rep. JPRS 63321.)

Carpenter, D. O. (1967) Temperature effects on pacemaker generation, membrane potential, and critical firing threshold in *Aplysia* neurons. *J. Gen. Physiol.* **50**:1469.

Casterline, J. L., and C. H. Williams (1969) The effect of pesticide administration on serum and tissue esterases of rats fed diets of varying casein, calcium, and magnesium content. *Toxicol Appl. Pharmacol.* **15**:532.

Chamness, A. F., H. R. Scholes, S. W. Sexauer, and J. W. Frazer (1976) Metal ion content of specific areas of the rat brain after 1600 MHz radiofrequency irradiation. *J. Microwave Power* **11**:333.

Chang, B. K., A. T. Huang, W. T. Joines, and R. S. Dramer (1978) The effect of microwave radiation (1.0 GHz) on the blood–brain barrier in dogs. *Proc. Biol. Eff. E. M. Waves.* XIX Gen. Assembly. Int. Union Radio Sci., Helsinki.

Chizenkova, R. A. (1967) Brain biopotentials in the rabbit during exposure to electromagnetic fields. *Fiziol. Zh. Akad. Nauk. UKR SSR (Moscow)* **53**:514.

Chizenkova, R. A. (1969) Background and induced activity of neurons of the optical cortex of a rabbit after the action of a SHF field. *Zh. Vyssh. Nernv. Deyat. im. I. P. Pavlova* **19**:495.

Chou, C. A. (1975) The Effects of Electromagnetic Fields on the Nervous System. Ph.D. dissertation, University of Washington, Seattle.

Clawson, C. C., J. F. Hartmann, and R. L. Vernier (1966) Electron microscopy of the effect of gram-negative endotoxin on the blood–brain barrier. *J. Comp. Neurol.* **127**:183.

Cleary, S. F. (1977) Biological effects of microwaves and radiofrequency radiation. In: *CRC Critical Reviews in Environmental Control*, Vol. 7, C. Straub (ed.). Chemical Rubber Co., Cleveland, pp. 121–165.

Cohen, M. E., and P. D. White (1972) Neurocirculatory asthenia. *Mil. Med.* **137**:142.

Cole, K. S. (1968) Membrane capacity. In: *Ions, Impulses, and Membranes*, C. A. Tobias (ed.). University of California Press, Berkeley, p. 12.

Cornish, H. H. 1971 Problems posed by observations on serum enzyme change in toxicology. In: *CRC Critical Reviews in Toxicology*, Chemical Rubber Company, Cleveland, p. 81.

Crone, C. (1963) The permeability of capillaries in various organs as determined by use of the indicator diffusion method. *Acta Physiol. Scand.* **58**:292.

Crone, C. (1965) The permeability of brain capillaries to non-electrolytes. *Acta Physiol. Scand.* **64**:407.

Czerski, P. (1975) Experimental models for the evaluation of microwave biological effects. *Proc. IEEE* **63**:1540.

de Seguin, L., and G. Castelain (1947) Action of ultrahigh frequency radiation (wavelength 21 cm) on temperature of small laboratory animals. *C. R. Acad. Sci.* **224**:1662.

Dodge, C., and S. Kassel (1966) Soviet Research on the Neural Effects of Microwaves. ATD Report 66-133, Library of Congress, Washington, D.C.

Dolina, L. A. (1961) Morphological changes in the central nervous system due to the action of centimeter waves on the organism. *Arkh. Patol.* **23**:51.

Drogichina, E. A., M. N. Sadchikova, M. N. Snegova, G. V. Konchalovskaya, and K. T. Glotova (1966) Autonomic and cardiovascular disorders during chronic exposure to superhigh frequency electromagnetic fields. *Gig. Tr. Prof. Zabol.* **10**:13.

Dumansky, Y. D., and M. G. Shandala (1974) The biological action and hygienic significance of electromagnetic fields of superhigh and ultrahigh frequencies in densely populated areas. In: *Biological Effects and Health Hazards of Microwave Radiation*, P. Czerski, K. Ostrowski, M. L. Shore, C. Silverman, M. J. Suess, and B. Waldesjog (eds.). Polish Medical Publishers, Warsaw, pp. 289–293.

D'Yachenko, N. A. (1970a) Changes in thyroid function with chronic exposure to microwave radiation. *Gig. Tr. Prof. Zabol.* **14**:51.

D'Yachenko, N. A. (1970b) Impact of SHF electromagnetic radiation on the functional state of the myocardium. *Voen. Med. Zh.* **2**:35.

Edelwejn, Z. (1968) Attempted evaluation of the functional state of brain synapses in rabbits exposed chronically to the action of microwaves. *Acta Physiol. Pol.* **19**:791.

Edelwejn, Z., and S. Haduch (1962) Electroencephalographic studies on persons exposed to microwave. *Acta Physiol. Pol.* **13**:431.

Ekel, G. J. (1974) Use of conditioned reflex methods in Soviet behavioral toxicology research. In: *Behavior Toxicology*, C. Xintaras, B. L. Johnson, and I. de Groat (eds.). HEW Publ. (NIOSH) 140, pp. 74–126.

Frey, A. H., S. R. Feld, and B. Frey (1975) Neural function and behavior: Defining the relationship. *Ann. N.Y. Acad. Sci.* **247**:433.

Fröhlich, H. (1977) Possibilities of long- and short-range electric interactions of biological systems. *Neurosci. Res. Program Bull.* **15**:67.

Fukalova, P. P. (1964) The sensitivity of olfactory and optic analyzers in persons exposed to the effect of constantly-generated SW and USW. *Tr. Nii Gig. Tr. Prof. AMN SSR* (*Moscow*) **2**:144.

Gillard, J., B. Servantie, G. Bertharion, A. M. Servantie, and J. K. C. Obrenovitch (1976) Study of the microwave-induced perturbations of the behavior by the open-field test in the white rat. In: *Biological Effects of Electromagnetic Waves,* Vol. I, C. C. Johnson and M. L. Shore (eds.). HEW Publ. (FDA) 77-8010, p. 693.

Ginzburg, D. A., and M. N. Sadchikova (1964) Changes in the electroencephalogram under the continuous action of radiowaves. *Tr. Gig. Prof. AMN SSSR* (*Moscow*) **2**:126.

Goldstein, L., and Z. Sisko (1974) A quantitative electroencephalographic study of the acute effects of X-band microwaves in rabbits. In: *Biological Effects and Health Hazards of Microwave Radiation.* P. Czerski, K. Ostrowski, M. L. Shore, C. Silverman, M. J. Suess, and B. Waldeskog (eds.). Polish Medical Publishers, Warsaw, pp. 128–133.

Goncharova, N. N., V. B. Karamyshev, and N. V. Maksimenko (1966) Occupational hygiene problems in working with ultrashort-wave transmitters used in TV and radio broadcasting. *Gig. Tr. Prof. Zabol.* **10**:10.

Gordon, Z. V. (1958) Questions on work hygiene related to the effect of a SHF-field. *Zh. Gig. Tr. Prof. Zabol.* **6**:14.

Gordon, Z. V. (1960) The problem of the biological action of UHF. *Tr. Nii Gig. Tr. Prof. USSR* **1**:65.

Gordon, Z. V. (1964) Problems of industrial hygiene and the biological action of various ranges of radio-waves. *Herald Acad. Med. Nauk* **19**:42 (JPRS 27032).

Gordon, Z. V. (1966) Biological Effect of Microwaves in Occupational Hygiene. Izd. Med., Leningrad (TT 70-50087, NASA TT F-633, 1970).

Gordon, Z. V. (1970a) Occupational health aspects of radio-frequency electromagnetic radiation. In: *Ergonomics and Physical Environmental Factors.* Occupational Safety and Health Series, No. 21, International Labour Office, Geneva, p. 159.

Gordon, Z. V. (1970b) Biological Effects of Microwaves in Occupational Hygiene. Israel Program for Scientific Translations, Jerusalem, pp. 56–66.

Gordon, Z. V., Y. A. Lobanova, and M. S. Tolgskaya (1955) Some data on the effect of centimeter waves (experimental studies). *Gig. Sanit.* **12**:16.

Grinbarg, A. G. (1959) VHF–HF therapy in certain affections of the peripheral nervous system. *Kazan. Med. Zh. USSR* **40**:59.

Grodsky, I. T. (1975) Possible physical substrates for the interaction of electromagnetic fields with biologic membranes. *Ann. N.Y. Acad. Sci.* **247**:117.

Gruneau, S. P., K. J. Oscar, M. T. Falker, and S. I. Rapaport (1982) Absence of microwave effect on blood–brain barrier permeability to [^{14}C]sucrose in the conscious rat. *Exp. Neurol.* **75**:299.

Gunn, S. A., T. C. Gould, and W. A. D. Anderson (1961) The effect of microwave radiation on morphology and function of rat testis. *Lab. Invest.* **10**:301.

Gvozdikova, Z. M., V. M. Anan'yev, I. N. Zenina, and V. I. Zak (1964) Sensitivity of the rabbit central nervous system to a continuous (non-pulsed) ultrahigh frequency electromagnetic field. *Byull. Eksp. Biol. Med.* **58**:63.

Hardy, J. D. (1973) Posterior hypothalamus and the regulation of body temperature. *Fed. Proc.* **32**:1564.

Johnson, C. C., and A. W. Guy (1972) Non-ionizing electromagnetic wave effects in biological materials and systems. *Proc. IEEE* **60**:692.

Karamyshev, V. B. (1966) Physiological–hygienic characteristics of the working conditions of television and radio station personnel. In: *Questions of Work Hygiene and Occupational Pathology in the Chemical and Mechanical Engineering Industries*. Reports of the Scientific Session of the Institute, Ukr. Gos. Inst. Patol. Gig. Tr., Kharkov, p. 106.

Kevork'yan, A. A. (1948) Working with ultrahigh frequency impulse generators from the standpoint of labor hygiene. *Gig. Sanit.* **4**:26.

Kholodov, Y. A. (1963) Changes in the electrical activity of the rabbit cerebral cortex during exposure to a UHF–HF electromagnetic field. Part 2. The direct action of the UHF–HF field on the central nervous system. *Byull. Eksp. Biol. Med.* **56**:42.

Kholodov, Y. A. (1964) The influence of a VHF–HF electromagnetic field on the electrical activity of an isolated strip of cerebral cortex. *Byull. Eksp. Biol. Med.* **57**:98.

Kholodov, Y. A. (1966) *The Effect of Electromagnetic and Magnetic Fields on the Central Nervous System*. Nauka, Moscow, p. 283 (NASA TT-F-465).

Kitsovskaya, I. A. (1960) An investigation of the interrelationships between the main nervous processes in rats on exposure to SHF fields of various intensities. *Tr. Nii Gig. Tr. Prof. AMN SSSR* **1**:75.

Kitsovskaya, I. A. (1968a) The effect of radiowaves of various ranges on the nervous system (sound stimulation method). In: *On the Biological Effect of Radiofrequency Electromagnetic Fields*. Moscow, p. 81.

Kitsovskaya, I. A. (1968b) The influence of low-intensity microwaves on indices characterizing the state of cholinergic processes. In: *Work Hygiene and the Biological Effect of Radiofrequency Electromagnetic Waves*. Moscow, p. 71.

Klimkova-Deutschova, E. (1974) Neurologic findings in persons exposed to microwaves. In: *Biological Effects and Health Hazards of Microwave Radiation*, P. Czerski, K. Ostrowski, M. L. Shore, C. Silverman, M. J. Suess, and B. Waldeskog (eds.). Polish Medical Publishers, Warsaw, p. 268.

Kolesnik, F. A., and V. M. Malyshev (1967) The problem of clinical observation of injuries caused by SHF electromagnetic fields. *Voen. Med. Zh.* **4**:21.

Letavet, A. A., and Z. V. Gordon (eds.) (1960) *The Biological Action of Ultrahigh Frequencies*. Inst. Labor Hygiene and Occupational Diseases, Acad. Med. Sci., Moscow (JPRS 12471, 1962).

Lin, J. C., and M. F. Lin (1980) Studies on microwave and blood–brain barrier interaction. *Bioelectromagnetics* **1**: 313.

Livanov, M. N., A. B. Tsypin, Y. G. Grigoriev, U. G. Kruschev, S. M. Stepanov, and A. M. Anen'yev (1960) The effect of electromagnetic fields on the bioelectric activity of cerebral cortex in rabbits. *Byull. Eksp. Biol. Med.* **49**:63.

Lobanova, Y. A., and A. V. Goncharova (1971) Investigation of conditioned-reflex activity in animals (albino rats) subjected to the effect of ultrashort and short radio-waves. *Gig. Tr. Prof. Zabol.* **15**:29.

Lobanova, Y. A. and Z. V. Gordon (1960) The study of olfactory sensitivity in persons exposed to SHF. *Tr. Nii Gig. Prof. AMN SSR* **1**:52.

Lorenzo, A. V., I. Shirahige, M. Liang, and C. F. Barlow (1972) Temporary alteration of cerebrovascular permeability to plasma protein during drug induced seizures. *Am. J. Physiol.* **223**:268.

McAfee, R. D. (1961) Neurophysiological effect of 3 cm microwave radiation. *Am. J. Physiol.* **200**:192.

McAfee, R. D. (1963) Physiological effects of thermode and microwave stimulation of peripheral nerves. *Am. J. Physiol.* **203**:374.

McKee, A., C. H. Dorsey, D. L. Eisenbrandt, and N. E. Woden (1980) Ultrastructural observations of microwave-induced morphologic changes in the central nervous system of hamsters. *Bioelectromagnetics* **1**:206.

Marha, K. (1963) Biological effects of RF electromagnetic waves. *Prac. Lek.* **15**:387.

Marha, K., J. Musil, and H. Tuha (1968) *Electromagnetic Fields and the Living Environment.* State Health Publishing House, Prague (Transl. SBN 911302-13-7, San Francisco Press, 1971).

Merritt, J. H., R. H. Hartzell, and J. W. Frazer (1975) The effect of 1.6 GHz on neurotransmitters in discrete areas of the brain. SAM-TR-76-3, USAF School of Aerospace Medicine, Aerospace Medical Division, pp. 1–11.

Merritt, J. H., A. F. Chamness, R. H. Hartzell, and S. J. Allen (1977) Orientation effects on microwave-induced hyperthermia and neurochemical correlates. *J. Microwave Power* **12**:167.

Merritt, J. H., A. F. Chamness, and S. J. Allen (1978) Studies in blood–brain barrier permeability after microwave-radiation. *Radiat. Environ. Biophys.* **15**:367.

Minecki, L., and R. Bilski (1961) Histopathological changes in internal organs of mice exposed to the action of microwaves. *Med. Pr.* **12**:337.

Mishchenko, L. I. (1968) The effect of a UHF electromagnetic field on acetylcholine exchange in the brain of rats. In: *Material of the Ukrainian Republic Conference of Industrial-Health Inspectors and Scientists.* Session of the Kharkov Institute of Work Hygiene and Occupational Diseases, Kiev, p. 135.

Mishchenko, L. I. (1969) The effect of an ultrahigh frequency electromagnetic field on carbohydrate exchange in the brain of rats. *Byull. Eksp. Biol. Med.* **68**:56.

Muratov, V. I., and A. P. Turaeva (1972) Changes in the cardiovascular system under the chronic influence of an SHF field. *Voen. Med. Zh.* **1**:22.

Myers, R.D., and D. H. Ross (1981) Radiation and brain calcium: A review and critique. *Neurosci. Biobehav. Rev.* **5**:503.

Nair, V., and L. J. Roth (1964) Effect of x-irradiation and certain other treatments on blood–brain barrier permeability. *Radiat. Res.* **23**:249.

Nikogosyan, S. V. (1960) Effect of SHF on cholinesterase activity in blood serum and organs in animals. In: *The Biological Action of Ultrahigh Frequencies,* A. A. Letavet and Z. V. Gordon (eds.). Acad. Med. Sci., Moscow, p. 81 (JPRS 12471).

Nikogosyan, S. V. (1964) A study of the activity of cholinesterase in blood serum and in organs of animals under the chronic influence of microwaves, p. 43; The effect of 10-cm waves on the amount of nucleic acids in the organs of animals, p. 66. In: *The Biological Effect of Radiofrequency Electromagnetic Fields.* Works of the Laboratory of Radiofrequency Electromagnetic Fields, Institute of Work Hygiene and Occupational Diseases, AMN SSR, Moscow.

Nikogosyan, S. V. (1971) Functional condition of certain analyzers in persons subjected to the influence of radiowaves. *Gig. Truda. Prof. Zabol.* **7**:49.

Nikogosyan, S. V., and I. A. Kitsovskaya 1968 The altered activity of cholinesterase in the CNS of animals in various functional states under the influence of low intensity decimeter waves. *Gig. Tr. Prof. Zabol.* **5**:5.

Novitskii, Y. I., Z. V. Gordon, A. S. Presman, and Y. A. Kholodov (1971) *Radio Frequencies and Microwaves, Magnetic and Electrical Fields* (NASA TT F-14.021)

Oldendorf, W. H. (1949) Focal neurological lesions produced by microwave irradiation. *Proc. Soc. Exp. Biol. Med.* **72**:432.

Oldendorf, W. H. (1970) Measurement of brain uptake of radio-labeled substances using a tritiated water internal standard. *Brain Res.* **24**:372.

Oldendorf, W. H. (1971) Brain uptake of radiolabeled amino acids, amines, and hexoses after arterial injection. *Am. J. Physiol.* **221**:1629.

Oldendorf, W. H. (1974) Blood–brain barrier permeability to drugs. *Annu. Rev. Pharmacol.* **14**:239.

Olsson, Y., and T. S. Reese (1969) Inaccessibility of the endoneurium of sciatic nerve to exogenous proteins. *Anat. Rec.* **163**:319.

Oscar, K. J. (1980) Interaction of Electromagnetic Energy with Absorptive Material by Thermally Inducing Elastic Stress Waves. Ph.D. thesis, American University, Washington, D.C.

Oscar, K. J., S. P. Gruneau, M. T. Folker, and S. I. Rapoport (1981) Local cerebral blood flow after microwave exposure. *Brain Res.* **204**:220.

Oscar, K. J., and T. D. Hawkins (1977) Microwave alteration of the blood–brain barrier system of rats. *Brain Res.* **126**:281.

Osipov, Y. A. (1965) *Occupational Hygiene and the Effects of Radio-Frequency Electromagnetic Fields on Workers.* Meditsina Press, Leningrad, pp. 78–103.

Paulsson, L. E., Y. Hamnerius, and W. G. McLean (1977) The effects of microwave radiation on microtubules and axonal transport. *Radiat Res.* **70**:212.

Pavlov, I.P. (1927) *Conditioned Reflexes.* Oxford University Press, London.

Pazderova, J. (1968) Effects of electromagnetic radiation of the order of centimeter and meter wavelength on human's health. *Prac. Lek.* **20**:447.

Pazderova-Vejlupkova, J. (1981) Update on epidemiology: Europe. Presented at the XXth Assembly of URSI, Washington, D.C.

Petrov, I. R. (ed.) (1970) *Influence of Microwave Radiation on the Organism of Man and Animals.* Meditsina Press, Leningrad (NASA TT F-708, 1971).

Pickard, W. F., Y. H. Barsoum, and F. J. Rosenbaum (1980) Is the Characean plasmalemma a radiofrequency rectifier? Presented at the 2nd Annual Meeting of the Bioelectromagnetics Society, San Antonio.

Pinneo, L. R., R. Baus, R. D. McAfee, and J. D. Fleming (1962) *The Neural Effects of Microwaves.* RADC-TDR 62-231. Tulane University, New Orleans, p. 24.

Portela, A., O. Llobera, S. M. Michaelson, P. A. Stewart, J. C. Perez, A. H. Guerrero, C. A. Rodriguez, and R. J. Perez (1975) Transient effects of low-level microwave irradiation on bioelectric muscle cell properties and on water permeability and its distribution. In: *Fundamental and Applied Aspects of Nonionizing Radiation,* S. M. Michaelson, M. W. Miller, R. Magin, and E. L. Carstensen (eds.). Plenum Press, New York, pp. 93–127.

Presman, A. S. (1965) The effect of microwaves on living organisms and biological structures. *Usp. Fiz. Nauk.* **86**:263.

Presman, A. S. (1968) *Electromagnetic Fields and Life.* Izd-vo Nauka, Moscow (Transl. Plenum Press, 1970).

Preston, E., and G. Prefontaine (1980) Cerebrovascular permeability to sucrose in the rat exposed to 2450 MHz microwaves. *J. Appl. Physiol.* **49**:218.

Preston, E., E. J. Vavasour, and H. M. Assenheim (1978) Effect of 2450 MHz microwave irradiation on permeability of the blood–brain barrier to mannitol in the rat. In: *Symposium on Electromagnetic Fields in Biological Systems.* IMPI, Ottawa, Canada, p. 5 (abstract).

Preston, E., E. J. Vavasour, and H. M. Assenheim (1979) Permeability of the blood–brain barrier to mannitol in the rat following 2450 MHz microwave irradiation. *Brain Res.* **174**:109.

Raichle, M. E., J. O. Eichling, and R. L. Grubb (1974) Brain permeability of water. *Arch. Neurol.* **30**:319.

Raichle, M. E., J. O. Eichling, M. G. Straatmann, M. J. Welch, K. B. Larson, and M. M. Ter-Pegossian (1976) Blood–brain barrier permeability of ^{14}C-labeled alcohols and ^{15}O-labeled water. *Am. J. Physiol.* **230**:543.

Rapoport, S. I., K. Ohno, W. R. Fredericks, and K. D. Pettigrew (1978) Regional cerebrovascular permeability to ^{14}C sucrose after osmotic opening of the blood–brain barrier. *Brain Res.* **150**:653.

Reese, T. S., and M. J. Karnovsky (1967) Fine structural localization of a blood–brain barrier to exogenous peroxidase. *J. Cell Biol.* **34**:207.

Rene, A. A., J. L. Parker, J. H. Darden, and N. A. Eaton (1973) Effect of a supralethal dose of radiation on the blood–brain barrier. AFFRI Sci., Report SR73-2, AD762 411.

Rinder, L., and U. Olsson (1968) Vascular permeability changes in experimental brain concussion, part I and part II. *Acta Neuropathol.* **11**:183.

Rodzilsky, B., and J. Olszewsky (1957) Permeability of cerebral blood vessels studied by radioactive iodinated bovine albumin. *Neurology* **7**:279.

Rogussky, S. S., L. A. Ulitsky, B. N. Bartsevich, A. V. Il'yin, and V. I. Krivenko (1970) Results of dynamic observation of persons working in an environment influenced by an SHF field. *Voen. Med. Zh.* **6**:39.

Rupp, T., J. Montet, and J. W. Frazer 1975 A comparison of thermal and radio-frequency exposure effects on trace metal content of blood plasma and liver cell fractions of rodents. *Ann. N.Y. Acad. Sci.* **247**:282.

Sabbot, I., and A. Costin (1974) Effect of stress on the uptake of radiolabeled calcium in the pituitary gland and the brain of the rat. *J. Neurochem.* **22**:731.

Sadchikova, M. N. (1962) State of the nervous system under the influence of UHF. In: *The Biological Action of Ultrahigh Frequencies*, A. A. Letavet and Z. V. Gordon (eds.). Acad. Med. Sci. Moscow, p. 25.

Sadchikova, M. N., and K. V. Nikonova (1971) Comparative evaluation of the state of health of persons working under conditions involving exposure to microwaves of different intensity. *Tr. Nii Gig. Tr. Prof. Zabol.* **15**(9):10.

Sadchikova, M. N., and A. A. Orlova (1958) Clinical picture of the chronic effects of electromagnetic microwaves. *Ind. Hyg. Occup. Dis.* **2**:16.

Schmidt, M. J., D. E. Schmidt, and G. A. Robison (1971) Cyclic adenosine monophosphate in brain areas: Microwave irradiation as a means of tissue fixation. *Science* **173**:1142.

Schwan, H. P. (1957) Electrical properties of tissue and cell suspensions. *Adv. Biol. Med. Phys.* **5**:147.

Schwan, H.P. (1971) Interaction of microwave and radiofrequency radiation with biological systems. *IEEE Trans. Microwave Theory Tech.* **MTT-19**:146.

Schwan, H. P. (1977) Electrical membrane potentials, tissue excitation, and various relevant interpretations. In: *Biologic Effects of Electric and Magnetic Fields Associated with Proposed Project Seafarer.* National Academy of Sciences, Washington, D.C., pp. 401–411.

Schwarz, G. (1962) A theory of the low-frequency dielectric dispersion of colloidal particles in electrolyte solutions. *J. Phys. Chem.* **66**:2636.

Seaman, R. L., and H. Wachtel (1978) Slow and rapid responses to CW and pulsed microwave radiation by individual *Aplysia* pacemakers. *J. Microwave Power* **13**:77.

Sercl, M., D. Jechova, M. Komrska, J. Kovarik, V. Kyral, H. Licha, J. Licky, S. Nettl, D. Simkiva, J. Slovicek, L. Urcha, L. Zdrahal, M. Tusl, S. Svorcova, and V. Kamt (1961) On the effects of cm electromagnetic waves on the nervous system of man: radar. *Sb. Ved. Pr. Lek. Fak. Karlovy Univ. Hradci Kralove* **4**:427.

Serdiuk, A. M. (1969) Biological effect of low-intensity ultrahigh frequency fields. *Vrach. Delo* **11**:108.

Servantie, B., G. Bertharion, R. Joly, A. M. Servantie, J. Etienne, P. Dreyfus, and P. Escoubet (1974) Pharmacologic effects of a pulsed microwave field. In: *Biological Effects and Health Hazards of Microwave Radiation*, P. Czerski, K. Ostrowski, M. L. Shore, C. Silverman, M. J. Suess, and B. Waldeskog (eds.) Polish Medical Publishers, Warsaw, pp. 36–45.

Servantie, B., A. M. Servantie, and J. Etienne (1975) Synchronization of cortical neurons by a pulsed microwave field as evidenced by spectral analysis of EEG from the white rat. *Ann N.Y. Acad. Sci.* **247**:82.

Shelton, W. W., and J. H. Merritt (1979) In vitro study of microwave effects on calcium efflux in rat brain tissue. *URSI Abstracts*, p. 338.

Shelton, W. W., and J. H. Merritt (1980) Efflux of $^{45}Ca^{++}$ from rat cortex tissue under microwave radiation. *Bioelectromagnetics* **1**:250A.

Sheyvekhman, B. Y. (1949) Effect of the action of a VHF–HF field on the aural sensitivity during application of electrodes in the zone of projection of the aural zone of the cortex (lamella of temporal bone). *Probl. Fiziol. Akust.* **1**:122.

Snyder, S. H. (1970) The effects of microwave irradiation on the turnover rate of serotonin and norepinephrine in rat brain. Annual Summary Report, Department of Pharmacology, Johns Hopkins University, p. 15.

Spackman, D. H., and V. Riley (1978) Studies of RF radiation effects on blood–brain barrier permeability using fluorescein and amino acids. *Proc. Biol. Eff. E.M. Waves.* XIX Gen. Assembly. Int. Union Radio Sci., Helsinki.

Stavinoha, W. B., B. Pepelko, and P. W. Smith (1970) Microwave radiation to inactivate cholinesterase in rat brain prior to analysis for acetylcholine. *Pharmacologist* **12**:257.

Stavinoha, W. B., M. A. Medina, J. Frazer, S. T. Weintraub, D. H. Ross, A. T. Modak, and D. J. Jones (1976) The effects of 19 megacycle irradiation on mice and rats. In: *Biological Effects of Electromagnetic Waves*, Vol. I, C. C. Johnson and M. L. Shore (eds.). HEW Publ. (FDA) 77-8010, pp. 431–448.

Stverak, I., K. Marha, and G. Pafkova (1974) Some effects of various pulsed fields on animals with audiogenic epilepsy. In: *Biological Effects of Microwave Radiation*, P. Czerski, K. Ostrowski, M. L. Shore, C. Silverman, M. J. Suess, and B. Waldeskog (eds.). Polish Medical Publishers, Warsaw, pp. 141–144.

Sutton, C. H., and F. B. Carroll (1979) Effect of microwave induced hyperthermia on the blood–brain barrier of the rat. *Radio Sci.* **14**:329.

Sutton, C. H., R. L. Nunnally, and F. B. Carroll (1973) Protection of the microwave-irradiated brain with body-core hypothermia. *Cryobiology* **10**:513.

Switzer, W. G., and D. S. Mitchell (1977) Long term effects of 2.45 GHz radiation on the ultrastructure of the cerebral cortex and on hematologic profiles of rats. *Radio Sci.* **12**:287.

Takashima, S., B. Onaral, and H. Schwan (1979) Effects of modulated RF energy on the EEG of mammalian brains. *Radiat Environ. Biophys.* **16**:15.

Taylor, E. M., and B. T. Ashleman (1974) Analysis of central nervous system involvement in the microwave auditory effect. *Brain Res.* **74**:201.

Thomas, J., L. Burch, and S. Yeandle (1979) Microwave radiation and chlordiazepoxide: Synergistic effects on fixed-interval behavior. *Science* **203**:1357.

Thompson, W. D., and A. E. Bourgeois (1965) Effects of Microwave Exposure on Behavior and Related Phenomena. Primate Behavior Lab., Aeromed. Res. Lab. Rep. Wright–Patterson AFB, Ohio (ARL-TR-65-20; AD 489245).

Tolgskaya, M. S. (1959) Morphological changes in animals exposed to 10 cm microwaves. *Vop. Kurortol. Fizioter. Lech. Fiz. Kul't.* **1**:21.

Tolgskaya, M. S., and Z. V. Gordon (1960) Changes in the receptor and interoreceptor apparatuses under the influence of UHF. In: *The Biological Action of Ultrahigh Frequencies*, A. A. Letavet and Z. V. Gordon (eds.). Acad. Med. Sci., Moscow, p. 104.

Tolgskaya, M. S., and Z. V. Gordon (1964) Comparative morphological characterization of the effects of microwaves of various wavelengths. *Tr. Nii Gig. Tr. Prof. AMN SSR* **2**:80.

Tolgskaya, M. S., and Z. V. Gordon (1973) *Pathological Effects of Radio Waves*. Meditsina Press, Moscow (Transl. Consultants Bureau, Plenum Press, 1973).

Tolgskaya, M. S., Z. V. Gordon, and Y. A. Lobanova (1960) Morphological changes in experimental animals under the influence of pulsed and continuous wave SHF-UHF radiation. *Tr. Nii Gig. Tr. Prof. AMN SSR* **1**:90.

Tomashevskaya, L. A., and Y. M. Makarenko (1967) The effect of a shortwave-electric field on certain biochemical processes in the organism. In: *Hygiene of Populated Areas*, Kiev, p. 38.

Tyagin, N. V. (1971) *Clinical Aspects of Irradiation in the SHF Range*. Meditsina Press, Leningrad.

Tyazhelov, V. V., R. E. Tigranian, and E. P. Khizhniak (1977) New artifact-free electrodes for recording of biological potentials in strong electromagnetic fields. *Radio Sci.* **12(6S)**:121.

Veninga, T. S. (1971) The significance of biogenic amines as radio-indicators in experimental animals with reference to man. In: *Biochemical Indicators of Radiation Injury in Man*. International Atomic Energy Agency, Vienna, p. 125.

Wachtel, H., R. Seaman, and W. Joines (1975) Effects of low intensity microwaves on isolated neurons. *Ann. N.Y. Acad. Sci.* **247**:46.

Ward, T. R., J. A. Elder, M. D. Jong, and D. Svendsgaard (1982) Measurement of blood-brain barrier permeation in rats during exposure to 245° MHz microwaves. *Bioelectromagnetics* **3**:371.

Williams, W. M., W. Hoss, M. Formanick, and S. M. Michaelson (1984a) Effects of 2450-MHz microwave energy on the blood-brain barrier to hydrophobic molecules. A. Effect on the permeability to sodium fluoride. *Brain Res. Rev.* **7**:165-170.

Williams, W. M., M. Del Cerro and S. M. Michaelson (1984b) Effects of 2450-MHz microwave energy on the blood-brain barrier to hydrophobic molecules. B. Effect on the permeability to HRP. *Brain Res. Rev.* **7**:171-181.

Williams, W. M., J. Platner, and S. M. Michaelson (1984c) Effects of 2450-MHz microwave energy on the blood-brain barrier to hydrophobic molecules. C. Effect on the permeability to [^{14}C]. *Brain Res. Rev.* **7**:183-190.

Williams, W. M., S-T. Lu, M. Del Cerro, and S. M. Michaelson (1984d) Effects of 2450-MHz microwave energy on the blood-brain barrier to hydrophobic molecules. D. Brain temperature and blood-brain barrier permeability to hydrophilic tracers. *Brain Res. Rev.* **7**:192-212.

Williams, W. M., S-T. Lu, M. Del Cerro, W. Hoss, and S. M. Michaelson (1984e) Effects of 2450-MHz microwave energy on the blood-brain barrier: An overview and critique of past and present research. *IEEE Trans. Microwave Theory and Techniques* **32**: 808-818.

Willis, J. A., S. T. Gaubatz, and D. O. Carpenter (1974) The role of the electrogenic sodium pump in modulation of pacemaker discharge of Aplysia neurons. *J. Cell. Physiol.* **84**:463.

Yakovleva, M. I., T. P. Shlyafer, and I. P. Tsvetkova (1968) On the question of conditioned cardiac reflexes and the functional and morphological status of cortical neurons under the action of SHF-UHF electromagnetic fields. *Zh. Vyssh. Nervn. Deyat. im. I. P. Pavlova* **18**:973.

Yamaura, I., and S. Chichibu (1967) Super-high frequency electric field and crustacean ganglionic discharges. *Tohoku J. Exp. Med.* **93**:249.

Yermakov, Y. V. (1969) On the mechanism of developing astheno-vegetative disturbance under the chronic effect of a SHF-field. *Voen. Med. Zh.* **3**:42.

Zeman, G. H., R. L. Chaput, Z. R. Glazer, and L. C. Gershman (1973) Gamma-aminobutyric acid metabolism in rats following microwave exposure. *J. Microwave Power* **8**:213.

11

Behavioral Effects

As previously indicated, microwaves can produce sensations of warmth and sound in humans. In other species, they also can serve as cues, they may be avoided, and they can disrupt ongoing behavior. These actions appear to be due to heat produced by energy absorption. The rate of absorption depends on the microwave parameters and the electrical and geometric properties of the subject. At "low levels" of exposure, microwaves can produce changes in behavior without large, or even measurable, changes in body temperature. Thermoregulatory behavior may respond to those "low levels" of heat, and thereby affect other behavior occurring concurrently. There are no reliable data demonstrating that behavioral effects of microwaves depend on any mechanism other than reactions to heat (Stern, 1980).

Studies have been conducted on the effects of MW/RF energies on the performance of tasks by trained rats, rhesus and squirrel monkeys (Sanza and de Lorge, 1977; de Lorge, 1976, 1977, 1978, 1979; D'Andrea et al., 1977, 1979; Lin et al., 1977; Gage, 1979; Galloway, 1975). All of the studies indicated that irradiation would suppress performance of the trained task, and that a power density/dose threshold for achieving the suppression existed. Depending on the duration and other parameters of exposure, the threshold power density for affecting trained behavior ranged from 5 to 50 mW/cm^2.

Justesen and King (1970) and King (1969) used a 2450-MHz CW multimodal resonating cavity system to investigate conditioned operant behavior in rats. In food-deprived rats, responding was maintained by a multiple fixed-ratio 40, extinction schedule. During the ratio component, every 40 responses produced a drop of dextrose solution, but during the extinction component, responses never produced a drop. Different stimulus conditions signaled the operation of the different components. Expected performances were observed during the component schedules, when tones or lights served as cues. However, when 2450-MHz microwaves, with simultaneous modulations of 60 and 12 Hz, replaced the tones or lights, they failed to function as cues over a range of exposure levels including those that could produce behavioral disruption. The investigators used a recurrent cycle of exposure, 5 min on and 5 min off, over a 30-min period at average absorbed energies of 3.0, 6.2, and 9.2 W/kg. The animal's performance usually stopped near the end of the 60-min test period during exposure with an energy absorption rate of 6.2 W/kg; at 9.2 W/kg, this effect occurred much earlier in the test period.

In a different study, under a different set of exposure conditions, rats were trained to respond for food in the presence of an auditory stimulus, but not in its absence (Johnson et al., 1977). Under this multiple schedule, responding during presentation of 918-MHz pulsed microwaves was similar to that occurring during the tone, but responding did not occur in its absence. Thus, the microwaves served as discriminative stimuli. These studies demonstrate that a cue function is not an intrinsic property of microwaves. Instead, such a function is an outcome that depends jointly on the behavioral and microwave parameters of the experiment (Stern, 1980).

Frey and Feld (1975) reported that rats avoid pulsed, but not CW, 1.2-GHz microwaves. It is quite possible that "microwave hearing" in this study facilitates acquiring such avoidance behaviors. If the rat is avoiding microwave-induced hearing, then the rat might avoid CW microwaves if another stimulus were presented along with them (Grove et al., 1979). Reported differences in behavioral effects between pulsed and CW microwaves may be controlled by the auditory consequences of the exposure (Stern, 1980). Rats apparently will avoid/escape pulsed but not CW microwaves at the same average power density. The auditory stimulus itself or in conjunction with the body heating might be aversive. Alternatively, but not necessarily mutually exclusive, is the likelihood that the auditory stimulus could provide a cue indicating the presence versus the absence of the microwaves that is more salient than the concomitant changes in temperature. Little work has addressed the significance of the cueing function of pulsed microwaves (Hjersen et al., 1979; Johnson et al., 1977). Finally, similar consequences of localized brain heating (if, indeed, that is the mechanism) could potentially produce other (behavioral) effects of exposure to microwaves (Lebovitz, 1973).

Some studies have examined the effect of microwaves on a behavioral baseline in which there is no explicit relationship between the behavior and the exposure to microwaves. The behavioral endpoint frequently is measured only during the absence of microwaves, usually in a different chamber. Here, the additional factors of handling and time since exposure intrude as potentially significant parameters that are often not reported (Stern, 1980).

Behavioral baseline studies include: open field behavior (Korbel,

1970), activity (Gillard et al., 1977; Hunt et al., 1975; Korbel, 1970; Mitchell et al., 1977; Roberti et al., 1975), swimming endurance (Hunt et al., 1975), food-maintained free operant behaviors (de Lorge, 1976, 1977; King, 1969; King et al., 1971; Mitchell et al., 1977; Thomas et al., 1975, 1977), and electric shock avoidance or escape (Mitchell et al., 1977; Roberti et al., 1975). Selection of the baseline often appears to have been arbitrary. The clearest index of microwave exposure is a cessation or reduction of responding, sometimes correlated with increases in colonic temperature (Stern, 1980).

Hunt et al. (1975), using a multimodal resonating cavity to expose rats to 2450 MHz pulsed, reported effects on exploratory activity, swimming, and discrimination performance of a vigilance task, after a 30-min exposure at about 6 W/kg. Lobanova (1960) exposed rats to 3000-MHz pulsed microwaves, after which the rats were tested for swimming time. A decrease in endurance was noted after exposure to power–time combinations ranging from $100 \, mW/cm^2$ for 5 min to $10 \, mW/cm^2$ for 90 min.

Roberti et al. (1975) measured the running time of rats in an electrifiable runway in which each subject was trained to peak performance. Exposure for 185 h at 10.7 GHz CW, 3 GHz CW, and 3 GHz pulsed, to $1 \, mW/cm^2$, caused no performance decrements. No change in baseline performance was noted when rats were irradiated with 3 GHz pulsed, for 17 days, with a power density of $25 \, mW/cm^2$.

In a study by D'Andrea et al. (1979), Long–Evans adult rats were exposed for 16 weeks to 915-MHz CW microwaves at an average power density of $5 \, mW/cm^2$. The resulting dose rate was 1.23 ± 0.25 S.E.M. mW/g. The animals were exposed 8 hr/day, 5 days/week, for a total of 640 hr (16 weeks) in a monopole above ground radiation chamber while housed in Plexiglas cages. Measures of spontaneous locomotor activity by both wheel revolutions and stabilimetric platforms indicated possible increases in activity after microwave exposure. Cortical EEG measured after microwave exposure also revealed no significant effects. Biweekly stabilimetric tests immediately after exposure revealed a significant depression of behavioral activity. Measures of locomotor activity based on revolutions of a running wheel, which were obtained during 12-hr periods between each 8-hr exposure, showed no significant effect of the exposure.

Lin et al. (1977) exposed rats to 918 MHz CW at 10, 20, or $40 \, mW/cm^2$ for 30 min. No effects on response rates were noted at the two lower levels, but at $40 \, mW/cm^2$ the animals' performance decreased after 5 min of exposure and ceased after about 15 min of exposure. The average energy absorption rate measured thermographically was $0.21 \, W/kg$ per incident mW/cm^2 or $8.4 \, W/kg$ absorbed at $40 \, mW/cm^2$.

Thomas et al. (1975) reported response-rate changes in rats exposed at between 5 and 20 mW/cm^2 to 2860 MHz CW and 9600 MHz pulsed. Response rates increased in five of ten tests, which suggested to the authors that "low-level" microwaves produce effects on the CNS.

de Lorge (1978) exposed rats, squirrel monkeys, and rhesus monkeys to 2450 MHz under far-field conditions. All animals were food deprived and performed on operant schedules for food reinforcement during the microwave exposures. Exposure sessions lasted 60 min and were repeated on a daily basis. Stable performance on the operant schedules was disrupted in all three species at power densities positively correlated with the body mass of the animals. When the averages of these power densities (28, 45, and 67 mW/cm^2) were plotted as a function of body mass (0.3, 0.7 and 5 kg), a semilog relationship was evident. Extrapolation along the resulting curve could permit prediction of the power densities needed to disrupt ongoing operant behavior in larger animals. The power densities associated with behavioral disruption approximated those power densities that produced an increase in colonic temperature of at least 1°C above control levels in the responding animals.

In these studies, the changes in behavior were observed as a consequence of exposure only when there were measured increases in core temperature. The simplest interpretation of such findings is that the thermal burden induced the change in behavior (de Lorge, 1979). These data support the need for scaling factors to extrapolate from small animals to larger species.

Galloway (1975) studied the performance of four monkeys irradiated by means of a 2450-MHz CW waveguide applicator (total absorbed power 10, 15, or 25 W) applied to the head. The duration of the exposure was 2 min or until convulsions began between 15 W and 25 W. Because of skin burns, only two subjects completed this series of experiments. Even with the severe exposures, there were no performance decrements in a discrimination task that the subjects performed immediately after the periodic exposures. Acquisition of a new task during the first ten trials of training was impaired at 25 W, which resulted in convulsions.

Diachenko and Milroy (1975) studied the effects of pulsed and CW microwaves on operant behavior in rats trained to perform a lever pressing response on a DRL (differential reinforcement of low rate) schedule. The rats were tested immediately after a 1-hr daily exposure to 2450 MHz at 1, 5, 10, and 15 mW/cm^2. No behavioral effects were found at these levels; however, the subjects exposed to 10 mW/cm^2, while showing no significant decrement in performance, did show obvious signs of heat stress.

A pharmacodynamic approach has been taken by some investigators in the study of microwave exposure effects on the CNS and on behavior

(Baranski and Edelwejn, 1968; Edelwejn, 1968; Thomas and Maitland, 1979). Following exposure to 10-cm pulsed microwaves, altered sensitivity to neurotropic drugs was noted. Decreased tolerance of rabbits to pentylenetetrazol and increased tolerance to strychnine were observed after a single exposure to 20 mW/cm^2. Repeated exposures at 7 mW/cm^2 produced a decreased tolerance to pentylenetetrazol, strychnine, and acetophenetidin (Baranski and Edelwejn, 1968).

Servantie *et al.* (1974) reported that exposure of rats to 3000 MHz at 5 mW/cm^2 for several days resulted in an altered reaction to pentylenetetrazol. Using curarelike compounds, a neuromuscular site of action for this microwave effect was implicated. Edelwejn (1968) observed alterations in the effects of chlorpromazine and/or D-tubocurarine on EEG recordings in rabbits repeatedly exposed to 7 mW/cm^2. The author concluded that synaptic structures at the level of the brain stem are affected by microwaves.

Thomas and Maitland (1979) investigated the effects of pulsed 2.45 GHz at 1 mW/cm^2 in combination with dextroamphetamine on behavior in rats. Both acute and repeated exposures modified the normal dose–effect function so that the maximum drug effect was obtained at lower microwave exposures. In another study, chlordiazepoxide-induced changes in the behavior of rats were enhanced by simultaneous exposure to 2450-MHz microwaves, pulsed at 500 Hz with a pulse width of 2 μsec, at a power density that did not itself affect the baseline performance (Thomas *et al.*, 1979). Unfortunately, the energy absorption rate was not specified, nor were there any attempts to replicate the observation with thermal controls.

Galloway and Waxler (1977) employed a serotonin-depleting drug (fenfluramine) to investigate the effect of 2.45-GHz CW microwaves at integral dose rates of 1–15 W. Combinations of the drug and microwaves at an integral dose rate of 15 W resulted in behavioral deficits whereas the drug or microwaves alone at up to 15 W failed to produce this effect. With respect to drugs such as dextroamphetamine and fenfluramine, their influence on thermal regulation may be significant in these results.

BEHAVIORAL THERMOREGULATION

That microwaves can affect behavior under certain conditions should not be surprising. We know that heat produces numerous reactions in animals, many of which serve to regulate body temperature. Some of these reactions are behavioral (Carlisle, 1970; Corbit, 1970; Hainsworth, 1967; Hamilton, 1963; Roberts *et al.*, 1974; Satinoff and Henderson, 1977). Temperature change can control behavior just as other stimuli such as sights, sounds, odors, and so on. Although temperature change can elicit behavioral reactions, it can also serve as a discriminative, or signaling stimulus, or as a stimulus to be sought, e.g., heat from the sun on a cool day, or to be avoided, e.g., heat from the sun on a hot day. Since microwaves produce heat, and we already know that heat can serve multiple functions in the control of behavior, it seems surprising that most behavioral studies of microwaves have not attempted a systematic analysis to determine the extent to which microwaves can influence these functions. Adequate interpretations of behavioral effects of microwaves require this information (Stern, 1980). It should be understood, however, that the capability for quantifying behavioral thermoregulatory motivation in animal experiments, where physiological variables could be freely manipulated, is relatively recent. Unlike physiological thermoregulation in which quantification of responses was made possible by early advances in thermometry, the development of operant conditioning techniques for precise measurement of thermoregulatory behavior is less than 25 years old.

Most of the research on the nervous system and behavior has been carried out in rodents and other small animals. Behavior among animal species reflects adaptive brain–behavior patterns. Behavioral thermoregulation is seen as an attempt to maintain a nearly constant internal thermal environment. Changes in body temperature bring about not only autonomic drives but also behavioral drives (Stolwijk, 1977). That microwaves can influence behavioral thermoregulation has been shown by Stern *et al.* (1979), Adair (1979), and Adair and Adams (1980). Behavioral responses are not necessarily manifestations of specific changes in the CNS and may be a function of direct or indirect action of microwaves on other body systems. However, they do indicate the existence of alterations in the animal's behavioral response patterns. Extrapolation of brain–behavior functions from lower animals to man is thus subject to many difficulties.

In assessing the significance of the reported behavioral changes, it is important to recognize certain fundamental factors. The resting metabolic rate for rats is approximately 7 W/kg. When the power input exceeds this level, disruption of behavior can be elicited. In most of the reports, alterations in the behavior of rats were observed with exposures at average energy absorption rates of 5 to 8 W/kg or greater, i.e., at similar exposure levels to those that produce increases in circulating corticosterone concentrations in rats (Lotz and Michaelson, 1978). Behavioral changes may be related to subtle heat alterations within the body. Heat may produce a general debilitating effect or decreased motivation for food, since it has been shown that rats maintained in hot environments eat less food (Hamilton, 1963) and rats showed decreased response and food reinforcement frequency on an operant schedule when the environmental temperature is 35°C, but not at 25°C. Behavioral responses may thus be influenced by the interaction of the organism with the environment.

The regulation of body temperature can be accomplished by complex patterns of responses of the skeletal musculature to heat and cold, which modify the rates of heat production and/or heat loss [e.g., by exercise, change in body conformation, change in the thermal insulation of bedding (rodents) or clothing (man), and by the selection of an environment that reduces thermal stress (Bligh and Johnson, 1973)].

Thermoregulation is part of a complex control system involving circulation, metabolism, and respiration, as well as neural structures. Temperature signals from cutaneous thermoreceptors reach the somatosensory region of the cerebral cortex. The main processing of thermal signals and generation of a controlling signal for the effector part of thermoregulation takes place in the hypothalamus (Ivanov, 1975).

Strategies or mechanisms to maintain body temperature in a narrow and desirable range in a complex and varying thermal environment are termed thermoregulatory, and fall into two main categories: voluntary behavioral adjustments, and involuntary physiological adjustments. The limits of effectiveness of involuntary physiological thermoregulation are rather narrow, and we must rely on behavioral thermoregulation over most of the range of environmental temperatures to which we are often exposed (Stolwijk, 1977).

Thermal motivation arises in situations of thermal stress. The uncomfortable feeling of excessive warmth creates a desire for temperature reduction; the unpleasant feeling of being too cold elicits the desire for temperature increase. By acting in such a way as to minimize thermal discomfort and maximize thermal comfort, the organism tends to escape from situations of thermal stress and locates itself in a physiologically neutral thermal environment, thereby solving the problem of physiological temperature regulation (Corbit, 1973).

Microwave-induced behavioral thermoregulation has been studied by Adair and Adams (1980) and Stern *et al.* (1979). In the study by Stern *et al.* (1979), a shaved rat was placed in a small chamber located in a dark refrigerated room. By pressing a lever, the rat could turn on a heat lamp for 2 sec. After a few sessions, the rat pressed the lever at a nearly constant rate for several hours. Then microwave exposures began. During a single session, the rat was exposed to 2450-MHz CW microwaves several times with a 15-min control period preceding each 15-min exposure. The incident power density varied between 5 and 20 mW/cm^2. The rate of turning on the heat lamp decreased as the power density increased. Statistical analyses confirmed that decrements in responding occurred at each power density. This experiment demonstrates that not only is behavior sensitive to changes in the thermal environment, but also that the behavioral adjustments serve a thermoregulatory function and do so in the absence of changes in, and in fact ensure the constancy of colonic temperature (Stern, 1980).

Similar results have been observed by Adair and Adams (1980) in a systematic replication with squirrel monkeys. In addition, in a variation of the procedure, a monkey increased its rate of responding during microwave exposure when it responded to cool itself in an otherwise hot environment. Thus, the microwaves need not suppress ongoing behavior. In neither experiment was there any sign of debilitation due to exposure to microwaves. Instead, the behavior showed an exquisite sensitivity to changes in thermal variables. This preparation represents a powerful tool for examining the functional significance of the absorption of microwaves as heat. Both its sensitivity and the importance of such regulatory functioning are reasons for using thermoregulatory behavior as a baseline in future studies of the behavioral effects of microwaves (Stern, 1980).

D'Andrea et al. (1978) reported that whiptail lizards placed in a 2450-MHz CW microwave gradient preferentially selected maximum microwave exposure (93 mW/cm^2) and thereby achieved some degree of body temperature regulation. On the other hand, when the lizards were allowed freedom to move beneath an infrared source, activity was greater and the regulated internal body temperature was 3°C higher than during microwave exposure. These results imply either inefficient microwave capture or perhaps an overriding effect of ambient temperature (unspecified) on thermoregulatory efficiency. However, it is clear that a microwave source can be utilized by a behaving organism as part of its thermoregulatory strategy (Adair and Adams, 1980). It should be noted, however, that the reported behavioral reactions are generally reversible upon cessation of exposure.

REFERENCES

Adair, E. R. (1979) Microwave modification of thermoregulatory behavior: Threshold and suprathreshold effects. *Bioelectromagnetics Symposium*, Seattle, p. 331.

Adair, E. R., and B. W. Adams (1980) Microwaves modify thermoregulatory behavior in squirrel monkey. *Bioelectromagnetics* **1**:1.

Baranski, S., and Z. Edelwejn (1968) Studies on the combined effects of microwaves and some drugs on bioelectric activity of rabbit CNS. *Acta Physiol. Pol.* **19**:37.

Bligh, J., and K. G. Johnson (1973) Glossary of terms for thermal physiology. *J. Appl. Physiol.* **35**:941.

Carlisle, H. J. (1970) Thermal reinforcement and temperature regulation. In: *Animal Psychophysics: The Design and Conduct of Sensory Experiments*, W. C. Stebbins (ed.). Prentice–Hall, Englewood Cliffs, N.J., pp. 211–229.

Corbit, J. D. (1970) Behavioral regulation of body temperature. In: *Physiological and Behavioral Temperature Regulation*, J. Hardy, A. P. Gagge, and J. A. J. Stolwijk (eds.). Thomas, Springfield, Ill., pp. 777-830.

Corbit, J. D. (1973) Thermal motivation. *Neurosci. Res. Program Bull.* **11**(4):317.

D'Andrea, J. A., O. P. Gandhi, and J. L. Lords (1977) Behavioral and thermal effects of microwave radiation at resonant and nonresonant wave lengths. *Radio Sci.* **12**(6S):251.

D'Andrea, J. A., O. Cuellar, O. P. Gandhi, J. L. Lords, and H. C. Nielson (1978) Behavioral thermoregulation in the whiptail lizard (*Cnemidophophorus tigris*) under 2450 MHz CW microwaves. In: *Proc. Biol. Eff. E.M. Waves.* XIX Gen. Assembly. Int. Union Radio Sci., Helsinki, p. 88.

D'Andrea, J. A., O. P. Gandhi, J. L. Lords, C. H. Durney, C. C. Johnson, and L. Astle (1979) Physiological and behavioral effects of chronic exposure to 2450 MHz microwaves. *J. Microwave Power* **14**:351.

de Lorge, J. (1976) Operant behavior and colonic temperature of Squirrel Monkeys (*Saimiri sciureus*) during microwave irradiation. NAMRL-1222, Naval Aerospace Medical Research Laboratory, Pensacola, Fla.

de Lorge, J. (1977) Operant behavior and colonic temperature of Squirrel Monkeys (*Saimiri sciureus*) during microwave irradiation. NAMRL-1236, Naval Aerospace Medical Research Laboratory, Pensacola, Fla.

de Lorge, J. (1978) Disruption of behavior in mammals of three different sizes exposed to microwaves: Extrapolation to larger mammals. In: *Electromagnetic Fields in Biological Systems*, S. S. Stuchly (ed.). IMPI, Edmonton, Canada, pp. 215-228.

de Lorge, J. (1979) Operant behavior and rectal temperature of squirrel monkey during 2.45 GHz microwave irradiation. *Radio Sci.* **14**:217.

Diachenko, J. A., and W. C. Milroy (1975) The effects of high power pulsed and low level CW microwave radiation on an operant behavior in rats. Naval Surface Weapons Center, Dahlgren Laboratory, Dahlgren, Va.

Edelwejn, Z. (1968) An attempt to assess the functional state of the cerebral synapses in rabbits exposed to chronic irradiation with microwaves. *Acta Physiol. Pol.* **19**:897.

Frey, A. H., and S. R. Feld (1975) Avoidance by rats of illumination with low-power nonionizing electromagnetic energy. *J. Comp. Physiol. Psychol.* **89**:183.

Gage, M. (1979) Behavior in rats after exposure to various power densities of 2450 MHz microwaves. *Neurobehav. Toxicol.* **1**:137.

Galloway, W. D. (1975) Microwave dose-response relationships on two behavioral tasks. *Ann N.Y. Acad. Sci.* **247**:410.

Galloway, W. D., and M. Waxler (1977) Interaction between microwave and neuroactive compounds. In: *Biological Effects and Measurement of Radiofrequency/Microwaves*, D. G. Hazzard (ed.). HEW Publ. (FDA) 77-8026, pp. 62-66.

Gillard, J. B., B. Servantie, G. Bertharion, A. M. Servantie, J. K. C. Obrenovitch, and J. C. Perrin (1977) Study of the microwave-induced perturbations of the behavior by the open-field test in the white rat. In: *Biological Effects of Electromagnetic Waves*, Vol. II, C. C. Johnson and M. L. Shore (eds.). HEW Publ. (FDA) 77-8010, pp. 175-186.

Grove, A. M., D. M. Levinson, and D. R. Justesen (1979) Attempts to cue successful escape from a highly intense microwave field by photic stimulation. In: *Bioelectromagnetics Symposium.* Seattle, p. 454.

Hainsworth, F. R. (1967) Saliva spreading, activity, and body temperature regulation in the rat. *Am. J. Physiol.* **212**:1288.

Hamilton, C. L. (1963) Interactions of food intake and temperature regulation in the rat. *J. Comp. Physiol.* **56**:476.

Hjersen, D. L., S. R. Doctor, and R. L. Sheldon (1979) Shuttlebox side preference during pulsed microwave and conventional auditory cues. In: *Electromagnetic Fields in Biological Systems*, S. S. Stuchly (ed.). IMPI, Edmonton, Canada, pp. 194-214.

Hunt, E. L., N. W. King, and R. D. Phillips (1975) Behavioral effects of pulsed microwave radiation. *Ann. N.Y. Acad. Sci.* **247**:440.

Ivanov, K. P. (1975) Temperature signalization and its processing in an organism. In: *Mechanisms of Information Processing in Sensory Systems.* Izdatel'stvo Nauka, Leningrad, p. 7.

Johnson, R. B., D. E. Myers, A. W. Guy, and R. H. Lovely (1977) Discriminative control of appetitive behavior by pulsed microwave radiation in rats. In: *Biological Effects of Electromagnetic Waves,* Vol. I, C. C. Johnson and M. L. Shore (eds.). HEW Publ. (FDA) 77-8010, pp. 238–247.

Justesen, D. R., and N. W. King (1970) Behavioral effects of low-level microwave irradiation in the closed space situation. In: *Biological Effects and Health Implications of Microwave Radiation,* S. F. Cleary (ed.). HEW Publ. BRH/DBE 70-2, p. 154.

King, N. W. (1969) The Effects of Low Level Microwave Irradiation Upon Reflexive, Operant, and Discrimination Behaviors of the Rat. Dissertation, University of Kansas (University Microfilms, Inc., Ann Arbor, 69-21, 540).

King, N. W., D. R. Justesen, and R. L. Clarke (1971) Behavioral sensitivity to microwave irradiation. *Science* **172**:398.

Korbel, S. F. (1970) Behavioral effects of low intensity UHF radiation. In: *Biological Effects and Health Implications of Microwave Radiation,* S. F. Cleary (ed.). HEW Publ. BRH/DBE 70-2, pp. 180–184.

Lebovitz, R. M. (1973) Caloric vestibular stimulation via UHF-microwave irradiation. *IEEE Trans. Biomed. Eng.* **20**:119.

Lin, J. C., A. W. Guy, and L. T. Caldwell (1977) Thermographic and behavioral studies of rats in the near field of 918-MHz radiations. *IEEE Trans. Microwave Theory Tech.* **MTT-25**:833.

Lobanova, Y. A. (1960) Survival and development of animals at various intensities and duration of SHF action. *Tr. Nii Gig. Prof. Tr. AMN SSR* **1**:61.

Lotz, W. G., and S. M. Michaelson (1978) Temperature and corticosterone relationship in microwave exposed rats. *J. Appl. Physiol.* **44**:438.

Mitchell, D. S., W. G. Switzer, and E. L. Bronaugh (1977) Hyperactivity and disruption of operant behavior in rats after multiple exposures to microwave irradiation. *Radio Sci.* **12(6S)**:263.

Roberti, B., G. H. Heebels, J. C. M. Hendricx, A. H. A. M. de Greef, and O. L. Wolthuis (1975) Preliminary investigations of the effects of low-level microwave radiation on spontaneous motor activity in rats. *Ann. N.Y. Acad. Sci.* **247**:417.

Roberts, W. W., R. D. Mooney, and J. R. Martin (1974) Thermoregulatory behaviors of laboratory rodents. *J. Comp. Physiol. Psychol.* **86**:693.

Sanza, J. N., and J. de Lorge (1977) Fixed interval behavior of rats exposed to microwaves at low power densities. *Radio Sci.* **12(6S)**:273.

Satinoff, E., and R. Hendersen (1977) Thermoregulatory behavior. In: *Handbook of Operant Behavior,* W. K. Honig and J. E. R. Staddon (eds.). Prentice–Hall, Englewood Cliffs, N.J., pp. 153–173.

Servantie, B., G. Bertharion, R. Joly, A. M. Servantie, J. Etienne, P. Dreyfus, and P. Escoubet (1974) Pharmacologic effects of a pulsed microwave field. In: *Biological Effects and Health Hazards of Microwave Radiation.* P. Czerski, K. Ostrowski, M. L. Shore, C. Silverman, M. J. Suess, and B. Waldeskog (eds.). Polish Medical Publishers, Warsaw, pp. 36–45.

Stern, S. (1980) Behavioral effects of microwaves. *Neurobehav. Toxicol.* **2**:49.

Stern, S., L. Margolin, B. Weiss, S. T. Lu, and S. M. Michaelson (1979) Microwaves: Effect on thermoregulatory behavior in rats. *Science* **206**:1198.

Stolwijk, J. A. J. (1977) Responses to the thermal environment. *Fed. Proc.* **36**:1655.

Thomas, J. R., and G. Maitland (1979) Microwave radiation and dextroamphetamine: Evidence of combined effects on behavior of rats. *Radio Sci.* **14:**253.

Thomas, J. R., E. D. Finch, D. W. Fulk, and L. S. Burch (1975) Effects of low level microwave radiation on behavioral baselines. *Ann. N.Y. Acad. Sci.* **247:**425.

Thomas, J. R., S. S. Yeandle, and L. S. Burch (1977) Modification of internal discriminative control of behavior by low levels of pulsed microwave radiation. In: *Biological Effects of Electromagnetic Waves,* Vol. I, C. C. Johnson and M. L. Shore (eds.). HEW Publ. (FDA) 77-8010, pp. 201-214.

Thomas, J. R., L. S. Burch, and S. S. Yeandle (1979) Microwave radiation and chlordiazepoxide: Synergistic effects on fixed-interval behavior. *Science* **103:**1357.

12

Neuroendocrine Effects

12.1. INTRODUCTION TO NEUROENDOCRINE PHYSIOLOGY

To maintain homeostasis, a mammal possesses two control mechanisms that react to changes in internal and external environments (stimuli or stress). These two control mechanisms are the neural and endocrine systems. Separation of endocrine from neural control is not always possible as neural signals are integrated at the hypothalamus to react to deviations in the internal or external environment. Hypothalamic–hypophysial–adrenocortical (HHA), hypothalamic–hypophysial–thyroidal (HHT), and hypothalamic–hypophysial–somatotropic (HHS) are three endocrine systems that participate in the "stress" response. Generally, they operate through a negative feedback mechanism.

The neuroendocrine system is an exquisitely sensitive organ and chemical system intimately involved with, and under the influence of the CNS. This system exhibits a profound influence on the body, often through the effects it has on the metabolism of various tissues. The neuroendocrine system in coordination with higher nervous centers is a major regulatory system in the body. The functional relationships of the neuroendocrine system follow a cybernetic pattern, with feedback mechanisms playing an essential role. These relationships in the endocrine system are distinguished by a hierarchy of activities, which consist of three levels of organization (hypothalamus, hypophysis, endocrine gland) in which overall output function, the secretion of hormones by the endocrine gland, is controlled by the balance of signals.

This balance is further modified by direct neural inputs from higher brain centers and peripheral nerves. A simplified block diagram indicating each level of organization and the known feedback and control pathways is shown in Fig. 12-1. The sensitivity of this system to perturbation is greatest at its highest level, the hypothalamus, where small chemical or electrical stimuli can produce significant alterations in the amount of hormones secreted by the endocrine gland. Thus, the neuroendocrine system forms a sensitive mode of analyzing responses of the endocrine system itself, and higher CNS centers under the influence

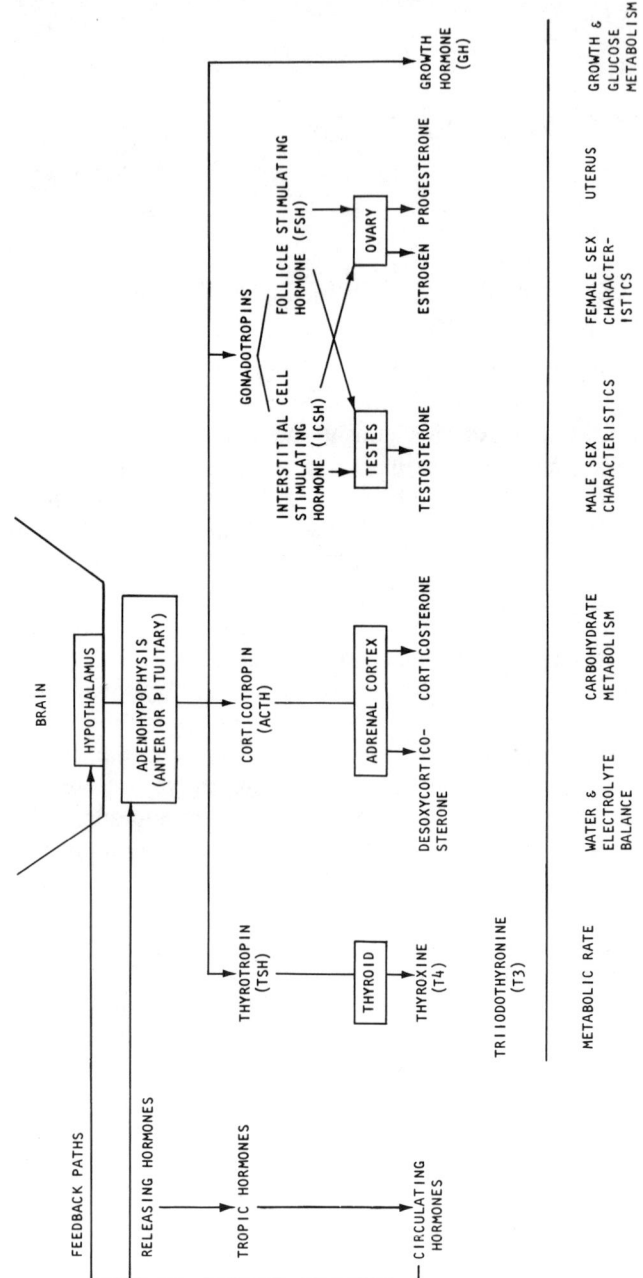

FIGURE 12-1. Neuroendocrine interrelationships.

of environmental changes and organismic readjustments. On this basis, it is reasonable to expect that alterations in the levels of the secretory products of these organs will occur in response to microwave exposure at some time–intensity relationship.

Over the past 40 years, the pathways of interaction and many interrelationships among the cerebral cortex, thalamus, midbrain, hypothalamus, hypophysis, and the various endocrine end organs have methodically been identified and clarified. During the last decade, with the advent of various laboratory methods such as radioimmunoassay for various hormones, refined electrostimulatory methodology, and a host of other analytical techniques, our knowledge and understanding of the neuroendocrine system has expanded remarkably. It is now a fairly accessible system for analysis by direct techniques of study.

Embryologically, the posterior lobe of the pituitary gland (neurohypophysis) develops from a region of the base of the brain called the diencephalon (later to become the hypothalamus), to which the posterior lobe remains attached directly, with neuronal interconnections. The anterior lobe of the pituitary gland (adenohypophysis) does not originate from neural tissues, but from an outpouching of the primitive embryo's mouth (stomodeum) called Rathke's pouch. It is connected to the hypothalamus by way of special vascular channels, called the pituitary portal system.

There is considerable evidence that the hypothalamus, which contains nuclei (groups of nerve cell bodies) and neuronal interconnections involved in the control and adaptation of the autonomic nervous system, various visceral functions, temperature regulation, feeding and mating impulses, and other activities, releases specific factors into the pituitary portal system that regulate the release of specific pituitary hormones. For certain pituitary hormones, there is evidence of the existence of specific releasing factor(s) and inhibiting factor(s), which originate in the hypothalamus.

In the body, endocrine organs and the humoral factors they release, act alone, in an integrative manner with one another, as well as through the coordinating mechanisms of the CNS. There is considerable interdependence and interrelationship between the various glands and hormones of this complex system that are not completely understood. It is recognized, nevertheless, that the neuroendocrine system is an exquisitely sensitive organ and chemical system intimately involved with and under the influence of the CNS, exhibiting a profound influence on the body, often through the effects it has on the metabolism of various tissues.

Endocrine balance is modified by direct neural input from higher brain centers and peripheral nerves. As an example, adrenergic neurons in the hypothalamus stimulate thyrotropin-releasing hormone (TRH) acting on the anterior pituitary to increase thyrotropin (TSH), which enters the general circulation to stimulate thyroid secretion of triiodothyronine (T_3) and thyroxine (T_4). T_3 and T_4 then act by negative feedback control on hypophysial TSH secretion.

There is evidence that suppression of central adrenergic tone is responsible for a reduction of growth hormone (GH) release. A specific growth-hormone-inhibiting factor (GIF) is present in the hypothalamus. GIF inhibits the release of GH and counteracts the effects of growth-hormone-releasing factor (GRF) from the hypothalamus. GRF acts on the anterior pituitary to release GH into the general circulation. GH acts on target tissue to increase glucose level (by decreased utilization) and nonesterified fatty acid levels (by mobilization) and to decrease the amino acid pool for protein synthesis. It is these substrates, especially glucose, that provide a feedback control on the hypothalamus for GH release. GH also acts directly by a short-loop negative feedback control on the hypothalamus and anterior pituitary. Physical stimuli, emotions, or any interference with the body's ability to maintain homeostasis (heat, cold, infections, toxins, lack of oxygen, injury) can result in the liberation of corticotropin-releasing factor (CRF), which in turn stimulates the release of adrenocorticotropic hormone (ACTH) from the anterior pituitary (hypophysis). ACTH then stimulates the secretion by the adrenal cortex of glucocorticoids, which are hormones related to the immune response.

Acting alone or in concert, the various components of the neuroendocrine system play a central role in the integrative activities known as homeokinesis. Normal integrative function of the body or those activities that result from stimuli within the individual or due to alterations in the physical environment are integrated or "linked" together by the reciprocal relationships of the CNS and the endocrine system.

The pathophysiological picture of "stress" has been characterized as the *general adaptation syndrome,* which develops in three stages, the alarm reaction, the stage of resistance, and the stage of exhaustion (Selye, 1946, 1950). The classic triad of the alarm reaction (adrenocortical stimulation, thymicolymphatic hypotrophy, and gastrointestinal ulcer) denotes the stereotyped response of the body to any demand that severely taxes the regulatory processes. The triad of the alarm reaction also points out the involvement of the hypothalamic–hypophysial–adrenocortical system and autonomic control. Only recently has the secretory pattern of adenohypophysial hormones (other than ACTH) been found to be involved in the nonspecific stress responses. It is now well established that in rats, acute stress inhibits GH secretion and stimulates ACTH (Matsuyama *et al.*, 1971) and prolactin release (Neill, 1970). In general, stress-induced hormonal changes are not related to the nature, but rather to the intensity and duration of the stressing agent.

Standard laboratory stressors can easily be found in the experimental procedures that are used in biomedical studies. Such commonplace procedures as handling, novelty of experimental environment and procedures, extreme environmental temperatures, forced muscular exercise, immobilization, transportation, noise, electrical shock, ether anesthesia, and so on can act as stressors under certain conditions. Great care must thus be exercised to ensure that the changes in hormone levels are a response to the specific stressor in question (i.e., electromagnetic fields) rather than to some extraneous factors.

Hypothalamic–adrenocortical interaction displays a diurnal rhythmicity. The interaction is intensified during "stress" to the point of changing or obliterating the diurnal pattern of secretion. Among the strongest of the stressful stimuli are surgery, anesthesia, cold, narcosis, burning, high environmental temperature, and rough handling or restraint. A new environment or new manipulation techniques alter the behavior patterns of animals to induce anxiety, avoidance behavior, and weight loss and thus could be interpreted as being "stressful." Therefore, investigation of the reactions of the endocrine axes to microwaves must be carefully designed and controlled, and investigations should be conducted in animals properly adapted to environmental conditions. For rats, the adaptation period should be at least 14 days (Grant *et al.*, 1971). Unless these factors are taken into consideration, it is not possible to eliminate stress reactions due to extraneous factors in experiments intended to investigate adrenal cortex function in relation to microwave exposure (Mikolajczyk, 1977). This is of paramount importance if one is interested in studying subtle indicators of microwave exposure, especially at lower intensities applied for long periods of time.

Neuroendocrine function and neurotransmitter activity react to alterations in internal or external environments to maintain homeostasis. Changes in hormone levels can result in modification of energy utilization, carbohydrate, fat, and protein metabolism, immune competence, and electrolyte balance. They can also modify perception, neural function, behavior, and mentality. The importance of these neuroendocrine factors is that they are slower and more persistent controllers of body functions than the quickly reactive neural mechanisms. Neuroendocrine functions are the controllers maintaining homeostasis of humans and animals in relation to diverse stimuli.

Functional alterations in the neuroendocrine system of both animals and humans exposed to MW/RF energies have been reported by several investigators. These include changes in the secretions of the pituitary gland, adrenal cortex, thyroid gland, and gonads. Certain investigators believe such changes result from stimulation of the hypothalamic–hypophysial system due to thermal interactions at the hypothalamic or immediately adjacent levels of organization, the hypophysis itself (pituitary), or the particular endocrine gland or end organ under study. According to other researchers, the observed changes have been interpreted to be the result of direct microwave interactions with the CNS. Regardless of which mechanism is responsible for the observed responses, there is no question that this highly integrated, extremely labile system, which is intimately linked to the CNS, has a great potential for study. On this basis, it is reasonable to expect that alterations in the levels of the secretory products of these organs will occur in response to microwave exposure at some time–intensity relationship since shifts of a few millidegrees may alter firing rates in hypothalamic cells (Nakayama *et al.*, 1963). On the other hand, brain temperature changes in the range of 0.1–2.0°C are possible with exercise and a consequence of certain environmental stresses (Baker and Chapman, 1977). In any case, one cannot consider neuroendocrine alterations as necessarily pathological because the function of the neuroendocrine system is to maintain homeostasis and hormone levels will fluctuate to maintain such organismic stability.

Several reviews (Michaelson, 1977; Michaelson *et al.*, 1975; Baranski and Czerski, 1976; Cleary, 1977; Lu *et al.*, 1980; Roberts *et al.*, 1986) have considered neuroendocrine responses in relation to microwave exposure.

12.2. NEUROENDOCRINE AND ENDOCRINE EFFECTS

Response of the endocrine system of rats to whole-body microwave exposure has been studied in recent years, but most of the reports are based on relatively short exposures at modest to high power densities (Lotz, 1979a,b; Lotz and Michaelson, 1978, 1979; Lotz and Podgorski, 1982; Guillet *et al.*, 1975; Guillet and Michaelson, 1977; Houk *et al.*, 1975; Travers and Vetter, 1976; Mikolajczyk, 1972, 1974, 1977; Lu *et al.*, 1977a,b, 1979a,b, 1981; Magin *et al.*, 1977a,b). A comprehensive review of neuroendocrine responses to microwave exposure has been presented by Lu *et al.* (1980).

12.3. HYPOTHALAMIC–HYPOPHYSIAL–ADRENAL RESPONSE

Several investigators have reported that biochemical and physiological changes resulting from microwave exposure suggest an adrenal effect.

According to Petrov and Syngayevskaya (1970), 3 and 24 hr after dogs were irradiated with 3000 MHz, 10 mW/cm^2, the corticosteroid content in their blood had increased by 100–150% above the original level. Serum potassium decreased by 5–10% and sodium increased by the same amount. They also noted that the susceptibility of rats to microwave exposure was sharply increased 1 week after bilateral adrenalectomy. Kirchev et al. (1959) reported that under the influence of an unspecified RF field (3–300 MHz), the weight of the adrenals increased as a result of hyperplasia, indicating adrenal stimulation.

Dumansky et al. (1972) reported that chronic exposure of animals to microwaves (CW or pulsed) is accompanied by reduced activity of blood cholinesterase, increased amount of 17-ketosteroids in the urine, reduced amount of ascorbic acid in the adrenal glands, and reduced weight of the adrenal glands. It should be noted, however, that blood cholinesterase activity is mostly "pseudocholinesterase," which has no correlation with acetylcholine activity, contrary to what the authors imply. Methods for adrenocortical function studies were not detailed.

Demokidova (1974) reported increased adrenal and pituitary gland weight in rats exposed to 69.7 MHz, 12 V/m, 1 hr/day for $1\frac{1}{2}$ months, and increased adrenal weight in infant rats exposed to 48 V/m, 4 hr/day for $1\frac{1}{2}$ months. Decreased weight of the adrenal glands was noted in infant rats exposed to 14.88 MHz, 70 V/m.

Schliephake (1960) observed an increase in 17-ketosteroids in the urine of humans "intentionally" exposed to "centimetric" microwaves (50 mW/cm^2, 10 min); in rats, a marked increase in the ascorbic acid content of the adrenal cortex was observed. The results of Leytes and Skurikina (1961) also indicated increased adrenocortical hormone production 1–2 hr after initiation of microwave exposure. It has been suggested that these results are an indirect indication of increased pituitary ACTH function.

In female mice exposed to 3000 MHz (10 mW/cm^2) twice daily for 5 months, the pituitary retained its gonadotropic function, although its activity was reduced in comparison to that of nonexposed animals (Bereznitskaya, 1968). Tolgskaya et al. (1972), in discussing the dynamics of changes in the neurosecretory function of the hypothalamus, noted the reversibility of the process upon termination of exposure.

Lenko et al. (1966) found that rabbits exposed to 3000 MHz (50–60 mW/cm^2) 4 hr daily for 20 days tended to show a decline in the amount of urinary 17-hydroxycorticosteroids at the beginning of exposure, followed by a gradual return to normal. No change was evident in the excretion of 17-ketosteroids in the urine.

In rats exposed to microwaves of varying intensity, no quantitative changes in corticosterone were found in the adrenals and blood plasma

(Mikolajczyk, 1972). Prepubescent hypophysectomized rats displayed no differences in adrenal growth rate when treated with pituitary homogenates collected either from rats exposed to microwaves or from control rats.

Rats exposed to 2450 MHz CW, 10 mW/cm^2 for 4 hr, showed no change in adrenal weight, phenylethanolamine-N-methyl transferase (PNMT) activity, or epinephrine level (Parker, 1973). After 16 hr of exposure (0.4°C increase in colonic temperature compared to controls), however, decrease in adrenal epinephrine (32%) was significant and PNMT activity was elevated (25%). There were no statistically significant differences ($p > 0.1$) in adrenal or plasma corticosterone levels between exposed and sham-exposed animals. It should be noted, however, that similar alterations in epinephrine levels can occur in rats subjected to a stressor such as immobilization or acute exposure to cold.

Michaelson *et al.* (1967) reported that exposure of dogs to 2880-MHz pulsed microwaves at power densities above 100 mW/cm^2 resulted in physiological responses indicative of adrenocortical stimulation, which was consonant with the concept of nonspecific "stress." It was suggested that microwaves of high power density can act as a "stressor" affecting regulatory and integrative homeokinetic activity resulting in an alteration in homeostasis.

Dumansky and Shandala (1974) reported adrenocortical changes in rats and rabbits chronically exposed (10–12 hr/day, 180 days) to 2 and 5 μW/cm^2, respectively. Petrov and Syngayevskaya (1970) suggested that the enhancement of corticosteroid activity during and after irradiation could be an adaptive reaction. Some animals develop inhibition of adrenocortical function (corticosteroid activity), attended by a decline in resistance to microwaves reflecting insufficient ACTH. Increased resistance may be related to an increase in the secretion of ACTH, which would also be an adaptive reaction of the organism. This is supported by the finding that the resistance of some animals to microwaves is slightly increased when ACTH is administered.

Lotz and Michaelson (1978) and Lu *et al.* (1980) reported that plasma corticosterone (CS) levels in rats exhibited a variable power density–threshold pattern of response, with a different threshold for 120-min exposure than for 30- or 60-min exposure to 2450 MHz CW (Fig. 12-2). For all these durations of exposure, a strong correlation was evident between mean colonic temperature and mean plasma CS levels (Fig. 12-2). The threshold power density was 50 mW/cm^2 for 30- or 60-min exposure, and 20 mW/cm^2 for 120-min exposure (Lu *et al.*, 1980). These thresholds occurred with whole-body SARs of 8.0 and 3.2 W/kg, respectively.

By sequential sampling, it was shown that in the rat, plasma CS increases within 15–30 min of the start of exposure to 2450 MHz and falls

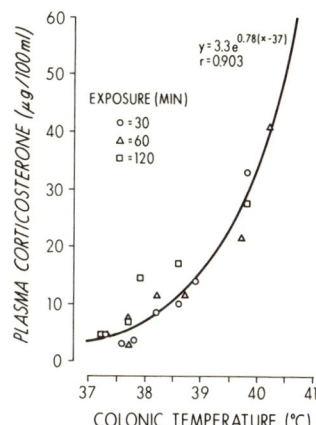

FIGURE 12-2. Correlation between plasma corticosterone level and colonic temperature in rats exposed to 2.45 GHz fields (Lotz and Michaelson, 1978).

sharply within 15–30 min after termination of exposure (Guillet et al., 1975). Thus, the adrenocortical response is transient.

In contrast to the pronounced adrenocortical response observed in intact rats, plasma CS levels in acutely hypophysectomized rats exposed to 60 mW/cm² for 60 min were below control levels (Lotz and Michaelson, 1979). The CS response to microwaves at 50 mW/cm² for 60 min was completely suppressed by 3.2 μg dexamethasone/100 g body wt) (Lotz and Michaelson, 1979). These results are consistent with the hypothesis that the stimulation of the adrenal axis in the microwave-exposed rat is a systematic, integrative process due to general hyperthermia. The results indicate that the microwave-induced CS response observed in rats is dependent upon ACTH secretion by the pituitary, i.e., the adrenal gland is not directly stimulated by microwave exposure. Adrenocortical function may be a sensitive, quantifiable indicator of the physiological compensation required of an animal exposed to microwaves.

Novitskii et al. (1977) studied the corticotropin-releasing factor (CRF) of the median eminence, ACTH of the hypophysis, and 11-oxycorticosteroid of the plasma in Wistar rats (180–230 g) exposed whole body to 0, 0.01, 0.1, 10, and 75 mW/cm² of 12.6-cm (2.6 GHz) microwaves with horizontal polarization for 30 min. Results indicated that the threshold intensity was 0.1 mW/cm² for increases in CRF, ACTH, and 11-oxycorticosteroid: peaking at 1 mW/cm². The finding suggested that the adrenocortical stimulation was a process mediated by the CNS.

It is important to recognize that the hypothalamic–adrenocortical interaction displays a diurnal rhythmicity. The interaction is intensified during "stress" to the point of changing or obliterating the diurnal pattern of secretion. In a study by Lu et al. (1977b) to assess the neuroendocrine responses to protracted exposure, adult rats were exposed to 2450 MHz CW at 1, 5, 10, or 20 mW/cm^2 for 1, 2, 4, or 8 hr. Exposure below 10 mW/cm^2 pushed the appearance of the peak colonic temperature to an earlier time of the day. In rats exposed to 20 mW/cm^2 for 8 hr, the serum CS increase was significantly inhibited from the expected circadian elevation. This inhibition of CS circadian elevation was also noted in rats exposed to 0.1 and 1 mW/cm^2 for 4 hr (Lu et al., 1981). A significant correlation between colonic temperature and CS level was found in sham-exposed rats sacrificed between 1230 and 1930 hr. Similar correlation was noted in rats exposed to 1 to 70 mW/cm^2 for 1 hr and sacrificed at 1230 hr, and rats exposed to 0.1 to 40 mW/cm^2 for 4 hr and sacrificed at 1530 hr. The temperature coefficient decreased sequentially among sham-exposed, 1-hr-exposed, and 4-hr-exposed rats, respectively, and was significantly lower in the 4-hr-exposed rats than in the sham-exposed rats. Thus, a dual action of microwaves on the hypothalamic–hypophysial–adrenocortical (HHA) axis was demonstrated in which low-intensity exposure of the rat (< 10 mW/cm^2) inhibited CS levels during the peak period of the CS circadian oscillation while higher-intensity exposure (> 20 mW/cm^2) stimulated CS secretion during any portion of the circadian periodicity.

In their study, Novitskii et al. (1977) suggested that increased HHA stimulation with increasing intensities from 0.01 to 1 mW/cm^2 (2.6 GHz) could be an indicator of an adaptive reaction of the organism to a harmful agent. The findings in repeated 30-min exposures to 2.6 GHz at 1 mW/cm^2 were considered to be evidence of "cumulative effect" and "exhaustion" by microwave exposure. However, the pattern of this HHA reaction could very well fit into the picture of the "general adaptation syndrome" (Selye, 1946).

Adrenocortical stimulation has been generally accepted to be a result of a stressor stimulus, i.e., a level of stimulation that requires bodily adjustment to counteract the insult. There is consistent evidence that microwave exposure of rats above 25 mW/cm^2 (4 W/kg) stimulates the HHA axis, and that this stimulation is modulated by the CNS. The existing evidence is contradictory for exposures below 25 mW/cm^2, suggesting stimulation in some cases, inhibition or no change in others. It may be that alterations in adrenocortical function at low exposure intensity are smaller than the magnitude of the daily oscillation of this system and are modified by their timing with respect to the normal biological periodicities (Lu et al., 1979a).

12.4. HYPOTHALAMIC–HYPOPHYSIAL–THYROIDAL RESPONSE

One of the major functions of the thyroid hormones is their effect on basal and resting metabolic rate and metabolic generation of heat in the tissues. Pituitary secretion of TSH has been shown to respond in a specific, metabolic pattern to extreme environmental temperature, and appears to respond in a nonspecific manner to other stressful stimuli. TSH secretion is under the control of the CNS, as are the secretions of the other adenohypophysial hormones.

The functional and structural integrity of the thyroid gland is essential for normal homeokinesis of the organism. Not only do the thyroid hormones act at the fundamental level of cellular metabolism by regulating cellular processes to maintain homeostasis, but the thyroid is also an integral member of the neuroendocrine system whose activity is dependent upon and responsive to functional disturbance in other members of the system.

The release of TSH by the anterior pituitary is regulated by an interaction between hypothalamic TRH, which stimulates TSH release, and the calorigenic ("metabolically active") thyroid hormones, T_4 and T_3, which suppress it. Of interest also is the indication that somatostatin (GH–RIH), the growth hormone-release-inhibiting hormone, may regulate TSH secretion by its inhibitory action on TSH release. Interest in this endocrine axis is, therefore, appropriate when considering the possible physiological perturbations of the thyroid as a consequence of microwave exposure.

The literature contains comparatively few experimental studies on the effect of MW/RF energies on the thyroid. In a study by Milroy and Michaelson (1972), rats exposed to microwaves in various regimens (2450 MHz CW, 1 mW/cm^2, continuously for 8 weeks, or 10 mW/cm^2, 8 hr/day for 8 weeks) showed no alterations in thyroid structure or function. On the other hand, Baranski et al. (1972) showed a stimulatory influence of 5 mW/cm^2 on the trapping and secretory function of the thyroid gland of rabbits. According to the authors, these functional changes were in agreement with altered histology of the thyroids.

In rats exposed for 16 hr to 2450 MHz CW at 10 to 25 mW/cm^2, tests of thyroid function in general showed no statistically significant deviations from the norm except that in animals with a 1.0 to 1.7°C increase in colonic temperature there was a reduction in the ability of the thyroid to concentrate iodide (Parker, 1973). Decreased thyroid gland weight was noted in infant rats exposed to 69.7 MHz, 48 V/m, 4 hr/day for 1½ months (Demokidova, 1974).

Indirect evidence has been obtained of some protective influence of lowered general and tissue metabolic rate following hypophysectomy on the time-related lethal exposure of rats to microwaves. Mikolajczyk (1974) found that the survival time of normal rats exposed to microwaves was largely a function of body mass; survival time per unit of body weight was significantly longer in hypophysectomized rats than in normal ones.

Shutenko and Shvayko (1972) found an increase in thyroid activity in animals subjected to a "prolonged exposure in a low-intensity" SHF field. Michaelson *et al.* (1967) reported transiently increased radioactive iodide uptake in dogs exposed to 1280- or 2880-MHz pulsed microwaves, 100–165 mW/cm^2.

Lu *et al.* (1977a) reported that serum T_4 levels were transiently elevated in rats after exposure to 2.45 GHz at 1 mW/cm^2 for 4 hr. This transient increase was not accompanied by changes in serum TSH (Lu *et al.*, 1977b). Magin *et al.* (1977a,b) demonstrated that localized thyroid exposure (2.45 GHz) that resulted in thyroid temperature elevation can stimulate thyroid secretion in the absence of pituitary influence.

Levels of thyroid hormone were found by Vetter (1975) to decrease as the power density of 2.45-GHz microwaves increased from 5 to 25 mW/cm^2. Lu *et al.* (1977a) also noted decreased T_4 levels in rats exposed to 2.45 GHz at 20 mW/cm^2 for 4 to 8 hr.

The thyroid depression apparently reflects inhibition of hypophysial TSH secretion as evidenced by decreased TSH prior to and accompanied by the decreases in serum T_4 in rats exposed to 2.45-GHz CW microwaves at 10 mW/cm^2 for 1 and 2 hr and 20 mW/cm^2 for 2 hr and 8 hr (Lu *et al.*, 1977b). Lotz *et al.* (unpublished observations) investigated TSH levels in rats exposed to 2.45 GHz at 13 to 60 mW/cm^2 for 30, 60, and 120 min. Their results indicated that a 30-min exposure did not affect the TSH levels. Depressed TSH levels were noted in rats exposed at 30 mW/cm^2 (SAR 4.8 W/kg) or higher for 60 min and 13 mW/cm^2 (SAR 2.1 W/kg) or higher for 120 min. Plasma thyroid hormone levels were not studied. A high correlation between decreases in serum T_4 and TSH was also reported in rats exposed to 2.45 GHz, 8 mW/cm^2, 8 hr daily for up to 20 days (Travers and Vetter, 1976),

Stimulation of thyroid function apparently to counteract the influence of decreased TSH, could be revealed in rats exposed to a relatively high power density (2.45 GHz, 70 mW/cm^2) for 1 hr (Lu *et al.*, 1981) or in rats with TSH obliterated by T_3 at the time of exposure to 2.45 GHz at 40 mW/cm^2 for 2 hr (Lu *et al.*, 1979a).

It has been reported that microwave-exposed workers develop an enlarged thyroid gland as well as increased radioactive iodine uptake, but in some cases without clinical symptoms of hyperfunction (Smirnova and Sadchikova, 1960). None of the reported alterations in thyroid function were irreversible or resulted in morbidity. D'Yachenko (1970) described the results of a study of thyroid function in 38 men who operated microwave equipment (centimeter band) for 3 to 15 years. Enhanced ^{131}I uptake by the thyroid was found, which was attributed to secondary effects resulting from radiation-induced disturbances of the sympathetic nervous system in the vicinity of the hypothalamus. Denisiewicz *et al.* (1970) did not find significant disturbances in thyroid function among

142 men exposed to power densities of 10 μW–1 mW/cm^2 while servicing microwave equipment.

Perturbation of the thyroid gland may be the result of an indirect effect, the thermal stress on the body producing a hypothalamic–hypophysial response. This is consistent with microwave-induced thermal stimulation of hypothalamic–hypophysial–thyroidal (HHT) activity (Michaelson et al., 1961). These changes in thyroid activity could be the result of increased TSH and/or increased metabolic activity of the thyroid gland due to heating. McLees and Finch (1971), after reviewing the experimental animal data indicating an increased radioactive iodide uptake by the thyroid following microwave exposure, point out that temperature elevation and heat stress have been associated with alterations in radioactive iodine turnover rate. The HHT axis has been shown to be sensitive to environmental temperature (Collins and Weiner, 1968). Differences in rate of temperature change or alteration in thermal gradients in the body would also result in qualitative differences in endocrine response.

Thus, there appear to be two types of action of microwave exposure on the HHT axis, i.e., local thyroid stimulation and axial inhibition. The local thyroid stimulation is, in contrast to the ACTH-dependent adrenocortical stimulation, caused by high-intensity microwave exposure. The inhibition of the HHT axis by thermogenic microwave exposure is a homeostatic reaction to the increased heat load.

12.5. GROWTH HORMONE

A secretory product of the pituitary is the polypeptide, growth hormone (GH) or somatotropin (STH). It has been shown that fasting, various forms of physical and psychological stress, onset of sleep, arginine infusion, alterations of protein intake, changes in plasma glucose levels, and administration of L-dopa, glucagon, or vasopression affect pituitary production of plasma GH levels (Martin, 1973).

GH circulates in the plasma in an unbound form and has ubiquitous sites of action, unlike its adenohypophysial counterparts, TSH and ACTH, which rely on their target gland secretory products for effect. Among its actions, GH antagonizes the effects of insulin, in that it inhibits cellular uptake of glucose (glucose-sparing or diabetogenic effect), and it causes the release of free fatty acids from tissue storage depots.

In the human and certain nonhuman primates, a variety of stresses, both physical and psychological may produce an acute GH release. The concomitant stresses in the rat are known to effect reduction in plasma

GH levels (Brown and Reichlin, 1972). Pulsatile bursts of GH secretion occur for apparently inexplicable reasons that are not associated with any changes in plasma metabolites that affect or are affected by GH secretion (glucose, free fatty acids, or circulating amino acids).

It appears that GH is regulated by a specific releasing factor (GRF) and a specific inhibiting factor (GIF) that originate in the hypothalamus, whereas ACTH and TSH have only a releasing factor. The absence of inhibiting factors for TSH and ACTH can probably be best explained by the fact that these hormones have specific target tissues, which in turn produce hormones that act via a negative feedback to the hypothalamus. GH, which possesses no specific target tissue, requires some mechanism to control its production. This control is achieved via the concentration of circulating metabolites, integrated with higher center inputs that affect hypothalamic GIF or GRF release when appropriate. It is interesting and significant to note that this area of the hypothalamus, located in the medial basal area, together with the lateral hypothalamus, also functions as a final integrative center for energy balance and food intake. Also, these areas are intimately associated with the region of the hypothalamus involved in temperature regulation (Schally *et al.*, 1973; Martin, 1973).

In the rat (8 to 12 weeks old) exposed to 2.45-GHz microwaves, GH response is altered at various power densities (Michaelson *et al.*, 1975). At $13\,\text{mW/cm}^2$ there is an increase in GH whereas at $36\,\text{mW/cm}^2$ serum GH drops after 60 min of exposure, to significantly low levels. Lotz *et al.* (1977) noted the threshold intensity for GH inhibition to be $50\,\text{mW/cm}^2$ (SAR $8.0\,\text{W/kg}$) for rats exposed to $2.45\,\text{GHz}$ CW for 30 amd 60 min. With exposure for 2 hr at $13\,\text{mW/cm}^2$ (SAR $2.1\,\text{W/kg}$) or higher, GH levels were lower than among sham-exposed rats with progressively lower GH at each successively higher power density. Part of this sensitivity may be attributed to the higher GH levels in the 2-hr-sham-exposed rats than among 30- or 60-min shams suggesting the possible stress effect of routine confinement of small experimental animals even in the absence of restraint. The significance of this report (Lotz *et al.*, 1977) is that the GH levels were determined in the same rats as those used for the CS study (Lotz and Michaelson, 1978).

12.6. NEUROENDOCRINE/METABOLIC CORRELATIONS

While hypothalamic–hypophysial–adrenocortical activation and hypothalamic–hypophysial–growth hormone inhibition can be viewed as nonspecific stress reactions, hypothalamic–hypophysial–thyroidal (HHT) depression may be considered as a specific reaction. The acute reaction of the HHT axis to thermogenic levels of microwaves is to lower the hormone affecting resting metabolic rate. Phillips *et al.* (1975) have shown that the decreases in the resting metabolic rate of male rats were dependent on the quantity of absorbed energy. The threshold at 6.5 W/kg was approximately equal to the resting metabolic rate.

Ho and Edwards (1977a,b) measured oxygen consumption in mice irradiated with 2.45 GHz at various SARs of 1.6 to 44.3 W/kg in a waveguide exposure system and found that the animals compensated homeostatically to a SAR of 10.4 W/kg or greater by a decrease in metabolic rate to compensate for thermal loading, but not at 1.6 or 5.5 W/kg. There was no detectable colonic temperature increase at or below 10.4 W/kg, but there was a 0.5°C increase at 23.6 W/kg and a 1.0°C increase at 44.3 W/kg. Normal metabolic activity was resumed following cessation of exposure. These results suggest that the mouse compensates for large doses of microwaves by adjusting its metabolic rate downward to compensate for the thermal load.

12.7. NEUROENDOCRINE ACTIVITY AND CARDIOVASCULAR FUNCTION

In the mammal, adjustment of the cardiovascular system is one of the principal mechanisms for regulating thermal inputs into the body. Thermoregulation, however, is complicated by multiple neural and hormonal pathways acting on the cardiovascular system. Perturbations of neuroendocrine function may modify the response of the cardiovascular system to thermal inputs.

The effect of small thermal inputs or altered body temperatures on the cardiovascular system has received only limited attention. The response to heat stress has been shown to include an increase of blood flow to the skin and an increase of cardiac output principally through increased heart rate. At a more detailed level of cardiovascular response, experimental data are sparse and tend to be conflicting. Neuroendocrine function influences mammalian systems such as the cardiovascular system in response to thermal stress. Thus, the necessity for studying temperature responses as well as neuroendocrine function in combination with studies of cardiovascular system responses is obvious.

12.8. LOCALIZED EXPOSURES

An important consideration with regard to cranial exposure to microwaves is the resonant absorption of microwaves in the skull (Shapiro et al., 1970; Kritikos and Schwan, 1972; Johnson and Guy, 1972; Lin et al., 1973). If such focusing and hot spots should occur in the brain, and there is a likelihood of stimulation of effects on the hypothalamus itself or significant alteration in the thermal milieu of the hypothalamus, then slight reaction of the hypothalamus can be monitored by studying various components of the neuroendocrine system.

Rosenthal (1973) reported that in patients subjected to cerebral electrotherapy or electrosleep by the application across the head of low-intensity 100-Hz pulses, 1-msec duration, a transient rise in serum T_4 was observed that was not accompanied by a change in T_3. Some patients also showed increases in urinary catecholamines and 17-ketosteroids. If neuroendocrine changes should occur from exposure to electromagnetic energy by local application to the head, then with the present availability of radioimmunoassays that can measure extremely small quantities of serum hormone levels, these can be used to monitor the possible perturbation of the HHT or HHA relationships.

One of the recent developments providing a strong basis for the study of the neuroendocrine system with MW/RF exposure is the field of psychosomatic medicine and its attempts to explain or to correlate mood changes in individuals with certain endocrine parameters known to be under neural control by indirect pathways that change with varying mood states (Mason, 1968; Curtis, 1972). Such relationships should be considered in the context of the reported effects of "low-level" microwave exposure. Can these effects be a result of feedback from end organs or endocrine glands to the pituitary and/or hypothalamus?

The foregoing indicates that investigators have to be aware of the effects of body temperature on pituitary hormones so that precise biological effects can be allocated specifically to microwave exposure; threshold intensities can vary in relation to what is considered to be the normal range in sham-exposed or unexposed populations of animals. As an example, pituitary nonspecific stereotyped reactions could occur in rats exposed to $50 \, mW/cm^2$ of 2.45 GHz (SAR 8.0 W/kg) for 1 hr. TSH adjustments of rats to an increased thermal load could occur at $10 \, mW/cm^2$ (SAR 1.6 W/kg).

Gandhi (1975) reported that RF energy near the scaled half-wave resonant frequency for the human of 68 MHz can produce hot spots in the lower neck of human figurines with an SAR of approximately 31 W/kg for a vertically polarized $10 \, mW/cm^2$ incident power density. The model presented by Magin et al. (1977a,b) can serve to predict the biological effects of microwaves when hot spots occur in the neck region.

de Lorge (1978) plotted the relationship between body weight and power densities at which disruption of ongoing operant behavior occurred with rats, squirrel monkeys, and rhesus monkeys as a basis for interspecies comparison. Although comparable studies for neuroendocrine parameters have not been made, Lotz (1979a) found that rats responded to 1.29 GHz (2-μsec pulse, 0.001 duty cycle) by increased CS levels at 15 mW/cm^2 for 30 min or longer. The same pulsed microwave exposure (1.29 GHz) was without effect on adrenocortical and GH secretion in the adult male rhesus monkey exposed at 20, 28, and 38 mW/cm^2 for 8 hr (Lotz, 1979b; Lotz and Podgorski, 1982). The increases in rectal temperature were 0.6, 1.0, and 1.5°C, respectively. These differences may suggest that neuroendocrine function of the rhesus monkey is more stable during thermogenic microwave exposure. This illustrates the difference in the response of a given species of animal to various frequencies and the resulting difference in energy deposition and distribution.

12.9. CONCLUSION

The acute effects of microwaves on hypothalamic–hypophysial function are: generally increased ACTH secretion, decreased TSH secretion, and decreased GH secretion. These stereotyped changes can be observed simultaneously in rats acutely exposed to 2.45-GHz microwaves at 50, 60, or 70 mW/cm^2 for 1 hr (Lu *et al.*, 1981). The characteristics of these changes in hypothalamic hormones constitute the pattern of stress reactions of animals. Because of their physiological significance, these biological endpoints of microwave effects can serve as meaningful criteria for hazard evaluation if sufficient care has been incorporated into the design of chronic or repeated exposure experiments.

In the present state of the art, endocrine activity cannot be separated from the functional state of the neural network. The influence of endocrine function on body metabolism is also longer lasting than that due to neural disturbances. In spite of the obvious importance of this subject, only sparse and sometimes insufficiently documented data are available. Nonspecific stress reactions to microwave exposure have to be isolated from extraneous factors that are usually associated with experimental procedures. Furthermore, evaluation of a given endocrine parameter involves not only its perturbation, but also its recovery or manifestation of delayed response if such should occur.

The neuroendocrine data are consistent with the hypothesis that the adenohypophysial responses are the integral results of CNS processing of multiple signals from many body locations, such that no single localization of absorbed energy is pivotal to the onset of a response. Factors such as circadian rhythmicity, stimulus intensity, and interspecies differences are important in determining the pattern of these responses. Thus, in addition to further studies to characterize the basic neuroendocrine response to microwave exposure, studies are needed to determine the physiological mechanism or mechanisms by which this regulatory system is affected during microwave exposure.

Evidence indicates that neuroendocrine effects are induced by microwave exposure with a threshold intensity of exposure required for the onset of the response. The level of that threshold is yet unclear due to conflicting reports. The response appears to be a nonspecific stress reaction in the case of the adrenocortical and GH changes, but it is apparently a metabolically specific response to increased energy input in the case of the pituitary–thyroid changes.

The effects of MW/RF exposure on endocrine function are generally consistent with both immediate and long-term responses to thermal input and to nonspecific stress, which can also arise from thermal loading. The long-term response of animals to whole-body RF exposure at thermally significant levels is a decrease in the level of pituitary TSH in the blood plasma, followed by a decrease in the level of T_4.

Changes in plasma levels of CS and GH are typical reactions of animals to nonspecific stress. Such results emphasize the great care that is required in performing experiments to ensure that the changes in hormone level do not result from stress caused by handling of the animals or novelty of the experimental situation.

Although some studies indicate that microwave exposure can be manifested by endocrinopathy or hormonal changes, the nature of microwave interactions with endocrine organs is not known. Evidence suggests that microwave energy can act as a "stressor" in that it may affect the integrative and regulatory mechanisms of the body, which would result in altered homeokinesis. Studies indicate HHA and HHT effects can be induced at relatively high exposure levels for the particular animal species.

Some investigators believe such changes are caused by stimulation of the hypothalamic–hypophysial system due to thermal interactions at the hypothalamus, or the particular endocrine gland or end organ under study. Other workers interpret the observed changes as effects of direct microwave interactions with the CNS.

Collins and Weiner (1968) point out that although the pattern of endocrine involvement in physiological adjustments of the homeotherm exposed to high-temperature conditions has been examined, the evidence available is in some respects insufficient. Moderate or gradual heating appears to be associated with reduced thyroid hormone and adrenocorticoid output: suppression of thyroid activity is accompanied by an increase in metabolic rate. They note that thyroid activity measured both by ^{131}I uptake and release and by histological changes is generally found to be decreased in a wide variety of experimental animals exposed to moderately warm (27–34°C) environments. Rapid or marked elevation of body temperature, however, induces an increased oxygen consumption; a few animal experiments indicate that this rise is accompanied by an increase in thyroid activity. In the blood, the level of 17-hydroxycorticosteroids is raised when body temperature is elevated rapidly enough.

The hypothalamus exerts a central influence on thermoregulatory processes, and when temperature is increased, this structure assumes control over and in integration of food and water intake, metabolic rate, osmoregulation, growth, and reproduction. Because neuroendocrine function is an integration of numerous underlying chemical and biological processes (Shizume and Okinaka, 1964), caution is required in interpreting the significance of changes in the endocrine system induced by MW/RF exposure.

Several components of the neuroendocrine system have been shown to be critically sensitive to environmental temperature (Collins and Weiner, 1968; Brown-Grant et al., 1954; Dempsey and Astwood, 1943; Johnson et al., 1966). Thus, reported low-power-density microwave-induced neuroendocrine perturbations could be a manifestation of sensitivity to small changes in peripheral temperature or selective stimulation of any component of the neuroendocrine system through alteration of thermal gradients in the body.

The effect of microwave exposure on neuroendocrine function may be an indirect one; the thermal stress on the body might produce a hypothalamic–hypophysial response. Some studies suggest that treatment with microwave intensities that cause whole-body temperature to rise, suppress the hormone-producing functions of the anterior pituitary, whereas intensities that do not increase rectal temperature apparently enhance hormone production (Petrov and Syngayevskaya, 1970).

Since moderate heat conditioning raises the functional activity of the adrenal cortex (Stefanovskaya and Klochkova, 1969), the reported enhancement of corticosteroid activity during and after microwave exposure could be an adaptive reaction (Petrov and Syngayevskaya, 1970). Alterations in epinephrine levels have been noted to occur in rats subjected to a stressful situation, such as immobilization (Kvetnansky et al., 1970) or acute exposure to cold (Leduc, 1961).

With regard to "stress" and adaptation, it should be emphasized that a new environment or new manipulation techniques can alter animals' behavioral patterns, namely by inducing anxiety, avoidance behavior, and weight loss, and thus could be interpreted as being "stressful." Therefore, investigations of neuroendocrine response to microwave exposure must be carefully designed and controlled and should be conducted in animals properly adapted to environmental conditions. Unless this is taken into consideration, it is not possible to eliminate stress reactions due to extraneous factors in experiments intended to investigate neuroendocrine function in relation to microwave exposure. This is of paramount importance in studying subtle indicators of microwave exposure, especially at lower intensities for long periods of time (Roberts et al., 1986).

It should be noted that behavior is not a simple process, but is the expression of various effects in different systems. It is important to realize that temperature input signals arise in many body structures among which the following have been identified experimentally: (1) the preoptic–anterior hypothalamus; (2) posterior hypothalamus; (3) midbrain, medulla, motor cortex, and thalamus; (4) spinal cord; (5) skin, respiratory tract; and (6) viscera. All of these except the motor cortex and thalamus have been shown to evoke behavioral and/or physiological responses to changes in local temperature. These two areas have been identified as locations of cells having firing rates with high temperature coefficients but which do not seem capable of evoking thermoregulatory activity by local temperature changes alone (Hardy, 1973).

Stress is known to cause the secretion of CRF, which stimulates the pituitary to release ACTH, which in turn causes the adrenal gland to release CS, a hormone carried back to the pituitary to shut off the release of further ACTH. Both active and passive types of avoidance behavior are potentiated by ACTH and reduced by CS.

Changes in deep body temperature influence both neural and hormonal thermoregulatory mechanisms by altering the activity of central thermodetectors in the anterior hypothalamus (Swenson, 1970). There is no doubt that studies of microwave bioeffects and attempts to extrapolate to the human should recognize the importance of thermal gradients and species differences with regard to brain circulation and regulation of brain temperature, since the hypothalamus, the controller of thermal regulation, is located in this area.

Specific organ or tissue systems may "function" at a significantly different rate if local thermal gradients are altered. Within a few degrees, nerve fiber transmission rates are temperature dependent (Currier and Nelson, 1969). The hypothalamic center can be influenced experimentally by direct heating; the threshold for direct heat activated is an increase in temperature of 0.5 to 0.6°C (Fischer and Solomon, 1958).

The distribution of heat induced by microwaves in the body and particularly the brain has been of interest to various investigators (Lin et al., 1973; Johnson and Guy, 1972; Shapiro et al., 1970; Kritikos and Schwan, 1972) using models and confirming the results by animal experimentation. As Larsen et al. (1973) have pointed out, brain temperature is not uniform within the confines of the meninges. There is a gradient of approximately 0.5°C between surface and deep brain structures (Delgado and Hanai, 1966). Further, the brain regions that are directly sensitive to temperature (i.e., central thermodetectors) and control peripheral thermoregulatory mechanisms during heat stress are located in the preoptic–anterior hypothalamus (Magoun et al., 1938).

Von Euler (1950) has shown that a temperature elevation of 0.1°C in the preoptic–anterior hypothalamus results in the generation of a 100-mV steady potential in that structure. Peripheral evidence of heat loss mode processing by central thermoregulators occurs with a temperature elevation of about 0.5 to 1°C in the preoptic–anterior hypothalamus (Ström, 1961).

Careful review and analysis of available information on effects of microwave exposure are consistent with a pattern of neuroendocrine involvement in the many physiological adjustments of the organism relative to increased body temperature or alterations in thermal gradients within the body that could affect any individual or combination of components in the hierarchical neuroendocrine system. Much more refined and sophisticated studies are required at various exposure levels to determine energy distribution patterns and the relation to subtle responses before firm statements can be made about microwave-induced effects on the neuroendocrine system.

REFERENCES

Baker, M. A., and L. W. Chapman (1977) Rapid brain cooling in exercising dogs. *Science* **195**:781.
Baranski, S., and P. Czerski (1976) *Biological Effects of Microwaves*. Dowden, Hutchinson & Ross, Stroudsburg, Pa.
Baranski, S., K. Ostrowski, and W. Stodolnik-Baranska (1972) Functional and morphological studies of the thyroid gland in animals exposed to microwave irradiation. *Acta Physiol. Pol.* **23**:1029.
Bereznitskaya, A. N. (1968) The effect of 10-centimeter and ultrashort waves on the reproductive function of female mice. *Gig. Tr. Prof. Zabol.* **9**:33.
Brown, G. M., and S. Reichlin (1972) Psychologic and neural regulation of growth hormone secretion. *Psychosom. Med.* **34**:45.
Brown-Grant, K., C. Von Euler, G. W. Harris, and S. Reichlin (1954) The measurement and experimental modification of thyroid activity in the rabbit. *J. Physiol. (London)* **126**:1.
Cleary, S. F. (1977) Biological effects of microwaves and radiofrequency radiation. In: *CRC Critical Reviews in Environmental Control*, Vol. 7, C. Straub (ed.). Chemical Rubber Company, Cleveland, pp. 121–165.
Collins, K. J., and J. S. Weiner (1968) Endocrinological aspects of exposure to high environmental temperatures. *Physiol. Rev.* **48**:785.
Currier, D. P., and R. M. Nelson (1969) Changes in motor conduction velocity induced by exercise and diathermy. *Phys. Ther.* **49**:146.
Curtis, G. C. (1972) Psychosomatics and chronobiology: Possible implications of neuroendocrine rhythms. *Psychosom. Med.* **34**:235.

Delado, J. M. R., and T. Hanai (1966) Intracerebral temperature in freely moving cats. *Am. J. Physiol.* **211**:755.

de Lorge, J. (1978) Disruption of behavior in mammals of three different sizes exposed to microwaves: Extrapolation to larger mammals. In: *Electromagnetic Fields in Biological Systems*, S. S. Stuchly (ed.). IMPI, Edmonton, Canada, pp. 215–228.

Demokidova, N. K. (1974) The effects of radiowaves on the growth of animals. In: *Biological Effects of Radiofrequency Electromagnetic Fields*, Z. V. Gordon (ed.). JPRS 63321.

Dempsey, E. W., and E. B. Astwood (1943) Determination of the rate of thyroid hormone secretion at various environmental temperatures. *Endocrinology* **32**:509.

Denisiewicz, R., E. Dziuk, and M. Siekierzynski (1970) Evaluation of thyroid function in persons occupationally exposed to microwave radiation. *Pol. Arch. Med. Wewn.* **45**:19.

Dumansky, Y. D. and M. G. Shandala (1974) The biological action and hygienic significance of electromagnetic fields of superhigh and ultrahigh frequencies in densely populated areas. In: *Biological Effects and Health Hazards of Microwave Radiation*, P. Czerski, K. Ostrowski, M. L. Shore, C. Silverman, M. J. Suess, and B. Waldeskog (eds.). Polish Medical Publishers, Warsaw, pp. 289–293.

Dumansky, Y. D., A. M. Serdyuk, C. I. Litvinova, L. A. Tomashevskaya, and V. M. Popovich (1972) Experimental research on the biological effects of 12-centimeter low-intensity waves. In: *Health in Inhabited Localities*, Ed. II, Kiev, p. 29.

D'Yachenko, N. A. (1970) Changes in thyroid function with chronic exposure to microwave radiation. *Gig. Tr. Prof. Zabol.* **14**:51.

Fischer, E., and S. Solomon (1958) Physiological responses to heat and cold. In: *Therapeutic Heat and Cold*, S. H. Licht (ed.). E. Licht, New Haven, Conn., p. 116.

Gandhi, O. P. (1975) Conditions of strongest electromagnetic power deposition in man and animals. *IEEE Trans. Microwave Theory Tech.* **MTT-23**:1021.

Grant, L., P. Hopkinson, G. Jennings, and F. A. Jennre (1971) Period of adjustment of rats used for experimental studies. *Nature (London)* **232**:135.

Guillet, R., and S. M. Michaelson (1977) The effect of repeated microwave exposure on neonatal rats. *Radio Sci.* **12**(6S):125.

Guillet, R., W. G. Lotz, and S. M. Michaelson (1975) Time-course of adrenal response in microwave-exposed rats. In: *Proceedings of the 1975 Annual Meeting of USNC/URSI*, p. 316.

Hardy, J. D. (1973) Posterior hypothalamus and the regulation of body temperature. *Fed. Proc.* **32**:1564.

Ho, H. S., and W. P. Edwards (1977a) Oxygen-consumption rate of mice under differing dose rates of microwave radiation. *Radio Sci.* **12**(6S):131.

Ho, H. S., and W. P. Edwards (1977b) Dose rate and oxygen consumption rate in mice confined in a small animal holder during exposure to 2450 MHz. *Radiat. Environ. Biophys.* **14**:251.

Houk, W. M., S. M. Michaelson, and D. E. Beischer (1975) The effects of environmental temperature on thermoregulatory, serum lipid, carbohydrate, and growth hormone responses of rats exposed to microwaves. In: *Proceedings of the 1975 Annual Meeting of USNC/URSI*, p. 309.

Johnson, C. C., and A. W. Guy (1972) Non-ionizing electromagnetic wave effects in biological materials and systems. *Proc. IEEE* **60**:692.

Johnson, H. D., M. W. Ward, and H. H. Kibler (1966) Heat and aging effects on thyroid function of male rats. *J. Appl. Physiol.* **21**:689.

Kirchev, K., P. Eftinova, and S. Sichev (1959) Some experimental data on the effects of a UHF electric field on the adrenals. In: *Problems of Physiotherapy and Health Reports*, Moscow, pp. 81–88.

Kritikos, H. N., and H. P. Schwan (1972) Hot spots generated in conducting spheres by electromagnetic waves and biological implications. *IEEE Trans. Biomed. Eng.* **BME-19:**53.

Kvetnansky, R., V. Weise, and I. Kopin (1970) Elevation of adrenal tyrosine hydroxylase and phenylethanolamine-N-methyl transferase by repeated immobilization of rats. *Endocrinology* **87:**744.

Larsen, L. E., R. A. Moore, and J. Acevedo (1973) An rf decoupled electrode for measurement of brain temperature during microwave exposure. In: *Proceedings of the 1973 IEEE G-MTT International Microwave Symposium,* Boulder, p. 262.

Leduc, F. (1961) Catecholamine production and release in exposure and acclimatization to cold. *Acta Physiol. Scand.* **53**(Suppl. 183):1.

Lenko, J., A. Dolatowski, L. Gruszecki, S. Klajman, and L. Januszkiewicz (1966) Effect of 10-cm radar waves on the level of 17-ketosteroids and 17-hydroxycorticosteroids in the urine of rabbits. *Przegl. Lek.* **22:**296.

Leytes, F. L., and L. A. Skurikina (1961) The effect of microwaves on the hormonal activity of the adrenal cortex. *Byull. Eksp. Biol. Med.* **52:**47.

Lin, J. C., A. W. Guy, and G. H. Kraft (1973) Microwave selective brain heating. *J. Microwave Power* **8:**275.

Lotz, W. G. (1979a) Adrenocortical response in rats exposed to 1.29 GHz microwaves. Presented at *Bioelectromagnetics Symposium,* Seattle.

Lotz, W. G. (1979b) Thermal and endocrinological effects of microwave exposures on rhesus monkeys. Presented at *Bioelectromagnetics Symposium,* Seattle.

Lotz, W. G., and S. M. Michaelson (1976) Temperature and corticosterone relationship in microwave exposed rats. *J. Appl. Physiol. Respir. Environ. Exercise Physiol.* **44:**438.

Lotz, W. G., and S. M. Michaelson (1979) Effects of hypophysectomy and dexamethasone on the rat's adrenal response to microwave irradiation. *J. Appl. Physiol. Respir. Environ. Exercise Physiol.* **47:**1284.

Lotz, W. G., S. M. Michaelson, and N. J. Lebda (1977) Growth hormone levels of rats exposed to 2450-MHz (CW) microwaves. In: *International Symposium on the Biological Effects of Electromagnetic Waves,* Airlie, Va., p. 39 (Abstr.).

Lotz, W. G., and R. P. Podgorski (1982) Temperature and adrenocortical response in rhesus monkeys exposed to microwaves. *J. Appl. Physiol.* **53:**1565.

Lu, S.-T., N. J. Ledba, and S. M. Michaelson (1977a) Effects of microwave radiation on the rat's pituitary–thyroid axis. In: *International Symposium on the Biological Effects of Electromagnetic Waves,* Airlie, Va., p. 37 (Abstr.).

Lu, S.-T., N. J. Lebda, S. M. Michaelson, S. Pettit, and D. Rivera (1977b) Thermal and endocrinological effects of protracted irradiation of rats by 2450 MHz microwaves. *Radio Sci.* **12**(6S):147.

Lu, S.-T., N. J. Lebda, S. Pettit, and S. M. Michaelson (1979a) Modification of microwave biological end-points by increased resting metabolic heat load in rats. Presented at *Bioelectromagnetics Symposium,* Seattle.

Lu, S.-T., S. Pettit, and S. M. Michaelson (1979b) Dual action of microwaves on serum corticosterone in rats. Presented at *Bioelectromagnetics Symposium,* Seattle.

Lu, S.-T., W. G. Lotz, and S. M. Michaelson (1980) Advances in microwave-induced neuroendocrine effects: The concept of stress. *Proc. IEEE* **68:**73.

Lu, S.-T., N. J. Lebda, S. Pettit, and S. M. Michaelson (1981) Microwave-induced temperature corticosterone, and thyrotropin interrelationships. *J. Appl. Physiol. Respir. Environ. Exercise Physiol.* **50:**399.

McLees, B. D., and E. D. Finch (1971) Analysis of the Physiologic Effects of Microwave Radiation. U.S. Nav. Med. Res. Inst., Bethesda (Project MF12.524:015-0001B, Rep. No. 3).

Magin, R. L., S.-T. Lu, and S. M. Michaelson (1977a) Stimulation of dog thyroid by local application of high intensity microwaves. *Am. J. Physiol.* **233:**E363.

Magin, R. L., S.-T. Lu, and S. M. Michaelson (1977b) Microwave heating effect on the dog thyroid. *IEEE Trans. Biomed. Eng.* **BME-24:**522.

Magoun, H. W., F. Harrison, J. R. Brobeck, and S. W. Ranson (1938) Activation of heat loss mechanisms by local heating of the brain. *J. Neurophysiol.* **1:**101.

Martin, J. B. (1973) Neural regulation of growth hormone secretion. *N. Engl. J. Med.* **288:**1384.

Mason, J. W. (1968) Overall hormonal balance as a key to endocrine organization. *Psychosom. Med.* **30**(Part II):791.

Matsuyama, H., A. Ruhmann-Wemhold, and D. H. Nelson (1971) Radio immunoassay of plasma ACTH in intact rats. *Endocrinology* **88:**692.

Michaelson, S. M. (1977) Endocrine and biochemical effects. In: *Microwave and Radiofrequency Radiation*, M. Suess (ed.). World Health Organization, Regional Office for Europe, Section 7, pp. 18–23.

Michaelson, S. M., R. A. E. Thomson, and J. W. Howland (1961) Physiologic aspects of microwave irradiation of mammals. *Am. J. Physiol.* **201:**351.

Michaelson, S. M., R. A. E. Thomson, and J. W. Howland (1967) *Biologic Effects of Microwave Exposure.* Tech. Rep. RADC-TR-67-461, Griffiss AFB, Rome Air Development Center, Rome, N.Y.

Michaelson, S. M., W. M. Houk, N. J. Lebda, S.-T. Lu, and R. Magin (1975) Biochemical and neuroendocrine aspects of exposure to microwaves. *Ann. N.Y. Acad. Sci.* **247:**21.

Mikolajczyk, H. (1972) Hormone reactions and changes in endocrine glands under influence of microwaves. *Med. Lotn.* **39:**39.

Mikolajczyk, H. (1974) Microwave irradiation and endocrine functions. In: *Biological Effects and Health Hazards of Microwave Radiation*, P. Czerski, K. Ostrowski, M. L. Shore, C. Silverman, M. J. Suess, and B. Waldeskog (eds.). Polish Medical Publishers, Warsaw, pp. 46–51.

Mikolajczyk, H. (1977) Microwave-induced shifts of gonadotropic activity in anterior pituitary glands of rats. In: *Biologic Effects of Electromagnetic Waves*, Vol. I, C. C. Johnson and M. L. Shore (eds.). HEW Publ. (FDA) 77-8010, pp. 377–383.

Milroy, W. C., and S. M. Michaelson (1972) Thyroid pathophysiology of microwave radiation. *Aerosp. Med.* **43:**1126.

Nakayama, T., H. T. Hammel, J. D. Hardy, and J. S. Eisenman (1963) Thermal stimulation of electrical activity of single units of the preoptic region. *Am. J. Physiol.* **204:**1122.

Neill, J. D. (1970) Effect of "stress" on serum prolactin and luteinizing hormone levels during the estrus cycle of the rat. *Endocrinology* **87:**1192.

Novitskii, A. A., B. F. Murashov, P. E. Krasnobaev, and N. F. Markozova (1977) The functional condition of the system hypothalamus–hypophysis–adrenal cortex as a criterion in establishing the permissible levels of superhigh frequency electromagnetic emissions. *Voen. Med. Zh.* **8:**53.

Parker, L. N. (1973) Thyroid suppression and adrenomedullary activation by low-intensity microwave radiation. *Am. J. Physiol.* **224:**1388.

Petrov, I. R., and V. A. Syngayevskaya (1970) Endocrine glands. In: *Influence of Microwave Radiation on the Organism of Man and Animals*, I. R. Petrov (ed.). Meditsina Press, Leningrad (NASA TT F-708, 1971, pp. 31–41).

Phillips, R. D., E. L. Hunt, R. D. Castro, and N. W. King (1975) Thermoregulatory, metabolic and cardiovascular response of rats to microwaves. *J. Appl. Physiol.* **38:**630.

Roberts, N. J., Jr., S. M. Michaelson, and S. T. Lu (1986) The biological effects of radiofrequency radiation: A critical review and recommendation. *Int. J. Radiat. Biol.* **50:**379.

Rosenthal, S. H. (1973) Alterations in serum thyroxine with cerebral electrotherapy (CET). *Arch. Gen. Psychiatry* **28:**28.

Schally, A. V., A. Akimura, and A. J. Kastin (1973) Hypothalamic regulatory hormones. *Science* **179**:341.
Schliephake, E. (1960) Endocrine influence on bleeding and coagulation time. *Zentralbl. Chir.* **85**:1063.
Selye, H. (1946) The general adaptation syndrome and the diseases of adaptation. *J. Clin. Endocrinol.* **6**:117.
Selye, H. (1950) *Stress.* Acta. Inc., Montreal.
Shapiro, A. R., R. F. Lutomirski, and H. T. Yura (1970) Induced fields and heating within a cranial structure irradiated by an electromagnetic plane wave. P-4458-1, Rand Corp., Santa Monica, Calif. *IEEE Trans. Microwave Theory Tech.* **MTT-19**:187, 1971.
Shizume, K., and S. Okinaka (1964) Control of thyroid function by the nervous system. In: *Major Problems in Neuroendocrinology,* E. Bajusz and G. Jasmin (eds.). Karger, Basel pp. 286–306.
Shutenko, O. I., and I. I. Shvayko (1972) Impact of low-intensity SHF radiation on the functional condition of the thyroid gland. In: *Industrial Health and the Biological Effect of Radio Frequency Electromagnetic Waves.* Material of the Fourth All-Union Symposium, Moscow, p. 52.
Smirnova, M. I., and M. S. Sadchikova (1960) Determination of the functional activity of the thyroid gland by means of radioactive iodine in workers with UHF generators. In: *The Biological Action of Ultrahigh Frequencies,* A. A. Letavet and Z. V. Gordon (eds.). Acad. Med. Sci., Moscow, pp. 47–49.
Stefanovskaya, N. V., and G. M. Klochkova (1969) Effect of hyperthermia on the reaction of the adrenal cortex of heat-conditioned animals. *Izv. Akad. Nauk Turkm. SSR Ser. Biol. Nauk* **4**:74.
Ström, G. (1961) Central nervous regulation of body temperature. In: *Handbook of Physiology,* Sect. I, Vol. II, J. Field, H. W. Magoun, and V. E. Hall (eds.). American Physiological Society, Washington, D.C., pp. 1173–1196.
Swenson, M. J. (ed.) (1970) *Duke's Physiology of Domestic Animals,* 8th edition. Cornell University Press, Ithaca, N.Y.
Tolgskaya, M. S., Z. V. Gordon, V. V. Markov, and R. S. Varonlov (1972) The influence of intermittent and continuous microwave irradiation on the hypothalamic neurosecretory function. In: *Gig. Tr. Biol. Deist. Elektromag. Radio Symp.,* Moscow, p. 34.
Travers, W. D., and R. J. Vetter (1976) Low intensity microwave effects on the synthesis of thyroid hormones and serum proteins. In: *Proceedings of the 1976 Annual Meeting of USNC/URSI,* pp. 91–92.
Vetter, R. J. (1975) Neuroendocrine response to microwave irradiation. *Proc. Natl. Electron. Conf.* **30**:237.
Von Euler, C. (1950) Slow temperature potentials in the hypothalamus. *J. Cell. Comp. Physiol.* **36**:333.

13

Cardiovascular Effects

Several investigators have reported that exposure of animals or humans to microwaves may result in direct or indirect effects on the cardiovascular system. Some have suggested that exposure to microwaves at intensities that do not produce appreciable heating may lead to functional changes that are observed with acute as well as chronic exposure. In other reports, however, no serious cardiovascular disturbances have been noted in man or animals as a result of exposure to microwaves (Edelwejn *et al.*, 1974).

Disturbances of the blood circulation that have been described in animals are evidenced by a change in blood flow (Richardson, 1954), usually an increase in flow that is proportional to both the intensity and the duration of exposure (Richardson *et al.*, 1950); a decrease is observed only in denervated extremities. These phenomena are related to vasodilation. Negative results, however, have been reported in studies of persons working with radar (Sacchitelli and Sacchitelli, 1960).

13.1. ANIMAL EXPERIMENTS

Increased heart rate has been observed in animals after exposure to power densities of 50–130 mW/cm^2 (1000–3000 MHz) for variable periods ranging from 10 to 140 min (Cooper *et al.*, 1962a,b; Marks *et al.*, 1961; Subbota, 1957). Soviet investigators have conducted numerous investigations on the influence of protracted or repeated exposures on the blood pressure of dogs, rabbits, and rats (Nikonova, 1964; Gordon, 1964). The results of these experiments have been reviewed by Subbota (1970) and Gordon (1966). Slowing of the heart rate is reported by some investigators with low (or what they consider "nonthermal") levels of microwaves (Tyagin, 1957a,b), although others have reported increased heart rate with low-level microwave exposure over the dorsal aspect of rabbits (Presman and Levitina, 1962a,b).

13.1.1. In Vitro Preparations

Paff *et al.* (1962, 1963) described ECG changes in chick embryo hearts after irradiation with 24,000 MHz at 74, 167, and 478 mW/cm^2 for periods of a few seconds to 3 min at 38°C. Changes in S and T deflections, shortening of the QT wave, and slow heart rate were observed.

Japanese quail (*Coturnix coturnix japonica*) embryos 8–13 days old were exposed to pulsed and CW 2450-MHz microwaves at SARs of 0.3–30 mW/g to investigate the effect of the exposure on heart rate. No effects on heart rate were detected that could not be attributed to temperature changes (Hamrick and McRee, 1980).

Frey and Seifert (1968), using 1425-MHz pulsed microwaves, reported effects based on the time relationship between the phase of heart action and the moment of pulse action. Frog heart rate may be accelerated if the pulse occurs about 200 msec after the P deflection, i.e., simultaneously with QRS. In some experiments, arrhythmia followed sometimes by cardiac arrest, was observed. If the pulse occurs simultaneously with the P deflection, no arrhythmia may be induced. It may be provoked, however, if the pulse occurs concomitantly with the R deflection. The use of a metallic cable makes this experiment suspect.

Liu *et al.* (1976) could not demonstrate any microwave-induced change in heart rate, and concluded that the data reported by Frey and Seifert (1968) were artifactual. Chapman and Cain (1975) were also unable to obtain the results reported by Frey and Seifert.

Reed *et al.* (1977), using an isolated rat heart, induced bradycardia by exposing the preparation to 1.5 W/kg of 960-MHz CW microwaves. When parasympathetic and sympathetic nerves were blocked by atropine and propranolol, respectively, no significant bradycardia was seen. The investigators suggest a direct effect at the neuronal or synaptic level by microwave exposure.

Levitina (1964) reported that whole-body exposure of frogs may cause a decrease in the heart rate, and irradiation of the head, an increase. No effects were obtained by direct irradiation of the denervated heart *in situ*.

13.1.2. Whole-Body or Regional Exposure

Cooper *et al.* (1961, 1962a,b, 1965) exposed male albino rats (400–500 g) to 2.45 GHz, 80 mW/cm^2, 5 cm from the upper abdomen. Colonic temperature reached 40.5°C in 12 min at which time the exposure was interrupted. Six cardiac variables were measured prior to exposure and again at 40.5°C. Cardiac output and stroke volume increased 40–50%. Cardiac work increased over 50%. Heart rate and mean arterial blood pressure showed slight increases. The peripheral resistance fell by approximately 30%. A statistically significant change was calculated for cardiac output, stroke volume, and cardiac work. These animals were anesthetized with pentobarbital, which no doubt influenced cardiodynamic and thermoregulatory processes.

According to the authors, microwave hyperthermia (40.5°C) could increase cardiac output, stroke volume, and cardiac work. However, heart rate, systemic arterial pressure, and peripheral resistance did not change in the microwave-induced hyperthermic rats. Microwave hyperthermia in the vagotomized rats and rats with ganglionic blockage increased cardiac output by increased heart rate but not by stroke volume. Both vagotomy and ganglionic blockage reduced the usual increase of cardiac output in the control hyperthermic rats. Adrenalectomy eliminated the usual increase in cardiac output during hyperthermia, indicating the importance of adrenal participation in the adaptive mchanisms of the rat under thermal stress of microwaves. None of the procedures altered catecholamine content in the myocardium.

These results indicated the importance of sympatho-adreno-medullary activation during microwave-induced hyperthermia. It was concluded that acute cardiovascular response to microwave exposure may be independent of vagal control. However, a vagolytic effect of the anesthetic used may cast some doubt on the interpretation.

Gordon (1964, 1966) measured the blood pressure in rats repeatedly exposed at various microwave frequencies for 6–8 months. The blood pressure rose following 10 mW/cm^2, 3000-MHz exposures during the first 10 and 22 weeks, respectively. Millimeter and 10,000-MHz fields did not induce any response at this power density. Power densities of 40–100 mW/cm^2 were required to obtain a blood pressure effect at these wavelengths. Following the initial period of increase, the blood pressure returned to normal and after this dropped below initial values. Gordon points out that different effects are obtained following exposures to 10-cm pulsed or CW. CW irradiation at 10 mW/cm^2 did not influence the blood pressure during the initial 8 weeks of exposure, following which a drop in blood pressure was noted. Ten-centimeter pulsed exposures caused an initial increase, followed by a return to normal and subsequent decrease in blood pressure. Abrikosov (1958) also noted differences in blood pressure reponses to pulsed or CW exposures. Following such chronic experiments, the blood pressure returned to normal 8–10 weeks after termination of the irradiation.

Nikonova (1964) reported a monophasic hypotensive response in rats exposed to 0.5-MHz waves, 2 hr daily for 10 months. Soviet authors stress the hypotensive effects of prolonged microwave and meter-wave exposures. This effect is ascribed to interference with CNS function, cardiac function alterations being mediated through interaction with skin receptors.

Phillips *et al.* (1975) exposed male Wistar rats (430 g) in a resonant cavity to 2.45-GHz pulsed microwaves for 30 min at 0, 4.5, 6.5, and 11.1 W/kg. Immediately after exposure, colonic temperatures of rats were 38.6 ± 0.1°C (0 W/kg or 0 mW/cm^2), 40.1 ± 0.1°C (4.5 W/kg or 22.5 mW/cm^2), 40.5 ± 0.1°C (6.5 W/kg or 32.5 mW/cm^2), and 42.4 ± 0.2°C (11.1 W/kg or 55.5 mW/cm^2). Overcompensation of colonic temperature after exposure occurred at 6.5 and 11.1 W/kg. The increase in skin temperature was dependent on absorption rate. Decreased oxygen consumption rate after microwave exposure occurred in rats exposed to 6.5 and 11.1 W/kg. Cardiac function was studied 10 min to 5 hr after exposure. The threshold for bradycardia and irregular heart rate were noted in rats exposed to 6.5 W/kg or with colonic temperature of 40.5°C or higher. Transient incomplete heart block occurred in rats exposed to 11.1 W/kg only (colonic temperature 42.4°C). Both bradycardia and irregular heart rate were transient after exposure.

Levitina (1964) and Presman and Levitina (1962a,b) examined the influence of 10-cm pulsed or CW and 12.5-cm microwaves on the heart rate in rabbits exposed in the near field. At 7 to 12 mW/cm^2 CW or 3 to 5 mW/cm^2 pulsed (pulse width 1 msec, repetition rate 700 Hz), irradiation of the ventral part of the body to 10-cm waves caused cardiac deceleration; exposure of the head or vertebral column produced cardiac acceleration. Decreased heart rate was observed immediately upon exposure; acceleration was observed at its termination. The effects of pulsed exposure were more marked than those of CW irradiation. In a further series of experiments, the animals were exposed to CW energy for 20 min, twice per second, 0.1-sec duration at 700–1200 mW/cm^2 or to pulsed (1 msec, 700 Hz) at a mean power density of 350–380 mW/cm^2. Exposure of any arbitrarily selected region of the body caused cardiac deceleration. This effect could be abolished by local skin anesthesia. The authors concluded that cardiac acceleration following head and dorsal spinal cord exposure is caused by microwave interaction at the CNS level. The effects of exposure of the ventral side of the body are the result of skin receptor excitation. This is claimed to be the dominant effect of exposure to high power densities. No effects on heart rate were observed at 1 mW/cm^2.

Eight to fifteen experiments were done for each exposure area with two different pulsed microwaves. Criterion used for changes in heart rate was 10 beats/min from the control period of the given individual in the given experiment. Other than the inguinal region of males, all exposure areas induced a slowing of the heart rate (bradycardia). No significant difference in the effects between continuously and intermittently pulsed microwaves was noted. The bradycardia effect of microwaves could be prevented by subcutaneous anesthetization.

This report lacks the details and quantitative data for a sound evaluation. The statistics presented was an incidence of bradycardia in 8 to 15 experiments. The control experiment did not show any acceleration or slowing of the heart rate for more than 10 beats/min. Such comparison between control and exposed experiments appeared to be plausible. However, it was not clear when the bradycardia occurred. The incident power densities used were relatively high. Most of the effect on cardiac rhythm was slowing. This was in contrast to their previous report (Presman and Levitina, 1962a,b) in which a tachycardia was noted when the dorsal area of the heart was exposed. Statistical analysis cannot be used to evaluate the magnitude of changes. Therefore, the biological significance of changes cannot be compared to the magnitude of the time-dependent spontaneous variations in the heart rate other than during the period of experimentation.

In the report by Presman and Levitina (1962a,b), descriptions of experimental designs and statistical analysis were vague. Six different exposure protocols were used. Apparently, each rabbit was subjected to two repeated exposures in each protocol, preexposure control experiment and postexposure experiment. Sources of variations were individual variation, sequence of within treatment, sequence of treatments, number of treatments and duration of treatment. Statistical analysis failed to indicate the significance of main effect and other interactions, i.e., sequence and duration of treatment. Lumped data were presented. Data treatment was far from desirable. Each datum point presented was the difference between mean changes of exposed and control experiments, which were averaged differences between each datum and the averaged preexperiment control period. A range of 2 standard errors was presented. However, it was not clear how the standard errors were calculated. In the first experiment, electrocardiography was used for heart rate determination. In the second experiment, heart rate, respiration rate, and subcutaneous temperature were measured. Biologically, a stressed animal was used.

Results showed that $10 \, \text{mW/cm}^2$ did not induce a significant change in heart rate by analysis of variance. Threshold intensity for respiration rate was at $40 \, \text{mW/cm}^2$, subcutaneous temperature at $80 \, \text{mW/cm}^2$, and heart rate at $100 \, \text{mW/cm}^2$. At $10 \, \text{mW/cm}^2$, magnitude of change was 12 beats/min and 0.3°C in subcutaneous temperature. The latter was measured in the shielded area, and thus was not representative of the highest skin temperature noted.

Evaluation is hindered by the partial-body exposure used. The factor between whole-body and partial-body exposure was not clear. Apparently, the effect noted was a physiological response to increased body temperature since threshold of respiration rate and body temperature were both lower than threshold of heart rate change.

Birenbaum *et al.* (1975) correlated changes in heart rate with subcutaneous temperature increases in rabbits exposed for 1 hr to 2.4 GHz CW or 2.8 GHz pulsed. Experiment 1: Head exposure. Shielding was used over the rest of the body. Power densities were 0, 20, 40, 60, and 80 mW/cm^2. Data presented were without variability except during the control period. Linearized slope in the first 10 min of exposure was used to evaluate the changes in each parameter. Change per minute in the respiration rate, heart rate, and subcutaneous temperature were dependent on power density; increasing with increased power density. Respiration rate and heart rate changes per minute correlated with subcutaneous temperature.

Experiment 2: Whole-body exposure; comparison between CW and pulsed microwaves. Four rabbits were used; each exposed four times to CW and pulsed microwaves at 20 mW/cm^2. A 10-min preexposure control and 20-min exposure period were used. No differences between CW and pulsed microwaves on change per minute in heart rate, respiration rate, and subcutaneous temperature were noted.

Experiment 3: Whole-body exposure; comparison between CW microwaves and infrared at 0, 10, and 20 mW/cm^2. Respiration rate and heart rate responded similarly to both types of radiation. Infrared exposure induced a substantially higher subcutaneous temperature than microwave exposure at the same incident power density.

A restraint procedure was used for the rabbit. Metallic objects were present in the field; these were needles of ECG, needle thermistor temperature sensors, mercury column and strain gauge for respiration rate, and cable for ECG. Significant disturbance of the electromagnetic field can be expected especially when animals were exposed without shielding.

These experiments were not performed under a resting state as evident by a continuous decrease in all the physiological parameters studied in the sham-exposed experiment. A very large number of data points was collected: 4260 in experiment 1, 1536 in experiment 2, and 900 in experiment 3. Instead of an analysis of variance or analysis of covariance (to take into consideration preexposure variation), a least-squares rate of change per minute of exposure was used for comparison. It is not clear whether the value was a least-squares fit of the individual data or a least-squares fit of the mean value for each 10-min interval. It is very difficult to evaluate the significance of parameters studied due to these ambiguities in the data treatment.

Data were not presented by variation. Furthermore, no statistical test was performed on data presented in experiment 1. Therefore, threshold for each parameter was not clear. Body temperature-dependent changes in respiration rate and heart rate were clearly evident in experiment 1. In experiment 2, a t test was used. In experiment 3, no statistical test was performed. The quantitative data were described qualitatively.

It was evident that variation in the mean heart rate could be more than 10 beats/min during the initial period of experiment 1. Threshold intensity could not possibly be deduced from these experiments due to the deficiencies indicated. Estimated threshold may be between 20 and 40 mW/cm^2 for 1 hr if one accepts a linear change in heart rate. Respiration rate was about ten times the resting value. Therefore, these rabbits were under a severe stress at the time of the experiment.

According to Subbota (1970), the reaction to microwave-induced hyperthermia does not differ from responses observed in a hot environment or following infrared irradiation. A single exposure to a high power density causes increased blood pressure, heart rate, and respiration rate. Arrhythmia and ECG changes may appear. Local cardiac irradiation at 100–200 mW/cm^2 may cause bradycardia and amplitude changes in the R, S, and T waves.

Little change in arterial pressure was evident in rabbits chronically exposed to 2450 MHz, 10 mW/cm^2 (Subbota, 1970). However, hemodynamic shifts were in evidence even at 1 mW/cm^2. No hemodynamic shifts were observed beginning with the fourth or fifth treatment. When the rabbits were exposed to 50 mW/cm^2, the arterial pressure dropped, then recovered to its initial level after 1–2 hr. Characteristically, these effects were registered only after the first few microwave treatments, and later, as the treatments were repeated (once every 1–3 days), the arterial pressure change became smaller in degree until disappearing at the ninth or tenth treatment. The colonic temperature rise was 1–1.7°C after the first exposure, but 0.7–0.9°C after the ninth or tenth exposure.

In rabbits and dogs, whole-body irradiation (100–200 mW/cm^2) caused brief constriction and subsequent vasodilation; especially in the veins of the pia mater (Subbota, 1957). Tyagin (1957b) reported that dogs exhibited slowing of the heart rate with alteration in the ECG during exposure to 3000 MHz, 5 mW/cm^2. Fall in blood pressure, bradycardia, sinus arrhythmia, retardation of auricular and ventricular conduction, changes (usually a decrease) in the P and T deflections, and a broadening of the QRS complex were observed. More marked and persistent microwave-induced ECG changes were seen in dogs with experimentally induced myocardial infarction than in normal dogs.

After sedation with pentobarbital, dogs were subjected to 2.45 GHz for 15–140 min with a diathermy generator 1, 1.5, and 2 inches from the chest wall (Marks et al., 1961). The heart rate rose 15–30%. Changes in the T wave were observed. Throughout the procedure, an output power level of 125 W was used. Microscopic examination of the mediastinum revealed injury similar to any thermal injury in that area. Specific cardiac effects included engorgement of coronary arteries and intramyocardial arterioles. In a similar experiment, increase in heart rate was noted (Marks et al., 1961). Analysis of data for cardiac output, mean blood pressure, and peripheral resistance failed to show any significant changes.

Hemodynamic response of the dog exposed to thermogenic levels of 2800 MHz pulsed resembles that of acute heat stress as manifested by early hemodilution followed by hemoconcentration (Michaelson et al., 1967). As the exposure is prolonged, hemoconcentration becomes more evident. Dogs exposed at 165 mW/cm^2 (SAR 6.1 W/kg) show a body weight loss of 2.0%/hr. At 100 mW/cm^2 (SAR 3.7 W/kg) there is a weight loss of 1.25%/hr, and hemodilution occurs, as contrasted with hemoconcentration evident at 165 mW/cm^2.

This is a study on dogs under a clinical setting. Near-field and high-intensity microwaves ($>$100 mW/cm^2) were used to induce localized hyperthermia. From the extent of tachycardia and cutaneous burns, the temperature at the skin surface could be higher than 45°C and a 2–4°C increase in the heart temperature could be expected. Apparently, temperature, metabolic rate, cardiac output, arterial blood pressure, and serum enzymes were also studied.

Lu et al. (1974, 1975) reported shifts in temperature, blood flow, and blood pressure of anesthetized dogs exposed cranially to 2.5 GHz CW for 1 hr at power densities from 20 to greater than 100 mW/cm^2. Changes in heart rate correlated with tympanic temperature and rectal temperature. Contractility (dP/dt) correlated with tympanic and colonic temperature. Pulmonary and systemic blood pressure did not change with exposure. Increase in pulmonary and renal blood flow was noted. The effect of microwave exposure on heart rate could be influenced by the type of anesthetic used. As noted previously, Tyagin (1957a,b) reported ECG changes in dogs during partial-body exposures to 5 to 10 mW/cm^2.

In this context, McAfee (1971) has pointed out how data can be misinterpreted to be the result of some unknown effect of microwave radiation, when hyperthermal effects are not involved. In cats, when peripheral nerves are stimulated by a temperature of 45°C, adrenal medullary secretion occurs with a rise in blood pressure as a result of adrenal secretion (McAfee, 1963). McAfee (1961) questions whether experiments on the effects of microwave energy on heart rate are carefully controlled for this possibility.

13.1.3. Atherosclerosis

Since elevated blood pressure is known to enhance atherogenesis (Bronte-Steward and Hepinstall, 1954), Sparks et al. (1976) studied the effect of RF/MW energies on dietary atherosclerosis of rabbits. Sixteen New Zealand white rabbits were exposed to 2.45-GHz microwaves at a power density of 20–30 mW/cm^2, 4 hr/day, 5 days/week for 8 to 10 weeks. Exposed animals had serum cholesterol concentrations, aortic wall cholesterol concentrations, and percentage of intimal surface involved in atherosclerotic lesions that were not different from age- and weight-matched controls. Continuous RF irradiation (1 MHz) for 8 to 11 weeks with a field strength of 30 V/cm also failed to change these indices of atherogenesis. Of interest also is the report by Perovsky *et al.* (1969) of diminished atherogenesis and decreased serum cholesterol and aortic cholesterol content in rabbits exposed to microwaves.

13.1.4. Pharmacodynamics

Cooper *et al.* (1965) examined the influence of various drugs on the circulatory reaction at its peak level, i.e., 40.5°C colonic temperature. Pyridoxine or pyridoxal administration did not influence the blood pressure and heart rate increases; heart stroke volume remained at the initial level. Digitoxin administration did not influence the blood pressure and heart rate increases, prevented an increase in heart stroke volume, increasing it in control animals (Pinakatt *et al.*, 1965). Ouabain abolished the circulatory reaction in irradiated animals, increasing the cardiac stroke volume in control animals, while the blood pressure and heart rate remained unchanged (Pinakatt *et al.*, 1963). Reserpine administration, vagotomy, and pharmacological ganglioplegia diminished the reaction to microwave hyperthermia (Cooper *et al.*, 1962a). Striking results were obtained following bilateral adrenalectomy, which completely abolished the circulatory response to microwave exposure (Cooper *et al.*, 1962a). These results indicate the importance of the endocrine and autonomic systems in compensatory reactions to microwave-induced hyperthermia (Hauswirth and Kraemer, 1958; Roberts *et al.*, 1986).

13.1.5. Conclusion

Results of the animal experiments are summarized in Table 13-1. Acute microwave exposure could induce an increase in cardiac performance (cardiac output, stroke volume, and cardiac work), postexposure bradycardia, postexposure sinus arrhythmia, and postexposure incomplete heart block in rats. Increased heart rate was noted in rabbits and dogs. Altered T-wave axis was also noted in dogs. However, some experiments on dogs (Marks *et al.*, 1961) used a high-intensity regional exposure. Skin burns were noted. Therefore, the incident power density was well above 100 mW/cm^2 and the skin temperature above 45°C. A

TABLE 13-1
Effects of Acute Microwave Exposure in Experimental Animals

Effect observed	Species	Intensity, frequency, duration	Colonic temperature (°C)	References
Increased cardiac performance	Rat	80 mW/cm^2, 2.45 GHz, 12 min	40.5	Cooper et al. (1962a)
Postexposure bradycardia	Rat	6.5 W/kg, 2.45 GHz, 1 hr[a]	40.5	Phillipps et al. (1975)
Postexposure sinus arrhythmia	Rat	6.5 W/kg, 2.45 GHz, 1 hr[a]	40.5	Phillips et al. (1975)
Postexposure incomplete heart block	Rat	11.5 W/kg, 2.45 GHz, 1 hr[a] 100 mW/cm^2, 2.45 GHz, 20 min	42.4	Phillips et al. (1975)
Increased heart rate	Rabbit	? mW/cm^2, 2.45 GHz, 20 min	—	Kaplan et al. (1971)
Increased heart rate	Dog	? mW/cm^2, 2.45 GHz, 5–140 min[b]	—	Marks et al. (1961)
Altered T-wave axis	Dog	? mW/cm^2, 2.45 GHz, 15–140 min[b]	—	Marks et al. (1961)

[a] Exposure was done in a resonant cavity. The SAR appears to be low. Power density of 71 mW/cm^2 would be needed to induce a colonic temperature of 40.5°C at 2.45 GHz for 1 hr.
[b] Probably ≥ 100 mW/cm^2 as evidenced by skin burn.

pain sensation should be elicited at such high exposure level. The threshold intensity noted by Phillips et al. (1975) was 29 mW/cm^2 as converted from an absorption rate of 6.5 W/kg. However, the absorption rate was measured in a resonant cavity. The values presented appeared to be lower than the corresponding increases in colonic temperature. To induce a colonic temperature of 40.5°C in rats would require 71 mW/cm^2 for 1 hr. The net increment of the threshold temperature, 1.9°C, in rats would require an absorption rate of 9.05 W/kg or 39 mW/cm^2 in the far field of 2.45-GHz microwaves. Lu et al. (1974) noted in the dog that the heart rate increase was a linear function of tympanic temperature or rectal temperature.

13.2. REPORTED OBSERVATIONS IN THE HUMAN

Functional alterations in the cardiovascular system indicated by hypotonus, bradycardia, delayed auricular and ventricular conductivity, and decreased height of ECG waveforms in workers in RF/MW fields have been reported by Soviet investigators (Drogichina, 1960; Obrosov et al., 1963; Orlova, 1960; Osipov, 1952).

Decrease in blood pressure from microwave exposure has been

reported (Gordon, 1960; Gordon et al., 1963; Kevork'yan, 1948; Orlova, 1960; Sadchikova and Orlova, 1958). Apparently, the pressure rises slightly at first and then begins to fall (Aronova, 1961; Baronenko and Timofeva, 1959), an effect that can be pronounced and last for several weeks following exposure. Drogichina et al. (1966) have reported that in individual cases, the "angiodystonic" manifestations caused by chronic exposure to SHF (2450–10,000 MHz) may develop further into more serious autonomic and cardiovascular pathologies. These are characterized by a tendency to angiospastic reactions and cerebral autonomic vascular attacks accompanied by pronounced arterial pressure lability and coronary spasms with corresponding changes in ECG. Osipov (1965), however, points out that these changes do not diminish work capacity, and are reversible.

Obrosov et al. (1963) investigated the effect of microwaves on cardiovascular function in volunteer subjects. The power source was a 200-W generator. It radiated by a waveguide emitter of 11.5 cm, 7 cm from the surface of the skin for 10 min at a time. They noted decreased heart rate, increased P–Q interval, decreased T-wave deflection, decreased systolic and diastolic pressure, increased systolic and diastolic pressure, decreased oscillographic index, and increased skin temperature in the exposed and unexposed area. All these effects were transient. No cumulative effect was noted. The incident intensity used could have been well above 100 mW/cm^2. No control experiments or experiments on control subjects were used. Deficits in the physical characterization and statistical techniques rendered the report unsuitable to estimate a threshold for cardiovascular change.

Observations by Glotova and Sadchikova (1970) have suggested that the nature and seriousness of cardiovascular reactions to prolonged exposure to microwaves are closely related to changes in the autonomic nervous system, and depend on the organism's individual characteristics as well. Some patients continue for a considerable period to present only slight asthenic symptoms with sinus bradycardia and arterial hypotension, without signs of general or regional hemodynamic disturbances. Others develop autonomic vascular dysfunctions, often accompanied by signs of "hypothalamic insufficiency and angiospastic reactions" that lead in some cases to disturbances in cerebral and coronary blood circulation. This study shares the inadequacy of other reports from the Soviet Union in lack of a control population, inadequate assessment of environmental contamination, unknown population at risk, and biased statistics. Improvement over others was that criteria for certain parameters were presented. The study may be biased by the investigators since all the subjects were classified as persons with microwave-induced asthenia, with vegetative-vascular syndrome or were incapacitated by microwave exposure.

In general, this report appeared to study symptoms related to two major cardiovascular diseases, i.e., myocardial insufficiency and hypertension. However, the authors never attempted to isolate these two diseases. The most striking observation was that "symptoms were characterized by crisis or attack" and "cardiac pains developed when a history of neurosis was present." The last statement revealed that the population studied could be biased for microwave effects especially since persons with neuroses who were not exposed to microwaves were not used as reference controls. Symptoms related to coronary insufficiency could be found in this report. These included fainting spells, pallor, systolic murmur, radiating pains in the cardiac region, sensation of labored breathing and bronchial spasms (dyspnea), tachycardia, ECG T-wave changes, and extrasystole (premature contraction). These symptoms constituted more than 30% of the symptoms and signs in subjects suffering heart attack. Hypertension was indicated by systolic, diastolic, and mean arterial pressure.

Follow-up was done on only some subjects. No criterion for selection of these subjects was offered. This longitudinal study revealed development and progression of hypertension, coronary insufficiency, and reversibility of symptoms in some subjects after removal from microwave sources. Preexposure history and personal habits were not studied. All symptoms were called microwave-related ailments without any evidence for this. Study of relative risk is extremely important when these symptoms are not different from known diseases. The symptoms were not specific to microwave workers as evidenced in other reports. The present study never attempted to correlate the cause–effect relationships or dose rate–duration–effect relationships.

According to Sadchikova (1974), two basic syndromes of hemodynamic disturbances induced by changes in "regulatory reflex function" exist, dependent on the preponderance of excitability of sympathetic or parasympathetic vegetative nervous centers. Clinical syndromes are induced simultaneously with or immediately after hazardous occupational exposure. Both types of reactions may be observed among persons exposed to microwaves at intensity levels of a few mW/cm^2, for long periods of time. Neurocirculatory disturbances of a hypertensive character are related to the duration of exposure; vagotonic reactions occur during initial periods of work. Prolonged exposure induces progressive changes; interruption of exposure may induce a remission. Symptoms of "sympathicotonic vegetative circulatory disturbances" occur in persons exposed to low intensities of a few tens of $\mu W/cm^2$ with occasional exposures of up to $1\,mW/cm^2$. This report warrants detailed analysis because of the use to which it has been put with regard to the implication of "radiowave sickness" or microwave sickness.

This is a summary report of clinical studies made at the Institute of Industrial Hygiene and Occupational Disease, USSR. It shares the same ambiguities in biological instrumentation and microwave physical variables as Drogichina *et al.* (1966), Monayenkova and Sadchikova (1966), Glotova and Sadchikova (1970), and Sadchikova and Nikonova (1971), which are clinical reports from the same Institute. Two statements in this report indicate the arbitrary standards in the description of the exposed population—these are "upon close examination in the ward a complex of symptoms corresponding to microwave sickness was diagnosed only in those patients of the first group who began their work under the most unfavorable conditions. Its frequency in the whole group did not exceed *15 percent*" and "those in the first group (*1000*) were subjected to the influence of a power density of up to a few mW/cm^2." Italicized are key words from the reports of this Institute. The largest number of patients examined by this series of reports is 130 in the first group. These 130 patients appear to constitute the 15% of the 1000 exposed personnel. In reports from this Institute, the statistics were based on the occurrence of symptoms in the "sick" patients, since each individual symptoms should never exceed 15%, which was not the case in this series of reports. The prevalence of each symptom should therefore decrease accordingly.

In addition, it is unclear whether the 180 exposed subjects of the second group and 200 controls were sick patients or randomly selected subjects for the study. According to the authors' custom for reporting the occurrence of symptoms, these populations are probably "sick" subjects being admitted for in-hospital examinations. Therefore, the prevalence of symptoms in the population at large bears no meaning in the cause–effect relationship since it has no significance in the risk-related estimation.

The symptoms listed as autonomic vascular disorders were inhibited dermographism, dermographism, hyperhidrosis, bradycardia (upon examination), arterial hypotension, and arterial hypertension. The cardiac symptoms listed were cardiac pain, dullness of heart sound, systolic murmur, bradycardia (ECG), and lower deflection in ECG leads T_1 and T_2. In the report, Sadchikova (1974) stated that in the majority of those examined, a single abnormality in their health status *did not interfere with the usual rhythm of life and work*. Also stated is that in a number of cases, the abnormalities combined into a complex of symptoms that required medical care. It is not clear what the incidence of the symptom complex is, or what the longitudinal consequence of any given abnormality is.

Of interest is that those patients suffering from "microwave sickness" of 1 to 10 years' duration showed that, despite repeated therapeutic courses and temporary withdrawal from work with microwave sources, upon returning to previous work conditions, symptoms increased in severity, particularly among patients with moderately advanced and advanced stage of disease. In such patients, autonomic vascular disturbance dominated, crisis of cerebral and coronary insufficiency progressed, and development of ischemic heart disease and hypertension was observed. Apparently, temporary withdrawal from work with microwave sources also removed unidentified causative factors. However, no attempts were made to isolate other possible causative factors of "microwave sickness" to ensure that such sickness was indeed caused by microwaves.

The descriptions may be intended to show the predisposing symptoms leading to the development of cerebral and coronary insufficiency. The microwave workers appeared to be under much higher physiological and psychological strain than controls, judging from their higher rates of neurological symptoms such as feeling of heaviness in the head, tiredness, irritability, sleepiness, and partial loss of memory. A correlational study on the "neurological symptoms" to the cardiovascular symptoms may resolve some of the controversies regarding the specificities of the microwave-induced cardiovascular disorders.

The Institute must have enough patients suffering symptoms alleged to be "microwave sickness" in a population that had never been exposed to microwaves. A study of the clinical courses of these patients can be a good indicator of the specificity of "microwave sickness" and the progressive nature of such sickness.

Investigators from this Institute did not attempt a thorough investigation of the risks of "microwave sickness." Instead, they reported what they saw as "microwave sickness." The symptoms described were noted in populations not exposed to microwaves. This is invalid without a risk analysis. Contributing factors, predisposing factors, and personal biases have never been ruled out. The value of the report is thus questionable.

In the report by Drogichina *et al.* (1966), a group of 100 subjects (73 men, 27 women) was studied. They were between 21 and 40 years of age with unknown duration of exposure to "SHF" (USA designation: "microwaves") at several mW/cm^2. Symptomatic observations, tacho-oscillogram, "capillaroscopic analysis" (?), ballistocardiogram, and ECG were used to evaluate the subjects.

In 39 subjects, initial effects were mild asthenia and autonomic–vascular shifts. Pathological findings concerning the heart were not noted. In 61 subjects, moderately severe and severe symptoms were noted as angiodystonic syndrome and angiospastic reactions. Present were tachycardia (16 subjects, >90 beats/min) and unstable bradycardia (19 subjects, <60 beats/min). Hypotension (<100 mm Hg) was noted in 28% of subjects. The hypotension decreased in prevalence to 7% and was replaced by hypertension (17% higher than 140/90 mm Hg). Angiospastic symptoms were mentioned. Changes in tacho-oscillographic indices and capillaroscopic analysis and constriction of retinal arteries were also mentioned. However, data were not presented.

Chest pains (49), slight enlargement of cardiac borders (11), mute heart tones (7), and functional cardiac murmur (11) were noted. Lower T-wave (24) was noted but disappeared in 1 to 2 weeks in most subjects. Persistent lower T-wave was noted in four subjects with decreased cardiac contraction function.

In 15 subjects, severe symptom resulted in crisis. Symptoms were severe headaches, dizziness, constricting pain in the cardiac region, adynamic sensation of difficult breathing, skin pallor, hyperhidrosis, and fainting spells. At the height of an attack, blood pressure might rise or fall. Those with frequent attacks showed sinus tachycardia and ventricular extrasystoles. During crisis, half of the subjects experienced a downward displacement of the S–T segment and a lowering or even inversion of the T-wave. Localized precardial T-wave changes with constricting pains in the cardiac region could be interpreted as angiospastic phenomena (coronary insufficiency). Two case histories were presented.

The present report was from the Institute of Labor Hygiene and Occupational Diseases, Soviet Academy of Medical Sciences. The series of reports from this Institute appear to repeat observations on the same subjects. The exposed population in the report by Drogichina *et al.* (1966) was 100. One hundred and thirty were examined as reported in 1970 (Glotova and Sadchikova, 1970), 100 in 1971 (Sadchikova and Nikonova, 1971), 34 in 1966 (Monayenkova and Sadchikova, 1966), and 1000 in 1974 (Sadchikova, 1974). The prevalence of each symptom in these reports is, therefore, distorted. The diagnosis of the symptom complex (asthenia, and autonomic–vascular disorders) is distorted for the same reason especially since diagnostic criteria were never presented.

Another report by Sadchikova and Nikonova (1971) is a summary report on two groups of microwave workers. The first group (100 subjects; 83 men and 17 women) was exposed to microwaves of up to several mW/cm^2. The second group (115 subjects; 91 men and 24 women) was exposed to several tenths of a mW/cm^2. These exposure intensities could be higher with brief exposure. Duration of exposure was 1 to 10 years, predominantly 5 to 10 years. Other than ECG recording, methods of study were not clear. A control group was included, composed of 100 men belonging to similar occupations and working in this same plant but not exposed to electromagnetic waves or other deleterious industrial factors.

Prevalences of the symptom complex were compared among the three groups. These were neuroasthenic syndromes (high: 45%, low: 15.6%, control: 5%) and vegetative–vascular dysfunctions (high: 30%, low: 29.6%, control: 16%).

It appears that those in the high-exposure group were the same subjects reported by Glotova and Sadchikova (1970). All the comments pertaining to this group were the same in the two reports. In the high-exposure group, neurasthenic syndromes consisting of the disorders noted were present in 45% and vegetative–vascular dysfunctions in 30%. These values were 15.6 and 29.6% in the low-exposure group; 5 and 16% in the control group. These data tended to indicate that the low-exposure and control group showed predominantly vegetative–vascular dysfunctions. This is in contrast to the concept that progression of neurasthenic syndromes into vegetative–vascular dysfunctions was noted in subjects working in microwave fields, since the disorders, if noted, were far more advanced in the low-exposure and control group than the high-exposure group.

The symptoms listed occurred in both exposed and control populations except for the prolongation of QRS complex, which was noted in the controls. Ignoring the dermographism and hyperhidrosis for which the prevalence was not known, the prevalence of stabbing chest pains, bradycardia, prolongation of QRS complex, and slight T-wave changes was significantly higher in the high-exposure group than in the control group. The only observed increase in prevalence in the low-exposure group was bradycardia.

Since symptoms were not specific to microwave workers, an epidemiological study is necessary to demonstrate the shift of incidence or prevalence in the microwave-exposed population. The present investigation lacks such approach since the population at risk, exposure intensity, and duration of exposure were either very vague or not known. Apparently, insufficient care was used to match populations under study. It should be pointed out, however, that no serious cardiovascular disturbances were ever seen in man or experimental animals as the result of microwave exposure (Edelwejn *et al.*, 1974).

In this context, a report by Guskova and Kochanova (1975) of the Institute of Industrial Hygiene and Occupational Pathology (Moscow), USSR Academy of Medical Sciences, disputes earlier reports of the relationship of occupational diseases to electromagnetic radiation. According to these authors, it is very difficult to make etiological diagnoses of pathology of the circulatory system in the groups of workers dealing with sources of SHF radiation (tuning radio equipment or operators of radar stations) since such work requires a high degree of nervous and emotional tension and involves other deleterious factors. The incidence of hypertension with chronic exposure to SHF fields coincides with the findings of a screening of the population of Moscow according to WHO criteria. In addition to smoking and obesity, genetic background, or emotional stress, psychological personality factors that determine an individual's reactivity to environmental conditions are proven risk factors in development of cardiac ischemia.

Guskova and Kochanova (1975) suggest, when diagnosing cardiovascular pathology in individuals exposed to UHF, in addition to assessing working conditions, the general rules for analyzing etiological and pathogenetic causes should be followed. In each case, it is also imperative to take into consideration frequently encountered causes of cardiopathy. When investigating working conditions, this should not be limited to demonstration of a high level of UHF fields; one must also pay attention to the extent of nervous and emotional stress, related to occupation and environment as well as night shifts. "As for the effects of microwave radiation on onset of cardiovascular pathology, in our opinion it may take a certain place among other deleterious factors. However, for the time being there is no reason to relate development of disease to it alone."

Conclusion

Seven reports of clinical investigations conducted in the USSR are summarized in Table 13-2. However, five of the reports are from the Institute of Industrial Hygiene and Occupational Diseases. Although these reports are based on a common group of subjects, different details and treatment of data are noted throughout the five reports.

In general, these clinical reports are very slipshod in their environmental assessment. Usually, an arbitrary number of "several mW/cm^2" at a "superhigh frequency" was reported. Such numbers appeared to stem from or to reflect the USSR standard or lack of standard at the time. The standard apparently was not rigidly observed by persons exposed to electromagnetic energies. For a brief exposure, the intensity could be higher (Sadchikova and Nikonova, 1971). None of these reports point out or refer to the sources or methods for assessment of environmental contamination in spite of the fact that several factors should be taken into consideration for assessment of such contamination even if actual measurements cannot be made: these are power output, frequency and modulation of the sources, radiating facility, spatial relation of subjects to the power sources. Other factors that can affect field intensity and therefore absorption rate should be included. These are ground surface, shielding, presence of other objects, and spatial relationships between subjects and objects. Without this information, it is impossible to place any confidence in the quoted exposure levels. This is especially true when the work involved is production, testing, repair, and operation of MW/RF sources.

Different studies were performed. Parameters and symptoms studied are listed in Table 13-2. The most critical deficiency in these clinical

TABLE 13-2
Clinical Observations on Cardiac Function among Microwave Workers (USSR)[a]

System or parameter	Fofanov (1969)	Glotova and Sadchikova (1970)[*]	Sadchikova and Nikonova (1971)[*]	Drogichina et al. (1966)[*]	Medvedev (1973)	Monayenkova and Sadchikova (1966)[*]	Sadchikova (1974)[*]
Heart							
1. Chest pains in the cardiac region	—	present	present	present	—	present	present
2. Cardiac border	Normal	enlarged	—	enlarged	—	—	—
3. Systolic pressure	tendency to decrease	—	—	—	—	—	—
4. Functional systolic murmur	—	present	—	—	—	—	?
5. Increased heart rate (tachycardia)	present	present	—	present	—	—	—
6. Decreased heart rate (bradycardia)	present	present	present	present	present	present	present
7. Uneven heart rate (sinus arrhythmia)	present	—	—	—	—	—	—
8. U-wave in ECG	present	—	—	—	—	—	—
9. T-wave changes (decreased deflection, S-T depression, and inversion)	—	present	present	present	present	present	present
10. Prolonged intraventricular conduction	—	—	—	—	?	present	present
11. Prolonged intraauricular conduction	—	—	present	—	—	—	—
12. Incomplete heart block	present	—	—	—	?	—	—
13. Ventricular extrasystoles	—	present	—	—	—	—	—
14. Left ventricular overload	present	—	—	—	—	increased	—
15. Cardiac output	normal	increased decreased	—	—	—	decreased	—

CARDIOVASCULAR EFFECTS

16. Stroke volume	somewhat lower	—	—	—	—	—	—	—	—
17. Effective power	somewhat lower	—	—	—	—	—	—	—	—
18. Cardiac work	normal	—	—	—	—	—	—	—	—
19. Muffled heart tone	—	—	—	—	present	—	—	—	present
Systemic									
1. Mean arterial pressure	normal	no change	—	—	—	—	—	—	—
2. Systolic arterial pressure	normal	no change	—	increase and decrease	increase and decrease	increase	increase and decrease	—	increase and decrease
3. Diastolic arterial pressure	—	—	no change	increase	—	—	—	—	?
4. Dynamic arterial pressure	normal	—	—	increase	—	—	—	—	?
5. Lateral arterial pressure	normal	—	—	increase	—	—	—	—	?
6. Pulse wave velocity in elastic vessel	normal	—	—	—	—	—	—	—	—
7. Pulse wave velocity in myogenic vessel	normal	—	—	increase	—	—	increase	—	—
8. Pulse wave velocity ratio	normal	—	—	increase	—	—	increase	—	—
9. Elastic modulus	—	—	—	increase	—	—	increase	—	—
10. Constriction of retinal arteries	—	—	—	—	present	—	present	present	—
11. Peripheral resistance	—	—	—	—	—	—	increase	—	—
12. Abnormal correlation between peripheral resistance and cardiac output	—	—	—	—	—	—	present	—	—

[a] Asterisks indicate that investigators are from the same Institute.

reports is in the definition of the exposed population, which was variably defined without any description as to why some of these subjects were selected for certain evaluations while others were not. For example, the reports from the Institute of Industrial Hygiene and Occupational Diseases were studies of a group of subjects. The number of subjects varied, i.e., 100 (Drogichina *et al.,* 1966), 130 (Glotova and Sadchikova, 1970), 100 (Sadchikova and Nikonova, 1971), 34 (Monayenkova and Sadchikova, 1966), and 1000 (Sadchikova, 1974). If there are any significant findings in these clinical observations, how can one proceed to evaluate the risks involved without the actual size of the population or the population at risk? Do the numbers vary because of specific selection?

Control populations were rarely described. The control population, when given, is a match of the same age range in the same plant. As an example, one report (Medvedev, 1973) revealed a high occurrence of congenital disorders in their subgroup of exposed population. Socioeconomic backgrounds between control and exposed subjects were never matched.

In spite of the poorly defined criteria for exposed and control populations, the prevalence or incidence of symptoms is used. However, the percentage of subjects having a particular symptom is a biased measurement based on the total number of subjects included instead of the number of subjects in the exposed population. The biases in this particular group can be very clear if one considers a statement made by Sadchikova (1974): "Upon close examination in the ward a complex of symptoms corresponding to microwave sickness was diagnosed only in those of the first group who began their work under the most unfavorable conditions. Its frequency in the whole group did not exceed 15 percent." Therefore, a reduction of the prevalence of symptoms should be employed. The best estimate of the occurrence of bradycardia (<60 beats/min) would be 5.7%. This occurrence can be within the sampling error of a control population (Specter in *Handbook of Biological Data,* Saunders, Philadelphia, 1956).

These presentations were further biased by scoring the symptom complex into individual symptoms. This procedure tends to overemphasize the prevalence and severity of the individual symptom scored. It has been stated that in the majority of those examined, a single abnormality in the worker's health status did not interfere with the usual rhythm of life and work (Sadchikova, 1974). Subjects with a symptom complex of similar nature as the individual symptoms might be pronounced unfit for work. Apparently, an individual symptom assumes a different meaning in the health status from the same individual symptom of a symptom complex. Worst of all, the symptom complex of the "moderately severe" and "severe" form of "microwave sickness" was regularly described as a crisis or attack. The majority of symptoms described were those of coronary insufficiency (Drogichina et al., 1966). In fact, diagnosis of coronary insufficiency and coronary spasmatic reaction were made (Glotova and Sadchikova, 1970; Drogichina et al., 1966; Medvedev, 1973). Differentiation between individual symptoms and similar symptoms from a symptom complex should be made. For example, hypertension by itself is pathological and potentially harmful if it is confirmed to be persistent. Hypertension with ECG changes can be harmful since the symptom complex may indicate that decompensation has already occurred. Increased or decreased heart rate by itself can be a nonpathological physiological adjustment depending on criteria, method of measurement, and physical fitness while it is a pathological finding if it is accompanied by ECG changes.

Functional measurements were not done on every subject studied. Quantitative data were rarely given. The difference between control and exposed subjects was usually not significant if quantitative data were used. Routinely, a qualitative occurrence of symptoms based on quantitative data was used. This qualitative occurrence depends on the normal ranges and the reliability of measurement technique. Deviation from normal ranges was also noted in the control population. Therefore, a randomly selected control and exposed population became critically important in evaluation of effects. The occurrence of a particular symptom in the exposed population, usually, did not compare to the occurrence in the control population. If this comparison were done, the significant findings reduce to *stabbing chest pains, bradycardia, prolonged ORS,* and *T-wave changes* (Sadchikova and Nikonova, 1971), assuming the population sizes were reliable and randomly selected.

Since these clinical observations were apparently from three different groups of investigators, consistent observations in more than two groups may be accepted as possible changes. These were *tachycardia, bradycardia,* and *T-wave changes.* Four studies in the United States (*Am. J. Epidemiol.* **112:**39–53, 1980, and *Bull. N.Y. Acad. Med.* **55:**1182–1186, 1979), Poland (*Aeros. Med.* **45:**1143–1145, 1974), and Yugoslavia (*Aviat. Space Environ. Med.* **50:**396–398, 1979) failed to find significant increases or an effect–dose rate–duration relationship in cardiovascular diseases in exposed populations.

Thus, 19 cardiac parameters and symptoms in addition to 9 vascular parameters were studied clinically by investigators from the Soviet Union. These clinical investigations shared common deficiencies such as lack of definition of the exposed population, inadequate or lack of control population, and drifting criteria between quantitative measurements and qualitative prevalence of any given symptom. The standard style of reporting is occurrence of symptoms, in "sick" microwave workers. Pathological description of the cardiovascular disorders appeared to be coronary insufficiency. No attempt was made to isolate individual symptoms from the symptom complex of coronary insufficiency. Therefore, overemphasizing the severity and risks of a given symptom is apparent.

13.3. IMPLANTED ELECTRONIC CARDIAC PACEMAKER INTERFERENCE

Aside from the primary biological hazard of direct irradiation by RF/MW energy, there is a more subtle influence, which can affect users of electronic prosthetic devices such as cardiac pacemakers, and diagnostic medical equipment, e.g., electroencephalographs, electrocardiographs, electromyographs and so on. This effect is called electromagnetic interference (EMI), and it may cause a variety of malfunctions. EMI occurs when signals generated by one or more electronic or electromechanical devices adversely affect the operation of other electronic devices. The offending signals can be products of intended radiation, such as radio, television, and radar transmission, or unintended signals generated by internal combustion engine ignition systems, electric razors, electromechanical relay, and so on. The characteristic of electronic equipment that permits undesirable responses when subjected to EMI is called susceptibility and the technology that has evolved to solve the problems of EMI is called electromagnetic compatibility (EMC). EMI can be diminished or eliminated by separation, shielding, filtering, and proper installation (e.g., grounding).

Although electronic pacemaker interference is not a biological effect *per se,* it is included in an assessment of RF/MW bioeffects because EMI, if not suppressed, could result in serious complications.

Thousands of individuals today owe their lives and productive activity to the development and use of implanted electronic cardiac pacemakers. Because this life-sustaining instrument is a sensitive electronic device, its activity may be influenced by external factors. Awareness of such factors is essential to provide the knowledge required for future development of cardiac pacing and to provide the security for the individual so that he or she may derive the full benefits of this device.

13.3.1. Normal Cardiac Function

The normal heart is paced by electrical impulses originating in the sinoatrial node, located in the upper right quadrant of the right atrium.

These impulses travel through heart muscle fibers to initiate contraction of both atria. They also activate the atrioventricular (AV) node, located in the lower left quadrant of the right atrium. Thereafter, the impulses are rapidly conveyed to all parts of the left and right ventricles via specialized conduction tissues. From the AV node, the impulses enter the bundle of His, a thick sheaf of tissue running down the muscular wall between the ventricles. The bundle of His divides into the left and right bundle branches, which further divide to form the Purkinje network, whose fibers fan out over the inner surface of both ventricles.

Incomplete heart block, disease, or operative injury of the heart's conduction tissue blocks nerve impulse conduction from the sinoatrial node (the heart's natural pacemaker located in the right atrium) to the ventricles. The ventricles thus lose their normal rhythm and frequently cease beating entirely. Subsidiary natural pacemakers usually take over and maintain the heart beat at a very slow rate that is just enough to sustain life but does not permit normal activity.

13.3.2. The Electronic Cardiac Pacemaker

Normal heart rate can be restored and maintained by artificial pacemakers. The use of self-powered, completely implantable, transistorized, fixed-rate electronic cardiac pacemakers was first introduced by Chardack and co-workers in 1960.

There at present two principal types of pacemakers: (1) asynchronous, which operate at a fixed or externally adjustable rate independent of the patient's heart activity; and (2) synchronous, which are either stimulated or inhibited by the patient's heart signals. In the absence of a detected signal from the heart, the synchronous pacers operate in a fixed-rate (asynchronous) mode.

Demand or noncompetitive (synchronous) pacemakers may be of three types: (1) atrial triggered; (2) ventricular triggered; (3) demand or ventricular inhibited. These pacemakers monitor spontaneous cardiac activity and possess a sensing circuit capable of detecting P waves or R waves arising spontaneously. They contain electronic circuitry to sense electrical cardiac activity and to modify the output of the pacemaker should a natural electrical signal occur within a prescribed timing interval. Such pacemakers have the inherent risk that they may detect electrical activity from sources other than the heart, and their behavior may be modified by electrical interference.

13.3.3. Pacemaker Interference

Electronic cardiac pacemaker activity is subject to interference from a variety of electrical and RF fields. As new and more sensitive types of pacemakers are developed, the interference problem becomes more complex. Some environmental sources of RF energy include RF transmission such as from radio and television broadcasting; RF energy from microwave ovens and radar; carrier current on power transmission lines; magnetic fields around power transformers and conductors carrying electric current; and arcing and sparking electrical equipment such as power tools, commutator motors, and ignition systems of aircraft, automobiles, motorcycles, and lawn mowers. Medical equipment, such as diathermy, electrocautery, neurosurgical stimulators, and high-voltage radiation therapy units, are potential sources of electrical interference within the hospital.

The design of sensors is a science in itself. They must respond accurately to the impulses they are designed to sense without affecting the condition they are to measure. Generally, they cannot discriminate between significant and insignificant signals and may respond to surrounding electromagnetic fields as well as to physiological electrical signals.

Such sensitivity is inevitable since a probe or sensor responds to a physiological phenomenon. If the phenomenon is not electrical, a transducer converts it into an electrical signal. This signal is transmitted to an amplifier (usually through wire conductors but also by telemetry). The amplifier increases the level of its input signal, usually in several stages, and may modify, select, or analyze the signal at some stage. Studies by Mitchell and Hurt (1976) indicate that EMI is strongly dependent on frequency, pulse width, pulse repetition rate, E-field level and polarization.

The fixed-rate (asynchronous) pacemaker has a low-frequency oscillator designed to deliver pulses at a desired cardiac stimulation rate. Once implanted, such units are fairly insensitive to electrical interference, except when electrocautery is used within a few inches of the unit or RF diathermy is applied directly over the pacemaker site. Fixed-rate pacemakers are not affected by X irradiation, auto ignition systems, incandescent, fluorescent, or neon lights, television apparatus, electric shavers, household appliances, or power tools.

Noncompetitive pacemakers are susceptible to electrical interference when tested externally. Interference with externalized pacemakers by noncardiac electrical signals has been reported with practically every type of pacemaker. However, once implanted in the patient, the pacemaker is shielded by the body from most of the recognized electrical interferences. Nevertheless, with the increasing use of noncompetitive pacemakers, which depend for their function upon detection of the intracardiac electrical activity, the problems of interference are much more serious than with simple fixed-rate models.

Patients with pacemaker electrodes connected to external battery units are especially vulnerable to the induction of ventricular fibrillation by stray electric currents (Whalen et al., 1964). If small currents such as 60 Hz enter the electrode, and if the circuit is completed by grounding the patient through another electrical device such as an electrocardiograph, the current will pass through the heart and induce ventricular fibrillation. There is also a possibility of external pacemakers picking up RF waves (Lichter et al., 1965). The same is also theoretically possible with fully implanted units, but according to Chardack et al. (1965), the risk is remote.

Interference can intrude into the amplification system at any point, but the most significant effect on signal reliability occurs when interference occurs before much amplification has taken place. As a result, the interfering signal is amplified in direct ratio to amplification of the signal.

As noted by Siddons and Sowton (1967), there are two ways in which currents capable of producing ventricular fibrillation can reach patients being paced artificially: first, when an external pacemaker is connected to the main power line and is inadequately grounded; and second, when patients with internal pacemakers come close to apparatus emitting electromagnetic waves, which may be picked up by the pacemaker system.

With the increasing use of noncompetitive pacemakers that depend for their function upon detection of the intracardiac electrical activity, the problems of interference are potentially more serious than with simple fixed-rate models (Sowton et al., 1970). Interference may be encountered at much lower signal levels. Parker et al. (1969) suggest that interfering signals enter a pacemaker via its electrodes. One should not assume, however, that interference may not occur in some other part of the circuitry. Any interference signal entering the electronic circuitry of the noncompetitive pacemakers which mimics the electrical signal corresponding to a normal electrical depolarization of the heart may be interpreted by the pacemaker as a normal heart beat and cause changes in the pacemaker's output.

13.3.4. Clinical Reports

Lichter et al. (1965) cited two cases of ventricular fibrillation in patients with external pacemakers when a surgical diathermy apparatus was in use. They were able to show that in general the external pacemaker was adversely affected by shortwave diathermy, broadcasting stations, and neon lights.

Carleton et al. (1964) noted that a fixed-rate pacemaker was adversely affected by interference from small gasoline engines and by diathermy apparatus; Chardack *et al.* (1965) attributed this response to the fact that the pacemakers were not implanted. A powerful magnetic field has also been shown by Silver *et al.* (1965) to be capable of interfering with certain older types of pacemakers.

A patient with an external electrode making contact with the myocardium always risks developing ventricular fibrillation due to stray electric currents passing through the heart; the risk is greater when the electrode contact area is small (Weinberg *et al.*, 1962; Whalen *et al.*, 1964) probably because of the resulting high current density. This is particularly true of external pacemakers. The possibility of picking up RF waves is very real with some designs of external pacemakers (Lichter *et al.*, 1965). It is also theoretically possible with fully implanted pacemakers, although the electrical coupling is different when the unit is implanted, and the risk is remote (Chardack *et al.*, 1965). Models designed to receive power from outside might be expected to be the most susceptible.

King *et al.* (1970) reported interference of a cardiac pacemaker from a microwave oven. In this report, a 68-year-old man with an implanted pacemaker lost consciousness while near an operating microwave oven in a restaurant. In the hospital, he was intentionally placed 5 feet from a microwave oven. When the oven was turned on, the electrocardiographic (ECG) recording showed an artifact, believed to be due to the microwave signal. The pacemaker signal stopped, and an idioventricular rhythm began. Temporary syncopal symptoms were subsequently experienced by the patient. Three other patients with implanted pacemakers were similarly exposed to emission from a 2.45-GHz microwave oven. A patient with the same type of pacemaker as the first patient demonstrated a loss of the pacemaker signal; however, no symptoms developed. Different models implanted in two other patients were not affected. It should be noted that no ECG tracings were taken without the oven operating. This particular case report suggested that it is not the microwave oven *per se* but the type of pacemaker that should be of concern. Of three patients tested, only one demonstrated a blocking of pacing activity; the other two with a different type of pacemaker showed no change in pacemaker activity. An apparent high-frequency artifact was noted on an ECG taken at the time the microwave oven was operating. Careful review of the ECGs from the patient with suspected microwave-induced pacemaker dysfunction suggests that premature, intermittent battery failure may also have existed. Thus, it appears that any real or apparent interference of cardiac pacemakers by microwave ovens may not be a function of microwave oven leakage but related more directly to specific characteristics of the pacemaker. The mode-stirrer in the oven could be the interfering factor (Michaelson and Moss, 1971).

Hunyor et al. (1971) studied the effects of various electrical and microwave-producing devices on three patients with the same type of implanted cardiac pacemaker. Times of exposure and power densities were not given. A 2.45-GHz microwave source was aimed at various body parts including the area containing the pacemaker. A 27.12-MHz physiotherapy diathermy unit was tested at various distances (not given) from the patient and also when touching the patient's knee. Finally, patients were exposed at 5, 3, and 1 m from, and right next to, a 2.45-GHz microwave oven. The door of the oven was opened repeatedly during the exposure. Neither the oven nor the diathermy unit produced ECG changes in any of the patients. The diathermy unit, when placed directly on the knee, caused the pacemaker of two patients to increase to up to 136 beats/min. When not in direct contact with the patient, the diathermy unit had no effect on the pacemaker.

In an experiment by Röhl et al. (1975), cardiac pacemakers were implanted in several dogs and patients. The subjects were placed 1.2 km from a radar antenna operating at a frequency of 2.5 GHz, 400 pulses per sec (pps), 5-μsec pulse width. The radar antenna, which emitted a power density of 3.5 mW/cm^2, revolved once every 5.5 sec. No time of exposure was given. When exposed, only one of four unshielded, implanted pacemakers was not inhibited or triggered. Two implanted pacemakers that were shielded were not affected.

Lichter et al. (1965) reported the results of diathermy irradiation on anesthetized sheep and dogs connected to identical external cardiac pacemakers. All animals underwent chest surgery during which a diathermy unit operating at 500 kHz to 2.5 MHz was employed. Immediately, or a short time after the diathermy unit was brought near or used on the animals, ventricular fibrillation was noted. Fibrillation occurred when the diathermy active electrode touched tissue or when placed up to 33 inches from the animals. Fibrillation was not produced in two similar experiments where different model pacemakers were used. Lichter et al. proposed that the circuitry in the first model was constructed in such a way that the use of a diathermy unit could interfere with the pacemaker signal and produce fibrillation. In another experiment, when animals were irradiated by a unipolar microwave generator at 2.45 GHz and 125-W output power, fibrillation did not result.

Inadvertent radar-induced pacemaker interference has been documented (Yatteau, 1970). It appears that radar from a station 1 mile away suppressed and stimulated the pacemaker's pulse generator, which was located outside the body. Presumably, the radar signals were interpreted by the sensing circuit as ventricular activity, and caused inhibition of impulse formation. Radar stimulation of the demand pacemaker may have been due to a direct effect on the pulse generator.

D'Cunha et al. (1973) cited a case history of a 68-year-old man with a demand-type cardiac pacemaker. He began experiencing attacks of vertigo and fainting and, over a 6-month period, lost consciousness on six occasions. The attacks all occurred at his place of work next to a UHF television transmitter. Attacks did not occur at any other location. Measurements in the parking lot where the syncopal incidents appeared revealed field intensities at 6.63 mW/cm^2 at a frequency of 492 MHz. The distance between the TV antenna and the parking area was roughly 850 feet. When the pacemaker was modified with titanium shielding, pacemaker inhibition ceased and there were no further syncopal episodes.

In a study by Sowton et al. (1970), 41 patients with implanted noncompetitive pacemakers were investigated. A variety of domestic electrical equipment, an automobile, and a physiotherapy apparatus were each operated in turn at various distances from the patient. Interference effects on pacemaker function were assessed. They found no particular model of domestic equipment that was especially liable to interfere with pacemakers, nor any that was completely free from this complication. It was usually necessary for the pacemaker and the domestic appliances to be fairly closely approximated before any effect could be detected. The appliances investigated could be brought near enough to the pacemaker during normal use to produce interference effects, but a fairly minor movement would then separate the pacemakers from the interference source so that normal pacing resumed. In most instances, it was impossible to influence the pacemaker apart from the production of a single ectopic beat when the apparatus was switched on or off. It was felt that the risk to pacemaker patients from domestic appliances is very low.

Sowton et al. (1970) have pointed out that the risk of total inhibition can be avoided if the pacemaker reverts to asynchronous (fixed-rate) pacing in the presence of severe interference. These authors have reemphasized the dangers of diathermy apparatus and coil ignition engines to patients with certain types of implanted, noncompetitive pacemakers.

13.3.5. Laboratory Tests

The earliest tests of pacemaker interference were performed with the pacemaker outside the body. Mansfield (1966) has pointed out that results from tests of this type cannot be applied to patients with implanted pacemakers because the attenuation effect of the body and the difference in electromagnetic coupling greatly reduce the interference risk.

Furman et al. (1968) tested triggered (synchronous) and untriggered (fixed-rate, asynchronous) pacemakers *in vivo* and on the bench for sensitivity to RF signals and intracorporeal 60-Hz alternating current. All untriggered units were insensitive *in vivo* except for those designed to be controlled by RF signals. Triggered pacemakers such as demand and synchronous units exhibited greater sensitivity and greater reversion to inactivity, fixed-rate operation, or maximum synchronous rate in the presence of interference. Two demand units were unaffected by the interfering signals *in vivo*.

Mitchell (1975) reported on a series of tests to determine the thresholds for interference of cardiac pacemakers from radarlike pulses. The study indicated that field intensities of radarlike pulses above some threshold can disrupt normal pacemaker function. The pacemakers tested were most susceptible to interference at frequencies of 500–1000 MHz, with the interference threshold inversely proportional to pulse width. Fields with a pulse-recurrence rate of 1–10 pulses/sec and a peak above the pacemaker's interference threshold could stop the operation of a pacemaker. When the effective pulse-recurrence rate was greater than some inherent value (which depended on the particular device), the pacemaker would revert to an interference-rejection mode by operating at a fixed rate. It was noted in the report that operation of a pacemaker at a fixed rate is generally judged nonhazardous, whereas inhibition of the output of the device could be hazardous.

Pacemakers were tested with the Association for the Advancement of Medical Instrumentation technique of simulating implantation by placing the pacemaker in an 80 × 40 × 20-cm container made of 5-cm-thick plastic foam and filled with 0.03 M saline solution. The pacemaker and leads were placed so that there was 1 cm of solution between the pacemaker and the wall of the container. The "implanted" pacemaker was exposed under controlled laboratory conditions to circularly polarized 450-MHz fields with electric field strengths of up to 292 V/m. The pulse widths and pulse-repetition rates were varied between 1 μsec and 1 msec and between 2 and 40 pulses/sec, respectively. Table 13-3 summarizes the results of Mitchell's report pertaining to 450-MHz interference.

An adverse effect is defined when the pacemaker rate falls below 50 beats/min or exceeds 125 beats/min as a direct result of EMI. Susceptibility to EMI ranged from 8 V/m to over 300 V/m of the 23 pacemaker models tested. Results show a dramatic improvement of newer models, such as the American Optical 281143, over the older models AQ 281003 and 281013 and the Starr Edwards newer model 8116 over the older model 8114. The report indicated that, with design improvements in the newer models, the interference problem should be eliminated.

TABLE 13-3
Summary of Adverse-Effect Thresholds for Cardiac-Pacemaker Electromagnetic Interference (Simulated-Implant Condition Frequency, 450 MHz; Pulse Width, 1 msec)[a]

Pacemaker manufacturer and model number[b]	V/m (beats/min)			
	Pulse repetition rate (pulses/sec)			
	2	10	20	40
American Optical 281003	13(0)	—	15(0)	243(0)
281013	26(0)	—	26(0)	—
281143	>300	—	—	>300
Biotronik IDP44	141(0)	>300	>300	>300
Cordis Atricor 133C7	>300	>300	—	141(172)
Omni-Atricor 164A	>300	>300	—	>300
Stanicor 143E7	15(0)	15(0)	243(0)	>300
Omni Stanicor 162C	8(0)	9(0)	—	>300
General Electric A2072D	29(0)	207(125)	—	—
A2075A	23(0)	141(125)	—	—
Medcor 3-80A	29(0)	141(0)	141(0)	141(0)
Medtronic 5842	15(0)	—	15(0)	15(0)
5942	12(0)	—	12(0)	12(0)
5943	23(0)	—	19(0)	>300
5944	26(0)	26(0)	>300	>300
5950	>300	—	—	>300
5951	>300	—	—	>300
9000	10(0)	10(0)	10(0)	>300
Pacesetter BD-101	>300	—	—	>300
Starr Edwards 8114	23(0)	—	>300	—
8116	>300	>300	—	>300
Stimtech 3821	107(0)	114(0)	>300	—
Vitatron MIP-40-RT	93(0)	107(0)	243(0)	243(0)

[a] Data from Mitchell (1975). Adverse-effect threshold is assigned when pacemaker rate falls between 50 beats/min or exceeds 125 beats/min as a direct result of electromagnetic interference.
[b] It should be noted that because of the extremely rapid development and improvements in cardiac pacing, many of these models may be obsolete at the time of publication.

13.3.6. Control of Potential Hazards

To protect individuals wearing cardiac pacemakers and also to prevent unwarranted implication of factors that may interfere with the operation of the instrument, several points should be recognized.

Representative members from the various companies making pacemakers have met periodically with interested physicians (cardiologists and cardiac surgeons) to discuss problems associated with the manufacture, distribution, utilization, and evaluation of cardiac pacemakers. This group constitutes the Pacemaker Section of the Standards Committee of the Association for the Advancement of Medical Instrumentation, which discusses any and all real or potential problems related to the field of pacemaking and makes recommendations (not in any way binding) to the fabricators or users of these devices.

It is clear that, at worst, electromagnetic fields may cause some synchronous pacers to revert to the asynchronous mode. In those few patients where it might occur, reversion to fixed rate will not pose a significant risk of harm.

The fact that external interference can disrupt the normal operation of some cardiac pacemakers has been recognized almost since the first unit was placed in service, but at the same time, cardiologists have generally maintained that such interference is not clinically significant (Smyth *et al.*, 1974). Notwithstanding these facts, manufacturers recognize that the sources of potential interference are ever increasing and they include EMI as one of many design considerations in their newer devices (Mitchell *et al.*, 1975).

The solution to the problem of potential risk situations can be achieved by the use of improved pacemaker designs and/or implantation methods that are within the state of the art. Thus, proper selection by the cardiologist and/or appropriate attention to state-of-the-art factors of pacemaker design will eliminate any question with regard to electromagnetic field interactions.

It should be noted that under the Medical Devices legislation, the Food and Drug Administration (FDA) is responsible for regulating medical devices such as cardiac pacemakers to assure that these devices are safe and effective. All incidents of pacemaker failure are reported. The FDA is cooperating with the medical profession and the pacemaker industry to reduce the threat of EMI to pacemaker wearers.

There is no agreement among cardiovascular specialists about the seriousness (or sometimes even the existence) of the problems associated with prolonged operation in the interference protection mode. Brief periods of operation in this mode are acceptable as indicated by the wide acceptance of transtelephonic monitoring of cardiac patients in which, by the use of a magnet, the patient actually causes reversion, thus permitting the cardiologist to check the efficiency of the pacer by telephone. It can be estimated that we now have 250,000 patient asynchronous pacing hours per year experience with no evidence of complications having developed.

The interference problem is a complex one as new and more sensitive types of pacemakers are produced in a variety of forms by different manufacturers. A review of pacemaker interference phenomena indicates that the basic problem does not necessarily lie with the interference sources, but that the older pacemakers were not designed to adequately shield out external interference. The basic solution is the modification of pacemaker designs to suppress such interference. The reasonable, prudent, and feasible solution has been to introduce adequate EMI protection into future pacemakers. Studies by Mitchell and Hurt (1976) found that protective shielding is a major factor in preventing or reducing interference.

Studies by the Air Force and other groups indicated that standard EMC techniques could be applied in pacemaker manufacturing to improve the overall characteristics of pacemakers. The Air Force has recommended to the FDA that pacemakers be designed and tested to be compatible with a 450-MHz signal having a pulsed electric field strength of 200 V/m. In the past few years, the manufacturers have made remarkable progress in eliminating the potential EMI problem. At present, essentially all current state-of-technology pacemakers will meet or exceed the EMI threshold level of 200 V/m (Mitchell and Hurt, 1976).

To put the pacemaker situation in perspective, in spite of the fact that there are numerous "everyday" sources of potential EMI, there is not a single documented case in the history of implanted cardiac pacemakers where EMI has resulted in death or other serious consequences to the patient.

Conclusions

The electromagnetic radiation (EMR) emission from microwave ovens, a large number of electrical appliances (e.g., drills, saws, food mixers, hair driers, razors, vacuum cleaners), and the ignition of gasoline engines (e.g., powerboat motors, automobiles, lawn mowers) can cause pacemakers to exhibit reversion to fixed rate, inhibition (cutoff), and tachycardia. However, in almost all such cases the pacemaker must be within about 0.5 m of the source to be adversely affected. Thus, as in the case of microwave ovens, such sources of EMI are not considered a serious threat to most currently marketed pacemakers (Mitchell, 1975).

Fortunately, actual accidents are so infrequent that virtually all are reported. Most small motors (tools and appliances) have too low an output to be dangerous unless they are held directly over the pacemaker (unlikely). Larger signals, such as from on–off switches or arcing equipment (i.e., television sets), are short-term or intermittent and, except in automobile ignitions or razors, not likely to inhibit the pacemaker for more than a beat or two. Specificity further reduces incidence, so that only some pacemakers in some patients are affected by some equipment. The greater degree of vulnerability that could be anticipated with RF receivers has not, apparently, been an issue. In high-frequency interference, inhibition may be the carrier wave or a low-frequency modulation, which brings the impulse into the physiological rate range (microwave-oven mode stirrers). The most vulnerable environment, particularly for external pulse generators, is the hospital with its diathermy, cautery, cardioversion, and electroshock therapy, monitoring equipment, electric beds, and electrical life-support equipment (Escher, 1973).

Upon sensing external EMR, many pacemakers revert to a fixed rate sufficiently close to their demand rate that the user would not normally detect the change (Mitchell, 1975). Reversion to a fixed-rate pacemaker will not cause any cardiac problems and in fact represents a safety factor in the prevention of asystole.

Body shielding can significantly alter the EMI, particularly at frequencies greater than ~ 1 GHz. An individual can completely suppress the EMI by simply rotating his or her body 90–180° to place more body shielding between the pacemaker and the EMR source. Also, pacemakers exhibit immediate recovery to normal function as soon as the EMR signal is eliminated (Mitchell, 1975). The shielding effect of implantation varies from 2:1 to about 10:1, depending on frequency of EMI signal and depth of implantation of the pacemaker. Hardening of pulse generators to withstand 300 V/m is both possible and practical. This would provide ample safety margins for pacemaker patients.

Reported threshold values for electronic cardiac pacemaker EMI range from 8 V/m for the more sensitive devices to greater than 300 V/m for the less sensitive devices. Such EMI threshold values are further modified by the frequency and pulse width of the incident EMR signal. Maximum interference coupling appears to occur at frequencies between 100 and 500 MHz and the EMI threshold is inversely proportional to pulse width over the range from 1 μsec to several milliseconds. The ultimate biological effect is dependent on the characteristics of the EMR source, the proximity of the pacemaker user to the source, and the attenuation afforded by body shielding and orientation. Many manufacturers have recognized EMI as a potential bioeffects problem and have taken the necessary corrective actions to build devices with good EMC.

Continued awareness of potential interference conditions by manufacturers, physicians, and pacemaker users will eventually resolve this problem and serve as the basis for good EMC design for future medical prosthetic devices (Mitchell, 1975).

Reports of interference from household appliances, electric razors, and automobile ignition systems, such as were discussed earlier, no longer appear. This can primarily be related back to the fact that these types of complications occurred in the early use of synchronous pacemakers, above all, because the manufacturers had made no provision for interference. The Medtronic 5841 pacemaker, one of the first demand types, contained no protective mechanism against interference. It is therefore not astonishing that the literature reported over and over again on the failure of these pacemakers. The last unit of this type was delivered in 1970 and, at this time, it is most unlikely that any of them are still being implanted. The experiences with this pacemaker, from which the early information on interference was gathered, can no longer be regarded as typical for demand pacemakers (Irnich et al., 1974).

The problem of EMI, while not a major one, was important enough to evoke from the manufacturers several remedial changes in design including shielding, filtration of extraneous signals, and the provision of a "noise rate" or "interference mode" in which the pulse generator reverted to a fixed rate, often different from the basic rate, in the presence of strong EMI fields. These various improved versions constitute the second generation of demand pacemakers. A third generation later appeared, in which the entire pulse generator or its circuitry was enclosed in a stainless steel or titanium shell to further improve the shielding (Smyth et al., 1974).

According to Smyth et al. (1974) in their combined experience, comprising 2200 patients and perhaps three times as many pacemakers, there have only been ten documented cases of implanted pacemakers affected by EMI. None of the cases was serious and none fatal (Smyth et al., 1974). It is their belief that the action of environmental EMI on the patient with an implanted demand pacemaker does not constitute a clinical problem. They also note that to preserve this status, continued vigilance is needed by physician, manufacturer, and government regulatory agencies (Smyth et al., 1974).

REFERENCES

Abrikosov, I. A. (1958) A Pulsed UHF Electric Field—A New Factor of Physiotherapy. Dissertation, Medgiz, Moscow.

Aronova, S. B. (1961) On the problem of the mechanism of action of a pulsed UHF field on arterial pressure. *Vopr. Kurortol. Fizioter. Lech. Fiz. Kult.* 3:243.

Baronenko, V. A., and K. F. Timofeyeva (1959) Effects of high frequency electromagnetic fields on the conditional reflex activity and certain unconditioned functions of animals and man. *Fiziol. Zh. SSSR im. I.M. Sechenova* **45**:184.

Birenbaum, L., I. T. Kaplan, W. Metlay, S. W. Rosenthal, and M. M. Zaret (1975) Microwave and infrared effects on heart-rate, respiration and subcutaneous temperature of the rabbit. *J. Microwave Power* **10**:3.

Bronte-Steward, B., and R. H. Hepinstall (1954) The relationship between experimental hypertension and cholesterol-induced atheroma in rabbits. *J. Pathol. Bacteriol.* **68**:407.

Carleton, R. A., W. Sessions, and J. S. Graettinger (1964) Environmental influence on implantable cardiac pacemakers. *J. Am. Med. Assoc.* **190**:938.

Chapman, R. M., and C. A. Cain (1975) Absence of heart rate effects in isolated frog heart with pulsed modulated microwave energy. *J. Microwave Power* **10**:411.

Chardack, W. M., A. A. Gage, and W. Greatbatch (1960) A transistorized, self-contained, implantable pacemaker for the long term correction of complete heart block. *Surgery* **48**:643.

Chardack, W. M., A. A. Gage, A. J. Federico, G. Schimert, and W. Greatbatch (1965) Five years' clinical experience with an implantable pacemaker: An appraisal. *Surgery* **58**:915.

Cooper, T., T. Pinakatt, and A. W. Richardson (1961) Effect of microwave-induced hyperthermia on the cardiac output of the rat. *Physiologist* **4**:21.

Cooper, T., T. Pinakatt, M. Jellinek, and A. W. Richardson (1962a) Effects of adrenalectomy, vagotomy and ganglionic blockage on the circulatory response to microwave hyperthermia. *Aeros. Med.* **33**:794.

Cooper, T., T. Pinakatt, M. Jellinek, and A. W. Richardson (1962b) Effects of reserpine on the circulation of the rat after microwave irradiation. *Am. J. Physiol.* **202**:1171.

Cooper, T., T. Pinakatt, M. Jellinek, and A. W. Richardson (1965) The effects of pyridoxine and pyridoxal on the circulatory responses of rats to microwave irradiation. *Experientia* **21**:28.

D'Cunha, G. F., T. Nicoud, A. H. Pemberton, F. F. Rosenbaum, and J. T. Boticelli (1973) Syncopal attacks arising from erratic demand pacemaker function in the vicinity of a television transmitter. *Am. J. Cardiol.* **31**:789.

Drogichina, E. A. (1960) Clinical aspects of the chronic influence of UHF on the human body. In: *The Biological Action of Ultrahigh Frequencies*, A. A. Letavet and Z. V. Gordon (eds.). Acad. Med. Sci., Moscow, pp. 29–31.

Drogichina, E. A., M. N. Sadchikova, G. V. Snegova, N. M. Konchalovskaya, and K. V. Glotova, (1966) Autonomic and cardiovascular disorders during chronic exposure to super-high frequency electromagnetic fields. *Gig. Tr. Prof. Zabol.* **10**:13.

Edelwejn, Z., R. L. Elder, E. Klimkova-Deutschova, and B. Tengroth (1974) Occupational exposure and public health aspects of microwave radiation. In: *Biological Effects and Health Hazards of Microwave Radiation*, P. Czerski, K. Ostrowski, M. L. Shore, C. Silverman, M. J. Suess, and B. Waldeskog (eds.). Polish Medical Publishers, Warsaw, pp. 330–331.

Escher, D. J. W. (1973) Types of pacemakers and their complications. *Circulation* **47**:1119.

Fofanov, P. N. (1969) Hemodynamic changes in individuals working under microwave irradiation. *Kardiologiya* **9**:124.

Frey, A. H., and E. Seifert (1968) Pulsed modulated UHF energy illumination of the heart associated with changes in heart rate. *Life Sci.* **7**:505.

Furman, S., B. Parker, M. Krauthamer, and D. J. W. Escher (1968) The influence of electromagnetic environment on the performance of artificial cardiac pacemakers. *Ann. Thorac. Surg.* **6**:90.

Glotova, K. V., and M. N. Sadchikova (1970) Development and clinical course of cardiovascular changes after chronic exposure to microwave irradiation. *Gig. Tr. Prof. Zabol.* **7**:24.

Gordon, Z. V. (1960) The problem of the biological action of UHF. *Tr. Gig. Tr. Prof. Zabol.* **1**:5.

Gordon, Z. V. (1964) Problems of industrial hygiene and the biological action of various ranges of radio-waves. *Herald Acad. Med. Nauk* **19**:42 (JPRS 27032).

Gordon, Z. V. (1966) Radiofrequency electromagnetic fields as a hygienic factor. *Gig. Tr. Prof. Zabol.* **10**:3.

Gordon, Z. V., Y. A. Lobanova, I. A. Kitsovskaya, and M. S. Tolgskaya (1963) Biologic effects of microwaves of low intensity. *Med. Electron. Biol. Eng.* **1**:67.

Guskova, A. K., and Y. M. Kochanova (1975) Some aspects of etiological diagnostics of occupational diseases as related to the effect of microwave radiation. *Gig. Tr. Prof. Zabol.* **3**:14.

Hamrick, P., and D. McRee (1980) The effect of 2450 MHz microwave irradiation on the heart rate of embryonic quail. *Health Phys.* **38**:261.

Hauswirth, C., and F. Kraemer (1958) Über die Wirkung von Mikrovellen auf das vegetative System. *Wien. Med. Wochenschr.* **108**:172.

Hunyor, S. N., R. Nicks, D. Jones, D. Coles, and J. Heath (1971) Interference hazards with Australian non-competitive ("demand") pacemakers. *Med. J. Aust.* **2**:653.

Irnich, W., J. M. T. de Bakker, and H.-J. Bisping (1974) Interference with cardiac pacemakers, sources of interference, pacemaker behavior, counteractions. *Biomed. Tech.* **19**:193.

Kaplan, I. T., W. Metlay, M. M. Zaret, L. Birenbaum, and S. W. Rosenthal (1971) Absence of heart-rate effects in rabbits during low level microwave irradiation. *IEEE Trans. Microwave Theory Tech.* **MMT-19**:168.

Kevork'yan, A. A. (1948) Working with ultrahigh frequency impulse generators from the standpoint of labor hygiene. *Gig. Sanit.* **4**:26. (ATD pp. 65–68, Library of Congress, Washington, D.C.)

King, G. R., A. C. Hamburger, P. Forough, S. J. Heller, and R. A. Carleton (1970) Effect of microwave oven on implanted cardiac pacemaker. *J. Am. Med. Assoc.* **22**:12.

Levitina, N. A. (1964) Effect of microwaves on the cardiac rhythm of rabbits during local irradiation of body areas. *Byull. Eksp. Biol. Med.* **58**:67.

Lichter, I., J. Borie, and W. M. Miller (1965) Radio-frequency hazards with cardiac pacemakers. *Br. Med. J.* **1**:1513.

Liu, L. M., F. J. Rosenbaum, and W. F. Pickard (1976) Insensitivity of frog heart rate to pulse modulated microwave energy. *J. Microwave Power* **11**:225.

Lu, S.-T., R. Bogardus, J. Cohen, J. Jones, E. Kinnen, and S. Michaelson (1974) Thermogenetic and cardiodynamic regulation in dogs cranially exposed to 2450 MHz (CW) microwaves. University of Rochester Atomic Energy Project Report No. UR-3490-441.

Lu, S., J. Jones, S. Pettit, N. Lebda, and S. Michaelson (1975) Neuroendocrine and cardiodynamic response of the dog subjected to cranial exposure to 2450 MHz microwaves. *Proc. Microwave Power Symp.*, p. 63.

McAfee, R. D. (1961) Neurophysiological effect of 3 cm microwave radiation. *Am. J. Physiol.* **200**:192.

McAfee, R. D. (1963) Physiological effects of thermode and microwave stimulation of peripheral nerves. *Am. J. Physiol.* **203**:374.

McAfee, R. D. (1971) Analeptic effect of microwave irradiation on experimental animals. *IEEE Trans. Microwave Theory Tech.* **MTT-19**:251.

Mansfield, P. B. (1966) ON interference signals and pacemakers. *Am. J. Med. Electron.* **5**:61.

Marks, J., E. T. Carter, D. T. Scarpelli, and E. Eisen (1961) Microwave radiation to the anterior mediastinum of the dog. Histologic and electrocardiographic observations. *Ohio State Med. J.* **57**:274.

Medvedev, V. P. (1973) Cardiovascular diseases in persons with a history of exposure to the effect of an electromagnetic field of extrahigh frequency. *Gig. Tr. Prof. Zabol.* **17**:6.

Michaelson, S. M., and A. J. Moss (1971) Environmental influences on cardiac pacemakers. *J. Am. Med. Assoc.* **216**:2006.

Michaelson, S. M., R. A. E. Thompson, and W. J. Quinlan (1967) Effects of electromagnetic radiation on physiological responses. *Aerosp. Med.* **38**:293.

Mitchell, J. C. (1975) Electromagnetic interference of cardiac pacemakers. *AGARD Lecture Series* No. 78, pp. 10-1–10-10.

Mitchell, J. C., and W. D. Hurt (1976) The Biological Significance of Radiofrequency Radiation Emission on Cardiac Pacemaker Performance. SAM-TR-76-4. Brooks AFB, USAF, AFSC, AMD, p. 13.

Mitchell, J. C., W. D. Hurt, and T. O. Steiner (1975) EMC design effectiveness in electronic medical prosthetic devices. In: *Fundamental and Applied Aspects of Nonionizing Radiation,* S. M. Michaelson, M. W. Miller, R. Magin, and E. L. Carstensen (eds.). Plenum Press, New York, p. 351.

Monayenkova, N. M., and M. N. Sadchikova (1966) Hemodynamic indices during the action of superhigh frequency electromagnetic field. *Gig. Tr. Prof. Zabol.,* **10**:18.

Nikonova, K. V. (1964) Effects of high frequency electromagnetic fields on blood pressure and body temperature of experimental animals. *Tr. Gig. Tr. Prof. Zabol. AMN SSR* pp. 61–65.

Obrosov, A. N., L. A. Skurikhina, and S. N. Safiulina (1963) Effect of microwaves on the cardiovascular system of a healthy person. *Vopr. Kurortol. Fizioter. Lech. Fiz. Kult.* **28**:223.

Orlova, A. A. (1960) Clinical aspects of changes in internal organs brought on by exposure to UHF. *Tr. Gig. Tr. Prof. Zabol.* **1**:36.

Osipov, Y. A. (1952) The influence of ultrahigh-frequency currents under industrial conditions. *Gig. Sanit.* **6**:22.

Osipov, Y. A. (1965) Measures of Protection, Therapy, and Prophylaxis to Be Taken during Work with Radio-frequency Oscillators. JPRS 32735.

Paff, G. H., W. B. Deichmann, and R. J. Boucek (1962) The effect of microwave irradiation on the embryonic chick heart as revealed by electrocardiographic studies. *Anat. Rec.* **142**:264.

Paff, G. H., R. J. Boucek, R. E. Nieman, and W. B. Deichmann (1963) The embryonic heart subjected to radar. *Anat. Rec.* **147**:379.

Parker, B., S. Furman, and D. J. W. Escher (1969) Input signals to pacemakers in a hospital environment. *Ann. N.Y. Acad. Sci.* **167**:823.

Perovsky, A. I., Y. S. Trotsenko, Y. S. Guz, E. S. Volkov, A. J. Barko, and T. N. Koshlyak (1969) The effect of superhigh frequency electromagnetic field on the course of experimental atherosclerosis. *Pat. Fiziol. Eksp. Ter.* **13**:64.

Phillips, R. D., E. L. Hunt, R. D. Castro, and N. W. King (1975) Thermoregulatory, metabolic and cardiovascular response of rats to microwaves. *J. Appl. Physiol.* **38**:630.

Pinakatt, T., T. Cooper, and A. W. Richardson (1963) Effect of ouabain in the circulatory response to microwave hyperthermia in the rat. *Aerosp. Med.* **34**:497.

Pinakatt, T., A. W. Richardson, and T. Cooper (1965) The effect of digitoxin on the circulatory response of rats to microwave irradiation. *Arch. Int. Pharmacodyn. Ther.* **156**:151.

Presman, A. S., and N. A. Levitina (1962a) The non-thermal effect of microwaves on the systolic rhythm of animals. Report I. The effect of non-pulsed microwaves. *Byull. Eks. Biol. Med.* **53**:39.

Presman, A. S., and N. A. Levitina (1962b) The non-thermal effect of microwaves on the rhythm of cardiac contractions in animals. Report II. Investigations of the effect of pulsed microwaves. *Byull. Eksp. Biol. Med.* **53:**41.

Reed, J. R., J. L. Lords, and C. H. Durney (1977) Microwave irradiation of the isolated rat heart after treatment with ANS blocking agents. *Radio Sci.* **12(6S):**161.

Richardson, A. W. (1954) Effect of microwave induced heating on the blood flow through peripheral skeletal muscles. *J. Phys. Med.* **33:**103.

Richardson, A. W., C. J. Imig, and B. L. Feucht (1950) The relationship between deep tissue temperature and blood flow during electromagnetic irradiation. *Arch. Phys. Med.* **31:**19.

Roberts, N. J., Jr., S. M. Michaelson, and S. T. Lu (1986) The biological effects of radiofrequency radiation: A critical review and recommendation. *Int. J. Radiat. Biol.* **50:**379.

Röhl, D., H. M. Laun, M. E. T. Hauber, M. Stauch, and H. Voight (1975) The effect of radar on cardiac pacemakers. *ISA Trans.* **14:**115.

Sacchitelli, F., and G. Sacchitelli (1960) On the protection of personnel exposed to radar microwaves. *Folia Med. (Naples)* **43:**1219.

Sadchikova, M. N. (1974) Clinical manifestations of reactions to microwave irradiation in various occupational groups. In: *Biological Effects and Health Hazards of Microwave Radiation,* P. Czerski, K. Ostrowski, M. L. Shore, C. Silverman, M. J. Suess, and B. Waldeskog (eds.). Polish Medical Publishers, Warsaw, pp. 261–267.

Sadchikova, M. N., and K. V. Nikonova (1971) Comparative evaluation of the state of health in persons working under conditions involving exposure to microwaves at different intensity. *Tr. Nii Gig. Tr. Prof. Zabol.* **159:**10.

Sadchikova, M. N., and A. A. Orlova (1958) Clinical picture of the chronic effects of electromagnetic microwaves. *Ind. Hyg. Occup. Dis.* **2:**18.

Siddons, H., and E. Sowton (1967) *Cardiac Pacemakers.* Thomas, Springfield, Ill.

Silver, A. W., G. Root, F. X. Byron, and H. Sandberg (1965) Externally rechargeable cardiac pacemaker. *Ann. Thorac. Surg.* **1:**380.

Smyth, N. P., V. Parsonnet, D. J. W. Escher, and S. Furman (1974) The pacemaker patient and the electromagnetic environment. *J. Am. Med. Assoc.* **227:**1412.

Sowton, E., K. Gray, and T. Preston (1970) Electrical interference in non-competitive pacemakers. *Br. Heart J.* **32:**626.

Sparks, H. V., D. L. Mossman, and C. L. Seidel (1976) Radio and microwave radiation and experimental atherosclerosis. *Atherosclerosis* **25:**55.

Subbota, A. G. (1957) Changes in respiration, pulse rate and general blood pressure during irradiation of animals with a UHF field. *Tr. Voyen. Med. Akad. Kirov* **73:**35.

Subbota, A. G. (1970) Nonthermal effects of microwaves. *Voyen. Med. Zh.* **9:**39.

Tyagin, N. V. (1957a) Changes in the blood of animals subjected to a UHF–SHF field. *Tr. Voyen. Med. Akad. Kirov* **73:**116.

Tyagin, N. V. (1957b) Electrocardiogram changes in dogs affected by SHF–UHF electromagnetic fields. *Tr. Voyen. Med. Akad. Kirov* **73:**84.

Weinberg, D. I., J. L. Artley, R. E. Whalen, and H. D. McIntosh (1962) Electric shock hazards in cardiac catheterization. *Circ. Res.* **11:**1004.

Whalen, R. E., F. Starmer, and H. D. McIntosh (1964) Electrical hazards associated with cardiac pacemaking. *Ann. N.Y. Acad. Sci.* **111:**922.

Yatteau, R. F. (1970) Radar-induced failure of a demand pacemaker. *N. Engl. J. Med.* **283:**1447.

14

Effects on Hematopoiesis and Hematology

A number of investigators have reported that the blood and blood-forming system are not affected by acute or chronic microwave exposure (Barron and Baraff, 1958; Daily, 1943; Drogichina *et al.*, 1966; Tyagin, 1957; Hyde and Friedman, 1968; Budd *et al.*, 1970; Spalding *et al.*, 1971). Effects on hematopoiesis have nevertheless been found by others (Petrov, 1970; Sadchikova and Orlova, 1958; Michaelson *et al.*, 1961, 1964, 1965, 1967; Kitsovskaya, 1964; Baranski and Czerski, 1966; Baranski, 1971, 1972; Goncharova *et al.*, 1966; Sacchitelli and Sacchitelli, 1960; Vacek, 1972; Czerski *et al.*, 1974a,b; Ivanov, 1962).

Analysis of these reports reveals divergence of results among studies and internal inconsistencies within certain studies. It does appear, nevertheless, that at high field intensities, well within the thermogenic range, hematopoietic and hemocytological shifts do develop which are comparable to those resulting from increased temperature within the body. Of significance also is the fact that adaptation is noted during multiple or chronic exposure or recovery occurs shortly after cessation of exposure.

14.1. IN VITRO STUDIES

Studies of the effects of microwave irradiation on the erthrocyte membrane have yielded conflicting results. In studies reported by Baranski *et al.* (1974) and Szmigielski (1975), red cell suspensions were exposed in thin-walled Plexiglas vials (2-cm diameter) to 3000 MHz CW at 1, 5, or 10 mW/cm^2 for 15–120 min. Granulocytes were exposed to 3000 MHz CW at 1 or 5 mW/cm^2 for 15–30 min. Increased permeability of erythrocyte membranes to hemoglobin was observed only after irradiation at 1 mW/cm^2 for 60 min. During the first 2 hr of irradiation at 1 mW/cm^2, no significant change in osmotic resistance of erythrocytes was observed. After 120 min of exposure, hemolysis occurred; at higher power densities, osmotic resistance decreased after 30 min.

Alteration in potassium metabolism was observed in erythrocytes exposed for 15 min at 1 mW/cm^2. An increase in the percentage of dead granulocytes was observed only in suspensions irradiated at 5 mW/cm^2. In reviewing these reports, it is important to note that the authors do not provide any statistics. Whether the differences noted are statistically significant is not clear because in many of these determinations the control samples show similar changes, albeit not to the same extent.

Transport and related properties of red cell membranes have been investigated. In these cases, K$^+$ transport was used as an endpoint. In the RBC, virtually all Na$^+$ and K$^+$ transport across the membrane is by the enzyme Na$^+$, K$^+$-ATPase. Ismailov (1971) exposed human RBCs to 1.0-GHz CW microwaves at a dose rate of 45 W/kg and found an increased efflux of K$^+$ and a concomitant increased influx of Na$^+$. The Na$^+$ influx was twice as large as the K$^+$ efflux. Exposures were carried out in a coaxial stripline for 30 min, with analysis of the ion content of the supernatant performed afterwards.

Baranski et al. (1971, 1974) observed greater leakage of both hemoglobin and K$^+$ from microwave-irradiated erythrocytes than from RBCs maintained at room temperature. In their experiments, rabbit RBCs were irradiated at 3 GHz with various power densities (1, 5, or 10 mW/cm^2). Similar results were obtained for human erythrocytes by Ismailov (1971) at a frequency of 1 GHz. Hamrick and Zinkl (1975) and Peterson et al. (1979) have performed similar experiments exposing RBCs at 2.45 GHz in the far field; dose rates were 3 to 57 W/kg, and about 200 W/kg, respectively. In neither investigation was there a difference between the K$^+$ efflux from microwave-exposed RBCs and conventionally heated RBCs with similar temperature histories, although Peterson et al. (1979) did find a difference between unexposed rabbit cells maintained at 25°C compared to those maintained at 37°C. This difference did not occur with human cells. Ismailov (1971) also used temperature controls, but he did not describe the composition of the solution in which the cells were suspended. Under some conditions, it is possible to reverse the Na$^+$, K$^+$-ATPase; however, Ismailov's (1971) controls behaved normally, indicating that no intervening factors confounded the controls.

Hamrick and Zinkl (1975) and Peterson et al. (1979) measured other endpoints as well. The former study looked at osmotic fragility of the RBCs and concluded that there was no difference. The latter paper gives data on hemoglobin release from RBCs, an indicator of membrane fragility. Again no differences were found between irradiated and heat-treated RBCs. Liu et al. (1979) similarly reported no significant differences in either K$^+$ efflux or hemoglobin release between microwave-treated RBCs and erythrocytes warmed to the same temperature by conventional heating techniques. These investigators irradiated rabbit RBCs at 2.45, 3, or 3.95 GHz with power densities of 10–58 mW/cm^2.

In this context, the effect of the shape and nature of the sample container, and of the depth of liquid on the actual field in the sample must be considered. Samples, containers, and the liquid in which the sample is suspended may act as dielectric lenses and/or reflectors and cause localized hot spots in the samples, which may render dosimetry inaccurate (Grant et al., 1974). If one were to consider watts per cubic centimeter in an absorber such as 5 cm^3 of water, 5 cal of heat energy would raise the temperature by 1°C. It is most likely, therefore, that thermal factors cannot be ignored in studies in which small sample volumes are used.

Ismailov (1978) also found increases in the electrophoretic mobility of human RBCs exposed under conditions identical to those in his study discussed previously. The electrophoretic mobility was measured at 10-min intervals after cessation of exposure. The mobility was found to peak at 30 min postexposure and return to baseline by about 60 min postexposure. The peak mobility decreased with shorter exposure durations (30, 15, 8, and 4 min). The mobility change also decreased as a function of energy absorption, disappearing between 5 and 10 W/kg. Although a change in the counterion distribution around the cell and possible conformational changes in the membrane proteins were studied as possible causes, it remains unclear why these phenomena peaked 30 min postexposure.

Passive ion transport in rabbit RBCs was examined by Olcerst et al. (1980) after exposure to 2.45 GHz CW at SARs of 100, 190, and 390 W/kg. The rabbit cells were treated with ouabain to inhibit active transport of Na^+ and K^+ by Na^+, K^+-ATPase. The exposures were conducted in a waveguide system in which the sample was placed in a cylindrical tube parallel to the E-field. Low-dielectric-constant organic coolant was circulated around the sample in a larger concentric cylinder to maintain the temperature of the sample under exposure. SARs were computed from measured forward and reflected power. The RBCs were preincubated with radioactive sodium and rubidium ion. Samples were exposed or heat-treated for 1 hr and the suspending medium analyzed for radioactivity. Graphs of the logarithm of the efflux versus inverse temperature were identical except at three transition temperatures where the exposed samples exhibited considerably higher efflux than the heated samples; however, no consistent differences between exposure levels could be established.

Peterson et al. (1979) also studied the effects of exposure throughout the range 12.5–18 GHz on K^+ efflux and hemoglobin loss by erythrocytes. Both conventionally heated and room temperature controls were employed in this study in order to facilitate comparison with earlier investigations (vide supra). Techniques were developed for irradiation of multiple samples, which assured that all erythrocytes in each RBC sample would be exposed to the same average power density. In addition, a technique was devised by which sample temperature could be continuously monitored by use of a relatively nonperturbing liquid crystal optic fiber (LCOF) temperature probe (Rozzell et al., 1974). The results obtained from such carefully controlled experiments indicate that heating of rabbit erythrocytes above room temperature by either microwave energy or conventional techniques causes an increased loss of hemoglobin and K^+. However, the effects of microwave heating and conventional heating were indistinguishable at all frequencies and power levels studied.

Platelet-rich human plasma was irradiated *in vitro* with 2450-MHz microwaves at power densities from 10 to 20 mW/cm^2 (1.3 to 38 W/kg) for 30 min to 24 hr by Boggs et al. (1972), and the effects on blood coagulation were analyzed. There were no significant changes in platelet count, coagulation time, or clot strength at these power densities.

When human RBCs were warmed to 37°C by 2.45-GHz microwaves or by conventional heating, the amount of leakage of either hemoglobin or K^+ did not differ from that for RBCs maintained at room temperature. Human RBC membranes are apparently more resistant to both microwave heating and conventional heating than are rabbit RBC membranes. Any increased loss of either hemoglobin or K^+ from microwave-irradiated rabbit RBCs was thus attributed to thermal effects on RBC membrane stability or permeability.

Olcerst and Rabinowitz (1978) found no effect on aqueous cholinesterase exposed to 2450 MHz CW at up to 125 mW/cm^2 for 1/2 hr or 25 mW/cm^2 for 3 hr. No effect was found on cholinesterase activity in defibrinated rabbit blood exposed for 3 hr to 21, 35, or 64 mW/cm^2, 2450 MHz CW or pulsed. Under similar exposure conditions, there was no effect on release of bound calcium or magnesium from rabbit RBCs. The only significant changes in cholinesterase activity were seen when the absorbed power caused thermal denaturation of the protein.

Erythrocyte damage to blood units in Fenwal blood bags was examined after water bath warming and after warming by a microwave blood warmer operating at a frequency of 2450 MHz (Linko and Hynynen, 1979). Extracellular hemoglobin and potassium, hematocrit, osmotic fragility, and mean cellular volume were used as indicators of RBC damage. The results indicate that microwaves *per se* are not harmful to erythrocytes but that penetration of microwaves together with insufficient blood mixing during warming are the critical factors leading to hemolysis.

14.2. ANIMAL EXPERIMENTS

Mice subjected to 10,000 MHz pulsed microwaves at 450 mW/cm^2 for 5 min showed a decrease in erythrocytes, leukocytes, and hemoglobin immediately, and at 1 and 5 days (Gorodetskaya, 1964). Hematological recovery was evident 10 days after exposure. Qualitatively similar changes also occurred with convectional heat.

Prausnitz and Süsskind (1962) studied the pathology and longevity in male Swiss mice exposed to an average power density of 100 mW/cm^2, 9270-MHz pulsed RF (duty cycle = 0.001) for 4.5 min daily, 5 days/week for 59 weeks. The exposure produced an average colonic temperature rise of 3.3°C. This daily dose is stated to be one-half the LD_{50} for the mice. Originally, there were 200 irradiated mice and 100 control mice. Two series of sacrifices were performed during the irradiation period. At 7 months into the experiment, 5% of both groups were killed and at 16 months (within 1 month after final irradiation) 10% of each group were killed. Survivors were killed 4 months after the final irradiation; 50% of the control animals and 64% of the irradiated mice were still alive. Although the authors stated that the longevity of the mice did not appear to be affected, the intermittent sacrifice, termination of the experiment at an apparently arbitrary point, and the lack of statistical analyses of the survival data would not support this statement. Twenty-three percent of the animals were lost to the study by spontaneous death and autolysis prior to necropsy. The remaining 100 animals (40 controls, 60 experimentals) formed a "longevity" study group. One of the findings reported in this group was "cancer of the white cells" defined as monocytic or lymphocytic leukosis, or lymphatic or myeloid leukemia.

Leukosis was defined as a noncirculating neoplasm of the white cells, whereas leukemia was defined as a circulating leukosis. Data were grouped and reported as "leukosis," which is particularly unfortunate since the organs used to look for lymphoid infiltration did not include the liver and spleen—organs usually involved in this kind of reaction, and data on the differential composition of the blood cell types were not presented. Appropriate statistical analysis, however, revealed that the prevalence of "leukosis" in irradiated animals was not significantly different from that in the control animals for any of the sacrifice series data. According to modern criteria, it is highly unlikely that these indications would be considered "cancer of white blood cells," as suggested by the authors (Roberts and Michaelson, 1983).

These data are severely compromised by (1) the high loss of animals, (2) the differential loss of control animals due to infection, and (3) the premature sacrifice of all remaining animals to resolve a nonexistent paradox. Furthermore, comparing groups of animals that selected themselves (by dying prior to 19 months and being found in time for necropsy) is not appropriate for optimal statistical procedures for the design or analysis of experimental data.

In summary, because of numerous flaws in the biological protocol, the lack of statistical methodology in the design of the experiment and in the analysis of the results, as well as the questionable significance of what was reported, the study by Prausnitz and Süsskind does not provide evidence of leukemia or other morbidity as a result of chronic exposure to microwaves (Roberts and Michaelson, 1983).

Baranski (1972) did not succeed in observing the changes of "leucaemic character" such as reported by Prausnitz and Süsskind (1962) in guinea pigs exposed to 10,000 MHz CW, 3.5 mW/cm^2, 3 hr daily for 3 months.

Spalding et al. (1971) exposed adult female mice in a waveguide to 800 MHz, average incident power density 43 mW/cm^2 (est. SAR 12.9 W/kg) for 2 hr daily, 5 days/week for 35 weeks. No changes in erythrocytes, leukocytes, hematocrit, or hemoglobin concentration were evident, nor did the mean life span of control compared to exposed mice differ significantly. There were no changes in the peripheral blood picture of exposed mice, although a thermal burden was placed on these animals. Four mice died from "thermal effects" on the 33rd and 34th exposures.

Hyde and Friedman (1968) exposed anesthetized female CF-1 mice to 3000 MHz, 20 mW/cm^2, and 10,000 MHz, 17, 40, or 60 mW/cm^2 for up to 15 min. No significant effect on total or differential leukocyte count or hemoglobin concentration was noted immediately, 3, 7, or 20 days after exposure. There were no changes in femoral bone marrow other than a variable but slight increase in the eosinophil series of the exposed animals which was not reflected in peripheral blood counts.

Ragan and Phillips (1980) exposed female mice in the far field of an anechoic chamber to horizontal-polarization 2.88-GHz pulsed microwaves, 3–7.5 hr daily for 60–360 hr at an incident power density of 5 or 10 mW/cm^2. The mice were housed individually during exposures in Lucite containers and exposed in groups of eight. SARs were determined in animals with the long axis of the body oriented in the E, H, and K vectors. Mean SARs were 2.25 mW/g at 5 mW/cm^2, and 4.50 mW/g at 10 mW/cm^2. Five studies were performed at 5 mW/cm^2, and four at 10 mW/cm^2. For each exposure, littermate controls were sham-exposed. In two of five studies at 5 mW/cm^2 pulsed microwaves, there was a significant ($p > 0.01$ and < 0.05) increase in bone marrow cellularity compared to the sham-exposed groups, but in the other three exposures at 5 mW/cm^2 no significant effect was observed. Differences were occasionally seen in the erythrocyte, leukocyte, platelet, and reticulocyte measurements from microwave-exposed groups, but were not statistically significant when appropriate tests were used. No effect on bone marrow hematopoietic colony-forming units (CFU) was revealed by CFU-agar assay techniques following exposure of mice to 5 mW/cm^2 pulsed microwaves. In one of four exposures to 10 mW/cm^2 pulsed microwaves, there was a significant ($p < 0.05$) increase in CFU-agar colonies. No exposure-related histopathological lesions were found when numerous tissues were examined from mice exposed at 10 mW/cm^2 for 200–300 hr.

In mice subjected to 2450 MHz CW, 100 mW/cm^2 for 5 min, Rotkovska and Vacek (1972, 1975) noted an increase in leukocytes that lasted 3–4 days and stimulation of hematopoietic activity in the bone marrow and spleen with an increase in the hematopoietic stem cell pool. This is in contrast to a decrease in erythrocyte production in guinea pigs reported by Czerski (1975). In the mice exposed by Rotkovska and Vacek (1975), the colonic temperature rose 2.3°C. Exposure to convectional heat sufficient to raise the colonic temperature 2.5°C produced reactions that were qualitatively, although not necessarily quantitatively, similar. It is of interest that neither the erythrocyte count nor ^{59}Fe incorporation in the femur was significantly altered by this exposure.

Several studies have provided evidence that microwave exposure of X-irradiated mice results in an accelerated recovery of hematopoietic tissue and an increase in their rate of survival (Rotkovska and Vacek, 1977). Microwave exposure (2450 MHz, 100 mW/cm^2, 5 min) was used to modify X-irradiation damage of the hematopoietic system in the mouse. Compared with X-irradiated controls, microwave-treated mice manifested an increased number of surviving hematopoietic stem cells, heightened erythropoiesis and myelopoiesis, and increased rate of survival.

Increase in the number of hematopoietic endogenous colonies (ESC) in the spleens of X-irradiated mice after microwave exposure supports earlier observations of an elevation of the number of stem cells in the spleens of intact mice after microwave exposure alone (Rotkovska and Vacek, 1975). Results of both experiments indicate that microwaves may influence the intricate mechanisms that activate the pool of stem cells. Since ESC grow from the hematopoietic stem cells that survive X-irradiation, the increase in their number may be due either to an improvement of the repair of sublethal radiation damage of the irradiated stem cells, or to increased proliferation of the stem cells that survive X-irradiation. The course of changes in the number of ESC in experimental mice correlated to a considerable extent with changes in the number of ESC after dose-fractionation X-ray exposures. These changes have been explained as a manifestation of a decrease in the radiosensitivity of the hematopoietic stem cells during intercellular repair of radiation damage. An acceleration of the repair processes of radiation damage of hematopoietic cells appears to occur following exposure to microwaves and is dependent upon the stage of intracellular repair at the time of microwave exposure.

An analysis of rates of survival of mice (Rotkovska and Vacek, 1972; Thomson *et al.*, 1965) and dogs (Michaelson *et al.*, 1963) after exposure to combined X-ray and microwave energies suggests that a decrease in radiosensitivity of the animals could be due to a stimulating effect of microwaves on the hematopoietic system. Michaelson *et al.* (1963) had earlier reported that simultaneous exposure to X rays and microwaves (2800 MHz, pulse-modulated, 100 mW/cm^2) accelerated recovery of hematopoietic function in dogs. Lappenbusch *et al.* (1973) reported that exposure of X-irradiated (725 to 950 R) Chinese hamsters to microwaves (2450 MHz CW, 60 mW/cm^2 for 30 min) 5 min following X-irradiation significantly increased the X-ray LD$_{50/30}$ compared to X rays alone or microwave exposure followed by X rays. The radioprotective effect of microwaves was associated with a delayed drop in the number of circulating white blood cells, reduced period of low cell density, and complete replenishment of white blood cells within 30 days following the dual treatment. Exposure to microwaves alone or in combination with X-ray exposure increased the relative number of neutrophils, reduced the relative number of lymphocytes, and slightly increased the number of circulating RBCs. Animals exposed first to microwaves and then to X rays demonstrated more severe leukocyte changes than X-irradiated hamsters because leukocyte counts dropped faster and the animals developed leukopenia. The radioprotective effect of microwaves may be due to a thermal mechanism involving surviving bone marrow cells.

Smialowicz (1979) exposed mice to 2450 MHz CW at 30 mW/cm^2 (SAR 22 mW/g) for 30 min on 22 consecutive days. These mice showed no significant differences in circulating erythrocyte counts, total and differential leukocyte counts, hematocrit, and hemoglobin concentration compared to sham-controls. Under the conditions of this study, microwave exposure did not elevate the colonic temperatures of exposed mice significantly more than among sham-controls. In contrast, when mice were exposed to thermogenic (2 to 4°C rise in rectal temperature) levels with 16 MHz CW, 8610 mW/cm^2, decreased numbers of circulating lymphocytes and increased circulating neutrophils were observed immediately following exposure (Liburdy, 1977). This shift reached its peak 3 hr after exposure. Levels of circulating lymphocytes and neutrophils returned to normal from 55 to 96 hr following exposure. On the other hand, mice exposed to high temperatures in a vented, dry-air oven showed an increase in circulating lymphocytes and neutrophils for 12 hr following exposure. It appears, therefore, that the response of circulating leukocytes to thermal loads depends on thermal distributions in the body (Smialowicz, 1979).

Preskorn *et al.* (1978) compared the life span of sham-treated and irradiated mice injected with sarcoma cells at 16 days of age. These were the offspring of pregnant mice exposed for 20 min daily on days 11, 12, 13, and 14 of gestation in a multimodal cavity at an SAR of 35 W/kg.

The mean and maximum survival time of "irradiated mice with tumors" exceeded those of "nonirradiated mice with tumors" ($p < 0.05$). The average survival time of "irradiates without tumors" was also greater than "controls without tumors." When 50% of the controls had died, 67% of the irradiates were alive. The difference was not significant, however, and maximum life span was unaltered.

Kitsovskaya (1964) subjected rats to 3000-MHz pulsed microwaves according to the following schedule: 10 mW/cm^2, 60 min, 216 days; 40 mW/cm^2, 15 min, 20 days; 100 mW/cm^2, 5 min, 6 days. At 40 and 100 mW/cm^2, total erythrocyte, leukocyte, and absolute lymphocyte counts were decreased; granulocytes and reticulocytes were elevated. At 10 mW/cm^2, total leukocyte, and absolute lymphocyte counts were decreased, and granulocytes increased. Bone marrow examination revealed erythroid hyperplasia at the higher power levels. The blood did not return to its normal state for several months after the series of exposures was discontinued. Since details of the exposure are not available, one cannot pass judgment on this report. It should be noted, however, that these were pulsed exposures of sufficient power density–time combinations to result in increased body temperature. Such temperature elevation can result in hematological redistribution. Decreased leukocyte count and phagocytic activity had been reported in rats and rabbits exposed to 50 MHz, 0.5 to 6.0 V/m, 10 to 12 hr/day, 180 days (Serdiuk, 1969).

Pazderova-Vejlupkova and Josifko (1979) reported that in rats exposed to 24.4 mW/cm^2 of pulsed microwaves, recovery of lymphocyte depression was evident 2 months after exposure. They exposed male rats for 7 weeks (5 days/week, 4 hr/day) to 2736.5 MHz (395 Hz pulse-repetition frequency prf, pulse width 1.6 μsec, mean power density 24.4 mW/cm^2). The colonic temperature increased 0.5°C during exposure. Blood was taken prior to and at the end of the 1st, 3rd, 5th, and 7th weeks of irradiation, and the 1st, 2nd, 6th, and 10th weeks after irradiation. The parameters studied included hematocrit, differential and absolute leukocyte count, alkaline phosphatase activity in neutrophils, and body weight. The results were compared with data obtained from a control group of 20 animals and evaluated by Student's test at a significance level of 1%. In the second half of the irradiation period, the experimental animals exhibited significantly lower mean hematocrit values, lower number of leukocytes, and lower absolute number of lymphocytes. These changes disappeared gradually within 10 weeks after cessation of exposure. Alkaline phosphatase in neutrophils was significantly increased in the 1st week of irradiation and dropped transiently after the irradiation. In the postirradiation interval, experimental animals displayed a significant decline in rate of body weight increase. The other parameters did not differ from the controls.

The initial drop in hematocrit value in both control and irradiated animals can be attributed to blood loss from frequent blood withdrawal in very young rats. This decreased with increasing intervals between individual blood samplings and with the growth of animals during adolescence. Retarded increase in the hematocrit value of irradiated rats during their adolescence, beginning in the second half of the irradiation period and persisting for several weeks after irradiation, was reproducible and explained only as being brought about by the irradiation.

Hematological changes were reported in immobilized Sprague–Dawley rats exposed for 7.5 hr to 24,000 MHz pulsed, 24 mW/cm^2 (Deichmann et al., 1959, 1964). There was an immediate rise in erythrocyte count and hemoglobin, and a drop in number of total leukocytes. The leukopenia was due to a drop in lymphocytes. Erythrocyte and hemoglobin recovery were prompt but 1 week elapsed before the leukocytes had returned to the preexposure level. Similar exposure of Osborne–Mendel, CFN, and Fischer strain rats induced a significant leukopenia, lymphopenia, and neutrophilia after 7 hr of continuous exposure to 20 mW/cm^2 with recovery in 1 week; 10 min of continuous exposure to 20 mW/cm^2, and 3 hr of continuous exposure to 10 mW/cm^2 with recovery in 2 days. Effects on erythrocytes, hemoglobin, and hematocrit differed in the three strains used. In Osborne–Mendel and CFN rats, all values increased; in Fischer rats, they decreased. These animals were immobilized and experienced a colonic temperature increase that by itself would produce blood cell changes. However, the differences in response among strains of rats are interesting and illustrate the importance of strain differences.

Djordjevic and Kolak (1973) exposed rats to 2400 MHz CW at 10 mW/cm^2 for 2 hr daily for from 10 to 30 days. Body temperature in rats exposed under these conditions increased by 1°C within the first 30 min of exposure, and remained at this level through the exposure period. Hematocrit, hemoglobin concentration, and circulating erythrocytes in the exposed rats increased during the 30-day exposure, and fluctuations in the various leukocyte populations also fluctuated—changes that were thought to be due to the thermal effect of microwaves.

Djordjevic et al. (1977) exposed male rats to 2400 MHz CW at 5 mW/cm^2, 1 hr daily for 90 days. Before, during, and after the irradiation period, hematological examinations were carried out. The histological examinations of various organs and tissues of irradiated rats were carried out after the experimental period. No significant difference in any of the observed biological parameters was detected in experimental animals in comparison with controls. It is of interest that the authors noted leukocyte increase in the control animals and exposed rats during the exposure. There was no significant difference between exposed and control groups.

Switzer and Mitchell (1977) exposed female Sprague–Dawley rats to 2.45 GHz CW in a multimodal resonating cavity with resultant SAR of 2.3 mW/g. The rats were exposed simultaneously, but restrained individually in polystyrene cylinders. Animals were exposed 5 hr daily for a total exposure of 550 hr. Littermate controls were sham-exposed under similar handling and housing conditions. RBC counts of the microwave-exposed rats were significantly ($p < 0.05$) increased over those of the sham-exposed rats, but mean hemoglobin and volume of packed RBC values were not different between the two groups. Mean WBC counts of the exposed rats were slightly greater than in the sham-exposed group, but the difference was not statistically significant. Comparisons of leukocyte differential counts revealed no significant differences between the two exposure regimens, although lymphocyte concentrations were lower and monocyte counts were higher in the exposed rats.

Hamrick and MeRee (1975) exposed quail eggs for 24 hr on the second day of incubation to 2450 MHz CW at 30 mW/cm^2 (SAR 14 mW/g). At 24 to 36 hr after hatching, quails were examined for gross deformities, changes in organ weight, and hematological changes. No significant effects due to microwave exposure were detected.

Budd *et al.* (1970) investigated the sensitivity of the fetal rat's hematological system by *in utero* microwave irradiation. Pregnant Sprague–Dawley rats were exposed at 15 days of gestation for 8.5 min to whole-body 2450 MHz, 100 mW/cm^2. Under these conditions, the colonic temperature of the irradiated rats increased 4.2°C above that of the controls. Hematological factors were measured in the pregnant rats at 4 hr, 24 hr, and 5 days postirradiation (shortly before the fetuses were removed). Body and spleen weights, and hematological changes were measured in the fetal rats at gestation day 20. No significant differences were found between control and microwave-exposed pregnant rats in body weight, leukocyte count, erythrocyte count, hematocrit, or hemoglobin value. Microwave-irradiated fetuses had significantly lower spleen weight ($p < 0.05$), total leukocyte count ($p < 0.01$), and somewhat lower hemoglobin value ($p < 0.10$) than controls. No appreciable differences were observed between microwave-irradiated fetuses and their controls in body weight, ^{59}Fe uptake in blood, or fetal resorption. The lack of any effect in the fetus than that which has been reported is noteworthy.

Smialowicz (1979) exposed rats pre- and postnatally to 425 MHz CW at 10 mW/cm^2 4 hr daily for up to 40 or 41 days after birth. Because of growth of animals during this time, SARs ranged from 3 to 7 mW/g. Absolute neutropenia and relative lymphocytosis were observed in exposed compared to sham-exposed rats, but these changes were not consistently reproduced. Rats exposed under the same regimen but to 2450 MHz CW at 5 mW/cm^2 (SAR 1–5 mW/g) showed no difference in circulating erythrocyte count, total and differential leukocyte counts, hematocrit, and hemoglobin concentration when compared to sham-controls.

Baranski (1971, 1972) exposed guinea pigs to 3000 MHz, 3.5 mW/cm^2, CW and pulsed 3 hr daily for 3 months. No changes in the granulocyte blood series were found. In the lymphocyte system, mitotic disturbances and changes in nuclear structure were noted. Lymphocytosis was also reported. It should be noted, however, that a comparison of the absolute numbers of lymphocytes in various periods of the experiment showed considerable fluctuation even during the preirradiation period. For example, before irradiation the mean number of lymphocytes was 5000/cm^3 with a range of 2500–11,800. One week after irradiation, the mean was 12,500 with a range of 10,500–16,800. Four weeks after irradiation, the mean was 6800 for CW and 8000 for pulsed with a range of 5900–8200 for CW and 7100–10,200 for pulsed. Regrettably, the author did not make any comparisons with control animals that should have been handled the same way. Similar fluctuations could occur under normal conditions.

Czerski *et al.* (1974a,b) noted "perhaps the most interesting finding is that 74 hours of exposure to pulsed microwaves induced much more pronounced effects than exposure to CW of the same duration, the differences between both these groups being highly significant. On the other hand, 158-hour exposure to CW microwaves is very similar in effect to those of exposure to pulsed microwaves of half that duration." In discussing some observations on effects of microwave exposure on the circadian rhythm of mitosis of cells belonging to various hematopoietic cell lines, Czerski *et al.* (1974a,b) suggested "this may serve to stress the importance of taking into account the physiologic properties of cells, tissues, and organs when investigating microwave bioeffects and the danger of generalizations."

In a series of studies carried out by Czerski, Baranski, and associates (Czerski, 1975; Czerski *et al.*, 1974a,b), guinea pigs were exposed to 3000 MHz CW and pulsed at 3 mW/cm^2 for 2 hr daily. One group was exposed for a total of 74 hr (37 days) to CW microwaves. The second group was exposed similarly to pulsed microwaves. The third group was exposed for 158 hr (79 days) to CW. The hemoglobin level and hematocrit did not change significantly. It appears that erythrocyte production was significantly altered. The CW exposure produced a moderate decrease in RBC production; for the same exposure, pulsed microwaves produced a marked increase in RBC production. Quantitative differences were demonstrated between the effects of exposure to CW and pulsed microwaves under identical conditions of mean power density, frequency, and duration (Czerski, 1975).

Chou et al. (1978) exposed rabbits to 2.45-GHz CW or pulsed microwaves at an average power density of 1.5 mW/cm^2 for 2 hr daily for 3 months. The mean SAR was 0.5 mW/g. An additional group of six rabbits was sham-exposed. No significant differences between groups were seen in hematological profiles obtained monthly.

In order to assess the long-term effects of microwave irradiation, Guy et al. (1980) developed a special exposure system to expose four rabbits to 2450 MHz, 10 mW/cm^2 (max. SAR 17 W/kg) 23 hr daily for 180 days. Comparison with four sham-exposed rabbits revealed no significant effects in terms of colonic temperature, hematocrit, hemoglobin, WBC count, and blood-coagulation studies.

Ferri and Hagen (1975) exposed six rabbits to 2.45 GHz CW at an incident power density of 10 mW/cm^2, 8 hr daily, 5 days/week for 8–17 weeks. Their studies included six littermate controls that were sham-exposed and handled in a manner otherwise identical to the exposed group. No differences were observed in the two groups when weekly RBC and WBC counts were compared.

Siekierzynski (1972) exposed three groups of rabbits to 2.95-GHz CW and pulsed microwaves at an average power density of 3 mW/cm^2 for 2 hr daily. The first group was exposed for a total of 74 hr to CW microwaves, the second for 74 hr to pulsed microwaves, and the third for 158 hr to CW. No significant changes were observed in RBC count, hemoglobin concentration, or volume of packed RBCs. However, ferrokinetic studies revealed alterations in erythrocyte production. Serum iron levels were reduced significantly in all microwave-exposed rabbits; the plasma clearance of ^{59}Fe incorporated into erythrocytes was markedly reduced. The effects were most dramatic and were similar following the 74-hr pulsed and 158-hr CW exposures.

Yagi et al. (1974) applied 1450 MHz CW at 1.3 W/cm^2 to the legs of rabbits. Each exposure of 30 min duration was repeated five times daily for seven consecutive days. The authors found aplastic bone marrow as well as serious inflammation. This should not be unexpected. The exposure produced an increase in temperature of the femoral tissue to 39°C within the first 5 min, which was maintained at 42°C during the next 25 min. In other words, a tissue temperature increase of more than 5°C was induced. There is little doubt that the aplastic bone marrow is a result of thermal damage.

In dogs exposed whole-body to 2800 MHz pulsed, 100 mW/cm^2 (SAR 3.7 W/kg) for 6 hr, there was a marked decrease in lymphocytes and eosinophils (Michaelson, 1970; Michaelson et al., 1967, 1971). Colonic temperature increased 1°C. The neutrophils remained slightly increased at 24 hr postexposure, while eosinophil and lymphocyte values returned to normal levels. Following 2 hr of exposure at 165 mW/cm^2

(SAR 6.1 W/kg), there was a slight leukopenia and decrease in neutrophils with 1.7°C increase in colonic temperature. When the exposure was of 3 hr duration, leukocytosis was evident immediately after exposure and was more marked at 24 hr, reflecting the neutrophil response. After exposure to 1285 MHz pulsed, 100 mW/cm^2 for 6 hr, there was an increase in neutrophils. At 24 h the neutrophil level was still noticeably increased. Lymphocyte and eosinophil values were moderately depressed initially but at 24 hr slightly exceeded the initial value. Six hours of exposure to 200 MHz CW, 165 mW/cm^2, resulted in a marked increase in neutrophils and a mild decrease in lymphocytes. On the following day, the leukocyte count was further increased, and the lymphocytes markedly increased. Such shifts in the WBC picture are consistent with focal thermal lesions to be expected under these exposure conditions.

Comparison of leukocyte changes over a 60-day period after a 6-hr exposure at 100 mW/cm^2, 2800 or 1285 MHz, revealed that 1285 MHz had a slightly greater and more prolonged effect on leukocyte response. Recovery of neutrophils to the preexposure level occurred 1–2 weeks after 1285 MHz and within 1 week after 2800 MHz. A 25 to 40% lymphocyte increase from the preexposure level was noted from 1 day to 2 years after 1285-MHz exposure. The reticulocyte count was moderately diminished during this period. Lymphocytopenia from 2800 MHz was followed by recovery to 95% of the initial value in 24 hr and a gradual decrease to 54% of the initial value by 60 days.

Early and sustained leukocytosis in dogs exposed to thermogenic levels of microwaves may be related to stimulation of the hematopoietic system, leukocytic mobilization, or recirculation of sequestered cells. Eosinopenia and transient lymphocytopenia with rebound or overcompensation when accompanied by neutrophilia may indicate increased adrenal function (Michaelson *et al.*, 1961, 1964, 1968).

At 1285 MHz, animals were exposed to 20, 50, or 100 mW/cm^2 (SAR 0.9, 2.3, 4.5 W/kg), 6 hr/day, 5 days/week, for 2–4 weeks (Michaelson *et al.* 1971). There was no effect on food or water consumption while percent weight loss showed a direct correlation between power density and weight loss. There was a marked increase in neutrophils after each 6-hr exposure during the first week. Physiological adaptation was seen during the second week in that neutrophil increase was minimal. Neutrophil changes after 20 and 50 mW/cm^2 were variable and essentially similar to those seen in sham-exposed dogs. Leukocyte decrease was noted after exposure to 50 and 100 mW/cm^2 but not after 20 mW/cm^2. Reticulocyte changes were variable. A slight increase in reticulocytes occurred during the 4-week irradiation period at 50 and 100 mW/cm^2. The animals exposed to 20 mW/cm^2 appeared to be similar to the sham-exposed group. Hematological examinations in 20 mW/cm^2 exposed dogs up to 1 year after exposure did not reveal any changes significantly different from the preexposure level or the sham-exposed dogs.

At 24,000 MHz there was no effect on colonic temperature; however, at 1285 MHz (100 mW/cm^2) there was a marked increase in colonic temperature during each exposure for the first week (Michaelson et al., 1971). During the subsequent 3 weeks, temperature increases were moderate. A progressive lowering of the preexposure temperatures was evident as the number of exposures increased. This response suggested physiological adaptation. Exposure to 50 mW/cm^2 resulted in slight temperature increase. Again, progressive lowering of the preexposure temperature was noted. Exposure to 20 mW/cm^2 resulted in slight temperature decrease, which was consistent with that seen in sham-exposed animals for the same duration. Hematocrit, hemoglobin, RBC, total and differential WBC remained essentially unchanged. There was no change in total blood cholesterol and protein iodide values. There was, however, an increase in cholesterol esters, the significance of which was not clear.

These exposures constitute rather high SARs; i.e., at 2880 MHz, 165 mW/cm^2, SAR = 6.1 mW/g; 100 mW/cm^2, SAR = 3.7 mW/g. At 200 MHz, the SAR for 100 mW/cm^2 would be 15 mW/g. In essence, what these studies showed is that at 165 mW/cm^2, 2880 MHz pulsed, critical temperature, i.e., lack of isothermia, occurs at 60 min in the dog, in contrast to 10 min in the rabbit. Additivity was evident at increased ambient temperatures.

Richardson (1959) exposed anesthetized mongrel dogs weighing 11–18 kg to 2.45 GHz CW at average power densities of 158 and 197 mW/cm^2. The horn antenna was 5 cm above the skin over the region of the liver. Nine dogs were subjected to a single 10-min exposure, and the whole-blood clotting time determined immediately after. Preexposure clotting times were used as control values. Mean clotting time increased 1.7 min ($p < 0.01$), or approximately 27% over control values. This peak increase occurred 17 min after exposure, and the values returned to the control level within 30 min. Another series of studies employed three exposure periods of 10 min each on eight dogs, with a 5-min interval between the first and second exposures and 2 hr between the second and third exposures. After the first exposure, clotting time was increased 1.4 min over control values ($p < 0.02$), and then decreased 1.5 min after the second exposure as compared to preexposure values ($p < 0.01$). These values returned to control levels by about 60 min. Following the third exposure, there was again a decrease in clotting time of 1.7 min below the control value ($p < 0.01$). This latter study was repeated on another group of eight dogs subjected to the same procedures without microwave exposure. In this control study, there was only a slight, but statistically insignificant decrease in clotting time.

In a study by Krupp (1978), rhesus monkeys were exposed wholebody to 500 to 1270 mW/cm^2 of 15-, 20-, and 26-MHz energies. Each animal was exposed for up to 6 hr on at least two occasions. One or two years later an extensive series of hematological and clinical chemistry determinations was performed. None of these showed any significant departure from normal. No abnormalities were noted during the physical examinations. The SARs for 26-MHz exposures are 0.85, 0.275, and 1.7 mW/g for 500, 750, and 1000 mW/cm^2, respectively. The SARs for 20-MHz exposures are 0.73 and 1.22 mW/g for 750 and 1270 mW/cm^2, respectively. For 15-MHz exposures the SARs are 0.42 and 0.5 mW/g for 775 and 1025 mW/cm^2, respectively. There are certain deficiencies in this study, namely no preexposure values are given, the number of animals is small, and only one sample is available at one point in time.

Effects of microwaves on the circadian rhythm of precursors of granulocytes and erythroblasts (young RBCs) have been reported by Czerski *et al.* (1974a). In one of these experiments, guinea pigs were repeatedly exposed to 3000 MHz pulsed, 1 mW/cm^2, 4 hr daily for 14 days. No marked differences between control animals and irradiated ones were seen in the circadian rhythm of precursors of granulocytes and erythroblasts. In bone marrow stem cells, changes in both amplitude and phase of the circadian rhythm were seen depending on whether the animal was irradiated in the evening or the morning and these differed from the control groups. The statistical significance of these findings is questionable. To study this phenomenon, mice were given a single exposure of 3000 MHz pulsed, 0.5 mW/cm^2, for 4 hr. No significant differences between irradiated and control animals were noted in mitotic indices of granulocyte precursors and erythroblasts. There was some difference in mitotic index of bone marrow stem cells between exposed and control animals. According to the authors, the most significant aspect of this study is that microwave exposure affects only one group of cells, mitosis of the granulocytic and erythroblastic cell lines remaining unaffected or affected only to a slight degree. This may be interpreted as an indication that microwaves under these conditions did not interfere with the process of cell division (or rather of the cell cycle, RNA and DNA synthesis, and the mechanism of initiation of cell division) as such, but induced a response of stem cells probably dependent on physiological attributes of the cell group. The authors also caution that the designation "stem cells" as used by them is a loose one, based on morphological criteria only and pertaining to a heterogeneous group of cells.

It should be noted that the usual procedure in the laboratory was to irradiate the animals in groups of 25 in Plexiglas cages containing 25 (5 × 5) separate compartments placed in a quadrangle. Also, during each exposure session the animals did not receive any food or water. It is known that exposure of animals in close proximity to each other results in considerable field perturbation. In addition, restricting the animals' access to food and water for periods ranging up to 4 hr will introduce hemodynamic changes that could affect the determinations. On the other hand, a phase shift in the circadian rhythm of body temperature was observed by Lu *et al.* (1977) in rats exposed to 2450 MHz CW, 1 mW/cm^2, 1 to 8 hr.

14.3. REPORTED OBSERVATIONS IN THE HUMAN

There are few reports of RF/MW-induced hematological changes in man. In surveys of military and industrial radar personnel, inconsistent hematological changes have been reported (Barron and Baraff, 1958; Barron *et al.*, 1955; Daily, 1943; Haduch *et al.*, 1962; Lysina, 1965; Miro, 1962). Reticulocytosis has been noted in some studies (Sokolov and Ariyevich, 1960).

Lysina (1965) reported no significant difference in the circulating erythrocyte counts of 100 workers exposed to superhigh-frequency (SHF) fields but gave no information about frequency, intensity, or duration of the exposure. He observed slight increases in reticulocyte counts in exposed personnel but no change in leukocyte counts. In another report, Sokolov *et al.* (1974) examined 131 persons who had been exposed to "significant levels" (several mW/cm^2) in previous years to SHF fields, but specifics about the exposure conditions, frequency, intensity, duration, and so on, were not given. Sokolov *et al.* (1974) reported a significant decrease in circulating thrombocytes and leukocytes due to neutropenia and relative lymphocytosis, a tendency toward reticulocytosis, increased bone-marrow erythroblasts, and an increase in the number of circulating cells undergoing mitosis. These hematological effects, however, were reported as reversible, and cessation of exposure led to normal hematopoiesis in most subjects. These investigators found no reason to believe that hypoplastic changes or leukemia follow exposure to SHF fields.

Daily (1943) studied 45 men exposed to radar and high-frequency radiowaves for 2 months to 9 years but gave no frequency or intensity levels. Periodic physical and blood examinations for 13 months revealed values within the normal range. Barron *et al.* (1955) performed comprehensive physical examinations on radar personnel employed by an aircraft company. Two hundred twenty-six subjects with radar contact varying from occasional beam exposure to 4 hr a day and up to 13 years' exposure were observed, although the frequency and intensity of the fields to which these individuals were exposed are not given. The radar bands most commonly associated with airborne equipment were the "S" and "X" bands near 2900 and 9000 MHz, respectively. Radar personnel were grouped by years of exposure and compared to controls of similar age. A significant decrease of polymorphonuclear cells was found in 25% of the radar personnel as compared to 12% in the control group. A marked increase in monocytes (above 6%) and eosinophils (more than 4%) was detected in radar personnel, but the significance of these changes was not evaluated. Reexamination of 100 subjects after 6 to 9 months of incidental contact with both "S" and "X" band radar revealed changes in erythrocyte counts, leukocyte counts, and relative numbers of polymorphonuclear cells. Barron et al. (1955) found this ". . . paradoxical and difficult to interpret." In a later report, however, Barron and Baraff (1958) stated that the changes were due to a variation in a laboratory technician's interpretation.

Baranski and Czerski (1966) reported on the hematological examination of a large group of people occupationally exposed to microwaves. Group No. 1 had the lowest exposure; group No. 2, a somewhat higher exposure; group No. 3, engaged in repair and production of microwave generators, had significant exposure up to several mW/cm^2.

There was a distribution based on duration of employment, i.e., 1 year, 1–3 years, 3–5 years, and 5–10 years. The biological indicators used were hemoglobin, RBC count, total and differential WBC count, reticulocytes, platelets, and bone marrow aspirations in 19 individuals. There is no indication of frequency or power density; no exposure details are provided, nor dosimetry, statistics, controls, or correction for age.

The authors reported: no deviation in hemoglobin level; highest reticulocyte count was observed in the higher exposure group; WBC count was within normal limits regardless of the type of work and the job exposure; a small number of cases with lymphocytopenia was encountered (however, this number did not change in the groups having different types or work or different levels of job experience); 40 to 50% of the persons examined showed a moderate decrease in the platelet count, but there were no signs of hemorrhage. In the high exposure (i.e., several mW/cm^2) group, there was an absolute granulocytopenia and eosinophilia. There was a decrease in the platelet count. The percentage of persons with these changes increased with the number of years of employment.

Bone marrow aspirations were basically normal, except for a tendency toward an increase in reticulocytes. In persons with over 5 years of exposure (the higher exposure group), there was a correlation between the hematological changes, lens opacities, and neurasthenia.

In summary, in the group with the highest degree of exposure, three types of changes in the WBC picture were detected: (1) most frequently lymphocytosis associated with monocytosis, (2) granulocytopenia with monocytosis, (3) neutrophilic leukocytosis of a moderate degree within the normal limits.

In a follow-up report 10 years later, the peripheral blood picture did not demonstrate any abnormalities (Czerski and Siekierzynski, 1975). Lack of hematological changes in this group of occupationally exposed individuals (some exposed to power densities $> 10 \, mW/cm^2$) was also reported by Siekierzynski et al. (1974).

Zalyubovskaya and Kiselev (1978) evaluated 72 engineers. These individuals worked with millimeter wave generators for 1 to 10 years. The flux density apparently was sometimes as high as $1000 \, \mu W/cm^2$. A control group consisted of 30 persons who had no contact with microwave energy. The subjects were observed for 3 years and during the winter months were given periodic medical examinations. These workers had complained of fatigue, sleepiness, headache, and reduced memory capacity. Changes in pulse rate and blood pressure did not go beyond the normal physiological variation. There was a decrease in hemoglobin, RBCs, and a tendency toward hypercoagulability. There was a decrease in WBCs and an increase in lymphocytes. A decrease was noted in the number of reticulocytes and thrombocytes. The changes, however, were inconsistent.

Reports of effects in the human must be put in perspective. Epidemiological and incidence studies suffer from inadequate design and examinations as well as substantiating actual power levels and duration of microwave exposure. Although such studies are applicable to disorders in which there may be a major definable, etiological agent, it is essential that evaluation be made of the multiple environmental factors that may interact among themselves and with personal characteristics of the individual (Petrov, 1970). There is always the danger that real factors may be overlooked leading to false association with factors of initial interest.

A careful review of the literature on hematological effects of microwave exposure does not support the notion that hematopoiesis or circulating blood cells are influenced by the microwave fields of concern for man (i.e., $< 10 \, mW/cm^2$). In evaluating reports of hematological changes, one must be cognizant of the relative distributions of blood cells in a population of animals or humans and the thermal influence on these alterations. Early and sustained leukocytosis in animals exposed to thermogenic levels of microwaves may be related to stimulation of the hematopoietic system, leukocytic mobilization, or recirculation of sequestered cells. Eosinopenia and transient lymphocytopenia with rebound or overcompensation, when accompanied by neutrophilia, may be indicative of increased hypothalamic–hypophysical–adrenal function as a result of thermal stress (Michaelson, 1974)

Alterations in one hematological parameter (RBCs) without concomitant changes in dependent variables (hemoglobin and RBC mass) are characteristic of several reports in the microwave literature. It emphasizes the need for rigidly applied appropriate multivariate statistical analyses of data before implying a biological effect based on invalid statistical tests. Thermogenic levels of microwaves are required to produce hematopoietic changes in experimental animals. These changes are transient in nature and are qualitatively not different from those produced by other heating modalities. In regard to the human, it is essential that appropriate scaling factors be considered before one can extrapolate from small experimental animals to the human. There is no reason to believe that localized and intermittent exposure of the human to microwaves would produce significant hematological changes.

REFERENCES

Baranski, S. (1971) Effect of chronic microwave irradiation on the blood forming system of guinea pigs and rabbits. *Aerosp. Med.* **42:**1196.

Baranski, S. (1972) Effect of microwaves on the reactions of the white blood cell system. *Acta Physiol. Pol.* **23:**685.

Baranski, S., and P. Czerski (1966) Investigations of the behavior of corpuscular blood constituents in persons exposed to microwaves. *Lek. Woisk.* **42:**903.

Baranski, S., H. Ludwicka, and S. Szmigielski (1971) The effect of microwaves on rabbit erythrocyte permeability. *Med. Lotn.* **39:**75.

Baranski, S., S. Szmigielski, and J. Moneta (1974) Effects of microwave irradiation *in vitro* on cell membrane permeability. In: *Biological Effects and Health Hazards of Microwave Radiation*, P. Czerski, K. Ostrowski, M. L. Shore, C. Silverman, M. J. Suess, and B. Waldeskog (eds.). Polish Medical Publishers, Warsaw, pp. 173–177.

Barron, C. I., and A. A. Baraff (1958) Medical considerations of exposure to microwaves (radar). *J. Am. Med. Assoc.* **168:**1194.

Barron, C. I., A. A. Love, and A. A. Baraff (1955) Physical evaluation of personnel exposed to microwave emanations. *J. Aviat. Med.* **26:**442.

Boggs, R. F., A. P. Sheppard, and A. J. Clark (1972) Effects of 2450 MHz microwave radiation on human blood coagulation processes. *Health Phys.* **22:**217.

Budd, R. A., J. Laskey, and C. Kelly (1970) Hematological response of fetal rats following 2450 MHz microwave irradiation. In: *Radiation Bio-effects, Summary Report, January–December 1970*, D. M. Hodge (ed.). HEW, PHS, BRH Publ. BRH/DBE 70-7 (December), p. 161.

Chou, C. K., A. W. Guy, J. A. McDonald, and L. F. Han (1978) Effects of continuous and pulsed chronic microwave radiation on rabbits. In: *Proceedings of the 1978 Annual Meeting of USNC/URSI*, p. 96.

Czerski, P. (1975) Microwave effects on the blood-forming system with particular reference to the lymphocyte. *Ann. N.Y. Acad. Sci.* **247:**232.

Czerski, P., and M. Siekierzynski (1975) Analysis of occupational exposure to microwave radiation. In: *Fundamental and Applied Aspects of Nonionizing Radiation,* S. M. Michaelson, M. W. Miller, R. Magin, and E. L. Cartensen (eds.). Plenum Press, New York, p. 367.

Czerski, P. E., E. Paprocka-Slonka, M. Siekierzynski, and A. Stolarska (1974a) Influence of microwave radiation on the hematopoietic system. In: *Biological Effects and Health Hazards of Microwave Radiation,* P. Czerski, K. Ostrowski, M. L. Shore, C. Silverman, M. J. Suess, and B. Waldeskog (eds.), Polish Medical Publishers, Warsaw, pp. 67–74.

Czerski, P., E. Paprocka-Slonka, and A. Stolarska (1974b) Microwave irradiation and the circadian rhythm of bone marrow cell mitosis. *J. Microwave Power* **9**:31.

Daily, L. (1943) A clinical study of the results of exposure of laboratory personnel to radar and high frequency radio. *U.S. Nav. Med. Bull.* **41**:1052.

Deichmann, W. B., F. J. Stephens, Jr., M. Keplinger, and K. F. Lampe (1959) Acute effects of microwave radiation on experimental animals (24,000 megacycles). *J. Occup. Med.* **1**:369.

Deichmann, W. B., J. Maile, and K. Landeen (1964) Effect of microwave radiation on the hemopoietic system of the rat. *Toxicol. Appl. Pharmacol.* **6**:71.

Djordjevic, Z., and A. Kolak (1973) Changes in the peripheral blood of the rat exposed to microwave radiation (2400 MHz) in conditions of chronic exposure. *Aerosp. Med.* **44**:1051.

Djordjevic, Z., N. Lazarevic, and V. Djokovic (1977) Studies on the hematologic effects of long-term, low-dose microwave exposure. *Aviat. Space Environ. Med.* **48**:516.

Drogichina, E. A., M. N. Sadchikova, G. V. Snegova, N. M. Konchalovskaya, and K. V. Glotova (1966) Autonomic and cardiovascular disorders during chronic exposure to super-high frequency electromagnetic fields. *Gig. Tr. Prof. Zabol.* **10**:13.

Ferri, E. S., and G. H. Hagen (1975) Chronic low-level exposure of rabbits to microwaves. In: *Proceedings 1975 Annual Meeting of USNC/URSI,* p. 319.

Goncharova, N. N., V. B. Karamyshev, and N. V. Maksimenko (1966) Occupational hygiene problems in working with ultrashort-wave transmitters used in TV and radio broadcasting. *Gig. Tr. Prof. Zabol.* **10**:10.

Gorodetskaya, S. F. (1964) The influence of an SHF electromagnetic field on the reproduction, composition of peripheral blood, conditioned reflex activity, and morphology of the internal organs of white mice. In: *Biological Action of Ultrasound and SHF-UHF Electromagnetic Oscillations,* A. A. Gorodetsky (ed.). Nauk Dumka, Kiev, p. 80.

Grant, E. H., K. H. Illinger, B. Servantie, and S. Szmigielski (1974) Effects of microwave radiation at the cellular and molecular level. In: *Biological Effects and Health Hazards of Microwave Radiation,* P. Czerski, K. Ostrowski, M. L. Shore, C. Silverman, M. J. Suess, and B. Waldeskog (eds.). Polish Medical Publishers, Warsaw, pp. 324–325.

Guy, A. W., P. O. Kramar, C. A. Harris, and C. K. Chou (1980) Long-term 2450 MHz CW microwave irradiation of rabbits: Methodology and evaluation of ocular and physiologic effects. *J. Microwave Power* **15**:37.

Haduch, S., S. Baranski, and P. Czerski (1962) The influence of ultrahigh frequency radio waves on the human organism. In: *Human Problems of Supersonic and Hypersonic Flight,* A. B. Barbour and H. F. Whittingham (eds.). Pergamon Press, New York, p. 449.

Hamrick, P. E., and D. I. McRee (1975) Exposure of the Japanese quail embryo to 2.45-GHz microwave radiation during the second day of development. *J. Microwave Power* **10**:211.

Hamrick, P. E., and J. G. Zinkl (1975) Exposure of rabbit erythrocytes to microwave irradiation. *Radiat. Res.* **62**:164.

Hyde, A. S., and J. J. Friedman (1968) Some effects of acute and chronic microwave irradiation of mice. In: *Thermal Problems in Aerospace Medicine,* J. D. Hardy (ed.). Unwin, Ltd., Surrey, pp. 163–175.

Ismailov, E. S. (1971) Mechanism of the effect of microwaves on the permeability of erythrocytes for potassium and sodium ions. *Biol. Nauki* **3:**58.

Ismailov, E. S. (1978) Effect of ultrahigh frequency electromagnetic radiation on the electrophoretic mobility of erythrocytes. *Biophysics* **22:**510 (transl. of *Biofizika* **22:**493, 1977).

Ivanov, A. I. (1962) Changes of phagocytic activity and mobility of neutrophils under the influence of microwave fields. In: *Summaries of Reports, Questions of the Biological Effect of a SHF–UHF Electromagnetic Field.* Kirov Order of Lenin Military Medical Academy, Leningrad, p. 24.

Kitsovskaya, I. A. (1964) The effect of centimeter waves of different intensities on the blood and hemopoietic organs of white rats. *Gig. Tr. Prof. Zabol.* **8:**14.

Krupp, J. H. (1978) Long-term Follow-up of *Macaca Mulata* Exposed to High Levels of 15-, 20-, and 26-MHz Radiofrequency Radiation. SAM-TR-78-3, Brooks AFB, Texas, p. 6.

Lappenbusch, W. L., L. J. Gillespie, W. M. Leach, and G. E. Anderson (1973) Effect of 2450 MHz microwaves on the radiation response of X-irradiated Chinese hamsters. *Radiat. Res.* **54:**294.

Liburdy, R. P. (1977) Effects of radio-frequency radiation on inflammation. *Radio Sci.* **12**(6S):179.

Linko, V., and K. Hynynen (1979) Erythrocyte damage caused by the Haemotherm^R microwave blood warmer. *Acta Anaesthesiol. Scand.* **23:**320.

Liu, L. M., F. G. Nickless, and S. F. Clearly (1979) Effects of microwave radiation on erythrocyte membranes. *Radio Sci.* **14**(6S):109.

Lu, S.-T., N. J. Lebda, S. M. Michaelson, S. Pettit, and D. Rivera (1977) Thermal and endocrinological effects of protracted irradiation of rats by 2450 MHz microwaves. *Radio Sci.* **12**(6S):147.

Lysina, G. G. (1965) Effect of ultrahigh frequency radiation on the formed elements of blood. *Gig. Sanit.* **30:**95.

Michaelson, S. M. (1970) Pathophysiological aspects of microwave irradiation. I. Thermal effects. *Non-Ioniz. Radiat.* **1:**169.

Michaelson, S. M. (1974) Thermal effects of single and repeated exposures to microwaves: A review. In: *Biological Effects and Health Hazards of Microwave Radiation.* P. Czerski, K. Ostrowski, M. L. Shore, C. Silverman, M. J. Suess, and B. Waldeskog (eds.). Polish Medical Publishers, Warsaw, pp. 1–14.

Michaelson, S. M., R. A. E. Thomson, and J. W. Howland (1961) Physiologic aspects of microwave irradiation of mammals. *Am. J. Physiol.* **201:**351.

Michaelson, S. M., R. A. E. Thomson, L. T. Odland, and J. W. Howland (1963) The influence of microwaves on ionizing radiation exposure. *Aerosp. Med.* **34:**111.

Michaelson, S. M., R. A. E. Thomson, M. Y. El Tamami, H. S. Seth, and J. W. Howland (1964) Hematologic effects of microwave exposure. *Aerosp. Med.* **35:**824.

Michaelson, S. M., R. A. E. Thomson, and J. W. Howland (1965) Comparative studies on 1285 and 2800 mc/sec pulsed microwaves. *Aerosp. Med.* **36:**1059.

Michaelson, S. M., R. A. E. Thomson, and J. W. Howland (1967) *Biologic Effects of Microwave Exposure.* Tech. Rep. RADC-TR-67-461, Griffiss AFB, Rome Air Development Center, Rome, N.Y.

Michaelson, S. M., R. A. E. Thomson, and W. J. Quinlan (1968) Effects of electromagnetic radiation on physiologic responses. *Aerosp. Med.* **39:**293.

Michaelson, S. M., J. W. Howland, and W. B. Deichmann (1971) Response of the dog to 24,000 and 1285 MHz microwave exposure. *Ind. Med.* **40:**18.

Miro, L. (1962) Hematological modifications and clinical disorders observed in persons exposed to radar waves. *Rev. Med. Aeronaut. (Paris)* **1**:16.

Olcerst, R. B., and J. R. Rabinowitz (1978) Studies on the interaction of microwave radiation with cholinesterase. *Radiat. Environ. Biophys.* **15**:289.

Olcerst, R. B., S. Belman, M. Eisenbud, W. W. Mumford, and J. R. Rabinowitz (1980) The increased passive efflux of sodium and rubidium from rabbit erythrocytes by microwave radiation. *Radiat. Res.* **82**:244.

Pazderova-Vejlupkova, J., and M. Josifko (1979) Changes in the blood count of growing rats irradiated with a microwave pulse field. *Arch. Environ. Health* **34**:44.

Peterson, D. J., L. M. Partlow, and O. P. Gandhi (1979) An investigation of the thermal and athermal effects of microwave irradiation on erythrocytes. *IEEE Trans. Biomed. Eng.* **BME-26**:428.

Petrov, I. R. (ed.) (1970) *Influence of Microwave Radiation on the Organism of Man and Animals*. Meditsina Press, Leningrad (NASA TT F-708).

Prausnitz, S., and C. Süsskind (1962) Effects of chronic microwave irradiation on mice. *IRE Trans. Bio-Med. Electron.* **BME-9**:104.

Preskorn, S. H., W. D. Edwards, and D. R. Justesen (1978) Retarded tumor growth and greater longevity in mice after fetal irradiation by 2450 MHz microwaves. *J. Surg. Oncol.* **10**:483.

Ragan, H. A., R. D. Phillips, R. L. Bushbom, R. H. Busch, and J. E. Morris (1980) Hematologic and immunologic effects of pulsed microwaves in mice. *Bioelectromagnetics* **4**:383.

Richardson, A. W. (1959) Blood coagulation changes due to electromagnetic microwave irradiations. *Blood* **14**:1237.

Roberts, N. J., Jr., and S. M. Michaelson (1983) Microwaves and neoplasia in mice: Analysis of a reported risk. *Health Phys.* **44**:430.

Rotkovska, D., and A. Vacek (1972) Effect of high-frequency electromagnetic fields upon haemopoietic stem cells in mice. *Folia Biol. (Prague)* **18**:292.

Rotkovska, D., and A. Vacek (1975) The effect of electromagnetic radiation on the hematopoietic stem cells of mice. *Ann. N.Y. Acad. Sci.* **247**:243.

Rotkovska, D., and A. Vacek (1977) Modification of repair of X-irradiation damage of hemopoietic system of mice by microwaves. *J. Microwave Power* **12**:119.

Rozzell, T. C., C. C. Johnson, C. H. Durney, J. L. Lords, and R. G. Olsen (1974) A nonperturbing temperature sensor for measurements in electromagnetic fields. *J. Microwave Power* **9**:241.

Sacchitelli, F., and G. Sacchitelli (1960) Protection of personnel exposed to radar microwaves. *Folia Med. (Naples)* **43**:1219.

Sadchikova, M. N., and A. A. Orlova (1958) Clinical picture of the chronic effects of electromagnetic centimeter waves. *Gig Tr. Prof. Zabol. (Moskow)* **2**:16.

Serdiuk, A. M. (1969) Biological effect of low-intensity ultrahigh frequency fields. *Vrach. Delo* **11**:108.

Siekierzynski, M. (1972) The influence of microwave radiation on iron metabolism in rabbits. *Med. Lotn.* **39**:53.

Siekierzynski, M., P. Czerski, H. Milczarek, A. Gidynski, C. Czarnecki, E. Dziuk, and W. Jedrzesczak (1974) Health surveillance of personnel occupationally exposed to microwaves. II. Functional disturbances. *Aerosp. Med.* **45**:1143.

Smialowicz, R. J. (1979) Hematologic and immunologic effects of non-ionizing electromagnetic radiation. *Bull. N.Y. Acad. Med.* **55**:1094.

Sokolov, V. V., and M. N. Ariyevich (1960) Changes in the blood under the influence of SHF-UHF on the organism. *Tt. Gig. Tr. Prof. AMN SSR* **2**: 43.

Sokolov, V. V., I. A. Gribova, and N. A. Chulina (1974) State of the blood system under the influence of SHF fields of various intensities and in radiowave sickness. In: *Biological Effects of Radiofrequency Electromagnetic Fields*, Z. V. Gordon (ed.). National Technical Information Service, Springfield, Va., pp. 63–71.

Spalding, J. F., R. W. Freyman, and L. M. Holland (1971) Effects of 800-MHz electromagnetic radiation on body weight, activity, hematopoiesis and life span in mice. *Health Phys.* **20:**421.

Switzer, W. G., and D. S. Mitchell (1977) Long-term effects of 2.45 GHz radiation on the ultrastructure of the cerebral cortex and on hematologic profiles in rats. *Radio Sci.* **12:**287.

Szmigielski, S. (1975) Effect of 10 cm (3 GHz) electromagnetic radiation (microwaves) on granulocytes *in vitro. Ann. N.Y. Acad. Sci.* **247:**275.

Thomson, R. A. E., S. M. Michaelson, and J. W. Howland (1965) Modification of X-irradiation lethality in mice by microwaves (radar). *Radiat. Res.* **24:**631.

Tyagin, N. V. (1957) Change in the blood of animals subjected to a SHF–UHF field. *Tr. Voen. Med. Akad. Kirov* **73:**116.

Vacek, D. R. A. (1972) Effect of high-frequency electromagnetic field upon haemopoietic stem cells in mice. *Folia Biol. (Prague)* **18:**292.

Yagi, K., R. Ueyama, S. Kurohane, N. Hiramine, H. Ito, and S. Umehara (1974) Harmful effects of microwave radiation on the bone marrow. In: *Biological Effects and Health Hazards of Microwave Radiation*, P. Czerski, K. Ostrowski, M. L. Shore, C. Silverman, M. J. Suess, and B. Waldeskog (eds.). Polish Medical Publishers, Warsaw, pp. 75–88.

Zalyubovskaya, N. P., and R. I. Kiselev (1978) The effect of radio-waves of a millimeter frequency range on the body of man and animal. *Gig. Sanit.* **43:**35.

15

Effects on Immune Responses

In recent years, considerable interest has developed on the relationship between microwave exposure and alteration of the immune response. The immune system is a physiological defense against a large spectrum of pathogens, including bacteria, viruses, fungi, parasites, tumors, toxins from organisms, and miscellaneous chemical substances. There is considerable adaptability and redundancy in the immune system. Thus, many perturbations of the immune response may not have clinical significance (Roberts, 1983). The immune response is initiated by the introduction of a foreign substance, called an antigen. The immune system can respond specifically and nonspecifically to challenge. It can recognize nonspecifically (as nonself) an offender that the host has not encountered previously. The responsive cells can produce antigen-specific or nonspecific mediators that recruit other immunocompetent cells. In fact, recruitment of cells and so-called "arming" or activation of cells are major features of the immune response. The true immune system consists of cells that are specialized for defense, broadly classified into phagocytic cells and lymphoid cells, and cell-derived humoral substances such as antibodies and complement (Roberts, 1983; Roberts *et al.*, 1986).

Because of the emphasis placed on the "hazard" aspects of the reports of lymphoblastoid transformations and immunological consequences of microwave exposure, it is important to place this in perspective. In essence, the reports do not negate the thermal influences of microwave energy absorption. If the reports are confirmed, they may not necessarily be indicative of a hazard, but actually portend an exciting and important possibility for therapy of infectious diseases or cancer which have been shown to be influenced by hyperthermia.

Lymphoblastoid transformation, *in vitro*, after free-field exposure to 3000-MHz pulsed microwaves, $7 \, mW/cm^2$ for 4 hr daily and $20 \, mW/cm^2$ for 15 min daily, 3 to 5 days, has been reported (Stodolnik-Baranska, 1974). At this power density, the temperature of the media increased after 15 min by 0.5°C, and after 20 min, 1°C. Changes in the mitotic index depended on exposure time. Although a 5-min exposure did not influence the proportion of dividing cells, slight differences compared with controls were observed after 10- and 15-min exposures and significant differences were seen following 3- and 4-hr exposures.

Changes in phagocytic activity have been reported to occur when rats are exposed to 14.88 MHz, 100 V/m, 4 hr/day, for 10 months (Volkova and Fukalova, 1974).
changes and either duration of exposure or incident power were noted.

Shandala et al. (1977) exposed rats, guinea pigs, and rabbits to 2.38 GHz at 10, 50, or 500 μW/cm^2 for 30 days. Lymphoblastoid transformations, stimulated by mitogens, were studied at various times during the 30-day exposure period. Exposure at 500 μW/cm^2 resulted initially in stimulation of transformation, followed by suppression. The phagocytic ability of guinea pig leukocytes was determined after exposure of guinea pigs to microwaves. At 10 μW/cm^2 the phagocytic index was elevated and at 500 μW/cm^2 was suppressed, as compared to control values. There was a reduced incidence of anaphylaxis in sensitized, microwave-exposed guinea pigs subsequently challenged with equine serum. Of particular interest is the reported finding of antibrain and antiliver antibodies in the three species exposed to power densities $\geq$ 500 μW/cm^2. The authors conclude that exposure to these low power densities can result in a primary lesion of the immune system, and may also result in autoimmune disease. Unfortunately, the authors provided no description of methods used in these assays, or whether appropriate sham-exposed groups were used.

Smialowicz (1976) examined the proliferative capacity of lymphocytes that are responsible for cellular immune responses (T cells) and humoral immune responses (B cells) following 2450-MHz exposure *in vitro*. Cultured mouse spleen cells were maintained at 37°C during exposure to 2450 MHz CW in the far field of an anechoic chamber for 1, 2, or 4 hr at an absorbed dose rate of 19 mW/g. The ability of mouse spleen lymphocytes to undergo blast transformation in response to mitogens that selectively stimulate either T or B cells was measured by the incorporation of [^{3}H]thymidine into DNA. No consistent difference was found between the blastogenic response of exposed (10 mW/cm^2, 19 W/kg, 1 to 4 hr) and control cells.

Mice exposed to 2450 MHz (CW), 5 to 35 mW/cm^2 (SAR 4 to 25 mW/g), for 1 to 22 consecutive days (15 to 30 min/day) showed no consistent significant alterations in several parameters including mitogen-stimulated response of T and B spleen lymphocytes, numbers of T- and B spleen lymphocytes, and primary antibody response of mice to sheep erythrocytes (Smialowicz et al., 1979b).

Smialowicz et al. (1979a) exposed rats *in utero* and neonatally through 40 days of age (4 hr/day, 7 days/week) in a controlled environment to either 2450 MHz (CW, 5 mW/cm^2, SAR 1 to 5 mW/g) or

425 MHz (CW, 10 mW/cm^2, SAR 3 to 7 mW/g). At 40 days of age, significant increases in the response of lymphocytes from exposed rats to *in vitro* stimulation with several mitogens were observed in several experiments. While these results have not been consistently reproduced, the trend in the results suggest that chronic exposure during fetal and neonatal development may change either the frequency or the responsiveness of lymphocyte subpopulations. The biological significance of these observed changes is unknown. The mechanism by which these changes are initiated may be related to a thermally induced stress response. Similar responses have been observed in animals following prolonged exposure to nonspecific stressors (Monjan and Collector, 1977).

Hamrick (1973) examined the response of mammalian lymphocytes exposed to 2450 MHz CW in cultures at 20 mW/cm^2 (7 mW/g) for 48 hr. Changes in the stimulation caused by phytohemagglutinin (PHA) under control and exposed conditions were studied. No effects of exposure were detected. Also, no effect on DNA was found at power densities as high as 67 to 160 mW/g (~200–300 mW/cm^2). It was concluded that 2450-MHz CW microwave exposure has very little, if any, effect other than that of heating on the secondary structure of DNA as determined by comparison of thermal denaturation curves.

Prince *et al.* (1972) reported that 30-min exposure to high-intensity fields of 26.6 MHz at 1.32 W/cm^2 increased the mitotic potential of certain populations of circulating nonhuman primate lymphocytes. These findings were accompanied by substantial tissue heating, i.e., 2.4 and 4.6°C rectal and surface temperature increases.

In an attempt to extend these observations, Lovely *et al.* (1979) initiated a series of studies employing a temperature-controlled RF-exposure culture cup that also provides for well-defined RF-field conditions. They attempted to determine if cultured nonhuman primate lymphocytes exposed to intense (E = 500 V/m; H = 4.4 A/m; SAR = 400 W/kg) 30-MHz fields would yield significantly higher mitotic figures than sham-exposed control samples of cultured lymphocytes, while the temperature of the cultures under both conditions was held at 37 ± 0.5°C. The results indicated that exposure of cultured lymphocytes, obtained from *Macaca mulatta,* to 500 V/m, 30 MHz produced no evidence of cell death, damage, or interference with mitotic activity, whether stimulated by PHA or unstimulated, immediately following, 24 to 48 hr after exposure.

In many of the studies on microwave effects, especially *in vivo,* varying conditions of exposure have been used, often with sufficient power density that thermal effects may be the predominant, if not the only, factor. This variation in application of microwaves may account for much of the diversity in data regarding the effects of such treatments on components of the hematopoietic system (Baranski, 1972; Czerski, 1975). Changes in phagocytic activity have been reported to occur when rats are exposed to 14.88 MHz, 100 V/m, 4 hr/day, for 10 months (Volkova and Fukalova, 1974).

Czerski *et al.* (1974a,b) have reported that inbred Swiss mice, immunized with sheep red blood cells (SRBC) and exposed 2 hr/day for 6 or 12 weeks to 0.5 mW/cm^2, 2950 MHz, showed increased serum hemagglutinin titers and antibody-producing cells in lymph node homogenates. The increase was greater in mice exposed 6 weeks than in those exposed 12 weeks. The serum hemagglutination titers against SRBC were also greater following either of the microwave exposure regimens than in the control group. However, the data presented do not include estimates of variances; therefore, it is not possible to establish the statistical significance of these tests. Apparently, the number of "lymphoblastoid" cells in lymphs was increased after microwave exposure.

Czerski (1975) exposed rabbits 2 hr daily for 6 months to pulsed 2.95-GHz microwaves at 2 mW/cm^2, and found an approximate 20-fold increase in spontaneous blastic transformation of peripheral blood lymphocytes in culture compared to control blood. The transformation and mitotic indices were also higher in PHA-stimulated cultures of lymphocytes from irradiated animals. The maximum increase occurred after 1 or 2 months' exposure, and then returned to control values.

Szmigielski *et al.* (1975) exposed rabbits to 3.0-GHz microwaves 5 hr daily for 6 to 12 weeks. The animals were then infected with virulent *Staphylococcus aureus*. Following infection, both the control and 6-week-exposed groups developed a marked granulocytosis, whereas no granulocytic response was observed in those rabbits exposed for 12 weeks. This was accompanied by a reduced bone marrow granulocyte reserve in both microwave-exposed groups, and a decrease in serum lysozyme levels. Nitroblue tetrazolium reduction, a measure of granulocyte function, was not decreased by microwave exposure. These results would suggest that microwave exposure may result in a decreased marrow reserve of granulocytes, but no alteration in the functional capacity of circulating granulocytes.

According to Czerski (1975), initial response and subsequent recovery during protracted exposure may indicate that after a period of response, the animals become adapted to the microwaves. The phenomenon of physiological adaptation or decreased reaction as a result of repeated exposure to microwaves has also been reported by others (Michaelson, 1974; Michaelson *et al.*, 1967; Petrov, 1970; Phillips *et al.*, 1975; Gordon, 1966; Baranski and Czerski, 1976).

Krupp (1977) exposed mice to 2.6 GHz at power densities of 10, 15, and 20 mW/cm² for various time durations and then sensitized them to SRBC. The spleens were collected and assayed for plaque-forming cells (B lymphocytes). There was an increase in plaque-forming cells when the exposures resulted in colonic temperature increases of $\geq 3.0°C$.

Baranski (1972) exposed adult guinea pigs 3 hr/day for 3 months to 3.5 mW/cm² of 3000-MHz microwaves and found an increase in lymphopoiesis over controls as indicated by increased incorporation of [^{3}H]thymidine and increased mitotic indices. No differences could be detected between pulsed and CW microwaves of the same average power level. Twofold increases in lymphocyte numbers were found in the spleen and lymph nodes.

Szmigielski et al. (1976) exposed mice to 3.0 GHz in the far field of an anechoic chamber for 2 hr daily at 40 mW/cm² for 2 to 14 days. At various times before and after microwave exposure, the mice were infected with herpes or vaccinia viruses to evaluate the course of the disease. Microwave exposure after vaccinia infection markedly reduced the number of dermal lesions. In mice infected with herpes and subsequently exposed to microwaves, the survival rate was much higher, and the incidence of encephalitis much lower, as compared to the control mice.

The effect of both local and systemic heating on transplanted tumors has been studied by Szmigielski et al. (1977) and Szmigielski and Janiak (1977). In both Guerin's epithelioma-bearing rats, and mice transplanted with sarcoma 180, microwave hyperthermia, whether local or systemic, reduced the tumor mass as compared with sham-irradiated, tumor-bearing controls. Based on enhancement of T-lymphocyte and macrophage reactions, the authors feel that immunostimulation is important in the hyperthermic inhibition of tumor growth.

Huang et al. (1977) reported that lymphocytes from Chinese hamsters exposed to from 5 to 45 mW/cm², 2450 MHz CW, for 15 min daily for 5 days showed changes in blastic transformation and mitosis. No chromosomal aberrations were evident. These studies noted increased but reversible transformation of lymphocytes (without mitogenic stimulation), related to the power density, but a decreased proportion of mitogen-stimulated cells in mitoses. Unstimulated, but microwave-exposed, lymphocytes showed a dose-related increase in the transformation index, which at 30 mW/cm² was approximately four times greater than in control cultures. At 45 mW/cm², blastic transformation fell to a level between those at 0 and 5 mW/cm². Repeated observations after irradiation indicated a progressive return to control-level transformations over a 5- to 10-day period. When lymphocytes were stimulated into mitoses with PHA, there was a microwave dose-dependent decrease in the mitotic indices. A thermal effect within a range that might normally be managed and dissipated by the animals could not be excluded. These investigators called attention to the changes over a range of body temperatures of less than 2°C and suggested that such limited hyperthermia might be of considerable interest to investigators of immunological effects of microwave radiation.

Microwaves have been reported to induce an increase in the frequency of complement receptor-bearing lymphoid spleen cells in mice (Wiktor-Jedrzejczak et al., 1977b). Although the significance of this has not been fully assessed, it may represent a maturation of B lymphocytes to a stage with expression of an activation structure.

Wiktor-Jedrzejczak et al. (1977a,b) exposed adult male mice to 2450 MHz CW at an absorbed dose of 12 to 15 mW/g for 30 min in an environmentally controlled waveguide facility and then measured the function of different classes of lymphocytes in vitro. A constant and substantial air flow inside the chamber maintained the ambient temperature at 25°C. Colonic temperature differences (after exposure relative to before exposure) ranged from -0.1°C to -0.05°C. Such exposure failed to produce any detectable changes in function of T lymphocytes or increase in DNA, RNA, or protein synthesis, as measured by incorporation of [^{3}H]thymidine, [^{3}H]uridine, and [^{3}H]leucine by spleen, bone marrow, and peripheral blood lymphocytes in vitro. However, the maturation of B lymphocytes from the spleen of exposed mice was stimulated. Consistent with this effect on B lymphocytes are the results reported by Czerski (1975) and Czerski et al. (1974a,b).

Smialowicz et al. (1979b) investigated lymphocyte function in mice exposed to 2450 MHz daily (15 or 30 min) for up to 22 consecutive mornings to power densities ranging from 5 to 35 mW/cm^2 (SAR 4 to 25 mW/g, 22°C, 50% humidity, 25 m^3 air flow/min). Colonic temperatures, taken prior to and immediately following exposure, showed no significant increase in exposed relative to sham-exposed animals on a given day or at a given power density. There were no differences between exposed and control animals in peripheral blood cell parameters (erythrocyte count, hemoglobin, hematocrit, leukocyte count, differential or absolute count of lymphocytes and polymorphonuclear leukocytes), or in frequencies of T or B lymphocytes in the spleen. There were no differences in B and T lymphocyte transformation responses to several mitogens, nor were there differences in DNA synthesis, between cells from exposed and control animals, in the absence of mitogen stimulation. The antibody response (plaque-forming cell assay after immunization with SRBC) did not differ between cells from exposed and control animals, nor did exposure cause a difference in spontaneous antibody production.

MW/RF-induced hyperthermia in mice has been associated with

transient lymphopenia and neutrophilia (Liburdy, 1976, 1977) with a relative increase in splenic T and B lymphocytes (Liburdy, 1979), and with decreased *in vivo* local delayed hypersensitivity (Liburdy, 1978, 1979). The latter was not affected by a comparable increase in core temperature produced by warm air. Reduced thymic mass and cell density (Liburdy, 1979), suppressed inflammatory response (Liburdy, 1976, 1977), and suppressed allograft transplant rejection (Liburdy, 1978) have been reported. Such alterations in lymphocyte distribution and function are concomitant with a state of immunosuppression. Qualitatively similar changes can be induced by administration of synthetic glucocorticoids or corticosterone (Liburdy, 1979). In fact, Liburdy (1979) reported elevated plasma corticosterone levels in mice following exposure to MW/RF energy sufficient to cause hyperthermia. A similar response has been reported by Lotz and Michaelson (1978), who showed a correlation between microwave-induced body heating and corticosterone levels in the blood of rats. These studies suggest that exposure to microwaves of sufficient intensity results in stimulation of the hypophysial–adrenal axis, which could affect the immune system (Liburdy, 1979; Roberts *et al.*, 1986).

It would appear, thus, that MW/RF exposure initially causes a general stimulation of the immune system, but if the exposure continues, the stimulatory effect disappears, suggesting a phase of adaptation to continued MW/RF exposure. There is a body of literature on the influence of heat *per se* on immunity. Significant influences of microwaves on immune responsiveness would be expected on the basis of the known effects of hyperthermia. Although there has been some uncertainty as to whether fever enhances host resistance to infection (Atkins and Bodel, 1972; Bennett and Nicastri, 1960), more recent evidence suggests that fever may enhance survival after infection in an animal model (Kluger *et al.*, 1975). Cell-mediated immunity plays a role in defense against facultative intracellular bacteria (Frenkel and Caldwell, 1975), viruses (Mandell, 1975), and certain other infectious agents. Roberts and Steigbigel (1977) have shown that increased temperature (38.5°C) enhanced human lymphocyte response to mitogen (PHA) and antigen (streptokinase–streptodornase) and enhances but does not accelerate certain bactericidal functions of human phagocytic leukocytes.

Studies performed with mice as the experimental subject require special consideration in this context. The mouse is a relatively inefficient thermal regulator. In contrast to other species, the mouse has been shown to remain afebrile or become hypothermic in response to infectious or inflammatory challenges that evoke febrile responses in humans (Larson *et al.*, 1939), even though the mouse has a similar system for endogenous pyrogen production and response (Bodel and Miller, 1976). One therefore has to be cautious in assessing the mechanisms of microwave exposure related to alterations in immune processes (Robert, 1983). It may be that if microwaves do in fact increase the proportion of lymphocytes undergoing transformation, this may not in itself be harmful but actually beneficial. The immune system has a considerable redundancy and adaptability (Roberts, 1983). Perturbations of the immune system may not have clinical significance (Stossel, 1979). It has not yet been established that microwave-induced immunological reactions exist independent of thermal effects. It is conceivable that such thermal effects, especially if not exceeding the limits of the subject's physiological regulatory systems, could be beneficial rather than detrimental (Roberts, 1979; Roberts et al., 1986).

Conclusion

There is a lack of convincing evidence for RF/MW effects on the hematological and immunological systems without some form of thermal involvement. The reported effects of RF/MW energies on these systems are comparable to those resulting from a stress response involving the hypothalamic–hypophysial–adrenal axis or following administration of glucocorticoids.

REFERENCES

Atkins, E., and P. Bodel (1972) Fever. *N. Engl. J. Med.* **286**:27.

Baranski, S. (1972) Effect of microwaves on the reactions of the white blood cell system. *Acta Physiol. Pol.* **23**:685.

Baranski, S., and P. Czerski (1976) *Biological Effects of Microwaves*. Dowden, Hutchinson & Ross, Stroudsburg, Pa.

Bennett, I. L., Jr., and A. Nicastri (1960) Fever as a mechanism of resistance. *Bacteriol. Rev.* **24**:16.

Bodel, P., and H. Miller (1976) Pyrogen from mouse macrophages causes fever in mice. *Proc. Soc. Exp. Biol. Med.* **151**:93.

Czerski, P. (1975) Microwave effects on the blood-forming system with particular reference to the lymphocyte. *Ann. N.Y. Acad. Sci.* **247**:232.

Czerski, P. E., E. Paprocka-Slonka, M. Siekierzynski, and A. Stolarska (1974a) Influence of microwave radiation on the hematopoietic system. In: *Biological Effects and Health Hazards of Microwave Radiation*, P. Czerski, K. Ostrowski, M. L. Shore, C. Silverman, M. J. Suess, and B. Waldeskog (eds.). Polish Medical Publishers, Warsaw, pp. 67–74.

Czerski, P., E. Paprocka-Slonka, and A. Stolarska (1974b) Microwave irradiation and the circadian rhythm of bone marrow cell mitosis. *J. Microwave Power* **9**:31.

Frenkel, J. K., and S. A. Caldwell (1975) Specific immunity and nonspecific resistance to infection: Listeria, protozoa, and viruses in mice and hamsters. *J. Infect. Dis.* **131**:201.

Gordon, Z. V. (1966) Biological Effect of Microwaves in Occupational Hygiene. Izd. Med., Leningrad (TT 70-50087, NASA TT F-633, 1970).

Hamrick, P. E. (1973) Thermal denaturation of DNA exposed to 2450 MHz CW microwave radiation. *Radiat. Res.* **56**:400.

Huang, A. T., M. E. Engle, J. A. Elder, J. B. Kinn, and T. R. Ward (1977) The effect of microwave radiation (2450 MHz) on the morphology and chromosomes of lymphocytes. *Radio Sci.* **12**:173.

Kluger, M. J., D. H. Ringler, and M. R. Anver (1975) Fever and survival. *Science* **188**:166.

Krupp, J. H. (1977) The relationship of thermal stress to immune response in mice exposed to 2.6 GHz radio-frequency radiation. In: *Proceedings of the 1977 Annual Meeting of USNC/URSI*, Airlie, Va., p. 143.

Larson, W. P., R. N. Bieter, M. Levine, and W. F. McLimans (1939) Temperature reactions in mice infected with pneumococci. *Proc. Soc. Exp. Biol. Med.* **42**:649.

Liburdy, R. P. (1976) Effects of radiofrequency radiation on peripheral vascular permeability. *Annu. Meet. Int. Union Radio Sci.*, Amherst, Mass. (Abstr.)

Liburdy, R. P. (1977) Effects of radio-frequency radiation on inflammation. *Radio Sci.* **12**(6S):179.

Liburdy, R. P. (1978) Suppression of allograft rejection by whole-body microwave hyperthermia. *Fed. Proc.* **37**:1281.

Liburdy, R. P. (1979) Radiofrequency alters the immune system: Modulation of T- and B-lymphocyte levels and cell-mediated immunocompetence by hyperthermic radiation. *Radiat. Res.* **77**:34.

Lotz, W. G., and S. M. Michaelson (1978) Temperature and corticosterone relationship in microwave exposed rats. *J. Appl. Physiol.* **44**:438.

Lovely, R. H., T. J. Sparks, A. W. Guy, and C. K. Chou (1979) Radiofrequency Field Exposure of Cultured Lymphocytes from Macaca mulata. Final Report SAM-TR-79-25, USAF School of Aerospace Medicine, Brooks AFB, Texas.

Mandell, G. L. (1975) Effect of temperature on phagocytosis by human polymorphonuclear neutrophils. *Infect. Immun.* **12**:221.

Michaelson, S. M. (1974) Effects of exposure to microwaves: Problems and perspectives. *Environ. Health Perspect.* **8**:133.

Michaelson, S. M., R. A. E. Thomson, and J. W. Howland (1967) Biologic Effects of Microwave Exposure. Tech. Rep. RADC-TR-67-961, Griffiss AFB, Rome Air Development Center, Rome, N.Y.

Monjan, A. A., and N. I. Collector (1977) Stress-induced modulation of the immune response. *Science* **197**:307.

Petrov, I. R. (ed.) (1970) *Influence of Microwave Radiation on the Organism of Man and Animals*. Meditsina Press, Leningrad (NASA TT F-708).

Phillips, R. D., E. L. Hunt, R. D. Castro, and N. W. King (1975) Thermoregulatory, metabolic and cardiovascular response of rats to microwaves. *J. Appl. Physiol.* **38**:630.

Prince, J. E., L. H. Mori, J. W. Frazer, and J. C. Mitchell (1972) Cytologic aspects of RF radiation in the monkey. *Aerosp. Med.* **43**:759.

Roberts, N. J., Jr. (1979) Temperature and host defense. *Microbiol. Rev.* **43**:241.

Roberts, N. J., Jr. (1983) Radiofrequency and microwave effects on immunological and hematopoietic systems. In: *Biologic Effects of Low-Energy Electromagnetic Fields*, M. Grandolfo, S. M. Michaelson, and A. Rindi (eds.). Plenum Press, New York, pp. 429–459.

Roberts, N. J., Jr., and R. T. Steigbigel (1977) Hyperthermia and human leukocyte functions: Effects on response of lymphocytes to mitogen and antigen and bactericidal capacity of monocytes and neutrophils. *Infect. Immun.* **18**:673.

Roberts, N. J., Jr., S. M. Michaelson, and S. T. Lu (1986) The biological effects of radiofrequency radiation: A critical review and recommendation. *Int. J. Radiat. Biol.* **50**:379.

Shandala, M. G., M. I. Rudnev, G. K. Vinogradov, N. C. Belonoshko, and N. M.

Goncharova (1977) Immunological and hematological effects of microwaves at low power densities. In: *Proceedings of the 1977 Annual Meeting of USNC/URSI*, Airlie, Va., p. 85.

Smialowicz, R. J. (1976) The effect of microwaves (2450 MHz) on lymphocyte blast transformation *in vitro*. In: *Biological Effects of Electromagnetic Waves*, Vol. I, C. C. Johnson and M. L. Shore (eds.). HEW Publ. (FDA) 77-8010, pp. 472–483.

Smialowicz, R. J., J. B. Kinn, and J. A. Elder (1979a) Perinatal exposure of rats to 2450 MHz (CW) microwave radiation: Effects on lymphocytes. *Radio Sci.* **14**(6S):47.

Smialowicz, R. J., M. M. Riddle, P. L. Brugnolotti, J. M. Sperazza, and J. B. Kinn (1979b) Evaluation of lymphocyte function in mice exposed to 2450 MHz (CW) microwaves. In: *Electromagnetic Fields in Biological Systems*, S. S. Stuchly (ed.). IMPI, Edmonton, Canada, pp. 122–152.

Stodolnik-Baranska, W. (1974) The effects of microwaves on human lymphocyte cultures. In: *Biological Effects and Health Hazards of Microwave Radiation*, P. Czerski, K. Ostrowski, M. L. Shore, C. Silverman, M. J. Suess, and B. Waldeskog (eds.). Polish Medical Publishers, Warsaw, pp. 189–195.

Stossel, T. P. (1979) Introductory overview/tutorial on immunology. In: *Program for Control of Electromagnetic Pollution of the Environment: The Assessment of Biologic Hazards of Nonionizing Electromagnetic Radiation*, Fifth. NTIA Report 79-19, p. C-23.

Szmigielski, S., and M. Janiak (1977) Alteration of cell-mediated immunity by local microwave hyperthermia (43°C) of Guerin epithelioma. In: *Proceedings of the 1977 Annual Meeting of USNC/URSI*, Airlie, Va., p. 141.

Szmigielski, S., J. Jeljaszewicz, and M. Wiranowska (1975) Acute staphylococcal infections in rabbits irradiated with 3 GHz microwaves. *Ann. N.Y. Acad. Sci.* **247**:305.

Szmigielski, S., M. Luczak, M. Janiak, M. Kobus, and B. Laskowska (1976) Effect of 3 GHz microwaves on experimental viral infections in mice (herpes, vaccinia). In: *Proceedings of the 1976 Annual Meeting of USNC/URSI*, Amherst, Mass., p. 117.

Szmigielski, S., G. Pulverer, W. Hryniewicz, and M. Janiak (1977) Inhibition of tumor growth in mice by microwave hyperthermia, Streptolysis S and colcemide. *Radio Sci.* **12**(6S):185.

Volkova, A. P., and P. O. Fukalova (1974) Changes in certain protective reactions of an organism under the influence of SW in experimental and industrial conditions. In: *Biological Effects of Radiofrequency Electromagnetic Fields*, Z. V. Gordon (ed.). JPRS 63321, pp. 168–174.

Wiktor-Jedrzejczak, W., A. Ahmed, P. Czerski, W. M. Leach, and K. W. Sell (1977a) Immunologic response of mice to 2450 MHz microwave radiation: Overview of immunology and empirical studies of lymphoid spleen cells. *Radio Sci.* **12**(6S):209.

Wiktor-Jedrzejczak, W., A. Ahmed, K. W. Sell, P. Czerski, and W. M. Leach (1977b) Microwaves induce an increase in the frequency of complement receptor-bearing lymphoid spleen cells in mice. *J. Immunol.* **118**:1499.

16

Biochemical Effects

Various types of metabolic/biochemical alterations have been reported to result from exposure of experimental animals and humans to MW/RF fields. Such effects generally appear to be reversible and no well-defined characteristic response pattern has been determined; nor is it known whether the changes are direct or indirect effects of exposure.

Although the reliability or relevancy of many of these studies, especially those performed before 1975, is questionable, they should be reviewed since biochemical indicators of exposure to these radiant energies could possibly provide a useful basis for hazard evaluation and early diagnosis of extremes of exposure. If there is a sensitivity to low levels, biochemical alterations become important. To be of any value, biochemical substances destined to function as indicators of the extent of injury in the human should fulfill a number of criteria, which can be summarized as follows (Veninga, 1971):

1. Substances of endogenous origin must show alterations with respect to either their release or their metabolism following exposure of the organism. These alterations might ultimately lead to changes in the excretion rate either of the native substances or of their metabolites or of both.
2. The alterations should be detectable early and their determination should not be too complicated.
3. Changes in components that are detectable only after high levels of exposure should be considered as less valuable, since they may be a reflection of other interacting factors, or even of gross stressful insult of a totally nonspecific nature.
4. The alterations should be demonstrable in several mammalian species in order to justify comparison with the human at least whenever sufficient data for the human are not available.
5. The alterations should show a certain degree of specificity with regard to the exposure as well as to the method of their determination.

Experimental data should be expressed in a way that supports the interpretation proposed (Gerber and Altman, 1970). Biochemical changes can be of significance for the organism as a whole and/or for a certain organ only. Alterations in the biochemistry of an organ may represent changes at the level of single cells but, more frequently, reflect changes in the cell population of the organ. It should be noted that no organ has a uniform cell population.

16.1. ENZYME ACTIVITY

Enzymes vary considerably in tissue distribution, with some being rather restricted in occurrence while others apparently occur in all cells. Those enzymes that carry out special reactions in various tissues tend to be more restricted in distribution (Cornish, 1971). Enzyme changes are investigated (1) to detect early physiological or biochemical changes in response to insult to the body, (2) to localize the site or sites of action with respect to organ damage, (3) to interpret changes in serum enzymes as they relate to effects on the whole animal.

Investigations on enzymes exposed *in vitro* to electromagnetic fields of various frequency ranges have shown changes in activity (Bach, 1965; Takashima, 1966). These results were obtained under a variety of conditions. There are indications, however, that temperature rise might be a dominant factor (Takashima, 1966).

In vivo studies by Baranski (1972) and Nikogosyan (1962) on cholinesterase activity have suggested that tissue and blood activity of this enzyme may be affected by microwave radiation. However, *in vitro* studies by Olcerst and Rabinowitz (1978) and Belkhode *et al.* (1974) on the activity of cholinesterase and glucose-6-phosphate dehydrogenase following microwave exposure *in vitro* have been negative. In these studies, at power levels of up to $100\,mW/cm^2$, microwaves had no effect on enzyme activity when the temperature was not allowed to increase during microwave exposure. However, enzyme activity was measured subsequent to microwave exposure rather than during microwave irradiation.

Bach (1965) reported that α-amylase was inactivated after exposure to 12–16 MHz. Exposure of guinea pigs to microwaves of relatively high intensity for 5–10 min led to a significant reduction in amylase and lipase activity, and an initial increase followed by a decrease in the amount of glutathione (Sacchitelli and Sacchitelli, 1956, 1958). Microwaves of 2450 MHz increased the phosphorylase activity in rats muscles (Kirchev *et al.*, 1961).

The effect of RF energy on enzyme activity was investigated in rabbits (Chirkov, 1964). In the first series of experiments, the animals were subjected to a single 20-min exposure to frequencies of 9.5 or 27 MHz at field strengths of 1–20 V/cm. There was a reduction in blood catalase and peroxidase activity. Another series of experiments involved multiple exposures of the head to 9.5 MHz at a field strength of 20 V/cm for 20 min daily (a total of ten exposures at 2-day intervals). There was a biphasic change in enzyme activity 5–150 min after exposure—a reduction after the first exposure and an increase after the subsequent ones. The enzyme activity returned to normal within 2–12 days after termination of exposure.

Reports in the Eastern European literature (Baranski, 1972; Nikogosyan, 1962; Revuts'kiy and Edel'man, 1964) have suggested a direct effect of microwave exposure on acetylcholinesterase activity. These earlier studies served as the basis for the *in vitro* experiments of Olcerst and Rabinowitz (1978) and Belkhode et al. (1974) (*vide supra*) who examined the *in vitro* effects of microwave radiation on enzymes. However, these investigators (Olcerst and Rabinowitz, 1984; Belkhode et al., 1974) could not demonstrate an effect on enzyme activity following microwave radiation. A significant change in enzyme activity was observed only when microwaves caused thermal inactivation of enzymes (Olcerst and Rabinowitz, 1978). However, such thermal effects probably would not occur in *in vivo* experiments (Baranski, 1972; Nikogosyan, 1962) because of the body's homeostatic thermoregulatory mechanisms. Furthermore, microwave effects on enzymes that are not due to enzyme inactivation may be reversible, and thus may not be demonstrable by protocols that measure enzyme activity subsequent to, but not during, microwave exposure.

In studies by Galvin et al. (1981), the enzyme rate was measured during exposure to microwaves, the sample temperature being maintained at 37°C. The data from these experiments indicate there was no significant difference between control and irradiated acetylcholinesterase and creatine phosphokinase activities.

Malyshev and Tkachenko (1972) found that exposure to 2.45 or 10 GHz at intensities of 25 to 1000 $\mu W/cm^2$ decreased the proteolytic activity of the mucous membrane of the small intestines of experimental animals, whereas the invertase and ATPase activities increased. Reduced synthesis of macroglobulin and macroglobulin antibodies resulted from exposure of experimental animals to 50 $\mu W/cm^2$. Serum glutamic oxaloacetic transaminase (SGOT), glutamic pyruvic transaminase (SGPT), lactic dehydrogenase (LDH), and creatine phosphokinase (CPK) levels were not affected in rhesus monkeys exposed to 19.27 MHz for up to 4 hr daily for 13 days at 115 mW/cm^2 (Mitchell and Gass, 1971).

Study of oxidative enzymes in various tissues of animals after exposure to microwaves in the ranges of 3000 and 10,000 MHz suggests that microwaves influence the activities of succinic acid dehydrogenase and cytochrome oxidase (Moskalyuk, 1957; Syngayevskaya, 1970). Exposure of rats to 10,000 MHz, 30–40 mW/cm^2, for 30 min (0.7–1.2°C colonic temperature rise) produced a slight suppression of the oxidative enzymes (succinic acid dehydrogenase and cytochrome oxidase), while irradiation not accompanied by a temperature rise increased the activities of these enzymes. Oxidative processes were sharply reduced after the animals had been exposed to the same frequency (10,000 MHz) at 150–170 mW/cm^2. Succinic acid dehydrogenase activity was reduced almost 50% in the myocardium, kidneys, liver, and brain; cytochrome oxidase activity was down 40% in the heart, liver, and kidneys and down 24% in the brain.

In these experiments, the colonic temperature of the rats increased 4–5°C within 12 min of exposure. Almost no suppression of the activity of these enzymes was observed on exposure (to 150–170 mW/cm^2) of anesthetized animals, whose colonic temperatures rose only by 1.5–2.5°C, while it had risen 4–5°C in unanesthetized animals irradiated under the same conditions. More marked changes in the activity of succinic acid dehydrogenase and cytochrome oxidase were observed on exposure of the animals to 3000 MHz than to 10,000 MHz at the same power densities and exposure times. Syngayevskaya (1970) has suggested this may be due to inhibition of the CNS from the anesthetic, accompanied by suppression of metabolic (oxidative) processes. It should be pointed out, however, that anesthesia will reduce body temperature, and this hypothesis may not be justified.

Changes have been noted in ATP, ADP, and inorganic phosphorus content in the liver, heart, skeletal muscle, and brain of rats exposed to 3000 MHz microwaves at intensities (between 10 and 100 mW/cm^2, for 65 min (Syngayevskaya, 1970). Exposure to "low-intensity" (10 mW/cm^2) microwave energy, for which the animals did not showed increased colonic temperature, produced a marked decrease in ATP content, along with an increase in ADP and inorganic phosphorus in the organs studied. The ATP/ADP ratio decreased, while the total content of ATP and ADP increased by as much as 15% compared with the control. It is doubtful a 15% increase is of biological significance.

Kolodub and Yevtushenko (1972) studied rats exposed to pulsed fields at 24 and 72 kA/m (7 kHz, pulse width 130 msec, and interpulse interval of 10 sec, 15 daily exposures for 3 hr). Rats were also exposed daily for 1½ hr, at 24 kA/m for 1½, 3, and 6 months. The authors found a reduction of ATP and creatine phosphate (CP). With the acute multiple exposures (72 kA/m), the level of CP decreased by 27% on the average in the brain tissue, and 30% in the skeletal muscles. Under conditions of chronic exposure to 24 kA/m, the reduction of CP was 23.8, 55.4, and

26.4% in the brain tissue, 29.3, 59.3, and 40.8% in the heart, and 39.9, 44.9, and 29.2% in the skeletal muscles at $1\frac{1}{2}$, 3, and 6 months, respectively. Simultaneously, an accumulation of ADP and AMP was detected. In the liver, the levels of ADP and AMP increased by 156 and 120%, respectively, in the brain tissue by 20.4 and 66.5%, and in the heart by 57.7 and 36%.

Thermal microwave intensities (2000–3000 MHz, 100 mW/cm^2) that caused an increase in body temperature (to 40–40.5°C) in rabbits resulted in increased ATP and ADP in the liver, skeletal muscles, and brain (Syngayevskaya, 1970). An increase in inorganic phosphorus content was observed simultaneously. In heart muscle, on the other hand, the ATP content decreased, but the inorganic phosphorus content increased. When the animals were moribund, a substantial decrease in ATP was observed, along with increases in ADP and AMP in the tissues and organs studied. (It should be noted that ATP generally decreases in the moribund state.) Inorganic phosphorus increased, sometimes to a greater degree than would be possible as a result of degradation of ATP to ADP and AMP; this may also indicate that degradation of CP took place without compensation by synthesis. The total content of ATP and ADP and their ratio showed a decrease. The studies of Moskalyuk (1957), on the other hand, indicated that ATPase activity increased under such irradiation with marked suppression of cytochrome oxidase.

In unanesthetized rabbits, succinic acid dehydrogenase and cytochrome oxidase activities were slightly affected, while in anesthetized rabbits (in which the basal metabolism had been lowered) exposure in a RF field raised the tissue respiration activity to normal levels (Kardashev, 1957).

In contrast to the above, Shtemler (1968) reported an *in vitro* experiment investigating the direct effect of exposure to 3000 MHz on catalase and cholinesterase. There was no evidence of a direct effect of 3000 MHz on these enzymes.

16.2. METABOLISM

16.2.1. Carbohydrate and Lipid Metabolism

A 4–5°C colonic temperature increase and a blood sugar increase of 40–45% were noted in rabbits exposed to centimeter (3000–10,000 Hz) microwaves, 125 mW/cm^2, 20 min (Syngayevskaya, 1970). Change in the character of the blood sugar curves (hyper- and hypoglycemia), and an increase in blood epinephrine were observed after exposure of animals to microwaves (3000–10,000 Hz) at both low (<10 mW/cm^2) with no "*marked*" temperature rise and high (> 10 mW/cm^2, with a rise in colonic temperature) intensities. The degree of the alteration depended on the wavelength and intensity of the energy. The blood sugar levels rose by 18, 36, and 22%, respectively, within 15–20 min after termination of exposure of rabbits to centimeter, decimeter, and meter waves with no resultant temperature rise (Syngayevskaya *et al.*, 1962).

Multiple exposures of rabbits to 3000 MHz of "high intensities" (>10 mW/cm^2), for 5–15 min daily resulted in a reduction in the synthesis of glycogen (Dainotto *et al.*, 1962).

Schliephake (1935) observed a 20–60% rise in blood sugar over the initial level in rabbits upon exposure of the upper abdomen and head to 2450- and 27-MHz fields. When only the head of the rabbit was irradiated, blood sugar rose by 90–100%. Faitel'berg-Blank (1964, 1965) reported increased absorption of glucose in isolated intestine when the epigastric region of dogs was subjected to 2450 MHz for 10 min. Syngayevskaya *et al.* (1962) noted that when dogs were subjected to centimeter waves for 1 min at 50 mW/cm^2, a 28–35% decrease in glucose absorption occurred. It should be emphasized that these results were obtained with 50 mW/cm^2 exposure, which unquestionably induces a thermal load on the rabbit.

In another study by Faitel'berg-Blank (1963), a 60-W UHF generator (apparently 40 MHz) with electrodes 0.5 to 1 cm from the skin surface was maintained so that maximum heating of gastric and intestinal mucosa could be obtained. Exposure was for 10 min. The author found increased absorption of water, glucose, glycine, and chlorides from the stomach and intestines. The responses could be a result of increased blood flow to the stomach and intestines. Because dosimetry was not presented, one cannot determine if this is a realistic phenomenon.

Hepatic gluconeogenesis was enhanced in rabbits an hour after 1000–3000 MHz, 1 mW/cm^2, and 300 Hz, 3 mW/cm^2; increasing 67 and 56% respectively, after administration of glucose (2 g/kg) as compared to control animals given the same amount of glucose (Syngayevskaya *et al.*, 1962). Blood sugar increased in anesthetized rabbits when they were exposed to "thermal" microwave intensities, but the picture differed from the curve obtained on exposure of unanesthetized rabbits. A small blood-sugar increase (10–18%) persisted as long as the anesthetic was effective.

Bud'ko (1964) studied the effect of 0.5-kHz to 3.0-MHz RF on carbohydrate metabolism in the rabbit by measuring the blood sugar level. Only the head or the liver region of the animal was exposed to 15 V/cm for 20 min. Exposure of the head caused much greater changes than exposure of the liver region. At the lower frequencies the sugar level was increased; at the higher frequencies it was reduced. Within this frequency range the magnitude of the effect was practically independent of frequency. In all cases, the sugar level began to return gradually to normal 20–30 min after exposure and reached a normal level in 60–90 min.

In humans, Bartonicek and Klimkova-Deutschova (1964) reported a disturbance of carbohydrate metabolism as a result of chronic exposure to "low-intensity" centimeter waves. Blood and urinary glucose were increased in 75% of the subjects and the blood sugar curves had a prediabetic form. Hasik and Mikolajczyk (1960), however, reported that in healthy individuals exposed to RF energy, only slight changes were observed in the levels of glucose, cholesterol, and lipids in the blood, but a pronounced decrease in all three components among diabetics.

Leites and Skurikhina (1961) exposed rats for 10 min at 100 mW/cm^2, 3000 MHz. At different times (1 hr to 14 days) after irradiation, the ascorbic acid and lipid content of the adrenal cortex was determined. It was found that during the first day after exposure the amount of these substances was reduced to 70% of normal; on the next day it rose to the normal level and subsequently exceeded the normal level by 6–7%. There was a return to normal in 2 weeks. Similar changes were observed in rats after a 5-min exposure to 10,000 MHz, 400 mW/cm^2 (Gorodetskaya, 1961).

In a report by Deficis et al. (1976), mice were exposed to 2450 MHz, 15 hr daily for 9 days at 1 to 3.3 mW/cm^2. Variation in serum triglyceride level was determined. There was no change in this level at 1 mW/cm^2, but at 1.5 and 3.3 mW/cm^2 there was an increase. Under these conditions the SAR would be 0.67 to 2.22 mW/g. Not much information was presented in this abstract. It should be noted that the animals were anesthetized the day before sacrifice. No irradiation characteristics details of data, or information on quality control were presented.

16.2.2. Protein Metabolism

Syngayevskaya et al. (1962) reported that the levels of 8 of 16 amino acids (cystine, lysine, arginine, glutamine, glycine, glutamic acid, tryptophan, phenylalanine) increased substantially in the blood serum of dogs and rabbits exposed to 300 to 3000 MHz, 3 mW/cm^2, 30 min. The levels of tyrosine and leucine decreased, while those of the remaining amino acids were not substantially changed.

Janes et al. (1969) reported altered protein synthesis and protein catabolism in hamsters subjected to 2450-MHz microwaves of unspecified power density which, however, was high enough to result in death due to hyperthermia. There was an apparent decreased amino acid incorporation in the liver 80 min after exposure, returning to normal at 20 hr.

Protein synthesis in the testes rose significantly from 80 min to 20 hr postexposure. The authors qualify these results by pointing out that the mechanism may be mediated through a rise in body temperature. It has been suggested that hyperthermia results in decreased protein synthesis and increased protein catabolism.

Rabbits and rats subjected to 3000 MHz, 10 mW/cm^2, 1 hr/day for 4–8 months, showed changes in the serum proteins, blood urea nitrogen, urinary amino acid and decrease in RNA content in the liver, brain, and spleen (Nikogosyan, 1967). In other studies, a single exposure of rats reduced the activity of both ribonuclease and deoxyribonuclease, but increased the level of both nucleic acids (especially RNA). Ten to twenty exposures resulted in a decrease in albumin and an increase in γ-globulin; 60 to 190 exposures produced a decrease in α- and γ-globulin and liver RNA and an increase in albumin.

The data are internally inconsistent. The author does not differentiate between results in rats and rabbits. Initially there was a decrease in albumin and an increase in γ-globulin, which was followed by an increase in albumin and a decrease in α- and γ-globulin. No information on physical parameters or dosimetry was presented. The methodology for NPN and amino acid determination is antiquated. No information was presented on specimen (i.e., blood, urine) collection, or environmental control.

An increase in the RNA level in the lymphocytes of workers using HF generators has been reported (Smurova *et al.*, 1962). Fibrinolytic activity was observed to increase in young and decrease in older persons following exposure to microwaves applied to the head (Benetato and Dumitresku-Papachadzhi, 1964).

16.3. HISTAMINE RELEASE

The effect of shortwave diathermy on the histamine content of various organs of the mouse was studied by Valtonen (1968). The histamine content of skin (abdominal skin and ear tip), skeletal muscle, blood, liver, kidney, and lung were measured by a fluorometric method 1/4, 1, and 4 hr after the treatment. Some changes in the histamine content of the tissues were observed, but the only significant change was a slight increase in the histamine content of skin. The author suggested that the "histaminelike" effect in the tissues caused by shortwave diathermy is due to the heat induced in the tissues.

Hildebrandt (1941) treated the chest or extremity of a dog with a shortwave apparatus (ca. 8.6 MHz) for 30 min. The histamine content of the blood increased after 1 hr and reached its maximum 2 to 3 hr after the treatment. Several hours later the histamine content was still considerably increased.

In rabbits exposed to 3000 MHz, 10 mW/cm^2, for 1 hr daily, the histamine content varied in the first 5 months, periodically increasing and decreasing, but remaining above the preexposure level (Gel'fon, 1964). Increase in the histamine content of the blood has been reported in individuals exposed to various RF/MW frequencies (Presman, 1968). A decrease in the histamine level in individuals exposed "briefly" to electromagnetic fields in the 13.56-MHz range has also been reported (Revuts'kiy and Edel'man, 1964).

16.4. CLINICAL CHEMISTRY, SERUM PROTEINS, ELECTROLYTES

Dose-dependent transient elevations in serum glucose, blood urea nitrogen (BUN), and uric acid were reported by Wangemann and Cleary (1976) following far-field exposure of rabbits to 2.45 GHz for 2 hr at intensities of 5, 10, and 25 mW/cm^2 with no detectable difference between CW and pulse-modulated exposures of equivalent average power density. There was an increase in colonic temperature of 1.7 to 3.0°C at 10 and 25 mW/cm^2. Calcium, inorganic phosphate, glucose, BUN, uric acid, cholesterol, total protein, alkaline phosphatase, lactic dehydrogenase (LDH), and serum glutamic oxaloacetic transaminase (SGOT) were measured. Glucose showed an increase initially with return to normal at 24 hr. BUN and uric acid increased at 25 mW/cm^2. At 24 hr postexposure, focal hemorrhagic lesions were seen grossly and mild to moderate tubular nephrosis was seen on histopathology. No pathology was seen 2 weeks after exposure.

At 5 and 10 mW/cm^2 (0.5 to 2 mW/g for both frequencies), thermally induced reactions were not evident, but at 25 mW/cm^2, which is 3 mW/g for 1.7 GHz and 2.5 mW/g for 2.45 GHz, evidence of thermal injury was present.

The authors did not feel that the pulsed and CW results could be compared directly, because the exposure conditions were different. The observed results were those that would be expected from heat stress. Animals exposed at 25 mW/cm^2 for 2 hr showed a significant increase in colonic temperature, the temperature increase being 1.7 and 2.9°C for pulsed and CW exposures, respectively. Those animals exposed at 10 mW/cm^2 showed mild evidence of heat stress, such as peripheral vasodilation, but not a significant increase in colonic temperature.

A study of the effects of microwaves on serum chemistry values was reported by Lovely *et al.* (1977), who exposed rats to 918-MHz, CW microwaves in a circularly polarized waveguide 10 hr/day for 13 weeks at 2.5 mW/cm² (~1.04 W/kg). There were no colonic temperature changes. Blood sampled after 4, 8, and 12 weeks showed no differences in most parameters of serum chemistry, i.e., sodium, potassium, chloride, BUN, carbon dioxide, and glucose. During the 11th week, serial assessments were made of colonic temperature and behavior, but neither demonstrated a significant effect. Serum corticosterone levels at 910 hr of exposure gave no indication of alteration. Neither one nor two bottle preference test for saccharin solution suggested any effect of irradiation.

There is a question as to the biological methods and techniques used. Although sufficient information is provided to adequately replicate such a study, factors such as use of ether anesthesia for blood sampling, night exposure, ignoring diurnal variation, and pooled AM and PM samples could constitute confounding factors. According to the authors the SAR is 1.04 W/kg. The authors reported a significant difference in the serum calcium values at the end of the 12-week exposure. However, this is most probably a spurious result, because the calcium levels in the sham-irradiated animals were decreased from previous values, while the levels in the irradiated animals remained unchanged from earlier values.

The effect of 3000-MHz microwaves on plasma electrolytes in rats after chronic exposure has been reported by Kulakova (1968). Animals exposed at 40 mW/cm² for 1 hr daily showed an increase in the Ca^{2+} content of the blood plasma after six exposures. During this time the Na^+ and K^+ contents were unaltered. Rats were also exposed for 2 months at 40 mW/cm², while various solutions of salts (KCl, NaCl, $CaCl_2$) were introduced into the diet. The author noted changes in salt requirements. Data characterizing ion shifts in the dialysate and urine suggested that a change occurs in the electrolyte composition, which was not the same at different periods of chronic exposure.

Exposure of rats for 15 min to pulsed 2.86 GHz at intensities of 5, 10, 20, 50, or 100 mW/cm² resulted in statistically significant changes in serum albumin and phosphorus levels only at 100 mW/cm² (Fulk and Finch, 1972). There was no change in serum glucose levels in rats exposed to 2.86- and 0.43-GHz pulse-modulated fields at an average power density of 5 mW/cm². Single or repeated exposures of rabbits to 3 or 10 GHz at intensities of 5 to 25 mW/cm² resulted in alterations in serum albumin/globulin ratio (Swiecicki and Edelwejn, 1963a,b).

Grigor'yan (1969) reported that after RF/MW exposure of animals the serum albumin content was reduced, but the β- and γ-globulin increased. The ratio of protein fractions in heart muscle changed more markedly with exposure at 40 than at 6 mW/cm².

Plasma proteins were decreased and plasma chlorides increased in dogs exposed daily for 6 hr at 50 mW/cm², 1280 MHz (Michaelson et al.,

1967). Immediately following each exposure there was an increase in plasma chlorides; venous CO_2 content was mildly decreased. When exposure was extended to 5 weeks, changes in pre- and post-exposure venous CO_2 content were essentially negligible, and the values were comparable to those noted prior to the first microwave exposure. There were no significant changes in blood glucose, NPN, plasma BUN, or calcium levels.

Rhesus monkeys were exposed to 10.5 MHz, 200 mW/cm^2 for 1 hr; 19.27 MHz, 170 mW/cm^2 for 4 hr, and 13 consecutive days, 4 hr each day at a power density of 115 mW/cm^2; and 26.6 MHz, 100 mW/cm^2 for 1 hr (Mitchell and Gass, 1971). Serum glucose, BUN, total serum protein, and serum sodium and potassium levels were fairly consistent throughout the study. Statistical analysis demonstrated that there was no influence of RF exposure on any of these values. Serum albumin, α-globulin, β-globulin, and γ-globulin levels remained within the normal range. Glucose, BUN, protein, and major electrolytes appeared within normal limits and indicated no gross pathological processes.

A decrease in γ-globulin and an increase in the α- and β-globulin of the blood serum with a simultaneous increase in the activity of SGOT have been reported in mice exposed to 10,000 MHz, 100 mW/cm^2 (Grzesik et al., 1960). It is known that this enzyme participates in transamination processes, which are closely related to metabolic functions of the liver. It should also be recognized that this enzyme level increases with tissue destruction, which can occur with 100 mW/cm^2.

A decrease in albumin content and an increase in γ-globulin were observed in the blood serum of rabbits after 10–20 1-hr exposures to 3000 or 10,000 MHz, 10 mW/cm^2, with no change in colonic temperature (Nikogosyan, 1962). Total serum protein remained unchanged, but the albumin/globulin ratio decreased. After 40 to 60 exposures, the α- and β-globulin levels decreased without any pronounced changes in overall serum proteins. Rabbits exposed to low-frequency (3–300 MHz) fields displayed a decrease in albumin and an increase in globulin fractions (Singatulina, 1961). Restoration of the original level occurred after 20 days. In rabbits exposed to 13.2–13.6 MHz with an unmodulated field strength of 25 V/m, there was a marked decrease in serum albumin and γ-globulins and a depression of total serum protein with no marked change in the albumin/globulin ratio (Subbota and Grebenshechnikova, 1967).

Alteration of serum proteins has been reported in individuals chronically exposed to RF fields of "low intensity" (Gel'fon and Sadchikova, 1964; Syngayevskaya, 1962). In 50% of the investigated subjects, the total protein content was increased—mainly due to the increase in the amount of globulins, as indicated by the change in the albumin/globulin ratio. The reliability of such findings has been disputed (Pazderova, 1968; Pazderova-Vejlupkova, 1981).

REFERENCES

Bach, S. A. (1965) Biological sensitivity to radio-frequency and microwave energy. *Fed. Proc.* **24**(Suppl. 14):22.
Baranski, S. (1972) Histological and histochemical effect of microwave irradiation on the central nervous system of rabbits and guinea pigs. *Am. J. Phys. Med.* **51**:182.
Bartonicek, V., and E. Klimkova-Deutschova (1964) Some biochemical changes in workers exposed to centimeter waves. *Cas. Lek. Cesk.* **103**:26.
Belkhode, M. L., D. L. Johnson, and A. M. Muc (1974) Thermal and athermal effects of microwave radiation on the activity of glucose-6-phosphate dehydrogenase in human blood. *Health Phys.* **26**:45.
Benetato, G., and E. Dumitresku-Papachadzhi (1964) Changes in the fibrinolytic activity of blood plasma under the influence of U.H.F. radiation in the hypothalamic region in various age groups. *Rev. Roum. Fiziol.* **1**:125.
Bud'ko, L. N. (1964) Dynamics of carbohydrate metabolism in isolated liver of white rats on exposure to electromagnetic fields of different frequencies, p. 31; Change in blood carbohydrate content due to the action of electromagnetic vibrations of audio- and radio-frequency on organisms, p. 73. In: *Some Questions of Physiology and Biophysics*. Trudy Otdeleniya, Voronezh, Izd-vo Voronezh Univ.
Chirkov, M. M. (1964) The effect of the energy of electromagnetic radiation of the acoustic spectrum on catalase activity of blood. In: *Some Questions of Physiology and Biophysics*. Trudy Otdeleniya, Voronezh, Izd-vo Voronezh Univ., p. 25.
Cornish, H. H. (1971) Problems posed by observations of serum enzyme changes in toxicology. *CRC Crit. Rev. Toxicol.* **1**:81.
Dainotto, F., D. Tognazzi, and A. Violanti (1962) Study of the glycolytic fractions of skeletal muscle in experimental animals treated with microwaves. *Policlinico Sez. Med.* **69**:270.
Deficis, A., J. C. Dumas, S. Laurens, and G. Plurien (1976) Variation of serum triglyceride rate under the action of electromagnetic waves—Power level influence. *J. Microwave Power* **11**:136.
Faitel'berg-Blank, V. R. (1963) Absorptive activity of stomach and intestine under the influence of a UHF electric field. *Fed. Proc.* **22**(Transl. Suppl.):T-301–T-305.
Faitel'berg–Blank, V. R. (1964) Effect of high-frequency waves of centimeter wavelength on the absorptive activity of the stomach and intestine. *Byull. Eksp. Biol. Med.* **57**:45.
Faitel'berg-Blank, V. R. (1965). Variation in mechanism of gastric and intestinal absorptive activity upon exposure to SHF–UHF radiowaves (in the centimeter range). *Fiziol. Zh. SSSR im. I.M. Sechenova* **51**:372.
Fulk, D. W., and E. D. Finch (1972) Effects of microwave irradiation *in vivo* on rabbit blood serum. Report No. 5, Project MF 51.524.0015-001BD7X. Naval Medical Research Institute, Bethesda.
Galvin, M. J., D. L. Parks, and D. I. McRee (1981) Influence of 2.45 GHz microwave radiation on enzyme activity. *Radiat. Environ. Biophys.* **19**:149.
Gel'fon, I. A. (1964) The effect of 10-cm waves of low intensity on the histamine content of the blood of animals. In: *Biological Effect of Radio-Frequency Electromagnetic Fields*. Inst. Ind. Hyg. Occup. Dis., Acad. Med. Sci., Moscow, p. 68.
Gel'fon, I. A., and M. N. Sadchikova (1964) Protein fractions and histamine in the blood under the effect of radiowaves of various ranges. In: *The Biological Effect of*

Radio-Frequency Electromagnetic Fields. Institute of Work Hygiene and Occupational Diseases, AMN SSR, Issue 2, Moscow, p. 133.

Gerber, G. B., and K. I. Altman (1970) General aspects of radiation biochemistry. *Radiation Biochemistry,* Vol. 2. Academic Press, New York, p. 9.

Gorodetskaya, S. F. (1961) The effect of 3-centimeter radiowaves on the functional state of the adrenal cortex. *Fiziol. Zh. Akad. Nauk UKR SSR* **7:**672.

Grigor'yan, D. G. (1969) A study of proteins in the blood serum, heart muscle and brain of animals subjected to the effect of microwaves. *Vopr. Kurortol. Fizioter. Lech. Fiz. Kult.* **34:**510.

Grzesik, J., F. Kumaszka, and Z. Paradowski (1960) Influence of a medium-frequency electromagnetic field on organ parenchyma and blood proteins in white mice. *Med. Pr.* **11:**323.

Hasik, J., and Z. Mikolajczyk (1960) Retention of sugar, cholesterol and lipids in the blood of diabetics under the influence of short waves. *Pol. Tyg. Lek.* **15:**817.

Hildebrandt, F. (1941) The influence of shortwaves, diathermy and fango mud packs on the histamine content in the blood and tissues. *Arch. Exp. Pathol. Pharmakol.* **197:**148.

Janes, D. E., W. M. Leach, W. A. Mills, R. T. Moore, and M. L. Shore (1969) Effects of 2450 MHz microwaves on protein synthesis and on chromosomes in Chinese hamsters. *Non-Ioniz. Radiat.* **1:**125.

Kardashev, V. L. (1957) The influence of a pulsed ultra-high frequency electrical field on processes of biological oxidation under conditions of normal and experimental hypertonicity. *Vopr. Kurortol. Fizioter. Lech. Fiz. Kult.* **22:**37.

Kirchev, K., P. Eftimov, and G. Chernaev (1961) Investigation of the microwave influence on the glycogen content, the phosphorylase activity and the dry weight of the musculature, on the blood sugar, the total protein, and the inorganic phosphorus in the blood of white rats. In: *Proceedings of the Fifth International Biochemical Congress,* Section 24–26 (Moscow).

Kolodub, F. A., and G. I. Yevtushenko (1972) Biochemical aspects of the biological effect of a low-frequency pulsed electromagnetic field. *Gig. Tr. Prof. Zabol.* **6:**13 (JPRS 56583, 1972).

Kulakova, V. V. (1968) The effect of 10 cm waves on special forms of appetite and the electrolytic composition of the blood and urine in rats. In: *The Biological Action of Radio-Frequency Electromagnetic Fields.* Institute of Work Hygiene and Occupational Diseases, AMN SSR, Moscow, p. 112.

Leites, F. L., and L. A. Skurikhina (1961) The effect of microwaves on the hormonal activity of the adrenal cortex. *Byull. Eksp. Biol. Med.* **52:**47.

Lovely, R. H., D. E. Myers, and A. W. Guy (1977) Irradiation of rats by 918 MHz microwaves at 2.5 mW/cm^2: Delineating the dose–response relationships. *Radio Sci.* **12(6S):**139.

Malyshev, V. T., and M. I. Tkachenko (1972) Activity of ferments on the mucus membrane of the small intestine under the influence of an SHF field. *Physiology and Pathology of Digestion,* Kishinev, p. 186.

Michaelson, S. M., R. A. E. Thomson, and J. Howland (1967) Biologic Effects of Microwave Exposure. Tech. Rep. RADC-TR-67-461, Griffiss AFB, Rome Air Development Center, Rome, N.Y. Also: Radiation Control for Health and Safety Act of 1967; Hearings before the Committee on Commerce, U.S. Senate, 90th Congress, Second Session on S. 2067, S. 3211, and H.R. 10790, 1968, p. 1143.

Mitchell, J. C., and A. B. Gass (1971) Hematological and biochemical results from RF exposures at 10.5, 16.6, and 19.3 MHz. In: *Proceedings of the Department of Defense Electromagnetic Radiation Research Workshop.* Bur. Med. Surg., Dep. Navy, Washington, D.C., p. 1.

Moskalyuk, A. I. (1957) Effect of a SHF field on oxidation reduction processes in some rabbit tissues. *Tr. VMOLA* **73:**133.

Nikogosyan, S. V. (1962) Effect of UHF on cholinesterase activity in blood serum and organs in animals. In: *The Biological Action of Ultrahigh Frequencies,* A. A. Letavet and Z. V. Gordon (eds.). Acad. Med. Sci., Moscow, pp. 83–91 (JPRS 12471).

Nikogosyan, S. V. (1967) Changes in protein metabolism under chronic exposure to 10 cm low-intensity waves. *Byull. Eksp. Biol. Med.* **64:**56.

Olcerst, R. B., and J. R. Rabinowitz (1978) Studies on the interaction of microwave radiation with cholinesterase. *Radiat. Environ. Biophys.* **15:**289.

Pazderova, J. (1968) Effects of electromagnetic radiation of the order of centimeter and meter wavelength on human health. *Prac. Lek.* **20:**447.

Pazderova-Vejlupkova, J. (1981) Update on epidemiology: European studies. In: *URSI Annual Meeting,* Washington, D.C. (Abst.).

Presman, A. S. (1968) *Electromagnetic Fields and Life.* Izd-vo Nauka, Moscow (Transl. Plenum Press, 1970).

Revuts'kiy, Y. L., and F. S. Edel'man (1964) The effect of electromagnetic fields in the centimeter and meter ranges on the amount of biologically active substances in human blood. *Fiziol. Zh. Akad. Nauk. UKR SSR* **10:**379.

Sacchitelli, G., and F. Sacchitelli (1956) The action of radar microwaves on plasma lipases and serum amylase. *Folia Med. (Naples)* **39:**1037.

Sacchitelli, G., and F. Sacchitelli (1958) On the behavior of blood glutathione following irradiation with radar microwaves. *Folia Med. (Naples)* **41:**345.

Schliephake, E. (1935) *Shortwave Therapy: The Medical Uses of Electrical High Frequencies,* Actinic Press, London (English translation of German edition), Ed. 6, Gustav Fischer Verlag, Stuttgart, 1960.

Shtemler, V. M. (1968) The effect of radio-frequency electromagnetic field radiation on the activity of catalase and cholinesterase enzymes. In: *Work Hygiene and the Biological Effect of Radio-Frequency Electromagnetic Waves.* Collection of material of the Third All-Union Symposium, p. 175.

Singatulina, R. G. (1961) The effect of ultrahigh-frequency currents on protein fractions in blood serum. *Byull. Eksp. Biol. Med.* **52:**812.

Smurova, Y. I., T. Z. Rogovaya, A. S. Troitskiy, N. S. Laschenko, and N. D. Melnikova (1962) Problems of hygiene and health of workers in areas where high-frequency currents are used. *Gig. Tr. Prof. Zabol.* **5:**22.

Subbota, A. G., and A. M. Grebenshechnikova (1967) In: *Medical and Biological Problems of SHF Radiation.* Abstracts of Papers at 22nd Scientific–Technical Conference Dedicated to the 50th Anniversary of the Soviet Regime, Leningrad, p. 57.

Swiecicki, W., and Z. Edelwejn (1963a) The influence of 3 cm and 10 cm microwave irradiation on blood proteins in rabbits. *Med. Lotn.* **11:**54.

Swiecicki, W., and Z. Edelwejn (1963b) Electrophoresis of blood protein in rabbits exposed to acute irradiation with very high frequency electromagnetic waves. *Farm. Pol.* **19:**189.

Syngayevskaya, V. A. (1962) Some metabolic indices in the blood and urine of individuals following their exposure to SHF–UHF electromagnetic fields. *In: Summaries of Reports: Questions of the Biological Effect of SHF–UHF Electromagnetic Fields.* Kirov Order of Lenin Military Medical Academy, Leningrad, p. 52.

Syngayevskaya, V. A. (1970) Metabolic changes. In: *Influence of Microwave Radiation on the Organism of Man and Animals,* I. R. Petrov (ed.). Meditsina Press, Leningrad, p. 48 (NASA TT F-708).

Syngayevskaya, V. A., G. F. Pleskena-Sinenko, and O. S. Ignatyeva (1962) The effect of microwave radiation in the meter and decimeter wave ranges on the endocrine regulation of carbohydrate metabolism and the functional state of adrenal cortex in rabbits and dogs. In: *Summaries of Reports: Questions of the Biological Effect of*

SHF–UHF Electromagnetic Fields. Kirov Order of Lenin Military Medical Academy, Leningrad, p. 51.

Takashima, S. (1966) Studies on the effect of radio-frequency waves on biological macromolecules. *IEEE Trans. Biomed. Eng.* **BME-12:**28.

Valtonen, E. J. (1968) Effect of treatment with short wave diathermy on the histamine content of various organs. *Am. J. Phys. Med.* **47:**75.

Veninga, T. S. (1971) The significance of biogenic amines as radio-indicators in experimental animals with reference to man. In: *Biochemical Indicators of Radiation Injury in Man.* International Atomic Energy Agency, Vienna, p. 125.

Wangemann, R. T., and S. F. Cleary (1976) The in-vivo effects of 2.45 GHz microwave radiation on rabbit serum components. *Radiat. Environ. Biophys.* **13:**89.

17

The Common Integument (Skin)

From anatomical and physiological aspects, it is appropriate to consider the skin in a review of the pathophysiological consequences of exposure to RF/MW energy. Because the skin covers the entire body, it has the greatest potential for most immediate exposure; it also contains the nerve endings for thermal sensation of microwave energy and plays an important part in thermal regulation of animals.

17.1. ANATOMY AND PHYSIOLOGY

For detailed information on the anatomy and physiology of the skin, Montagna (1956), Rushmer *et al.* (1966), or standard anatomy or physiology texts should be consulted. Only those points pertinent to understanding the reaction of the skin and its structures in response to microwave exposure will be emphasized here.

The skin consists of the surface epithelium (epidermis) and underlying connective tissue (dermis). Beneath the dermis is the hypodermis, a layer of looser connective tissue containing variable amounts of fatty tissue. The epidermis is stratified squamous epithelium, ranging in thickness from 0.05 to 0.15 mm in most regions, but reaching thicknesses as great as 1.0 mm or more on palmar surfaces and even greater thicknesses on the soles of the feet. The structure of the epidermis is most typical in thick regions; i.e., in such regions the epidermis contains the four main strata of cells, from within outward, the germinal, granular, clear, and horny strata. Regions of thin epidermis may lack completely or nearly completely the granular or clear stratum or both, but they always contain the germinal and horny strata. The epidermis is completely avascular, being nourished by tissue fluid that infiltrates the intercellular spaces of the germinal stratum from capillaries in the underlying dermis (Rubin and Casarett, 1968).

Blood perfusing through the vessels in the dermis plays a major role in regulating body temperature. Free nerve endings are present in the dermis, Malpighian layer, or germinal stratum of the epidermis. These nerve endings overlap, branching and rebranching so that a single nerve fiber may serve many areas of the skin. As a consequence of the location and distribution of the nerve endings, the skin is responsive to all four classical modalities of sensation—pressure, pain, cold, warmth.

Application of heat to a peripheral nerve causes an increase in the pain threshold in the area it supplies. Heating of tissues has been shown to affect the gamma fiber activity in muscle (Fischer and Solomon, 1965). The resulting decrease in the sensitivity of the muscle spindle to stretch, as well as reflexes triggered through temperature receptors, may be the physiological basis for the clinically observed relaxation of muscle spasm following the application of heat.

Some physiological responses of temperature receptors seem more pronounced during rapid tissue temperature elevation (Dodt and Zotterman, 1952a,b); marked bursts of activity have been observed in nerve fibers leading from temperature receptors when the tissue temperature is changed rapidly. Such bursts of activity are not observed when the temperature change is gradual (Hensel, 1950; Hensel and Zotterman, 1951).

The region of the skin in which a temperature difference is considered to be established when warmth is experienced is very well innervated by a profuse arborization of fine, naked axoplasmic filaments. Weddell *et al.* (1954), Weddell (1960), Arthur and Shelley (1959), and Baker and Hall (1969) have described this rich innervation of the cutaneous tissues.

In warm-blooded animals, heat emission by conduction, radiation, and evaporation is of practical importance in heat regulation. Heat loss through the skin dominates; it normally accounts for 90% of the aggregate heat loss and, at high temperatures, is the primary mechanism for maintenance of body temperature. Likewise, the skin is dominant in the transfer of heat to the body from external radiation sources whenever the wavelengths involved cause appreciable effects in the skin itself. At optical wavelengths, the effects of exposure are concentrated almost entirely in the skin, with the exception of effects on other exposed organs, such as the eyes. At wavelengths in the microwave region, some effects occur in the skin and some in deeper tissue; the present discussion will be limited to those effects occurring in the skin.

As for any physical body whose surface may absorb incident radiation and thus manifest a surface temperature increase, skin temperature elevation caused by exposure to microwaves depends both on the physical properties at the wavelengths of the radiation involved and on the local thermal characteristics. Specifically, living skin's thermal conductivity (κ), density (ρ), and specific heat (c) determine the temperature elevation produced by heat liberated through absorption of incident radiant energy. The product of these three factors, $\kappa\rho c$, is the physiologically important quantity that determines the temperature elevation of the skin or other tissue upon exposure to nonpenetrating radiation. For very short exposure times, the $\kappa\rho c$ product of normal skin is the same as that for skin in which the blood flow has been stopped. However, for longer exposure of normal skin, blood flow increases through vasodilatation and cools the skin. This action takes from 20 sec to longer than 2 min to become effective, depending upon the initial state of the blood vessels in the skin. For the first 20 sec or more of exposure, the skin can be considered to have a $\kappa\rho c$ value of 110 to 130 × 10^{-5} cal^2/cm^4/°C^2/sec (Hardy, 1965).

The solar radiation spectrum extends from the near infrared at a wavelength of 18,500 Å, through the visible, to the far ultraviolet at a wavelength of 2900 Å. The amount and wavelengths of this spectrum reaching the earth's surface depend on the season, the latitude, the time of day, and atmospheric conditions. In terms of heat equivalent, the maximum aggregate of the spectrum energy is roughly 800 kcal/m^2/hr on a surface normal to the incident radiation (Hardy and Stoll, 1954). Most of the effects of solar radiation on the skin are well known, from sensations of heat due to infrared radiation, to photochemical action, mainly involving the pigment melanin, causing suntan or sunburn, due to ultraviolet radiation (about 3000 Å). Chronic exposure to sunlight produces deleterious effects such as accelerated aging and a variety of lesions, especially senile keratoses. Ultraviolet energy absorbed in the skin causes DNA alterations, which, if maintained by excessive exposure over many years, can be carcinogenic, leading to skin cancer (Urbach, 1969). "Sun worshippers" are then a subclass of persons deliberately exposing themselves to potentially harmful radiation; no such human or animal behavior has yet been observed for other radiation frequencies.

In particular, radiation at wavelengths longer than 3000 Å does not produce sunburn or related phenomena; the longer the wavelength, the less the energy involved is capable of evoking any of the effects so well documented for solar radiation. In fact, all evidence to date indicates that the only important actions of RF/MW energy on the skin are thermal. These seem to be the only nonspecific effects on the skin in contrast to the photochemical action of ultraviolet light or the ionizing effects of X rays. However, secondary to heating the skin, important physiological effects have been observed. Vasodilatation and constriction of cutaneous blood vessels can be stimulated as well as sensations of warmth, cold, and pain. These effects, in turn, can give rise to other reactions that affect the metabolism of the cells of the skin and thus influence its health (Hardy and Oppel, 1937; Lipkin and Hardy, 1954).

17.2. THERMAL PERCEPTION

Awareness of microwave exposure may be developed by several mechanisms, including cutaneous thermal sensation or pain. The physiology of thermal sensation and pain, which is essentially the basis for microwave perception, has been the subject of several studies. Several investigators have established the thresholds for microwave-induced thermal sensation and pain in man (Cook, 1952a,b; Hendler, 1968; Hendler *et al.*, 1963; Schwan *et al.*, 1966; Vendrick and Vos, 1958).

Sensations of warmth and cold are evoked by radiation exchanges between the skin and the environment (Hardy and Oppel, 1938). There seems to be no specific morphological substrate of thermoreceptors; the thermosensitive structures are a network of free nerve endings (Weddell, 1960; Bullock and Diecke, 1956; Sinclair, 1955). These nerve endings can be defined in two different ways: (1) by the specific sensation aroused by stimulation of a receptor and (2) by the response of a receptor to thermal changes (Hensel, 1963), as indicated by a change in action potential. These sensations, which are important as thermal detectors for regulating body temperature, are evoked when even the slightest change in skin temperature occurs (Hardy, 1965). However, subthreshold changes in skin temperature may occur without evoking thermal sensations. The role of these subthreshold changes in thermoregulation is unknown. On the other hand, marked alterations in rate and magnitude of change in skin temperature can occur without evoking the thermal sensations usually reported. Thus, precooled skin can be rapidly heated without evoking sensations of warmth.

In humans there are two types of thermoreceptors that transmit temperature stimuli as sensations of heat and cold: (1) caloreceptors transmit sensations of heat or warmth, lie deeper in the skin, and are less numerous than receptors for sensations of cold. These caloreceptors are more abundant on the forehead, cheeks, and palms than on the rest of the body surface. Ruffini endings are profuse in the eyelids, which are particularly sensitive to heat, and thus are classed as caloreceptors. (2) Frigidoreceptors transmit sensations of cold to the brain. They lie closer to the surface of the skin and are also more numerous than the caloreceptors.

At certain constant temperatures, thermoreceptors produce a steady discharge rate proportional to the temperature. The steady discharge of a single fiber has a maximum rate of 2 to 15 impulses/sec, which occurs between 38 and 43°C for so-called warm fibers (Hensel, 1963).

Weber (1846) proposed that the rate of change of skin temperature, dT_s/dt, was the effective stimulus for temperature sensation. Many investigators subsequently corroborated this hypothesis; under certain circumstances, a direct relationship could be established between dT_s/dt and temperature sensation. Hardy and Oppel (1937) and Hendler and Hardy (1960) made quantitative measurements of this relationship using infrared and microwave sources of radiant energy. Lele et al. (1954) suggest that sensation is caused by a difference in temperature between two different layers of the skin. Others (Hensel and Zotterman, 1951) suggest that at least three quantities (temperature, rate of change of temperature, and surface area) must be considered to adequately describe thermal stimulation. Therefore, temperature and its rate of change, rather than the spatial gradient, effect a change in the rate of the action potentials generated by the thermal receptors (Fischer and Solomon, 1965; Hendler et al., 1963).

With infrared, the threshold for warmth perception is reached when the skin is warmed at a rate of about 0.001–0.002°C/sec in the skin temperature range of 32–37°C. Because of spatial summation (effect of size of area of stimulation in altering the sensory threshold and the intensity of sensation), threshold and intensity of temperature sensation depend to a large extent on the size of the skin area undergoing temperature change. Similarly, the minimum time that the skin must be warmed before a temperature sensation is elicited, depends on the size of the area affected and on the density of the specific temperature receptors in that area.

By studying the rate at which the skin temperature increases during the early stages of exposure to thermogenic radiation, it is possible to calculate the thermal conductivity of tissues. Such experiments show, for example, that while thermal conductivity for ischemic tissues remains constant during exposure, tissues with no vascular occlusion have a thermal conductivity that increases very rapidly during exposure (Cook, 1952a,b).

Opel and Hardy (1937a,b) found that exposure of 7.5 cm^2 of the forehead to infrared at a power density of 6.7 mW/cm^2 causes a threshold sensation in 3 sec. This amount of energy gives a temperature increase of the order of 0.05°C a few tenths of a millimeter below the skin surface.

There are several studies that describe the cutaneous perception of microwave exposure. Hendler et al. (1963; Hendler, 1968) have presented the cutaneous receptor response of humans to 3000- and 10,000-MHz microwaves and far infrared. The forehead was selected for investigation of warmth sensation, since previous studies had shown that the temperature receptors in the skin of the forehead are relatively numerous and evenly distributed, so that it constitutes a low-threshold region of uniform temperature sensitivity (Oppel and Hardy, 1937a,b). Exposure power

TABLE 17-1
Stimulus Intensity and Temperature Increase to Produce a Threshold Warmth Sensation over a 37 cm^2 Forehead Surface Area[a]

Exposure time (sec)	3000 MHz Power density (mW/cm^2)	10,000 MHz Power density (mW/cm^2)	10,000 MHz Increase in skin temp. (°C)	Far infrared Power density (mW/cm^2)	Far infrared Increase in skin temp. (°C)
1	58.6	21.0	0.025	4.2–8.4	0.035
2	46.0	16.7	0.040	4.2	0.025
4	33.5	12.6	0.060	4.2	—

[a] Data from Hendler (1968) and Hendler et al. (1963).

densities of 3000- and 10,000-MHz microwaves, as well as far-infrared stimuli producing a threshold sensation of warmth, are summarized in Table 17-1 (Michaelson, 1972).

Calculations of the temperature gradient (dT/dx) occurring within the cutaneous layers and the infrared and microwave stimuli producing threshold sensation, revealed no consistency in these layers for either the infrared or microwave cases. For the range of exposure times used, it was found that for both infrared and microwave stimuli that are capable of evoking threshold sensations, a threshold of warmth is elicited when the temperature of a more superficial layer of subcutaneous tissue, about 200 μm below the skin surface, is increased about 0.01–0.02°C over the temperature of a deeper layer lying about 1000 μm below the surface (Hendler, 1968; Hendler et al., 1963).

Studies in humans indicate that when a 40 cm^2 area of the face is exposed to microwaves, thermal sensation can be elicited within 1 sec at power densities of 21 mW/cm^2 for 10,000 MHz and 58.6 mW/cm^2 for 3000 MHz. Within 4 sec, the threshold is lowered by approximately 50% i.e., 12.6 mW/cm^2 (10,000 Hz) and 33.5 mW/cm^2 (3000 Hz) (Hendler, 1968). On this basis, if the entire face were to be exposed, assuming uniform temperature sensitivity of the facial skin, the threshold for thermal sensation to 10,000 MHz would be 4–6 mW/cm^2 within 5 sec, or approximately 10 mW/cm^2 for a 0.5-sec exposure (Michaelson, 1972).

Schwan et al. (1966) found that when the forehead was exposed to 74 mW/cm^2 of 3000-MHz microwaves, the reaction time (the time that elapses before the person is aware of the sensation of warmth) varied between 15 and 73 sec. Warmth perception of 56 mW/cm^2 ranged between 50 sec and 3 min of exposure.

Vendrick and Vos (1958) and Eijkman and Vendrick (1961) also studied warmth sensation induced by infrared and microwaves in humans. Using 3000 MHz pulsed and infrared, it was shown that irradiating a 13 cm^2 area of the inner forearm with microwaves resulted in a threshold temperature rise of 0.4–1.0°C, depending on the subject, which is in agreement with the threshold temperature rise obtained with infrared at a depth of about 0.3–0.5 mm. For stimulus duration longer than 3–5 sec, a pronounced influence of the rate of change of temperature was found. The change in the temperature gradient caused by irradiation with microwaves is so small that, during exposure times of not more than about 10 sec, heat conduction is almost negligible. With a constant radiation intensity, therefore, temperature in the skin increases linearly with time. These authors suggest that a threshold sensation is obtained when the temperature of the warmth receptors is increased by a certain amount ΔT. For stimulus durations longer than 3–5 sec, the rate of change of temperature has a very pronounced influence. This is an adaptation phenomenon. These authors also described effects of "peripheral" and "central" adaptation, and related these to the electrophysiological findings in cats, which had been reported by Hensel and Zotterman (1951).

It should be pointed out that due to shape factors and nonuniform sensitivity, it is likely that the figures for threshold thermal sensation may be somewhat low, although the practical significance of corrections to these figures is probably small. In this context it is well to note that the subjects used for threshold sensation experiments may be well trained and particularly attentive to stimuli they could expect. Extraneous sensory stimuli may be removed or kept at some low, constant level. Consequently, these conditions are appreciably different from those to be expected in most practical situations, where "naive" personnel may be exposed to microwaves under very distracting circumstances. (Michaelson, 1972).

The experiments with microwave irradiation indicate that persistent warmth sensations may be experienced even after irradiation has ceased and the skin temperature is rapidly falling. This suggests the existence of an effective temperature difference between the subcutaneous tissue layers (Hendler *et al.*, 1963).

A comparison of the heating effects induced by infrared and microwave irradiation of skin suggests that establishment of a temperature difference between more superficial and deeper cutaneous layers is necessary to produce a temperature sensation. The fact that this difference must be established between layers lying about 800 μm apart is differentiated from the usual concept of a spatial temperature gradient (Hendler, 1968).

These data and other information on microwave sensation suggest that cutaneous perception of microwaves may provide a warning mechanism. There are several caveats, however, to this point. Microwave frequencies well above 3000 MHz will induce surface heating of the skin, which initiates the heat-regulating mechanisms of the body, in an attempt to institute effective cooling of the body surfaces. In addition, the surface heating stimulates the heat sensors of the skin surfaces and "alerts" the organism to dangerous heat levels, thereby bringing into play homeokinetic and adaptive mechanisms. Lower frequencies (below 1000 MHz) produce differentially greater heat in the subcutaneous fatty tissue, which has poor heat conductance. Therefore, a significant temperature rise may result before an adequate gradient is developed across the fatty layer to dissipate the heat by conduction and radiation.

17.3. PAIN PERCEPTION

The sensory receptors for pain are spread throughout the body, and three general types of pain can be recognized: superficial or cutaneous pain; deep pain from muscles, tendons, joints, and fascia; and visceral pain. Pain can be elicited by several kinds of stimulation: electrical, mechanical, thermal, and chemical. This indicates that the receptors are not necessarily specific for any particular kind of stimulation as may be the case with other cutaneous receptors. Much evidence points to the free nerve endings as the receptors for pain.

Pain conduction in medullated fibers proceeds at a rate of 14.45 m/sec, whereas unmyeliated fibers conduct at approximately 2 m/sec. By the careful mapping of certain cutaneous regions, a normal human adult has been shown to have the following approximate skin receptor ratios, which indicates that pain receptors are far more numerous than other tactile receptors (Oppel and Hardy, 1937b):

Estimated number		Ratio
30,000	Caloreceptors	2
250,000	Frigidoreceptors	13
4,000,000	Algesireceptors (pain)	200

Itching seems to result from rather minimal stimulation of the free nerve endings. It is also brought about as an aftereffect of the sharp sensation of pain. Like pain, it can be induced by electrical, chemical, or mechanical stimulation (Gilstrap et al., 1964).

Skin temperature apparently is the vital factor in determining pain when the skin is exposed to microwaves, though only in as much as this is a measure of the temperature of the thermal pain receptors below the skin surface (Cook, 1952a). Although spatial summation of warmth sense occurs, some investigators suggest summation is absent in the case of pain sensation; this appears to be based on experiments with irradiated areas of 10 cm^2 and less, in which the pain-producing intensity is independent of area (Hardy, 1965). Cook (1952a), on the other hand, showed that the intensities provoking pain, like those producing sensation of warmth, decrease with increasing exposed area. A physical explanation of both these phenomena, not involving spatial summation, is that the rate of heat transfer from the superficial tissues decreases with increasing exposed area. Thus, radiation intensities to produce either warmth or pain, decrease with increasing area. The temperature of the skin, and presumably that of the temperature receptors, can be changed and then maintained at some level, higher or lower than the initial level. Temperature sensation, which initially may be quite marked, gradually subsides, and the subject reports thermal neutrality. Since adaptation is such a prominent phenomenon in the study of thermal sensation, the actual temperature of the sensory endings may not be the sole determinant of sensation.

Pain threshold measurements can be influenced by such variables as the skin temperature prior to measurement and vasomotor tone (Bilisoly et al., 1954; Hardy et al., 1951; Wertheimer and Ward, 1952). It has been found that the first sensation of pain is perceived when a certain temperature threshold is exceeded at the pain receptors. It can be assumed that the skin temperature at which pain occurs is independent of the amount of blood flowing through the skin and of the skin temperature before the exposure (Lehmann et al., 1958). Investigations have demonstrated an appreciable individual variability of the pain threshold (Clark and Binda, 1956; Hardy et al., 1952) and the pain threshold varies from one area of the body to another (Lehmann et al., 1958). Hardy et al. (1951) and Wertheimer and Ward (1952) found, with infrared, that pain occurred when the temperature in the area of the pain receptors was between 44.1 and 44.9°C.

Using thermal radiation to determine pain threshold, Hardy et al. (1951) observed that the initial skin temperature was important. The pain threshold varies linearly with skin temperature up to 45°C, at which further stimulus is not required. This relationship indicates that pain threshold for any level of skin temperature represents that amount of energy required to raise the skin temperature to 45°C. Physiologically, this means that the pain threshold is dependent upon skin temperature alone and not upon the rate of change of internal thermal gradients; this temperature has a mean value of 44.5 ± 1.3°C (Hardy, 1965).

It has been shown that a skin temperature of 45°C is critical for evoking both pain and reflex responses, as stimuli evoking pain are the same as those eliciting flexor reflex responses in the spinal animal. Such stimuli giving rise to both pain and reflex activity, are termed "noxious" stimuli (Hardy, 1953). As the radiation intensity above threshold rises, increasing intensities of pain are perceived. There is a marked increase in pain between 44 and 52°C, after which the increase in pain becomes less. Maximal pain is perceived at a skin temperature of approximately 65°C (Hardy et al., 1947). It should be pointed out that the intensity of pain sensation does not depend solely on the peripheral excitation pattern sent from the pain receptors, but also on many other elements influencing the CNS at that time, such as suggestions, attitude, and other psychological factors (Wolff and Hardy, 1947).

Cook (1952a) investigated the pain threshold for 3000-MHz microwaves. All experiments were carried out at room temperature of 20 ± 1°C, and with minimal air circulation. As far as could be judged, the sensations of warmth and pain with microwave heating differed little from those felt when heating was produced by infrared radiation. The initial skin temperatures in these experiments were in the range of 31.5–33.5°C, and the average skin temperature rise required to achieve pain was 15.0°C. Apparently a thermal pain sensation is evoked when end-organs located approximately 1.5 mm below the skin surface reach a temperature of about 46°C.

The threshold for pain reaction to 3000-MHz exposure of a 9.5 cm^2 area of the forearm was found to range from 830 mW/cm^2 for exposures longer than 3 min to 3.1 W/cm^2 for a 20-sec exposure. If a larger area (53 cm^2) was exposed, the pain threshold for a 3-min exposure was 560 mW/cm^2 (Cook, 1952a). The threshold for pain sensation, as a function of exposure time, is shown in Table 17-2.

In attempting to relate threshold for pain sensation to microwave

TABLE 17-2
Threshold for Pain Sensation as a Function of Exposure Duration (3,000 MHz; 9.5 cm^2 Area)[a]

Power density (W/cm^2)	Exposure (sec)
3.1	20
2.5	30
1.8	60
1.0	120
0.83	>180

[a] Data from Cook (1952a).

exposure, differences in method of irradiation, exposed areas, anatomical sites, and also the nonuniform nature of the microwave power distribution combine to render difficult any detailed comparison. The results, however, support the concept that threshold sensation and pain occur when energy absorption (and corresponding temperature rise) in a critical thickness of superficial tissues exceeds a certain value. Thus, comparing the intensities tolerated by large areas, it is significant that although the tolerated intensity of 3000-MHz microwaves is over four times that of both short- and long-wave infrared radiation, the energy absorbed in all cases in the first 1.5 mm of tissue is approximately the same. Using 3000-MHz microwaves, 20% of the energy entering the skin is absorbed in this depth. The remaining 80% is absorbed below the skin but does not influence pain sensation. The energy absorption in a 1.5-mm depth is approximately 90 and 100% respectively, for short- and long-wave infrared. Thus, on this basis, there should be little difference in the tolerated intensities of the two types of radiant energies, which is in agreement with experimental findings (Cook, 1952a,b).

It is noteworthy that in normal skin, burning pain is produced by microwave exposure adequate to produce a skin temperature of approximately 46°C, regardless of other variables. Although the temperature gradient after painful exposure varies with energy penetration and exposure time, experiment shows that, except for very short exposures (about 3 sec or less), the gradient in the first few millimeters of tissues is small after both microwave and infrared exposures. The results of these studies suggest that thermal pain occurs at an approximately constant skin temperature for all thermogenic radiations (Cook, 1952a,b).

17.4. BIOCHEMISTRY

Laurence (1969) exposed sections of guinea pig skin to 9.6 GHz pulsed. An exposure to 6000 mJ/cm^2 reduced respiratory activity of the skin by 50%. According to the author, these respiration tests reflect the overall effect of pulsed microwaves on skin metabolism. Other experiments were carried out on specific aspects of skin biochemistry; these included the biosynthesis of skin collagen, sulfated mucopolysaccharide (intercellular components), phosphoprotein, phospholipid, and nucleic acid (intracellular components). There was no specific effect of pulsed microwaves on any of these processes.

Nieset *et al.* (1958) showed by means of irradiating frog skin *in vitro* that exposure for 10 to 20 min to 10,000 MHz (42 mW/cm^2) usually reduced ion transport. It was later found, however, that raising the skin temperature to 38°C usually blocked Na$^+$ transport.

17.5. PATHOLOGY (BURNS)

The appearance of lesions of the skin and underlying tissues from microwave exposure has been described (Addington et al., 1959; Boyle et al., 1950; Boysen, 1953; Essman and Wise, 1950; Howland and Michaelson, 1959; Keplinger, 1958; Michaelson et al., 1961, 1967; Osipov and Kalyada, 1964; Slabospitskiy, 1965a,b).

Coagulation necrosis of the skin of rats has been observed after exposure that produced a local temperature elevation to 50–55°C in the irradiated area (Essman and Wise, 1950). Skin lesions in rats and rabbits exposed to 10,000 MHz (50 mW/cm^2) have been described in detail by Slabospitskiy (1965a,b). Skin biopsy immediately after exposure revealed multiple hemorrhages, unevenly distributed, in foci of various sizes, chiefly at the boundary of the derma and the muscular layer. Most of the blood vessels were engorged. Leukocyte reaction was negligible; cellular infiltration, absent. Biopsy at 24 hr after exposure revealed more marked changes, such as damaged nerve fibers. Five days after exposure, brownish foci of mummified areas of necrosis of the skin were visible. Isolated areas of coagulation necrosis, penetrating to the subcutaneous tissue, were noted. Because of the depth of tissue injury, the microwave lesions of the skin could be compared with fourth-degree burns. According to the author, "higher temperatures from other thermal sources are needed for the development of burns comparable to those caused by microwaves. Minimally expressed symptoms of inflammation are a peculiarity of microwave effects." According to Osipov and Kalyada (1964), the skin temperature increase to 55 ± 3°C during a comparatively short interval (3 min) is apparently similar to that obtained by Slabospitskiy (1965a,b) and indicates that heat induction exceeded the rate of heat loss. Exposure to microwaves of the same intensity, but with skin heating reduced, did not produce pathological changes. Thus, the skin lesions appear to result from the action of heat as a consequence of the absorption of microwave energy.

Superficial and deep burns occasionally developed in dogs after exposure to 2800 MHz (pulsed) at 100 or 165 mW/cm^2 for 2 to 6 hr (Michaelson et al., 1961, 1967). Although the lesions occurred in various portions of the body, the lateral aspect of the rib cage seemed most susceptible to this injury (Figs. 17-1–17-3). A comparison was made of the response to 2800-MHz microwave exposure among normal dogs and those that had been previously exposed to X-irradiation (Michaelson et al., 1967). In normal dogs, 6 days elapsed before burns became evident. In dogs previously exposed to X-irradiation, burns appeared 10 days following exposure. The burns, in general, were deep, clean, and

THE COMMON INTEGUMENT (SKIN)

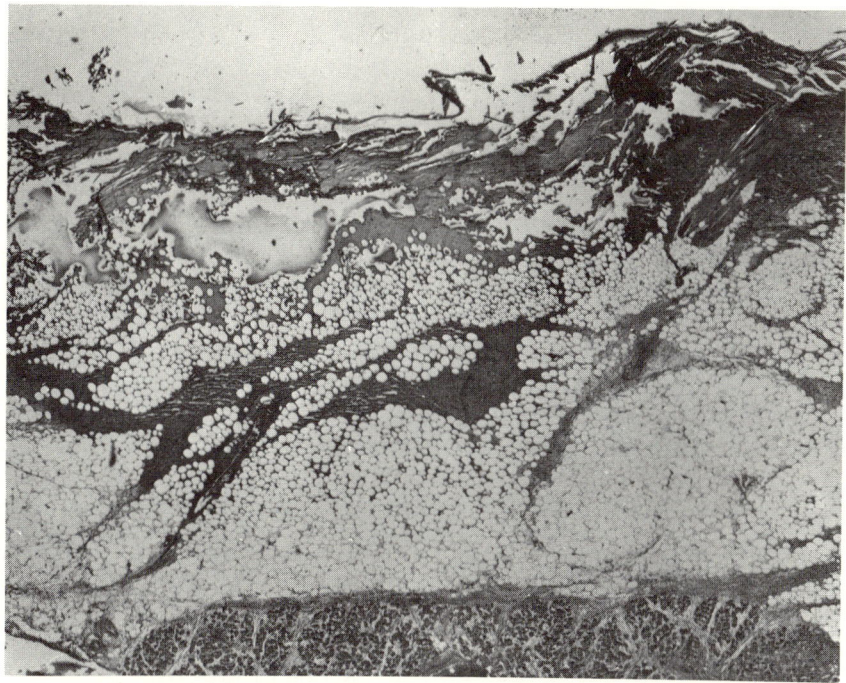

FIGURE 17-1. Histological section of burned and adjacent tissues from a normal dog 7 days after exposure to $100\,mW/cm^2$, 2800 MHz pulsed for 6 hr.

identical in appearance with a third-degree burn. Healing was slower in the X-irradiated dogs and was accompanied by considerable suppuration. No scarring or keloid development was noted.

Histological sections from areas with burns indicated that changes noted at the earliest postexposure times ($\frac{1}{2}$ hr, $1\frac{1}{2}$ hr, and 1 day) were mild and consisted of edema and congestion, which were, if anything, more marked in the deeper tissue (fat and muscle) than in the dermis. At 5 days, the normal dog showed moderate, focal necrosis in the dermis, vesiculation of the epidermis, and marked inflammatory and degenerative changes in the fat and muscle. The X-irradiated dog, at 7 days, showed extensive deep tissue destruction with ulceration and eschar formation. At 4 days, a dog that had not been X-irradiated also showed a deep ulcerating lesion, while an X-irradiated dog was normal. At 15 days, both normal and X-irradiated dogs had deep ulcerative lesions. It is noteworthy that between 5 and 15 days, degenerative muscle changes tended

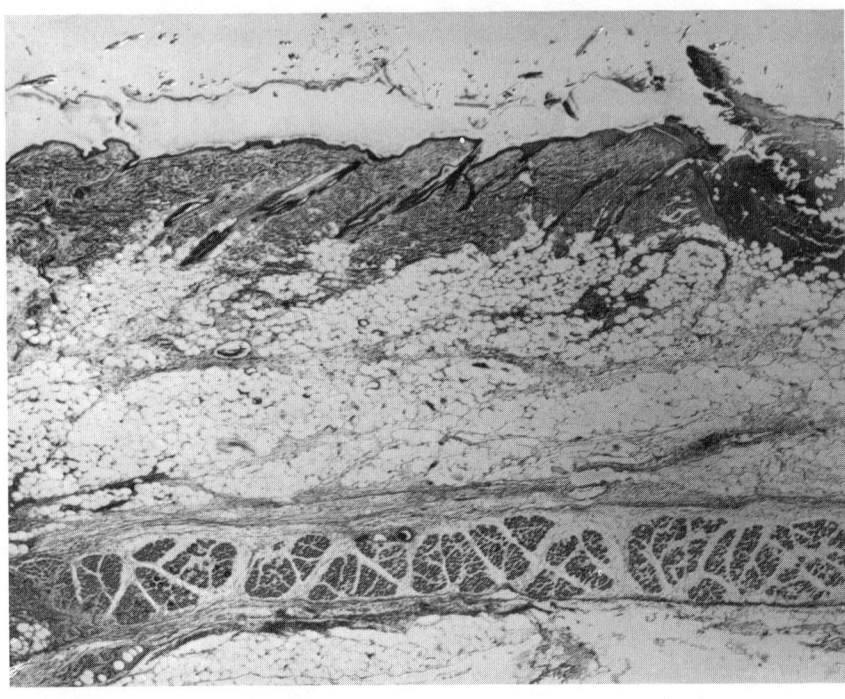

FIGURE 17-2. Histological section of burned and adjacent tissues from a normal dog 15 days after exposure to 100 mW/cm^2, 2800 MHz pulsed for 6 hr.

to be more severe at a considerable distance lateral to the area of more superficial damage (Michaelson et al., 1967).

Using 2450 MHz, Worden et al. (1948) also observed burns that appeared to be the result of energy reflected at the bone interface over the femurs of dogs. Engle et al. (1950) reported that horse muscle tissue was heated to a higher degree if bone was present under the muscle at a depth of 1 cm than if the bone had been removed. This observation also could be explained by reflection at the muscle–bone interface.

Worden et al. (1948) also attempted to determine the effect of microwave exposure on the temperature of tissue in which the blood supply was normal, as compared with ischemic tissue. They exposed the thighs of dogs to a microwave source maintained at 30 W at 2.5 cm (ca. 400 mW/cm^2). During the first 5 min of a 10-min exposure, temperature of ischemic tissues did not differ appreciably from the temperature of tissues with intact circulation; there was no evidence of burning.

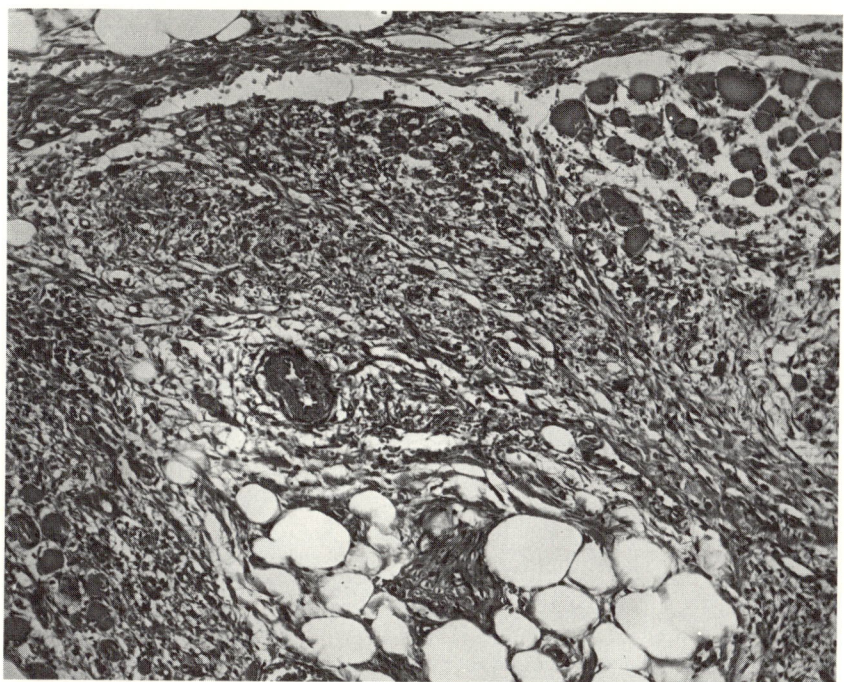

FIGURE 17-3. Muscle tissue beneath burned and adjacent tissues from a normal dog 15 days after exposure to 100 mW/cm^2, 2800 MHz pulsed for 6 hr.

However, after exposure of 15 or 20 min, the temperature of ischemic tissues rose higher than that of tissues with intact circulation. Moreover, in the presence of ischemia, four of the five animals exposed for 15 min were burned, as were all six of those exposed for 20 min. In no instance did burning occur when the circulation was intact and irradiation of the same animal at the same site was repeated for six consecutive periods of 20 min each. The highest temperature obtained when the circulation was intact was 44.6°C and there was no evidence of burning. After ischemic tissues had been exposed to microwaves for 20 min, the highest temperature was only 42.3°C, yet there was gross evidence of burning. Thus, temperature alone is not an indicator as to whether or not tissues will be burned. Duration of exposure and the presence or absence of the protective mechanism for dissipation of heat provided by the circulating blood are also factors. The skin and subcutaneous tissues, with circulation intact, were heated very rapidly and reached high values after 5 or

10 min of exposure. The temperature of superficial and deep muscle rose more slowly and all four layers reached a peak in 20 min. After 30 min of exposure, all of the temperatures dropped below the peak achieved at 20 min. It appears that factors that favor cooling become more effective after 20 min of exposure. Increasing circulation is largely responsible for this cooling effect.

In reviewing the preceding, it becomes apparent that skin lesions, due to microwave exposure, are a manifestation of a thermal response to energy absorption. Henriques (1947), Moritz and Henriques (1947), and Henriques and Moritz (1947) have shown that 45°C is critical in producing cutaneous burns; skin temperatures lower than 44–45°C do not, in general, produce a burn. It may be speculated that noxious stimulation results from chemical reactions in the skin, probably involving inactivation of cellular protein. The pain threshold is thereby determined as the lowest rate of inactivation of tissue proteins that, if sufficiently prolonged, will cause tissue damage. Pain is related to skin temperature only, whereas tissue damage is dependent upon both the skin temperature and the duration of the hyperthermic episode (Hardy, 1965).

REFERENCES

Addington, C. H., C. Osborn, G. Swartz, F. P. Fischer, and Y. T. Sarkees (1959) Thermal effects of 200 megacycles (CW) irradiation as related to shape, location, and orientation in the field. In: *Proceedings of the Third Annual Tri-Service Conference on Biological Effects of Microwave Radiating Equipments,* C. Süsskind (ed.). University of California, Berkeley, p. 10.

Arthur, R. P., and W. B. Shelley (1959) The innervation of human epidermis. *J. Invest. Dermatol.* **32:**397.

Baker, C. H., and R. J. Hall (1969) Cutaneous Sensitivity: A Review of Some Literature, Problems, and Approaches. Human Factors, Inc., Goleta, Calif., Technical Memorandum 21-69, AMCMS 5016.11.84400.

Bilisoly, F. N., H. Goodell, and H. G. Wolff (1954) Vasodilatation, lowered pain threshold and increased tissue vulnerability: Effects dependent upon peripheral nerve function. *AMA Arch. Intern Med.* **94:**759.

Boyle, A., H. F. Cook, and T. J. Buchanan (1950) Effects of microwaves: A preliminary investigation. *Br. J. Phys. Med.* **13:**2.

Boysen, J. (1953) Hyperthermic and pathologic effects of electromagnetic radiation (350 mc). *AMA Arch. Ind. Hyg. Occup. Med.* **7:**516.

Bullock, T. H., and F. P. J. Diecke (1956) Properties of an infrared receptor. *J. Physiol. (London)* **134:**47.

Clark, J. W., and D. Binda (1956) Individual difference in pain thresholds. *Can. J. Psychol.* **10:**69.

Cook, H. F. (1952a) The pain threshold for microwave and infrared radiation. *J. Physiol. (London)* **118:**1.

Cook, H. F. (1952b) A physical investigation of the heat production in human tissues when exposed to microwaves. *Br. J. Appl. Phys.* **3:**249.

Dodt, E., and Y. Zotterman (1952a) Mode of action of warm receptors. *Acta Physiol. Scand.* **26**:345.

Dodt, E., and Y. Zotterman (1952b) The discharge of specific cold fibers at high temperatures (the paradoxical cold). *Acta Physiol. Scand.* **26**:358.

Eijkman, E., and A. J. H. Vendrick (1961) Dynamic behavior of the warmth sense organ. *J. Exp. Psychol.* **62**:403.

Engle, J. P., J. F. Herrick, K. G. Wakim, J. H. Grindlay, and F. H. Krusen (1950) The effects of microwaves on bone and bone marrow, and on adjacent tissues. *Arch. Phys. Med.* **31**:453.

Essman, L., and C. Wise (1950) Local effects of microwave radiation on tissues in the albino rat. *Arch. Phys. Med.* **31**:502.

Fischer, E., and S. Solomon (1965) Physiological responses to heat and cold. In: *Therapeutic Heat and Cold*, 2nd edition, S. H. Licht (ed.). E. Licht, New Haven, Conn., p. 126.

Gilstrap, L. O., Jr., J. S. McNeil, L. P. Greenberg, and R. B. Spodak (1964) A Compilation of Biological Laws, Effects, and Phenomena with Associated Physical Analogs. Wright-Patterson AFB, Ohio.

Hardy, J. D. (1953) Thresholds of pain and reflex contraction as related to noxious stimulation. *J. Appl. Physiol.* **5**:725.

Hardy, J. D. (1965) Thermal radiation, pain, and injury. In: *Therapeutic Heat and Cold*, 2nd edition, S. H. Licht (ed.). E. Licht, New Haven, Conn., p. 157.

Hardy, J. D., and T. W. Oppel (1937) Studies in temperature sensation. III. The sensitivity of the body to heat and the spatial summation of the end organ responses. *J. Clin. Invest.* **16**:533.

Hardy, J. D., and T. W. Oppel (1938) Studies in temperature sensation. IV. The stimulation of cold sensation by radiation. *J. Clin. Invest.* **17**:771.

Hardy, J. D., and A. M. Stoll (1954) Measurement of the radiant heat load on man in summer and winter. *J. Appl. Physiol.* **7**:100.

Hardy, J. D., H. Wolff, and H. Goodell (1947) Studies on pain: Discrimination of differences in intensity of a pain stimulus as a basis of a scale of pain intensity. *J. Clin. Invest.* **26**:1152.

Hardy, J. D., H. Goodell, and H. G. Wolff (1951) Influence of skin temperature upon pain threshold as evoked by thermal radiation. *Science* **114**:149.

Hardy, J. D., H. G. Wolff, and H. Goodell (1952) *Pain Sensations and Reactions*. Williams & Wilkins, Baltimore.

Hendler, E. (1968) Cutaneous receptor response to microwave irradiation. In: *Thermal Problems in Aerospace Medicine*, J. D. Hardy (ed.). NATO, Unwin, England, p. 149.

Hendler, E., and J. D. Hardy (1960) Infrared and microwave effects on skin heating and temperature sensation. *IRE 12th Annual Conference on Electrical Techniques in Medicine and Biology* **7**:143.

Hendler, E., J. D. Hardy, and D. Murgatroyd (1963) Skin heating and temperature sensation produced by infrared and microwave irradiation. In: *Temperature—Its Measurement and Control in Science and Industry*, Vol. 3, J. D. Hardy (ed.). Reinhold, New York, p. 221.

Henriques, F. C., Jr. (1947) Studies of thermal injury. V. The predictability and the significance of thermally-induced rate processes leading to irreversible epidermal injury. *Arch. Pathol.* **43**:489.

Henriques, F. C., Jr., and A. R. Moritz (1947) Studies of thermal injury. I. The conduction of heat to and through skin and the temperatures attained therein. A theoretical and experimental investigation. *Am. J. Pathol.* **23**:531.

Hensel, H. (1950) Temperaturempfindung und intracutane Warmbewegung. *Pfluegers Arch. Gesamte Physiol. Menschen Tiere* **252**:165.

Hensel, H. (1963) Electrophysiology of thermosensitive nerve endings. In: *Temperature—Its Measurement and Control in Science and Industry*, Vol. 3, J. D. Hardy (ed.). Reinhold, New York, p. 191.

Hensel, H., and Y. Zotterman (1951) Quantitative Beziehungen zwischen der Entladung einzelner Kaltefasern und der Temperatur. *Acta Physiol. Scand.* **23:**291.

Howland, J. W., and S. Michaelson (1959) Studies on the biological effects of microwave irradiation of the dog and rabbit. In: *Proceedings of the Third Annual Tri-Service Conference on Biological Effects of Microwave Radiating Equipments*, C. Süsskind (ed.). University of California, Berkeley, p. 191.

Keplinger, M. L. (1958) Review of the work conducted at the University of Miami. In: *Proceedings of the Second Annual Tri-Service Conference on Biological Effects of Microwave Energy*, E. G. Pattishall and F. W. Banghart (eds.). University of Virginia, Charlottesville, p. 215.

Laurence, J. C. (1969) Effect of pulsed microwaves at X-band on skin metabolism. *Non-Ioniz. Radiat.* **1:**80.

Lehmann, J. F., G. D. Brunner, and R. W. Stow (1958) Pain threshold measurements after therapeutic application of ultrasound, microwaves, and infrared. *Arch. Phys. Med. Rehabil.* **39:**560.

Lele, P. P., G. Weddell, and C. W. Williams (1954) The relationship between heat transfer, skin temperature, and cutaneous sensitivity. *J. Physiol. (London)* **126:**206.

Lipkin, M., and J. D. Hardy (1954) Measurement of some thermal properties of human tissues. *Fed. Proc.* **13:**90.

Michaelson, S. M. (1972) Cutaneous perception of microwaves. *J. Microwave Power* **7:**67.

Michaelson, S. M., R. A. E. Thomson, and J. W. Howland (1961) Physiologic aspects of microwave irradiation of mammals. *Am. J. Physiol.* **201:**351.

Michaelson, S. M., R. A. E. Thomson, and J. W. Howland (1967) Biologic Effects of Microwave Exposure. Tech. Rep. RADC-TR-67-461. Griffiss AFB, Rome Air Development Center, Rome, N.Y.

Montagna, W. (1956) *The Structure and Function of Skin.* Academic Press, New York.

Moritz, A. R., and F. C. Henriques, Jr. (1947) Studies of thermal injury. II. Relative importance of time and surface temperature in causation of cutaneous burns. *Am. J. Physiol.* **23:**695.

Nieset, R. T., R. Baus, Jr., R. D. McAfee, J. T. Friedman, A. S. Hyde, and J. D. Fleming, Jr. (1958) Review of the work conducted at Tulane University. In: *Proceedings of the Second Annual Tri-Service Conference on Biological Effects of Microwave Energy*, E. G. Pattishall and F. W. Banghart (eds.). University of Virginia, Charlottesville, pp. 202–214.

Oppel, T. W., and J. D. Hardy (1937a) Studies in temperature sensation. I. A comparison of the sensation produced by infrared and visible radiation. *J. Clin. Invest.* **16:**517.

Oppel, T. W., and J. D. Hardy (1937b) Studies in temperature sensation. II. The temperature changes responsible for the stimulation of the heat end organs. *J. Clin. Invest.* **16:**525.

Osipov, Y. A., and T. V. Kalyada (1964) Temperature response of the skin during irradiation with microwaves of low intensity. JPRS 23287, p. 73.

Rubin, P., and G. W. Casarett (1968) Skin and adnexa. In: *Clinical Radiation Pathology*, Vol. 1. Saunders, Philadelphia.

Rushmer, R. F., K. J. K. Buettner, J. M. Short, and G. F. Odland (1966) The skin. *Science* **154:**343.

Schwan, H. P., A. Anne, and L. Sher (1966) Heating of Living Tissue. Report NAEC-ACEL-534, U.S. Naval Air Engineering Center, Aerospace Crew Equipment Lab., Philadelphia.

Sinclair, D. C. (1955) Cutaneous sensation and the doctrine of specific energy. *Brain* **78**:584.

Slabospitskiy, A. A. (1965a) Morphological changes in the skin of white rats exposed to centimeter range radio waves. In: *Problems of the Biophysics and Mode of Action of Radiation.* Transl. JPRS 34963, p. 89.

Slabospitskiy, A. A. (1965b) The mechanism of action of microwaves on the skin. *Fiziol. Zh. SSR im. I.M. Sechenova* **11**:225.

Urbach, F. (ed.) (1969) *The Biological Effects of Ultraviolet Radiation* (*with Emphasis on the Skin*). Pergamon Press, New York.

Vendrick, A., and J. Vos (1958) Comparison of the stimulation of the thermal sense organ by microwave and infrared radiation. *J. Appl. Physiol.* **13**:435.

Weber, 1846, cited by Hendler, E. (1968) Cutaneous receptor response to microwave irradiation. In: *Thermal Problems in Aerospace Medicine,* J. D. Hardy (ed.). NATO, Unwin, England, p. 149.

Weddell, G. (1980) Studies related to the mechanism of common sensibility. In: *Advances in Biology of Skin,* Vol. 1, W. Montague (ed.). Pergamon Press, New York, p. 112.

Weddell, G., W. Pallie, and E. Palmer (1954) The morphology of peripheral nerve terminations in the skin. *J. Microsc. Sci.* **95**:483.

Wertheimer, M., and W. D. Ward (1952) Influence of skin temperature upon pain threshold as evoked by thermal radiation—a confirmation. *Science* **115**:499.

Wolff, H. G., and J. D. Hardy (1947) On the nature of pain. *Physiol. Rev.* **27**:167.

Worden, R. E., J. F. Herrick, K. G. Wakim, and F. H. Krusen (1948) The heating effects of microwaves with and without ischemia. *Arch. Phys. Med.* **29**:751.

18

Cataracts and Other Ocular Effects

18.1. INTRODUCTION

Cataract is the best known of all eye diseases, but despite wide public awareness and research that has been devoted to elucidation of its etiology, knowledge of the biochemistry of the normal and pathological lens is still somewhat fragmentary. During the past 25 years, numerous investigations in animals and several surveys among human populations have been devoted to assessing the relationship between exposure to microwaves and subsequent development of cataracts. It is significant that of the many experiments on rabbits by several investigators using various techniques, power density >100 mW/cm^2 for 1 hr or longer appears to be the lowest time–power threshold in the frequency range of 2450 to 10,000 Hz. In other species of animals such as dogs and nonhuman primates, the threshold for experimental microwave-induced cataract appears to be even higher. Data that are presented to indicate nonthermal, cumulative, or direct cellular effects are equivocal. If one carefully reviews the human data that are presently available, little is added to our knowledge of microwave cataractogenesis.

Of interest is the statement by Shilyayev (1970), "on the basis of our present knowledge of the conditions under which experimental microwave cataract arises and of its diagnosis and treatment, it must be acknowledged that none of the cases of cataracts in man described in the literature is fully verified. Under normal working conditions, personnel are exposed at levels representing several orders of magnitude below the level with which the various changes in the lens are produced experimentally. It appears that damage to the lens from exposure to microwaves may occur very seldom (if at all), and then only under unusual circumstances."

18.2. ANATOMY AND PHYSIOLOGY OF THE EYE

In order to understand the complexity of cataracts and cataractogenesis, it is necessary to present a concise anatomy of the related structures affected in the eye with emphasis on the lens. The eyeball is very nearly spherical and lends itself to description by anterior and posterior poles, meridians through the poles, and an equator. It rests in the front half of the cavity of the orbit with only its anterior aspect exposed.

The outer surface of the eye is a tough, white tissue called the sclera. The sclera is essentially a support tissue that is somewhat elastic. The extraocular muscles are inserted into the sclera, and it is on this tissue that they actually pull to rotate the eye in the desired direction (van Pelt *et al.*, 1973).

The transparent cornea is thicker than the sclera and consists of a highly refractile modified connective tissue laminated between two thin limiting membranes. The cornea is the chief refracting surface of the eye because it separates media of such different indexes of refraction as air and aqueous humor. The cornea is actually a continuation of the sclera. It is transparent to light and has a greater curvature than the rest of the sclera. The transition between the cornea and the white sclera is rather sharp and is called the limbus. The cornea is the major light-focusing device of the eye (van Pelt *et al.*, 1973).

The cornea possesses several unique qualities (Dawson, 1963). First, it is wholly avascular, which requires that all nutrition diffuse inward from the surrounding limbic vascular plexus. Second, it is obviously transparent to at least the visible portion of the electromagnetic spectrum; it is transparent to electromagnetic energies over the range of wavelengths from about 320 to 1400 nm. Third, it is supplied with only freely ending sensory nerves, i.e., sensory nerve endings without a complex end organ. It is exquisitely sensitive to pain—a particle of sand in the eye is adequate demonstration of this. Damage to the corneal tissue may be accompanied by intense pain and partial clouding of vision. Unless damage is quite extensive, complete recovery of the tissue and vision usually occurs (van Pelt *et al.*, 1973).

The effectiveness of the corneal innervation has produced a tissue of such sensitivity that its role has been limited to the transduction of all stimuli into experiences of pain (Dawson, 1963). This limitation of the cornea's sensory capacity was described almost a century ago by the theorist von Frey (1895). Thus, the ending type that is found in this tissue must be responsible for sensations of pain only. In order to gauge pain, studies were done by Dawson (1963) on nondecerebrate cat corneas with specially outfitted thermistor probes utilizing direct infrared stimulation with a maximum output of $1 \text{ cal/cm}^2 \text{ sec}$. This output was termed "low intensity" as designated by Lele and Weddell (1956). The authors found that reports of cornea-localized "warm" were noted, with transfer rates of up to $2 \text{ cal/cm}^2 \text{ sec}$. Warm is defined as any elevation of tissue temperature of less than 10°C. The term "warm" is used relative to measured ΔT values rather than energy input. A threshold was defined as that corneal temperature increment (ΔT) at which the first neural response was seen or at which the first change in integrated response to stimulation occurred. Studies indicated that the cornea ΔT at which sensation first occurred was highly variable but ranged from a minimum of $\Delta T = 0.058°C$ to $\Delta T = 7.47°C$. Other data (Kenshalo, 1960) have established the corneal thermal pain threshold to be at 47°C, the cornea being less sensitive to changes in temperature than the skin or conjunctiva. These properties of sensitivity lend themselves to implications of corneal burns associated with infrared and microwave radiation.

The middle or uveal part of the eye consists of the choroid, the ciliary body, and the iris. The choroid is a vascular layer providing the blood supply to the retinal pigment epithelium and the outer half of the sensory retina adjacent to it. The ciliary body lies on the inner aspect of the sclera behind the sclerocorneal junction. The ciliary body is a wedge-shaped, flattened ring, about 5 to 6 mm wide. This body secretes aqueous humor and contains the smooth muscle responsible for the change in shape of the lens, causing accommodation. The iris is continuous peripherally with the ciliary body but is also attached to the cornea. It is a highly vascular pigmented structure that surrounds a central opening, the pupil, and controls the amount of light entering the eye. The pupil lies in front of the lens and is slightly off-center toward the nasal side.

The crystalline lens is a grossly transparent, biconvex structure located directly behind the iris and the pupillary aperture, and in front of the vitreous body. In the human it is approximately 10 mm in diameter and 4 mm thick. Its anterior and posterior surfaces meet at the equator. Its posterior surface has greater convexity than its anterior surface. The lens is held in position by the zonular fibers that insert into the lens capsule in a zone concentric with the equator and extend farther over the anterior than the posterior surface. The lens continues to form fibers throughout life. Old fibers are not desquamated, but they become compressed centrally to form an increasingly larger and more inelastic nucleus. Although grossly the lens appears brilliantly transparent, by microscopic examination it is seen to contain minute opacities and concentric areas of different indexes of refraction (Newell and Ernest, 1974).

Structurally the lens is composed of three parts: (1) the capsule entirely surrounding the lens, (2) the epithelium beneath the anterior capsule, and (3) a lens substance that consists of the cortex (newly formed soft fibers) and the nucleus (a dense central area of old fibers).

The lens capsule is a smooth, homogeneous, acellular structure. It is thickest on either side of the equator just central to the insertion of zonular fibers. It is divided into two layers: (1) a superficial layer composed of acid mucopolysaccharides, which constitutes the attachment of the zonule to the lens, and (2) the capsule proper, which is probably the basement membrane of the lens epithelium.

The epithelium is located directly under the anterior lens capsule. It consists of a single row of cuboidal cells of irregular shape and having numerous interdigitations. The lack of a posterior epithelium is the result of these cells having gone to form the primitive lens fibers during embryonic development. At the equator the cells are elongated and arranged meridionally in rows. This is the region where new lens fibers are constantly being formed; the cells themselves may be regarded as young lens fibers.

The lens substance consists of fibers embedded in an amorphous cement substance with a concentric construction similar to that of an onion. Each new fiber has its nucleus at the equator, and a long (10 mm), tapering, six-sided, ribbonlike process extends toward the anterior and posterior poles. The most recently formed fibers have their nuclei closest to the equator. As the fiber ages, the cell and its nucleus are pushed axially into the lens substance. This produces a "nuclear bow" of cell nuclei that approximately parallels the anterior lens surface. With further aging, the fiber nucleus degenerates, the cell fiber shrinks, and the fibers become compressed centrally. The nucleus of the lens, composed of cell processes, is inelastic, yellowish, and increases in size with aging. Hence, the basis is found for both definitions and progression that Duke-Elder (1972) and Albert and Scheie (1969) describe. The cement substance binding the lens fibers together is somewhat more abundant where the ends of the fibers meet each other. There is, therefore, formed a central strand in the axis between anterior and posterior poles of the lens fibers into sectors. These lines of separation, the lens sutures, are evident on the anterior and posterior lens surface as star-shaped figures, sometimes termed "lens stars". It is customary to differentiate between a softer superficial cortex and a harder central lens nucleus. The term "lens bow" occurs frequently in all literature concerned with the formation of cataracts. It is a term applied to the characteristic accurate distribution of epithelial nuclei in the region of the equator of the lens, as seen in meridional sections.

The eye contains three chambers: the anterior chamber, the posterior chamber, and the vitreous cavity. The anterior chamber is bounded anteriorly by the cornea, posteriorly by the front surface of the iris and lens, and peripherally by the angle recess. In the human, the anterior chamber is deepest in its central portion (3 mm) and shallowest at the peripheral insertion of the iris. It has a volume of slightly more than 0.1 ml.

The posterior chamber is bounded anteriorly by the iris, posteriorly by the front surface of the zonular fibers, medially by the lens, and laterally by the ciliary processes. Its volume in adults is about 0.06 ml. The aqueous humor secreted by ciliary processes flows from the posterior chamber through the pupil into the anterior chamber. From the anterior chamber the fluid escapes through the space of the iridocorneal angle into the canal of Schlemm and, hence, passes to the anterior ciliary vein. The aqueous humor contributes to the maintenance of intraocular pressure and supports the metabolism of the lens, which does not have a blood supply and thus has mainly an anaerobic metabolism. Additionally, the aqueous humor contributes to the nutrition of the cornea.

The vitreous cavity is surrounded by the retina and the optic nerve posteriorly. Anteriorly it is bounded by the zonule, the ciliary body, and the posterior surface of the lens. Its volume is 4.5 ml.

The vitreous is a transparent tissue that has many properties physically of a gel and fills the posterior parts of the eye. It has the shape of a sphere with a segment removed anteriorly to provide a hollowed-out space for the lens. The vitreous body, adjacent to this indentation, is described as the anterior hyaloid membrane. In the healthy eye, the vitreous body is in contact with the entire retina and is attached to the basement membrane of the retina by scattered collagenous filaments.

The retina is a membrane, surrounding the posterior part of the vitreous body, which consists of an outer pigmented layer and an inner neural layer. The axons of the rod and cone cells synapse upon the dendrites of bipolar cells that form the middle nerve cell layer of the retina. Beneath the retina the thin (10 μm) layer of cells, the pigment epithelium, contains a large quantity of melanin (pigment) granules. The pigment epithelium functions to absorb scattered light, stop reflection, and provide some physical support for the photoreceptor cells. Beneath the pigment epithelium is the choroid, a somewhat thicker (100–200 μm) tissue layer that is rich in blood vessels and nerves. It functions to provide nutrition for the retina and to convey nerves and blood vessels to the iris.

18.2.1. Definition of Cataract

Foremost among the difficulties in reviewing the subject of cataract is presenting a suitable and consistent definition of "cataract". Appleton (1973) illustrates a sensitivity to this problem by preferring to use the term "opacity". He notes type and character of opacities upon observation of his subjects. As to whether he views cataracts as defined as an opacity that interferes with vision, he replies, "How much constitutes interference? Anything below 20/20? Suppose an individual is capable of 20/15 in one eye and has a discrete opacity in it, does he have a cataract in that eye or not?" The implications become more impressive when thought is given to the fact that vision impairment cannot be used as a determining factor for animal lenses. Instead, a grading system is used.

According to Duke-Elder (1972), a cataract may simply be defined as any opacity in the lens. Albert and Scheie (1969) also define cataract as an opacification of the lens or its capsule. In this sense, almost every adult has cataracts, for some fine lens opacities are frequently visible during slit lamp biomicroscopic examination. Cataracts are not considered to be of serious clinical significance unless they interfere with vision. Newell and Ernest (1974) agree with this clinical definition. They feel that any loss of transparency of the lens must be designated as cataract. Sorsby (1972) classifies cataracts on an etiological basis but also believes it is often more convenient to define and classify cataracts by the effect on function—and this is determined by the situation and extent of the cataract, or by its degree of maturity. He states that when the fibers around the equator of the lens, which form the cellular part of the lens, are imperfectly formed or diseased, areas of opacity appear in the clear lens structure. These opacities he calls cataracts and the term is extended to include opacities that form in the capsule around the lens. He further states that an increase in life expectancy of the world population must invariably result in an increase in cases of senile cataract implying a steady progression of opacity. Duke-Elder (1972) also maintains that senile cataract may be looked upon as a normal sign of senescence, occurring to some degree in 65% of people in the sixth decade and in over 95% above 65 years of age. Albert and Scheie (1969) limit this progression with the condition that not all cataracts progress. Many opacities, particularly congenital ones, remain stationary. Most cataracts are bilateral, but the severity and rate of progression in each eye may vary. Cogan (1959) prefers a cataract to be defined as an abnormal opacification of the lens. The qualification "abnormal" is essential to distinguish it from the many stationary punctate spots that are commonly present in an otherwise normal lens and from the optical zones of reflectivity in the lens that are present normally and that increase with age without having the connotation of cataracts. It must be apparent that "abnormal" necessarily involves a judgment on the part of the examiner as to what is normal and what is not. Appleton (1973) aptly illustrated this fine line. Thus, whether a cataract is present or not may, in borderline cases, be equivocal and have to depend on the course of events for decision. This obviously affects an important factor of epidemiology—incidence, which will be discussed shortly. For the sake of convenience, a cataract can be defined as an opacity of the crystalline lens or of its capsule which may be developmental or degenerative, obstructing passage of light. The degenerative cataract is a manifestation of aging, systemic disease, certain therapeutic agents, trauma, or exposure to some forms of radiant energy.

18.2.2. Classification and Appearance

Among the many difficulties in cataract research is the problem of determining the number of different types or causes. By itself, age is not a rational basis for classifying cataracts, but it must be considered in making comparisons with normal lenses. Salit (1936) distinguished two types of lens pathology termed "cataract" (cortical) and "sclerosis" (nuclear). Cataractous lenses were classified as incipient, intumescent, and mature. Sclerotic lenses were graded partly on the basis of increasing nuclear color. Most investigators have classified human cataracts as posterior subcapsular, nuclear, or cortical. Some add a group with both nuclear and cortical opacities and some divide cortical cataracts into early or incipient, advanced or intumescent, and completely opaque. Such classification relies heavily on the judgment of the examiner, has no proven pathological basis, and does not allow for continuous variation (Barber, 1973).

Albert and Scheie (1969) and Sorsby (1972) elaborate somewhat on these classifications and provide adequate definitions. A nuclear cataract usually begins soon after the age of 40 as an extension of sclerosis of the nucleus of the lens. Yellow or brown pigment may be deposited. When very dark brown, the term *cataracta brunescens* or *nigra* is applied. Increasing optical density of the nucleus results in an increase in the refractive index and in myopia without any evidence of opacity formation (sometimes termed "second sight" because the patient can read without glasses once more). This is a very slowly developing type of cataract, and it may be a number of years before a patient's vision is poor enough to justify an operation. Little by little, however, a well-defined nuclear opacity is formed in the center of the lens which finally is replaced by a dense, homogeneous rigid nucleus. Little light can be transmitted through the cataract at this end stage and its large size and inability to mold may cause difficulties during extraction.

A cortical cataract manifests itself first as peripheral, wedge-shaped opacities ("water clefts") and as lamellar separations within the lens. The clefts extend into the pupillary area and are seen by focal illumination as radical gray or white bands. This type of lens change confines opacities to the cortical areas and is much more common than nuclear.

A posterior subcapsular cortical cataract or cupuliform cataract is an opacity in the posterior cortex just under the capsule. It is usually associated with a definite opacification within the posterior capsule. It is located centrally, and therefore seriously affects vision very early, so that the lens often must be removed when most of it is still clear.

Immature or incipient cataract is incomplete. The lens is only slightly opaque, the lens cortex being, for the most part, clear. When the entire lens is completely opaque, the cataract is said to be mature. After a cataract is complete, the osmotic effect of degenerated lens protein may cause the lens to swell. When the lens is extremely swollen, the cataract is called intumescent. This type of cataract can lead to secondary angle closure (acute) glaucoma.

A hypermature cataract is one in which degraded protein molecules are absorbed or escape, leaving behind a shrunken yellow lens and wrinkled capsule. A Morganian cataract is a hypermature cataract in which the cortex has become completely liquefied and the nucleus, with its greater density, settles inferiorly within the intact lens capsule. Complete and hypermature cataracts present dangers to the eye such as spontaneous dislocation of the lens and angle closure glaucoma.

Thus, essentially there are two stages in the development of cataracts. The first stage consists of the accumulation of water between the lens fibers and under the capsule. Separation of the lens fibers by water clefts and the formation of fluid vacuoles can be observed clinically. During this first stage, intumescent cataract may develop.

The second stage is the breakdown of the degenerating protein fibers. These fibers become granular, swell, and finally break down into rounded bodies composed of protein, which are called Morganian globules. They lie in spaces along with fluid amorphous granular substances, surrounded by fibers that are degenerating in their turn. The last fibers to turn opaque usually are the superficial fibers of the anterior cortex. The cataract has now matured. Maturity may be present indefinitely but sometimes hypermaturity may occur as described above. There are three complications: Morganian cataract, previously defined; calcification, in which the lens is converted into a calcareous mass due to widespread impregnation with calcium salts; and phacolytic reaction, in which there is a leakage of the products of cataract formation from the capsule into the surrounding ocular fluids. It is probable that the escape is due to minute holes or splits in the posterior lens capsule. The lens proteins are highly irritating and cause a violent intraocular reaction often associated with glaucoma.

18.2.3. Age Factors

The age-related phenomenon of presbyopia has long been ascribed to hardening of the nucleus, which has never been demonstrated in human lenses. This has led to the widely accepted but, according to Barber (1973), unfounded concept of sclerosis as a component of normal aging. Human cataract, therefore, is often considered to be the final result of such sclerosis, possibly accelerated by environmental, metabolic, or genetic factors. This idea is no longer tenable. The supposition that old human lenses are harder than young ones pervades the ophthalmic literature and probably is derived from demonstrable (pathological) hardness of advanced cataracts and the progressive dehydration with age observed in animal lenses, particularly in the nucleus. This, however, does not happen in normal human lenses.

In postmortem lenses, van Heyningen (1972) found no change in hydration with aging, and in lenses in which the nucleus was examined separately, there was no change in protein concentration from age 31 to 92. This has been confirmed by Satoh (1972), who found no change in protein concentration in postmortem lenses from 8 to 80 years.

Since in normal human lenses no processes of sclerosis involving lens proteins exist, any change in viscoelastic properties responsible for loss of accommodative function must involve changes in the lens capsule and/or cell membranes (Kikkawa and Sato, 1963; Fisher, 1971). Ball-and-socket type interdigitations have been demonstrated in normal lenses (Wanko and Gavin, 1961; Leeson, 1971; Dickson and Crock, 1972) and increase in complexity with aging.

In 1969, Waley listed three things known to increase with aging in human lenses: scattering of light, pigmentation, and insoluble protein content. At present, there is no evidence, obtained by artifact-free techniques, that demonstrates any increase of insoluble protein as percent of lens weight. There is evidence that increased light scattering (Mellerio, 1971) and increased pigmentation (Coren and Girgus, 1972) are directly proportional to increased thickness, and are, therefore, manifestations of growth rather than aging.

In very old normal lenses, light absorption due to increased thickness is appreciable, the absorbance being about 0.5 at age 80, although connected visual acuity may be normal (Coren and Girgus, 1972). Under such conditions, a much smaller degree of pathological opacification may be required to reduce vision than in younger lenses. From this point of view alone, it is reasonable to consider cataractogenesis as a manifestation of aging.

Peripheral opacities can be detected in lenses of most older subjects. Pirie (1968) noted that the incidence of cataract in such lenses is very low and Fisher (1973) has reported that peripheral, spokelike opacification is a manifestation of mechanical stress, which does not progress and should not be regarded as beginning cataract.

18.2.4. Mechanisms of Opacification

When considering mechanisms of opacification, it is necessary to consider the possibility that insolubilization of soluble protein occurs in cataracts because this mechanism has been so widely indicated as the cause of opacification. Harding (1969, 1972a,b) has shown that most of the insoluble protein obtained from rat and human lenses is artifactual, resulting from oxidation of protein sulfhydryl groups during aerobic homogenization. Pirie (1968) has shown that if formation of this artifact is prevented, no more insoluble protein is obtained by extraction of most human cataracts than from normal lenses. This conclusion has been confirmed by Auricchio and Testa (1972). In summary, there appear to be at least five well-documented changes that affect soluble proteins in human cataracts: (1) conformational changes; (2) oxidation of sulfhydryl; (3) photooxidative cross-linking and pigmentation; (4) dilution by hydropic swelling; and (5) loss of smaller molecules. These changes may coexist to variable degrees in morphologically different cataracts and, in addition, four other plausible but undemonstrated changes may occur: (1) aggregation to larger, light-scattering units; (2) increased binding to cell membranes; (3) inhibition of synthesis; (4) increased net proteolysis (Barber, 1973).

It has not yet been demonstrated that any of these changes is a direct cause of opacification, and indeed the available evidence suggests that derangement of cell membrane regularity and development of steep refractive index gradients between regions of high and low protein concentrations are more commonly responsible. Pathological swelling is a more plausible mechanism for producing such distortions than primary alteration of soluble protein. Swelling is probably initiated by changes of the transport or permeability functions of cell membranes, although osmotic swelling caused by accumulation of metabolites is possible. The fundamental cause of such changes is unknown for human cataracts, although many speculations have been made and animal experimentation has demonstrated many possibilities.

18.2.5. Incidence of Cataract

Cataract is a large and worldwide problem. Sorsby (1962) has estimated that $1\frac{1}{4}$ million people a year are affected. A WHO (1966) report on blindness in different countries shows widely varying percentages of blindness due to cataract. Table 18-1 shows that even in countries with well-developed medical services, approximately a quarter of those registered as blind are listed as blind from cataract. The incidence rises to between a third and a half in the Punjab plains of India and in Kenya

TABLE 18-1
Percent Blindness Due to
Cataract[a]

England and Wales	22
Israel	28
Ceylon	28
USA	22
Japan	8
Ghana	7
Kenya	46
India (Haryana)	39

[a] Data from WHO (1966).

while it is surprisingly less than 10% in Ghana and Japan where other causes of blindness prevail.

Caird (1973) has compiled epidemiological data concerning cataract incidence. Such statistics are of value in two main ways: they provide information about the size and importance of a medical problem and they also provide clues to the causes of disease. The validity of this type of information is subject to question unless there is consistency and certainty of diagnostic criteria and completeness of ascertainment.

Epidemiological information about cataract derives from three sources: statistics of blindness registration, population surveys, and data derived from cataract extraction. Each source presents its own problems.

International comparisons of statistics of blindness registration may suffer from variation in diagnostic criteria, arising from the fact that, unlike death, blindness is subject to different definitions. More difficulty arises from differing rules for the notification and registration of blindness. In some countries this is voluntary and in others, though technically mandatory, is known to be incomplete, especially by the elderly.

Remarkably few population surveys of cataract have been made, in the sense of studies of random samples of the general population rather than of patients presenting themselves to eye clinics. McGuiness (1967), studying a sample of the population of the Rhondda in South Wales, found that the frequency of lens opacities of all types was about 40% at the age of 40 and around 80% in the first half of the eighth decade. The frequency was somewhat higher in women than in men. In a study of several thousand eyes (population is not clearly stated), Fischer (1948) noticed a sharp increase in the frequency of lens opacities with age after the fifth decade; the 50% prevalence at about age 50 rose to 100% by age 80. He does not mention any sex difference.

The third set of epidemiological data about cataract is derived from the study of cataract extraction. There is some hazard in dealing with the

TABLE 18-2
Surveys of Lens Opacities[a]

Country	No. of subjects	Age	With cataract
USA	914	>20	57
Germany	313	>50	20
France	—	>45	15
Japan	296	>45	13
Jamaica	250	>20	11

[a] From Caird (1973).

results even though there is the advantage of dealing with events whose occurrence can certainly be determined. First, cataract extractions should be studied only in a clearly defined population. Before definite inferences about the frequency of cataract in any population group can be made, it is necessary to consider the relation between cataract extraction and lens opacities in the population as a whole. According to Caird (1973), no study has been made in normal people of the rate of either development or maturation of lens opacities. Second, inferences about cataract in the general population can only be derived from cataract extraction rates with some sort of correction for age and sex differences in indications for operation. It is difficult to see how such a correction could be made, and all that can usefully be done is to ascribe the existing differences in indications for operation.

Both these problems, therefore, make it difficult to compare population groups with regard to cataract extraction unless great care is taken to standardize for the population studies and to give some idea of what the visual indications for cataract extraction are. Table 18-2 presents reasonably reliable findings in five studies since 1935.

18.2.6. Etiology of Cataract

The essential problem in lens pathology is the formation of opacities and impairment of vision. Several different morphological manifestations of this process are now recognized, the most frequent being senile cataracts (Koch *et al.*, 1972). Pirie (1968) suggests that the term "senile" cataract be abandoned because it conveys a false sense of uniformity.

In many cases, known factors are responsible for a certain type of opacity and certain diseases are associated with some specific types of cataract, but understanding of pathophysiological processes that lead to lens opacities is still poor. Many studies done on the development of cataracts induced by nutritional, chemical, or physical means allow proposal of theories on cataractogenesis based on the morphological and

TABLE 18-3
Causative Factors of Cataracts

Aging
Congenital
Trauma
Electromagnetic radiation
Metabolic diseases (e.g., diabetes)
Drugs (phenylthiazines, miotics)

biological changes observed. In some cases, e.g., in cataracts resulting from the feeding of galactose to young rats or ionizing radiation exposure, satisfactory theories may be proposed. However, these findings are still of limited value in understanding the etiology of human cataracts (Tables 18-3 and 18-4).

Damaging agents can cause lens opacification in a number of different ways. Black et al. (1960) reported an increase in the incidence of posterior subcapsular opacities in patients with rheumatoid arthritis, and suspects that it was due to their long-term treatment with corticosteroids. Other investigators have established the cataractogenic effect of corticosteroids (Bettman et al., 1968; Cotlier and Becker, 1965; Cremer-Bartels et al., 1968).

TABLE 18-4
Etiology of Cataracts

Senile
  Nuclear: hard cataract
  Cortical: soft cataract
  Posterior subcapsular cortex (PSC): most common
Corticosteroids
  PSC
Mitotic drugs
  Anterior subcapsular cortex (ASC)
Phenylthiazines
  Star-shaped anterior capsular
Traumatic
  Contusion and/or concussion: PSC (long latency period)
  Rupture of lens capsule: PSC extending to whole lens
Diabetic
  Cortical ASC and PSC with snowflakes
Ionizing radiation
  Form initially at posterior pole. Have doughnut shape with clear center surrounded by opacity. Opacity spreads as in ordinary PSC opacity and ultimately lens becomes entirely opaque. Following initial signs, ionizing radiation cataracts do not differ from ordinary senile or other types of lens opacities.

In many cases a combination of toxic agents is needed to induce cataract formation. Pilocarpine used alone in experimental studies did not induce opacities (Koch *et al.*, 1972) but was effective when combined with other cataractogenic agents such as naphthalene (Hockwin *et al.*, 1964) or X-irradiation (Hockwin *et al.*, 1969/1970).

Clinical observations also suggest that surgical treatment of glaucoma may accelerate the formation of presenile cataracts. In order to test the hypothesis that impaired lens nutrition caused by loss of aqueous humor may act as a subliminal cataractogenic factor in the glaucomatous individual, rabbits were subjected to naphthalene feeding, together with puncture of the anterior chamber (Hockwin *et al.*, 1964, 1969/1970). This resulted in a significant acceleration of cataract development. Others (Axelsson, 1968, 1973; Muller *et al.*, 1956; Tarkkanen and Karjakainen, 1966) have discussed the possibility that local administration of miotics in glaucoma therapy may induce cataracts.

Dinitrophenol (DNP), once widely used as a reducing agent, has been found to cause cataracts in man with an incidence of 0.86% (Horner, 1942). Bettman (1946) concluded that metabolic abnormalities in genetically obese mice accounted for their susceptibility to DNP cataracts. In guinea pigs, lens opacities can be induced only by DNP in conjunction with a deficiency of vitamin A (Ogino and Yasukara, 1957). There are many examples of cataractogenesis due to combined toxic agents (Koch *et al.*, 1972). Many agents may be potentially injurious to the lens but not necessarily cataractogenic when applied alone to normal lenses. The additive hazards when combined provided insult sufficient to induce cataracts. It also appears that subliminal lens hazards can aggravate the course of other cataracts without producing a different morphological type.

Presently many questions are being raised about the possible causes of presenile cataracts, i.e., cataracts of a morphologically senile type at a presenile age. Becker (1877) theorized that senile opacities are a normal feature of aging that cannot be avoided if the individual lives long enough. But why do signs of senile cataracts appear in some people before senescence? Koch *et al.* (1972) purports that an accumulation of subliminal lens hazards may accelerate the onset of senile opacities. Muller *et al.* (1956) first started investigations into this problem when they noted presenile cataracts in several of their patients. Upon inquiring further, it was found that they had been exposed for some time to cataractogenic agents, although the morphology of the opacities at first seemed to exclude these agents as the cause of the cataract.

An important consequence of subliminal cataractogenesis is in the treatment of already existing eye diseases. Uveitis alone can cause complicated cataracts. If corticosteroid therapy is used, it could act as a subliminal lens hazard. This has implications in testing new drugs for not only long-term effects of use but also additive effects in relation to cataract formation.

Diabetics develop typical diabetic cataracts when young (Newell and Ernest, 1974). However, later in life these true diabetic opacities may no longer be found. Instead, they now develop cataracts of the senile type, but earlier and more frequently than nondiabetics. van Heyningen (1959, 1962) found that lenses of diabetic rats contained sorbitol, which is not present in normal lenses. Sorbitol was formed in the lens from glucose but only when there was a high blood sugar. Kinoshita *et al.* (1962) postulated and then proved that sorbitol in the lens increased osmotic pressure within the fibers. The fibers then swell and sometimes ultimately disrupt. This disruption of fibers and alterations of the lens metabolism led directly to lens opacity in experimental animals. Pirie and van Heyningen (1964) were able to apply the same mechanism to humans when they found that the lens of the human diabetic, whether cataractous or not, contains sorbitol, which is not present normally in the nondiabetic lens.

According to Pirie (1972), diabetics make up 13% of all patients at Oxford having a cataract extracted. This is much higher than the percentage in the adult population. There are two ways to delay or prevent the accumulation of sorbitol in the lens. One is to control the diabetes, since aldose reductase is active only when blood glucose is high. The other is to inhibit the enzyme. Burditt and Caird (1968) studied the relationship of diabetic control to lens opacities. They found that the frequency of lens opacities in diabetics was greater in those less well-controlled. In a small percentage there was actually regression in those who were better controlled. Thus, some evidence supports the view that the control of diabetes is related to frequency of lens opacities. Their study also provided evidence that bilateral lens opacities may disappear completely in as many as 10% of younger diabetics.

Cataracts in the pediatric age group represent a major ocular problem and account for some 11.5% of blindness in preschool children. Like so many ocular abnormalities, cataracts can be unique, or associated with other ocular problems or with systemic disorders (Albert and Scheie, 1969). The cataracts may be inherited but may also be a result of maternal infection during pregnancy. Metabolic and endocrine disorders, traumatic and other disturbances at birth may be additional causes of a congenital cataract (Liesmaa, 1972). Hereditary cataract is the most common etiological type, comprising about 25% (Albert and Scheie, 1969). Intrauterine infections (e.g., rubella) form the second largest group among etiological factors of congenital cataract. It is important to note that regardless of etiology, any congenital cataract, including the inherited variety, can either remain stationary or increase in severity as the child grows older. The types of cataracts are varied and there is no one characteristic type.

The last major category as a factor in cataract is trauma. A cataract may result from blunt injury to the eye. Rosette-shaped opacities, located in the anterior or posterior subcapsular region, are characteristic of this type of cataract, although lamellar cataracts and diffuse punctate opacities may also occur. In addition, contusion of the eye may give rise to a ring of pigment granules deposited on the surface of the anterior lens capsule. Penetrating injuries of the eye with a rent in the lens capsule usually result in total opacification of the lens. Occasionally, however, only a small localized area may opacify at the site of a capsular injury (Albert and Scheie, 1969).

"Glassblower's" cataract, an example of infrared cataract, is a true exfoliation of the lens. Thickening and lamination of the anterior lens capsule are seen clinically as a curling of the capsule, the free ends of which float in the anterior chamber. This is associated with characteristic posterior cortical opacities. Latency period can be from 1 year to many years. In a study by Frey *et al.* (1973), the interval between injury and surgery ranged from a few hours to 10 years. Since the lens lacks heat-dissipating mechanisms, such as circulating blood, the heat generated by absorption of infrared (IR) in the adjacent pigment cells of the iris and conducted into the lens, raises the temperature in the lens. Many years of exposure is usually required to produce these types of changes in the lens (Geeraets, 1970).

18.3. SPECTRAL TRANSMISSION OF THE OCULAR MEDIA

The transmission of the ocular media between 300 and 1400 nm has been measured by several investigators. Two studies are most often used, those of Geeraets and Berry (1968) and Boettner and Wolter (1962). Boettner and Wolter measured the spectral transmission of the cornea, aqueous, lens, and vitreous.

The primary hazard from optical radiation (UV, visible, IR) is exposure of the eye. This is particularly important in the visible and near-IR regions of the spectrum, but in the other regions there are also serious problems.

Excessive UV exposure produces photophobia accompanied by redness, tearing, conjunctival discharge, corneal surface exfoliation, and stromal haze. This is the syndrome of photokeratitis often called "snow blindness." In the UV C region (100 to 280 nm) and UV B region (280 to 315 nm), this photokeratitis is the primary result of excessive acute

CATARACTS AND OTHER OCULAR EFFECTS 575

exposure. In this region as well as in the UV A region (315 to 380 nm), photochemical cataracts will result from chronic, high-level exposures (Sliney and Freasier, 1973). The action of the UV radiation is photochemical rather than thermal, since the temperature rise from a hazardous exposure appears to be negligible.

In the visible region (beginning near 380 to nearly 750 nm), the cornea, lens, and associated eye media are largely transparent as they neither absorb nor scatter light to any great degree (Geeraets and Berry, 1968). Only a small fraction (5% or less) of the energy that passes through the eye media is used for vision. The greater part is absorbed in the pigment granules in the pigment epithelium and the choroid, i.e., behind the photoreceptors (the rods and cones). This energy that is absorbed is converted into heat. If this absorbed energy becomes too great, tissue damage (usually referred to as retinal burn) can develop (Vos, 1966). Until recently, only the sun was bright enough—and then only by prolonged viewing—to cause retinal burns. However, the availability of compact arc sources and lasers has greatly increased this danger.

There is little doubt that the temperature rise in the chorioretinal tissue is a major factor in causing threshold damage. But in recent years more evidence has become available that under some circumstances light as a visual stimulus can also cause permanent loss of visual function.

Another transition zone between corneal damage and retinal effects begins at the far end of the visible region and extends into the IR A region (750 nm to 1.4 μm). Retinal function can be disturbed from short-duration exposures, while chronic exposures can produce injury to both the retina and anterior parts such as the lens and vitreous. In the IR B region (1.4 to 2.5 μm), both lenticular and corneal damage are seen. The ocular media becomes opaque in the IR C region (2.5 μm to 1 mm) as the absorption by water, a major constituent of all cells, is very high in this region. Thus, the damage is primarily to the cornea, although lens damage has sometimes been correlated with IR radiation below 2.5 μm. The damage mechanism appears to be thermal, at least for the longer wavelengths. The CO_2 laser at 10.6 μm, in its action on all materials containing water, exemplifies the thermal nature of the damage. In the IR C region, as in the UV A and B regions, the threshold for damage to the skin is comparable to that for the cornea.

18.4. RADIATION CATARACTS

The eye is unusually sensitive to many forms of electromagnetic radiation. The occurrence of cataracts in the human has occupied a conspicuous place in discussions of ionizing radiation. According to Cogan (1959), it must not be construed that the lens has any mysterious vulnerability to these energies. Instead the relatively sluggish lens cells are actually refractory to irradiation as compared to the lymphatic, myelogenous, or other tissues that have a rapid turnover of cells. The practical importance of the lens hinges on the fact that opacification of the lens substance, which is what a cataract is, results in loss of useful visual functions, whereas opacification of tissue elsewhere would be of such little consequence that it would go unnoticed. As Cogan (1959) has pointed out, the eye is unusually sensitive to many forms of radiation. A brief description is in order. Certain portions of the eye are more susceptible to particular wavelengths. This susceptibility is due to the specific absorption by the anterior segment of the globe of particular bands of radiant energy and the transmission of other wavelengths by these structures to the interior of the eye. Thus, the long radio waves are readily transmitted through the globe (there is little if any absorption) and therefore do not give rise to any deleterious effects on the lens. However, the shorter waves (microwaves), of the order of several centimeters, can be harmful to the anterior half of the eye because of their heating effects (Lerman, 1962).

The penetration of IR rays is inversely proportional to their wavelength; the longer waves are absorbed mostly by the cornea and aqueous humor while the shorter wavelengths can easily reach the retina. The visible spectrum or white light is a mixture of wavelengths between 770 and 390 nm, and their degree of ocular penetration is directly proportional to their length. That is, there is much greater penetration of the red end of the spectrum than of the violet end. Most of the UV rays up to 320 nm are absorbed by the cornea, while the lens absorbs those between 320 and 390 nm. The vast majority of the Grenz rays (long-wavelength X rays) are absorbed by the cornea, but as one approaches the shorter end of the radiation spectrum, the penetrating powers of the rays are greater. Thus, the ordinary X ray with the potential of from 100 to 250 kV, which is employed most frequently in radiotherapy, is capable of penetrating the globe quite effectively. Gamma and cosmic rays and neutrons can penetrate the eye with ease, even more efficiently than X rays (Lerman, 1962).

There are several factors that might serve to enhance the susceptibility of the lens to the deleterious effects of radiation. Cogan (1950) noted that not only is the lens avascular, but it is located at least 2 mm or more from any blood supply, thus making it much less effective in dissipating heat as compared with most other tissues and organs. Since many forms of radiant energy are particularly associated with the production of heating, e.g., microwaves and IR waves, this factor may be an important consideration in the enhanced susceptibility of the lens to certain forms of radiation cataract. Another important consideration is the rather unique method of differentiation and growth that is present in the lens. The major metabolic activity, particularly oxidative respiration, occurs within the layer of epithelial cells located only in the anterior subcapsular region extending toward the equator. Thus, damage to this area may require a relatively lengthy latent period prior to the clinical manifestations of lenticular opacities. This might apply particularly to the effects of radiant energy on RNA and DNA (Lerman, 1962).

Cogan (1959) discusses an important aspect of the lens that is unique in the body and that may contribute to the irreversibility of cataracts or to the failure in effective repair of the damaged lens. This is the fact that the lens cells are, from an early stage in embryonic development, encased in a capsule that, for the entire life of the animal, prevents exchange at the cellular level with the rest of the body. Thus, the cells that have been damaged cannot get out of the lens (except by solubilization of their constituents) and wandering phagocytes cannot get into the lens. The scavenging process that is universally employed elsewhere in the body thus does not apply to the lens, and one would therefore infer that the lens is either handicapped in its reparative facilities or else has developed a compensatory process. The nature of this compensatory process, if it exists, has not been discovered. Much research has been done on the experimental production of X radiation and neutron cataracts. Cataracts that result from exposure to neutrons, X rays, and γ rays are all similar in appearance and structure. The characteristic appearance in early stages in the human appears to be that of a dot at the posterior pole of the lens. At this stage it causes no visual impairment. Progression of the cataract is characterized by extension of the opacity to a disk less strictly confined to the posterior pole. This is often accompanied by a curious clearing, relatively, of the center so that the opacity becomes doughnut shaped. At this time, several vacuoles appear just in front of the opacity. Opacities and vacuoles then occur in the anterior cortex of the lens; subsequently, opacification extends to the posterior cortex and eventually the entire lens (Cogan, 1959). These cataracts all exhibit latent periods before becoming visible, and they can occur with doses that do not necessarily produce any other clinically evident lesions. Furthermore, the greater the dose of these forms of energy, the shorter is the latent period, the more intense the damage to the lens, and the more rapid the progression of the opacities (Lerman, 1962). The minimal X-radiation dose for human cataract is generally accepted to be 500 to 600 R depending on the type of X rays employed (Cogan et al., 1954). These threshold values apply to localized exposure rather than whole-body radiation. Younger individuals are more susceptible to cataract formation from X-ray exposure.

The duration of the latent period between exposures of the lens and developments of cataracts is generally related inversely to the dose. With near-threshold dose, the cataract may take many years to appear (Cogan, 1959; Lerman, 1962). Also important is whether or not the cataract is progressive. Cogan (1959) followed several cases for years without noticeable increase in the opacification.

All hot bodies radiate in the IR, and radiate IR to other objects with lower surface temperatures. The direct damaging effect of the IR results from (1) an increase in temperature of the absorbing tissue that depends upon which wavelengths are absorbed, (2) the parameters involved in heat conduction and dissipation, (3) the total amount of energy delivered to the tissue, and the period over which the energy is supplied (Matelsky, 1968). The primary response to exposure to the IR wavelengths is a thermal one. The most prominent direct effects of short-wavelength IR radiations on the skin include acute skin burn, increased vasodilation of the capillary beds, and an increased pigmentation that can persist for long periods of time. The heat load imposed on the skin can be removed by the circulating blood or evaporation of moisture. The fact that the eye is less able to dissipate the heat and the focusing nature of its lens makes it the organ of major concern. Damage of the lens of the eye from IR has been the subject of considerable investigation over a period of many years. The term 'glassworkers" cataract has become generic for lenticular opacities found in individuals exposed to processes hot enough to be luminous.

Dunn (1950) of Corning Glass Company was unable to find evidence of any ocular disturbance among glassworkers who had been exposed for at least 20 years to IR of 2 cal-cm^2/min at 2000°K. Keatinge et al. (1955) were unable to find any posterior cortical changes in the eyes of iron-rolling mill workers exposed to 0.02–0.1 cal-cm^2/sec for an average of 17 years; however, there was a higher incidence of posterior capsular opacities. The evidence now favors the concept that the IR energies emitted from hot sources in industry are the agents responsible for IR cataractogenesis (Keatinge et al., 1955; Cogan et al., 1952; Goldmann, 1935).

The original mechanism postulated for the formation of IR radiation cataracts was the focusing of the rays on the posterior surface of the lens causing the maximum damage at that point. Vogt (1932) considered changes arising from increase in lenticular temperature and direct effects on the lens fibers. Changes in the lens are secondary to heating of the whole anterior segment of the eye. After the initial damage to the anterior portion, the cataract becomes well defined at the posterior surface of the cortex with successive degeneration of the posterior lens fibers (Michaelson, 1972).

Evidence has been presented indicating that heat *per se* in the absence of IR can produce cataracts. Goldmann (1935; Goldmann *et al.*, 1950) noted that elevation of temperature at the anterior portion of the lens is the prime etiological factor in glassblower's cataract.

The experimental production of IR cataracts, which requires heat much greater than the intensities to which humans are ordinarily exposed, indicates that the lesion results from a local thermal effect rather than from the absorption of specific rays by the lens fibers (Lerman, 1962). Langley *et al.* (1960) note that the lenticular lesions following the exposure of an animal to a cataractogenic dose of IR radiation are located adjacent to burned areas of the iris. These studies tend to confirm Goldmann's (1935; Goldmann *et al.*, 1950) observations that the lenticular changes occur secondarily to heating. That is, the IR rays are absorbed by the iris pigment epithelium and then converted to heat, thus damaging the adjacent lens epithelium (Michaelson, 1972).

18.5. EFFECTS OF MICROWAVES ON THE OCULAR LENS

The ocular lens is avascular and is located at least 2 mm or more from any blood supply, making it much less effective in dissipating heat than most other tissues and organs of the body. Since microwave absorption is associated with the production of heat, this is an important factor in the suggested susceptibility of the lens to higher power density microwave exposure (Michaelson, 1972, 1978).

18.5.1. Animal Experiments

Microwaves have been shown to produce cataracts in some experimental animals, the eyes of which were directly exposed to microwaves (Carpenter *et al.*, 1960a; Carpenter and van Ummersen, 1968; Daily *et al.*, 1950; Michaelson, 1972, 1978; Richardson *et al.*, 1951; Seth and Michaelson, 1965; Williams *et al.*, 1955; Zeller *et al.*, 1951).

In several studies, exposure of animals to various frequencies ranging from 200 to 5500 MHz at field intensities up to 150 mW/cm^2 did not produce eye damage; most of these exposures were whole-body (Addington *et al.*, 1958; Ely *et al.*, 1957; Howland and Michaelson, 1959; Michaelson *et al.*, 1961). Lubin *et al.* (1960) reported that lens changes did not occur in rabbits given 400-MHz whole-body exposure even if radiation times were extended to the lethal period. Addington *et al.* (1958) did not find any eye changes in guinea pigs, dogs, sheep, or mice following chronic whole-body exposures to 200 MHz CW. Some of these studies are summarized in Table 18-5.

TABLE 18-5
Ocular Effects of Far-Field Exposure to Microwaves

Effects	Species	Frequency (MHz)	Intensity (mW/cm^2)	Duration (days × min)	SAR (W/kg)	Reference
No ocular effects, including no lenticular changes	Rabbit	3000 (CW)	100, 200	1 × 15, 30	14, 28[a]	Appleton et al. (1975)
Acute ocular changes, e.g., hyperemia of lids and conjunctiva, miosis, anterior chamber flare, engorgement of iris vessels, and periorbital cutaneous burns. No lenticular changes			300, 400 500	1 × 15	42, 56[a] 70[a]	
Death			300 500	1 × 30 1 × 15	42[a] 70[a]	
No cataracts	Rabbit	385 (CW) 385 (CW) 468 (CW)[b]	60 30 60	10 × 15 10 × 90 10 × 20	48[a] 24[a] 8.1	Cogan et al. (1958)
No cataracts	Rabbit	2450 (CW)	10	5 × 480 (× 8–17 weeks)	15[a]	Ferri and Hagan (1976)
No ocular effects	Monkey (*Macaca mulatta*)	9310 (pulsed)	150	30–40 × 294–665[c]		McAfee et al. (1979)

[a] Estimated SAR values (according to Durney et al., 1978).
[b] Waveguide exposure.
[c] Total exposure time in minutes for the entire 30- to 40-day experimental period.

Whole-body exposure of dogs to 2800-MHz pulsed microwaves at a power density of 165 mW/cm² (SAR 6.1 W/kg) for 3 hr in a single exposure or as much as 6 hr daily over a 3-week period did not produce lenticular changes, the eyes being examined regularly for 4 years after irradiation (Michaelson et al., 1967). In another report by Michaelson et al. (1971), among dogs exposed to 1280 MHz pulsed at 20, 50, or 100 mW/cm², (SAR 4.5 W/kg) 6 hr/day, 5 days/week for periods ranging from 2 to 4 weeks, or to 24,000 MHz pulsed (24 mW/cm²), 400 min/day, 5 days/week or 16½ hr/day, 4 days/week for 20 months, periodic examination, for 12 months after cessation of exposure, by direct and indirect ophthalmoscopy and slit lamp did not reveal abnormalities of the lens or retina. In these exposures, the dogs could move around in their cages, and their eyes were never exposed directly for long periods.

Single or fractionated exposure of the eyes directly to 2800 MHz pulsed, 350 mW/cm² (SAR 13 W/kg) for 20 min did not result in permanent lenticular alteration in dogs. Exposure of the eyes directly to 700 mW/cm² (SAR 26 W/kg) of 2800-MHz pulsed microwaves for 20 min (single or fractionated) resulted in lens opacification involving the posterior lens capsule and posterior subcapsular cortex (Michaelson et al., 1967).

Exposure Threshold Values

Threshold for appearance of cataracts in the rabbit after a single exposure to 2450 MHz CW was originally established by Williams et al. (1955) to be 290 mW/cm² for a 90-min exposure and 600 mW/cm² for a 5-min exposure. Subsequently, Carpenter et al. (1960a) and Guy et al. (1975) reported time and power density threshold curves for cataract induction in rabbits by single exposures to near-field 2.45-GHz radiation which are similar in shape but are quantitatively different. The latter studies found lower threshold values than reported by Williams et al. (1955). This probably reflects differences in the method of irradiation and in techniques used to measure power density. In fact, Carpenter (1979) determined that his power densities were 50% higher than originally published.

Using 2450 MHz CW, Kramar et al. (1973) produced cataracts in rabbits at incident power levels of 200 mW/cm² applied locally to the eye for 30 min or more. Measurements and calculations indicate that under these conditions, the temperature at the posterior pole of the lens exceeds 46°C, which is above the denaturation point of protein.

It is important to note that in all studies in which cataracts (or lens opacities) were produced in rabbits, the animal's eye was directly "coupled" to the waveguide or within a few centimeters from the feed horn or antenna of the radiating device. In addition, in many of these studies the animals were anesthetized, which would influence the results by affecting thermal regulation in the eye.

Carpenter *et al.* (1960a) exposed one eye of anesthetized rabbits to microwaves in the near field; the unirradiated eye served as the control. The eyes were then examined at various intervals by opthalmoscope, slit-lamp biomicroscope, or both instruments. The earliest positive reaction in this type of study occurred within 24 to 48 hr after a cataractogenic exposure, with the appearance of one or two narrow translucent or milky bands in the posterior cortex of the lens, just under the capsule, which extended no farther than the lens equator. These bands could be seen by slit-lamp examination. If the ocular injury was minimal, no further change occurred and the cortical banding disappeared within a few days. Otherwise, in 2 to 4 days after exposure, small granules appeared in the posterior lens suture region. If a more intense reaction occurred, larger numbers of granules appeared over a larger area within the next few days, and small vesicles occasionally developed. These early changes sometimes developed further and became either well-defined circumscribed or diffuse opacities. Such lens changes remained as permanent ocular defects. In general, it has been found that microwave cataracts in rabbits involve only the posterior lens cortex, unless the exposure is so intense that the opacity extends throughout the lens. Guy *et al.* (1975) replicated Carpenter's work for single acute exposures with essentially the same results and also quantified the threshold of cataractogenesis in terms of SAR. It thus appears that the cataractogenic threshold for a 100-min exposure is 150 mW/cm^2 (138 W/kg peak absorption).

At exposure levels that cause cataracts, other ocular reactions such as swelling and chemosis of bulbar and palpebral conjunctivae, pupillary constriction, hyperemia of the iris and limbal vessels, and vitreous floaters and filaments occur. These, however, are transient and differ in severity with the intensity and duration of exposure. All these attest to the hyperthermic nature of the exposure.

In studies by Carpenter *et al.* (1972a),* rabbits exposed daily for 25 days to 2450 MHz CW, 150 mW/cm^2, in the near zone (1 hr/exposure) did not develop cataracts. With regard to possible age sensitivity, van Ummersen and Cogan (1965) reported that in the case of microwave-induced cataracts, the age of the animal has no bearing on the latent period and that there is no significant relationship between the age of the

---

* It must be noted that the power density calculated in the investigations of Carpenter, Kinoshita, Merola, and van Ummersen is approximately 50% higher than reported. This is due to a repeat measurement of the field with a more accurate instrument (Carpenter *et al.*, 1972a).

animal and the susceptibility of its lens to damage by microwave exposure.

Zaret (1964) and Birenbaum *et al.* (1969a,b) studied cataract production in rabbits exposed to CW and pulsed 5500-MHz microwaves. Lens opacities resulted after exposure to 390 mW/cm^2 for 34–37 min (Zaret, 1964). The average power causing an observable loss of transparency (in at least a portion of the lens) in 50% of the animals was defined as the "threshold" value (Birenbaum *et al.*, 1969a,b). Logarithmic time–threshold curves were obtained when the exposure times for cataract production were plotted against the corresponding "threshold" values for both CW and pulsed modalities. Carpenter *et al.* (1960a) obtained comparable time–threshold curves at 8200 and 10,000 MHz as Birenbaum *et al.* (1969a,b) using similar criteria for definition of "threshold" values. These studies indicate the 1-hr threshold to be above 400 mW/cm^2 for these frequencies.

Carpenter and van Ummersen (1968) also utilized a closed waveguide system and exposed the eyes of albino rabbits at frequencies in the range of 8000–10,000 MHz and reported production of anterior cortical cataracts. With a free-space radiation system, they reported production of posterior subcapsular cataracts, but only at power levels that were lethal unless the body was shielded. In the majority of these animals, skin burns were also produced.

Appleton *et al.* (1975) irradiated 30 New Zealand rabbits at 3000 MHz by direct exposure to the eye. The animals were divided into nine groups and exposed to increasing power density versus time. Groups I–IV received 100 or 200 mW/cm^2 for 15 or 30 min and exhibited no ocular changes during or immediately after exposure. Daily examinations for 14 days and weekly examinations for 1 month, followed by monthly examinations for 1 year, revealed no lenticular changes. Groups V, VII, and VIII were subjected for 15 min to 300, 400, or 500 mW/cm^2 and exhibited acute ocular changes during exposure, which consisted of hyperemia of lids and conjunctiva, miosis, anterior chamber flare, engorgement of iris vessels, and periorbital cutaneous burns. Subsequent examination revealed no lenticular abnormalities.

Group VI received 300 mW/cm^2 for 30 min and died during exposure. In addition, three of the six animals in group VII died immediately after exposure, and the three that did survive were greatly stressed. The (three) control animals did not exhibit ocular effects at the 1-year follow-up examination.

It is noteworthy that 1 year after a single microwave exposure, sufficient in intensity to cause both thermal cutaneous and acute gross ocular effects, no lens changes or cataracts were observed. Appleton (1975) states that experiments with rabbits have shown that daily

TABLE 18-6
Ocular Effects in Rabbits of Near-Field Exposure to Millimeter or Microwaves

Effects	Exposure conditions					Reference
	Frequency (GHz)	Intensity (mW/cm^2)	Duration (days × min)	SAR (W/kg)	
Cataract	5.5 (CW and pulsed)	470–785[a]	1 × 2–100	300–500[b]	Birenbaum et al. (1969a)
Cataract	0.8 (CW)	785[a]	1 × 25	500[b]	Birenbaum et al. (1969b)
	4.2 (pulsed)	785[a]	1 × 17	500[b]	
	4.6 (pulsed)	785[a]	1 × 15	500[b]	
	5.2 (pulsed)	500–785[a]	1 × 5–12	350–500[b]	
	5.4 (CW and pulsed)	500–785[a]	1 × 3–4	300–500[b]	
	5.5 (CW and pulsed)	500–785[a]	1 × 2–3	300–500[b]	
	6.3 (pulsed)	785[a]	1 × 5	500[b]	
Cataract	2.45 (CW)	180	1 × 240		Carpenter (1979)
		120–180	20 × 60		
No cataract	2.45 (CW)	75	20 × 60		Carpenter (1979)
Cataract	2.45 (CW)	295	1 × 30		Hagan and Carpenter (1976)
	10 (CW)	375	1 × 30		
No cataract; keratitis (inflammation of cornea)	35	~40	1 × 60	>175[d]	Rosenthal et al. (1976)
	107	~40	1 × 60	>238[d]	

[a] Estimate calculated by dividing the microwave power by the irradiated area ($d = 1.27$ cm) of the eye.
[b] Estimate based on the assumption that all the incident power was absorbed by the eye (2 g).
[c] Maximum SAR in the eye.
[d] Estimated SAR values for the cornea.

exposures over the course of a month to levels of microwaves that would be obvious to humans as sensation of heat on the skin (25 mW/cm^2) did not result in any detectable lens effect at the end of 1 year. These observations correlated well with the work of Kramar *et al.* (1975), Carpenter *et al.* (1960a), and Williams *et al.* (1955) at 2450 MHz, in which single microwave exposures of longer than 15 min were required for cataract production at power levels of 300 mW/cm^2 and above. In addition, single exposures at 200 mW/cm^2 for 30 min were not sufficient to cause cataracts (Appleton *et al.*, 1975).

Carpenter (1975) induced lens opacities with a single dose of 500 but not 400 mW/cm^2. According to his findings, if the human eye responds like the rabbit eye, the worries voiced by the public press over the incidence of opacities or cataracts from use of a microwave device, such as an oven, are unfounded (Carpenter, 1975). Hirsch (1975) concurs and adds that at 400 mW/cm^2, 3000 MHz, it took at least ten exposures to produce cataracts.

Guy *et al.* (1974) and Kramar *et al.* (1975) have shown that in rabbits exposed to 2450 MHz, threshold for cataract production was 150 mW/cm^2 for 100 min. The data suggest that the critical temperature for cataractogenesis is 43°C. These investigators also found that single potentially cataractogenic exposures will not injure the eye under conditions of controlled general hypothermia. They also found that exposure to 100 mW/cm^2, 2 hr/day for 8–9 days, produced no cataracts upon periodic examinations for 6 months after exposure. Guy *et al.* (1974) exposed rabbits to 918 MHz, 466 mW/cm^2 for 15 min and 117 mW/cm^2 for 100 min, with no evidence of cataract and concluded that the threshold for cataractogenesis is higher for this frequency than for 2450 MHz. Some of these studies are summarized in Table 18-6.

18.5.2. Biochemical Changes

Merola and Kinoshita (1961) reported decreased ascorbic acid content in the lens of rabbits 6 to 18 hr and decreased glutathione 24 to 48 hr after the eyes had been exposed to 2450 MHz, 280 mW/cm^2. Kinoshita *et al.* (1966) suggested that the decrease in ascorbic acid was not simply a thermal effect. They kept isolated rabbit lenses at 45°C for 8 min; this was the temperature attained in the eyes exposed to microwaves for that length of time. There was no effect upon the normal ascorbic acid level of these lenses. The authors suggest that lens permeability may be increased by microwave exposure and that this effect may be due to nonthermal properties of the energy, i.e., "metabolic imbalance."

18.5.3. Frequency Specificity

Most experimental cataract studies have been done at 2.45 GHz, but opacities in rabbit eyes have been reported after near-field exposures at 0.8, 4.2, 4.6, 5.2, 5.4, 5.5, 6.3, and 10 GHz (Birenbaum et al., 1969a,b; Hagan and Carpenter, 1976). In several studies, the cataractogenic potential of different frequencies was addressed. Hagan and Carpenter (1976) determined the relative effects of 2.45- and 10-GHz CW energies on the rabbit eye and concluded that the cataractogenic potential for single acute exposures is greater at the lower frequency. For both frequencies, the opacities were characteristically located in the posterior subcapsular cortex of the lens, although the initial appearance and subsequent development differed. These variations probably reflect differences in the pattern of absorbed microwave energy in the eye due to the different depths of penetration of the energy at these two frequencies.

Guy et al. (1974, 1975) measured the absorbed power distribution in rabbit eyes exposed to 918 and 2450 MHz and found the patterns to be significantly different. At 2450 MHz, the absorbed power was maximum in the vitreous body at a point midway between the posterior surface of the lens and the retinal surface. Peak absorption thus correlates well with the observation of irreversible changes in the posterior cortical lens only. Exposure to 918 MHz in a cavity resulted in relatively uniform absorption in the eye, but the maximum absorbed power was only about 25% of the peak absorption at 2450 MHz. Therefore, one would expect the threshold for cataractogenesis in rabbits exposed to 918 MHz to be considerably higher than the threshold for 2450 MHz. But more importantly, at 918 MHz under these conditions, peak absorption in the rabbit brain was 36% higher than in the eye.

Hagan and Carpenter (1976) and Guy et al. (1975) used exposure systems that applied microwave energy across an air space to the eye, and both groups reported posterior subcapsular cataracts. Birenbaum et al. (1969b) produced cataracts in the anterior cortex of rabbit lens with an exposure system that applied pulsed microwave energy to the corneal surface. Furthermore, as the frequency decreased from 6.3 to 5.2 to 4.6 to 4.2 GHz, longer exposure times at a constant field strength were required to produce lens defects. Under similar experimental conditions, even longer exposure times were required to induce cataracts at a lower frequency, i.e., 0.8 GHz, CW.

Rosenthal et al. (1976) examined the effects of 35 and 107 GHz on the rabbit eye. For both frequencies, keratitis occurred at lower intensities than required to produce any other demonstrable ocular effect such as lens injury or iritis. Irradiation at 107 GHz was more effective in producing immediate corneal damage, but this change generally disappeared by the next day, and was associated with marked injury to the corneal epithelium. Effects on the cornea correlate well with the pattern of microwave energy absorption, because most of the energy at these high frequencies is absorbed in the superficial regions of the eye. The earliest stage of keratitis or minimal corneal stromal injury was found to occur after 30-min exposure to an incident power density of 50 mW/cm^2 or after 60-min exposure at 25 mW/cm^2. Estimates of the power absorbed by the eye at 25 mW/cm^2 are 35 mW/g at 35 GHz and 47.5 mW/g at 107 GHz (Rosenthal *et al.*, 1976); the average SARs of a rabbit eye weighing 2 g are 17.5 and 23.8 W/kg. Since maximum absorption occurs in the outer structures of the eye, the SAR in the cornea is estimated to exceed the average SAR of the eye by more than an order of magnitude.

Although the above data cannot be directly compared because widely varying experimental procedures were used, these results indicate that the potential for cataract induction in rabbits is higher in the frequency range between 1 and 10 GHz than at either lower or higher microwave frequencies. At power densities that would cause cataracts at frequencies below 1 GHz and above 10 GHz, other ocular or tissue effects became significant. Rosenthal *et al.* (1976) found that 35 and 107 GHz primarily affected the outer structure of the eye, the cornea, for example; and at 918 MHz, Guy *et al.* (1974) showed that maximum energy absorption occurred in the brain and not in the eye.

18.5.4. Modulation Effects

Birenbaum *et al.* (1969a) found no substantial differences in the cataract threshold values for CW and pulsed 5.5-GHz energy and concluded that the average power density determines whether injury to the lens will occur.

18.5.5. Far-Field Exposures

In contrast to the acute, near-field exposures that can cause cataracts and other ocular effects, cataracts have not been produced in animals exposed to whole-body radiation in the far field. Cogan *et al.* (1958) found no cataracts 4 weeks after rabbits were exposed twice weekly for 5 weeks to whole-body 385-MHz radiation at 60 mW/cm^2 for 15 min or 30 mW/cm^2 for 90 min. No cataracts were observed 6 weeks after rabbits were irradiated at 468 MHz in a waveguide at 60 mW/cm^2 (8.1 W/kg) for 10 days (20 min daily). The exposures at both frequencies were near lethal levels.

Appleton *et al.* (1975) exposed anesthetized rabbits whole-body to 3000 MHz for 15 or 30 min at 100 or 200 mW/cm^2. No ocular changes were observed during or immediately after exposure. Daily examination for 14 days and weekly examination for 1 month followed by monthly exams for 1 year revealed no lenticular changes. During exposures at higher levels (300, 400, or 500 mW/cm² for 15 min), animals exhibited acute ocular changes consisting of hyperemia of lids and conjunctive, miosis, anterior chamber flare, engorgement of iris vessels, and periorbital cutaneous burns. Subsequent examinations at up to 1 year revealed no morphological lenticular abnormalities. It should be noted these power levels and durations were well above the cutaneous sensation level, because unanesthetized animals became heat stressed and struggled out of the field during a 15-min exposure at 100 mW/cm². Exposure at 300 mW/cm² for 30 min or 500 mW/cm² for 15 min was lethal to some of the rabbits during or immediately after irradiation.

Ferri and Hagan (1976) exposed unanesthetized rabbits to 2.45 GHz CW in the far field at 10 mW/cm², 8 hr/day, 5 days/week for 8 to 17 weeks. Weekly examination of the eyes showed no abnormal changes during the study, and no changes in the following 3 months.

McAfee *et al.* (1979) trained monkeys (*Macaca mulatta*) to expose their face and eyes to pulsed microwaves (9.31 GHz, 150 mW/cm²). Over a period of about 3 months, the animals were irradiated for 294 to 665 min during 30 to 40 daily sessions. No cataracts or corneal lesions were observed in these monkeys during a 1-year period following irradiation.

Conclusions

The following conclusions may be drawn from selected animal experiments on the cataractogenic potential of exposure to microwave energies:

1. Exposure to high-intensity microwaves could be cataractogenic.
2. For single acute exposures, the threshold intensity for lenticular opacity exceeds 100 mW/cm².
3. Multiple exposures below threshold for single acute exposures do not result in lens opacities.
4. The cataractogenic potential of microwaves varies with frequency; the most effective frequencies appear to be in the range 1 to 10 GHz.
5. Similar ocular effects are produced by CW and pulsed microwave energies of the same average intensity.
6. In contrast to the above conclusions, which are based on acute, near-field exposures to the eye or head, no cataracts have been reported in animals after far-field, whole-body exposures even at near-lethal intensities.

18.6. THERMAL ASPECTS OF MICROWAVE CATARACTOGENESIS

Most experimental evidence indicates that cataracts have been produced with single or multiple exposures at threshold power densities exceeding $100\,\text{mW/cm}^2$. This threshold is, in fact, a time–power threshold; i.e. the higher the power density, the shorter the time threshold and vice versa.

The experimental results indicate that radiation-induced temperature elevation may be essential for the cataractogenic effect of microwaves. Additional evidence for this position has been provided by Kramar et al. (1975), who reported that rabbits kept under general hypothermia during irradiation at known cataractogenic levels of 2.45 GHz (near-field) did not develop cataracts.

Exposure of the rabbit eye to RF/MW energies at sufficient power density and duration causes an immediate increase in intraocular temperature and, after a few days, opacities develop in the posterior subcapsular cortex of the lens (Kramar et al., 1975). Several experiments have been designed to directly test the cause-and-effect relationship between temperature increase and cataract formation. Kramar et al. (1975) exposed rabbit eyes to cataractogenic levels of microwaves while the animal's body was submerged in cold water. By this means, microwave-induced intraocular temperature was limited to less than 41°C, and no lens opacities developed. In a later experiment, Kramar et al. (1976) used heated water to produce ocular and colonic temperatures characteristic of those in rabbits exposed to a cataractogenic level of microwaves. Although the vicinity of the lens was heated to temperatures above those known to be associated with microwave-induced cataracts, no lens opacities were observed; however, the rate of ocular temperature rise was one-tenth the rate of increase with microwaves. Kramar et al. (1976) concluded that a combination of a sharp temperature gradient and a rapid rise in temperature following irradiation may be more traumatic to the lens than a critical temperature *per se.*

Carpenter et al. (1977) reported no posterior subcapsular cataracts in rabbits in which the eye was heated at the same rate, to the same extent, and for an equal period of time as it would experience during a cataracotogenic microwave exposure, by direct application of heat to the surface of the eye over a 6-week period. In addition, elevation of both retrolental and colonic temperatures to values characteristic of a cataractogenic microwave exposure by a combination of restricted body heat loss and irradiation of one eye to power densities slightly below the cataractogenic threshold produced cataracts in only three of ten rabbits. Carpenter et al. (1977) therefore concluded that the increase in intraocular temperature occurring during microwave irradiation is not the sole causative factor in microwave cataractogenesis.

The reason for the apparent disagreement between the conclusions of Carpenter et al. (1977) and Kramar et al. (1976) probably rests with the difficulty of duplicating by nonmicrowave heating techniques the temporal and spatial temperature profiles induced by microwave irradiation of the eye.

Strong evidence for heat being the causative factor in microwave cataracts is provided by the experiment of Kramar et al. (1975), which showed that cataracts were not produced in hypothermic rabbits receiving a cataractogenic microwave exposure. Presently, it is generally understood that intense exposure of the eye for substantial durations, i.e., 150 mW/cm^2 for 100 min, is necessary to induce cataracts in laboratory animals and that these exposure conditions cause death by hyperthermia if the entire animal is irradiated.

The possibility of a cumulative effect on the lens from repeated "subthreshold" exposures of the eyes to microwaves has been suggested in the rabbit by Carpenter et al. (1960b), Carpenter and van Ummersen (1968), Carpenter (1970). The cumulative effect of microwave radiation on rabbit cataractogenesis has been examined by repeatedly exposing the eye to power densities below the threshold for single acute exposures (Carpenter, 1979). For example, daily 1-hr exposures to 180 mW/cm^2 for 13 to 20 days were found to be cataractogenic in 8 of 10 animals, whereas a single exposure at this power density was not effective. At 150 mW/cm^2, 4 of 10 rabbits showed a positive response after 18 to 32 daily exposures. No cataracts were observed after 20 daily 1-hr exposures at 75 mW/cm^2.

In contradistinction to this view, however, most investigators point out that there is a critical intraocular temperature that must be reached before opacities develop. This temperature, as reported by various authors, ranges from 45 to 55°C. Obviously, no cumulative rise in temperature can occur if the intervals between exposures exceed the time required for the tissue to return to normal temperature. The cumulative effect to be anticipated, therefore, is an accumulation of damage resulting from repeated exposures each of which is individually capable of producing some degree of damage (Kalant, 1959). Baillie (1970) showed opacity production to be a temperature-dependent phenomenon. He failed to demonstrate a cumulative effect in dogs subjected to radiation during total-body hypothermia. The cataract that developed during the course of this study could only be explained on the basis of thermal coagulation of lens protein. It was found that dog lens protein coagulates at approximately 60°C. This agrees with results of Richardson et al. (1948) for the rabbit.

The question of a possible nonthermal effect is probably the area of greatest controversy in microwave effects in general. Carpenter has proposed a nonthermal cataractogenic effect while others feel that this has not been satisfactorily demonstrated. Carpenter (Carpenter et al., 1960b; Carpenter and van Ummersen, 1968; Carpenter, 1970) based his conclusion on three points: cataractogenesis appeared to be independent of (1) any fixed temperature limit, (2) the amount of temperature rise, and (3) the total duration of elevated temperature. His temperature measurements were made in the vitreous at the posterior pole of the lens. Baillie et al. (1970) demonstrated that a greater amount of heat was generated in the lens than in the vitreous humor. Baillie's work provides rather substantial evidence that cataractogenesis is a thermal effect in the dog.

Guy et al. (1974) and Kramar et al. (1973, 1975) studied rabbits exposed to near-zone 2450-MHz radiation at subthreshold levels when the retrolental temperature was kept below 41°C by means of general hypothermia. A computer model developed previously for predicting induced temperature distribution in normothermic rabbits was modified to account for the effect of hypothermia. Immediately after irradiation, slight tearing and pupillary constriction were found. These effects disappeared on the second day. The lenses of all the animals remained clear throughout the observation period of 2–3 months. The study of Guy et al. indicates that single potentially cataractogenic exposures of 2450 MHz at 5 cm will not injure the lenses of rabbits under conditions of controlled general hypothermia. Although a critical cataractogenic temperature has not been found, no lens opacities have been produced with retrolental temperatures below 41°C. Even with temperatures well above 41°C, the eye has to be exposed to these temperatures for a certain period of time before observable lens damage is found. It would appear that the increased temperature induced by the radiation, effective over a certain length of time, is essential for microwave cataractogenesis. The conclusion of Guy et al. substantiates the thermal factor in the formation of cataracts.

As an indicator of lens damage, Weiter et al. (1975) measured changes in ascorbic acid concentration in the lens. Kinoshita et al. (1966) had reported that the earliest detectable biochemical change in rabbit lenses after exposure to microwave energy is a decrease in ascorbic acid. This decrease precedes opacification of the lens. The use of whole lens tissue cultures by Weiter et al. (1975) allowed more accurate measurement of the power of incident microwave energy and excluded unwanted biological variables, such as different uveal blood flow rates in response to heat stress. In order to determine whether the decrease in lens ascorbic acid after microwave irradiation was thermal or nonthermal, effects of radiation modulation were reviewed. The average power, measured at the lens surface, of both pulsed and CW microwave radiation was identical. The time–temperature conditions during the experiment were also similar. The rationale was that for a nonthermal effect, peak power should be a significant factor in inducing lens damage; for a purely thermal phenomenon, average power should be the significant factor. The results showed that pulse-modulated and CW radiation resulted in *comparable* decreases in lens ascorbic acid. Weiter *et al.* conclude that a decrease in ascorbic acid is apparently a direct thermal effect of microwave radiation in rabbit lens culture, but were unable to find a critical threshold temperature for lens damage. Their results concur with those of Baillie (1970).

Nearly all of the reported effects of microwave radiation on the lens can be explained on the basis of thermal effect. The acute injury to the lens results in hydration of the lens fibers. This may be reversed if no further injury takes place, but with further insult protein denaturation results leading to permanent damage. The increased permeability of the capsule and increase in water content of the lens fit well with this theory and have been described as thermal effects. Decreased enzymatic activity may quite likely be due to thermal inactivation and result in alterations in metabolism. All of these effects could be fully reparable until the altered metabolism has produced a permanent opacification of the lens. Latent period and time–power thresholds would be in agreement with a mechanism of this nature. The evidence at present tends to suggest that the effect is thermal (Michaelson, 1978).

18.7. CONCEPT OF THRESHOLD AND CUMULATIVE EFFECT

The concept of thresholds is that although exposures may produce a response at some power density if experienced for a sufficient period of time, a power density duration exists for which no response of any kind may be expected no matter how long the exposure. Stated mathematically, the threshold concept is a *nonlinear* relationship between dose and response at the initiation of the response as opposed to a wholly linear nonthreshold response relationship that passes through the origin (Stokinger, 1972).

Adaptation represents the most cogent and convincing basis for the existence of threshold, first through homeostatic mechanisms that commonly find their ultimate expression in tolerance and development against noxious stimuli. Stated in more mechanistic terms, toxicity is the net result of two competing reactions; reaction 1, the toxic substance acts on the body; and reaction 2, the body reacts to the substance. These reactions are the general basis for the attempt of the body to maintain normality (homeostasis) in the face of noxious stimuli, resulting in the utilization of a certain finite amount (dose) of a noxious agent without production of a toxic effect, hence a threshold (Stokinger, 1972).

Carpenter et al. (1960b; Carpenter and van Ummersen, 1968) found the threshold cataractogenic power density/time parameter for 2450 MHz CW or pulsed to be 120 mW/cm^2 for 1 hr. These investigators have suggested the possibility of cumulative damage to the lens from repeated "subthreshold" exposures to microwaves. This concept is based on studies in which the eyes of rabbits were directly exposed to 2450 MHz at power densities ranging from 80 to 280 mW/cm^2.*

In order not to confuse the suggested "cumulative" effect with that recognized for ionizing radiation, it is important to define the cumulative effect produced by ionizing radiation to put this point in its proper perspective. Cumulative injury from exposure to ionizing radiation is a manifestation of the irreparableness of a certain fraction of the injury, which has been designated "residual radiation injury." Such residual radiation injury is additive with frequency of exposures and is not dependent on intervals between exposures once the full recovery potential has been realized (Blair, 1964). A cumulative effect is the accumulation of damage resulting from repeated exposures each of which is individually capable of producing some degree of damage. In other words, in the linear hypothesis for ionizing radiation, there is no concept of threshold for damage but rather any exposure produces some damage, no matter how limited in extent. Thus, many "small" exposures, even separated in time, may be equivalent to a large acute exposure if repair mechanisms are not effective or rapair time may be infinite.

Careful analysis of the work of Carpenter et al. (1960b; Carpenter and van Ummersen, 1968) as well as Williams et al. (1955) reveals that whenever cataracts are produced among animals subjected to different power densities, a *threshold* becomes obvious. This is an additional aspect of microwave exposure response that invalidates the concept of cumulative effect (Michaelson, 1978).

Carpenter and van Ummersen (1968) note that the cumulative cataractogenic effect of microwaves involves initiation of a chain of events in the lens, the end result of which is an opacity, and that this chain of events must be initiated by an adequate power density acting for a sufficient duration of time if it is to progress to the development of an

---

* It must be noted that the power density calculated in the investigations of Carpenter, Kinoshita, Merola, and van Ummersen is approximately 50% higher than reported. This is due to a repeat measurement of the field with a more accurate instrument (Carpenter et al., 1972a).

opacity. If either the power density or the duration of the exposure is below a certain threshold value, then the damage done to the lens is not irreparable and recovery can occur, provided sufficient time elapses before a subsequent similar episode. Most investigators agree that there is a critical intraocular temperature that must be reached before opacities develop. This temperature, as reported by various authors, ranges from 45 to 55°C. Obviously, no cumulative rise in temperature can occur if the intervals between exposures exceed the time required for the tissue to return to normal temperature. The cumulative effect to be anticipated, therefore, is the accumulation of damage resulting from repeated exposures each of which is individually capable of producing some degree of damage (Kalant, 1959; Michaelson, 1978).

Analysis of available data indicates that when the repeated exposures are near threshold and within the time frame of the latency, cataract does appear. When the time interval between exposures is longer than the latency period, the lesion does not appear, unless the power density/time relationship is *well* above threshold. The so-called "cumulative effect" is only a phenomenon confined to near-threshold exposures and of little practical significance in the context of thresholds for microwave-induced pathophysiological manifestations (Michaelson, 1978).

According to Zaret (1959), acute injury of the lens leads first to hydration, which is reversible providing no lens protein denaturation has taken place despite the fact that banding, striations, and opacification are evident. Hydration of lens fibers may last for many days. If the excess water leaves the lens before denaturation has occurred, no permanent residua result. If another thermal injury intervenes, however, at a time when the lens is partially damaged, there may be a summation of effect.

The concept of a cumulative effect remains controversial, especially since the investigators themselves (Carpenter *et al.*, 1960b) have never clearly stated what they mean by "cumulative." There are certain discrepancies in this assumption. Carpenter *et al.* (1960b) have noted that the latency for production of cataracts is 3–6 days and found that the lesion occurs only in the narrow range of power density/time relationships below single exposure thresholds. With repeated exposures of $100\,\text{mW/cm}^2$ for 1 hr/day for several days, cataracts did not develop (Carpenter *et al.*, 1974). These studies confirm that the cumulative effect is observed only at a power density close to the single-exposure threshold cataract level, i.e., in the range $100-180\,\text{mW/cm}^2$.

At frequencies between 2.45 and 10 GHz when rabbits are irradiated in a free field below lethal thresholds, the cataracts are all posterior and not anterior (Carpenter and van Ummersen, 1968). Carpenter (1970) has shown that anterior cataracts are found only if the eye is close (0–2 inches) to a small hole in a waveguide or a small antenna.

The acute thermal insult resulting from microwave exposure is the predominant mechanism responsible for the production of lenticular opacities. It appears that intraocular temperatures in the range of 45–55°C must be reached before opacities develop. Thus, cumulative effects of microwave exposure would not be anticipated unless each single exposure exceeded the critical threshold level necessary to produce some degree of injury. Based on the experimental evidence, the threshold level is greater than $100\,mW/cm^2$ applied for more than 1 hr. A latency period of several days is indicated for the development of cataracts. *No one has yet been able to produce cataracts, even by repetitive exposures, when the power density is below threshold* (Michaelson, 1978).

Thus, after 35 years of studies of the effects of microwaves on the ocular lens, primarily in the rabbit, the principal conclusions are:

1. The acute thermal insult from high-intensity microwave fields is cataractogenic if intraocular temperatures reach 45–55°C.
2. The microwave exposure threshold is between 100 and $150\,mW/cm^2$ applied for about 60–100 min.
3. There does not appear to be a cumulative effect from microwave exposure unless each single exposure is sufficient to produce some irreparable degree of injury to the lens.

18.8. PROBLEMS IN SIMULATION STUDIES AND EXTRAPOLATION TO THE HUMAN

That cataract can be produced in rabbits by exposure to microwaves is well established. Extrapolating interpreted results from animal studies to humans can have serious consequences. There are some reports of microwave-induced cataracts in the human. The interpretations and conclusions are often equivocal. The mechanism and conditions of exposure required for cataractogenesis in humans still remain a matter of speculation since microwave exposure appears to be quite difficult to assess dosimetrically (Neidlinger, 1971). Dosimetry is a significant problem for all those engaged in microwave research. How reliable are the field strength measurements and, more important, how much incident or re-reflected energy is actually being absorbed by the animals under test? Because their physical size approximates certain very short wavelengths, small animals such as rabbits, rats, and even dogs can absorb lethal amounts of energy from microwave fields that would not cause noticeable harm to humans.

In the performance of experimental studies on animals, it must be remembered that the changes in the organism depend to a major degree on the geometric dimensions of the animal, owing to the depth of penetration of microwave energy, which varies with wavelength. The experimental animal itself perturbs the microwave field, since it neither completely transmits or absorbs the energy incident upon it. Carpenter *et al.* (1972b) also found that the position of the animal in the field in relation to the position of the power source can change power density measurements by as much as 50%. They also determined that cages, animal restrainers, or supports made of plastic, other than expanded polystyrene, can perturb the field and thereby alter the conditions of the experiment; thus, the power density should be reported only as a measurement taken in the radiation field where the experiment is to be conducted and made in the absence of all perturbing factors, including the experimental animal. The size, shape, and orientation of the animal are unpredictable factors.

In much of the previous work on microwave induction of lens opacities, irradiations have been performed close to a dipole antenna with the eye positioned only a few inches from it. The near-zone radiation was largely confined to the animal's head with consequent difficulties in attempting to assess the level of microwave power acting on the eye. It does possess the advantage of limiting the radiation generally to the eye region. Far-zone radiation offers several advantages, including greater field uniformity and reliability and ease of power density measurements. However, a crucial disadvantage is that the whole body is subjected to radiation, and the resultant resonant heating may cause death from hyperthermia. Attempts to shield all but the target area by microwave-absorbent material alter the field unpredictably and thus preclude the advantages originally sought.

Carpenter *et al.* (1975) attempted to resolve this dilemma by placing a dielectric lens in the far zone and concentrating radiation on the eye positioned a short distance behind it. In this manner, the animal's body can be subjected to a relatively weak field, which, by the focusing action of the lens, is increased severalfold in the eye. The radiation was approximately 7–13 times greater than that to which most of the body of the animal was subjected. Their measurements show that the field behind a dielectric lens is less affected by the presence of the experimental subject in comparison to far-field exposure.

In principle, one could use an experimental protocol sufficiently large to demonstrate that "virtual safety" is obtained. The use of extremely large numbers of animals to establish safety may well be self-defeating. The almost certain occurrence of unusual syndromes in one or more of a large number of test animals, despite the fact that these may have arisen spontaneously, will require admitting the possibility that they may be attributable to treatment (Mantel and Bryan, 1961). Often the publication of preliminary results or incomplete studies, by their very nature, stimulates misinterpretation by unsophisticated abstractors and writers who in turn influence public opinion. In contrast, properly designed and completed experimental studies will only be benefitted by being subjected to proper scientific criticism.

It is essential to define the conditions under which animal experimental data may be seriously considered as significant with respect to human health hazard. It is essential that such experiments be conducted using properly acceptable methodology to ensure acceptable results.

REFERENCES

Addington, C., F. Fischer, R. Neubauer, C. Osborn, Y. Sarkees, and G. Swartz (1958) Review of work conducted by the University of Buffalo: Studies on the biological effects of 200 mc. In: *Proceedings of the Second Annual Tri-Service Conference on Biological Effects of Microwave Energy*, E. G. Pattishall and F. W. Banghart (eds.). University of Virginia, Charlottesville, p. 189.

Albert, D. M., and H. G. Scheie (eds.) (1969) *Adler's Textbook of Ophthalmology*, 8th edition. Saunders, Philadelphia, p. 22.

Appleton, B. (1973) Results of clinical surveys for microwave ocular effects. HEW Publ. (FDA) 73-8031.

Appleton, B. (1975) Comment. *Ann. N.Y. Acad. Sci.* **247**:133.

Appleton, B., S. Hirsch, and P. V. K. Brown (1975) Investigation of single-exposure microwave ocular effects at 3000 MHz. *Ann. N.Y. Acad. Sci.* **247**:125.

Auricchio, G., and M. Testa (1972) Some biochemical differences between cortical (pale) and nuclear (brown) cataracts. *Ophthalmologica* **164**:228.

Axelsson, U. (1968) Glaucoma, miotic therapy and cataract. *Acta Ophthalmol.* **46**:83, 99, 831.

Axelsson, U. (1973) Miotic-induced cataract. *Ciba Found. Symp.* **19**:249.

Baillie, H. D. (1970) Thermal and nonthermal cataractogenesis by microwaves. In: *Biological Effects and Health Implications of Microwave Radiation*, S. Cleary (ed.) HEW, PHS, BRH/DBE 70-2, p. 59.

Baillie, H. D., A. Heaton, and D. Pal (1970) The dissipation of microwaves as heat in the eye. In: *Biological Effects and Health Implications of Microwave Radiation*, S. Cleary (ed.). PHS, BRH/DBE 70-2, p. 85.

Barber, W. (1973) Human cataractogenesis: A review. *Exp. Eye Res.* **16**:85.

Becker, O. (1877) Pathologie und therapie des Linsen-systems. In: *Handbuch der Gesamter Augenheilkunde*, Vol. VI, A. Graefe und T. Saemisch (eds.). Sect. 5, p. 157.

Bettman, J. W. (1946) Experimental dinitrophenol cataract. *Am. J. Ophthalmol.* **29**:1388.

Bettman, J. W., W. E. Fung, R. G. Webster, P. O. Nuyes, and N. J. Vincent (1968) Cataractogenic effects of corticosteroids in animals. *Am. J. Ophthalmol.* **65**:581.

Birenbaum, L., M. Grosoff, S. W. Rosenthal, and M. M. Zaret (1969a) Effects of microwaves on the eye. *IEEE Trans. Biomed. Eng.* **BME-16**:7.

Birenbaum, L., I. T. Kaplan, W. Metlay, S. W. Rosenthal, H. Schmidt, and M. M. Zaret (1969b) Effect of microwaves on the rabbit eye. *J. Microwave Power* **4**:232.

Black, R. L., R. B. Oglesby, L. von Sallman, and J. J. Bunim (1960) Posterior subcapsular cataracts induced by corticosteroids in patients with rheumatoid arthritis. *J. Am. Med. Med. Assoc.* **174**:166.

Blair, H. A. (1964) The constancy of repair rate and of irreparability during protracted exposure to ionizing radiation. *Ann. N.Y. Acad. Sci.* **114**:150.

Boettner, E. A., and J. R. Wolter (1962) Transmission of the ocular media. *Invest. Ophthalmol.* **16**:776.

Burditt, A. F., and F. L. Caird (1968) Natural history of lens opacities in diabetics. *Br. J. Ophthalmol.* **52**:433.

Caird, F. I. (1973) Problems of cataract epidemiology with special reference to diabetes. *Ciba Found. Symp.* **19**:281.

Carpenter, R. L. (1970) Experimental microwave cataract: A review. In: *Biological Effects and Health Implications of Microwave Radiation*, S. Cleary (ed.). HEW, PHS, BRH/DBE 70-2, p. 76.

Carpenter, R. L. (1975) Comment. *Ann. N.Y. Acad. Sci.* **247**:154.

Carpenter, R. L. (1979) Ocular effects of microwave radiation. *Bull. N.Y. Acad. Med.* **55**:1048.

Carpenter, R. L., and C. A. van Ummersen (1968) The action of microwave radiation on the eye. *J. Microwave Power* **3**:3.

Carpenter, R. L., D. K. Biddle, and C. A. van Ummersen (1960a) Biological effects of microwave radiation with particular reference to the eye. *Proc. Third. Int. Conf. Med. Electron.* **3**:401.

Carpenter, R. L., D. K. Biddle, and C. A. van Ummersen (1960b) Opacities in the lens of the eye experimentally induced by exposure to microwave radiation. *IRE Trans. Med. Electron.* **7**:152.

Carpenter, R. L., E. S. Ferri, and G. J. Hagan (1972a) Lens opacities in eyes of rabbits following repeated daily irradiation at 2.45 GHz. *International Microwave Power Institute Symposium*, Ottawa.

Carpenter, R. L., E. S. Ferri, and G. J. Hagan (1972b) Perturbation of the microwave field by experimental animal and apparatus in biological research. In: *International Microwave Power Institute Symposium*, Ottawa, p. 196.

Carpenter, R. L., G. J. Hagan, and E. S. Ferri (1975) Use of a dielectric lens for experimental microwave irradiation of the eye. *Ann. N.Y. Acad. Sci.* **247**:154.

Carpenter, R. L., G. J. Hagan, and G. L. Donovan (1977) Are microwave cataracts thermally caused? In: *Biological Effects and Measurement of Radiofrequency/Microwaves*, D. G. Hazzard (ed.). HEW Publ. (FDA) 77-8026, pp. 352–379.

Cogan, D. (1950) Lesions of the eye from radiant energy. *J. Am. Med. Assoc.* **142**:145.

Cogan, D. (1959) Radiation cataracts in man. In: *Symposium on the Delayed Effects of Whole-Body Radiation*, B. B. Watson (ed.). Johns Hopkins Press, Baltimore, pp. 59–66.

Cogan, D., D. D. Donaldson, and A. B. Reese (1952) Clinical and pathological characteristics of radiation cataract. *Arch. Ophthalmol.* **47**:55.

Cogan, D. G., S. I. Fricker, M. Lubin, D. D. Donaldson, and H. Hardy (1958) Cataracts and ultra-high frequency radiation. *AMA Arch. Ind. Health* **18**:299.

Coren, S., and J. S. Girgus (1972) Density of human lens pigmentation: *In vivo* measures over an extended age range. *Vision Res.* **12**:343.

Cotlier, E., and B. Becker (1965) Topical corticosteroids and galactose cataracts. *Invest. Ophthalmol.* **4**:806.

Cremer-Bartel, G., O. Hockwin, K. Ganter, and H. Werry (1968) Additionskatarakt nach Corticosteroid-applikation bei Galactose-gefutterten ratten. *Ber. Dtsch. Ophthalmol. Ges.* **69**:436.

Daily, L., K. G. Wakim, J. F. Herrick, E. M. Parkhill, and W. L. Benedict (1950) The effects of microwave diathermy of the eye: An experimental study. *Am. J. Ophthalmol.* **23**:1241.

Dawson, W. W. (1963) The thermal excitation of afferent neurones in the mammalian cornea and iris. In: *Temperature—Its Measurement and Control in Science and Industry,* Vol. 3, J. D. Hardy (ed.). Reinhold, New York, p. 199.

Dickson, D. H., and G. W. Crock (1972) Interlocking patterns on primate lens fibers. *Invest. Ophthalmol.* **11**:809.

Duke-Elder, S. (ed.) (1972) *System of Ophthalmology Series,* Vol. 11. Mosby, St. Louis, p. 63.

Dunn, K. L. (1950) Cataract from IR rays. "Glassworkers cataract"—A preliminary study on exposures. *Arch. Ind. Hyg. Occup. Med.* **1**:166.

Durney, C. H., C. C. Johnson, C. W. Barber, H. Massoudi, M. F. Iskander, J. L. Lords, D. K. Ryser, S. J. Allen, and J. C. Mitchell (1978) Radiofrequency Radiation Dosimetry Handbook, 2nd edition. Tech. Rep. SAM-TR-78-22, USAF School of Aerospace Medicine, Brooks AFB, Texas.

Ely, T. S., D. E. Goldman, J. Hearon, R. B. Williams, and H. M. Carpenter (1957) Heating Characteristics of Laboratory Animals Exposed to Ten-Centimeter Microwaves. U.S. Nav. Med. Res. Inst. (Res. Rep. Proj. NM 001-056.13.02). *IEEE Trans. Biomed. Eng.* **BME-11**:123 (1964).

Ferri, E. S., and G. J. Hagan (1976) Chronic low-level exposure of rabbits to microwaves. In: *Biological Effects of Electromagnetic Waves,* Vol. I, C. C. Johnson and M. L. Shore (eds.). HEW Publ. (FDA) 77-8010, pp. 129–142.

Fischer, F. P. (1948) Senescence of the eye. In: *Modern Trends in Ophthalmology,* Second Series, A. Sorsby (ed.). Butterworths, London, p. 54.

Fisher, R. F. (1971) The elastic constants of the human lens. *J. Physiol. (London)* **212**:147.

Fisher, R. F. (1973) Human lens fibre transparency and mechanical stress. *Exp. Eye Res.* **16**:41.

Frey, T., D. Friendly, and D. Wyatt (1973) Re-evaluation of monocular cataracts in children. *Am. J. Ophthalmol.* **76**:381.

Geeraets, W. J. (1970) Radiation effects on the eye. *Ind. Med.* **39**:441.

Geeraets, W. J., and E. R. Berry (1968) Ocular spectral characteristics as related to hazards from lasers and other light sources. *Am. J. Ophthalmol.* **66**:15.

Goldmann, H. (1935) The genesis of the cataract of the glass blower. *Ann. Ocul.* **172**:13; *Am. J. Ophthalmol.* **18**:590.

Goldmann, H., H. Koenig, and F. Maeder (1950) The permeability of the eye lens to infrared. *Ophthalmologica* **120**:198.

Guy, A. W., J. C. Lin, P. O. Kramar, and A. F. Emery (1974) Quantitation of Microwave Radiation Effects on the Eyes of Rabbits at 2450 MHz and 918 MHz. Scientific Report No. 2 (January).

Guy, A. W., J. C. Lin, P. O. Kramar, and A. F. Emery (1975) Effect of 2450 MHz radiation on the rabbit eye. *IEEE Trans. Microwave Theory Tech.* **MTT-23**:492.

Hagan, H. J., and R. L. Carpenter (1976) Relative cataractogenic potencies of two microwave frequencies (2.45 and 10 GHz). In: *Biological Effects of Electromagnetic Waves,* Vol. I, C. C. Johnson and M. L. Shore (eds.). HEW Publ. (FDA) 77-8010, pp. 143–155.

Harding, J. J. (1969) Nature and origin of the insoluble protein of rat lens. *Exp. Eye Res.* **8**:147.

Harding, J. J. (1972a) Conformational changes in human lens proteins in cataract. *Biochem. J.* **129**:97.

Harding, J. J. (1972b) The nature and origin of the urea-insoluble protein of human lens. *Exp. Eye Res.* **13**:33.

Hirsch, S. E. (1975) Comment. *Ann N.Y. Acad. Sci.* **247**:133.

Hockwin, O., H. K. Muller, and U. Blaser (1964) Nachweis von Philocarpin im Kammer-wasser von Kaninchenaugen mit Hilfe der Polarographie. *Albrecht von Graefes Arch. Ophthalmol.* **167**:459.

Hockwin, O., T. Okamoto, H. D. Bergeder, W. Klein, L. Ferrari, and W. Streit (1969/1970) Genesis of cataracts: Cumulative effects of subliminal noxious influences. *Ann. Ophthalmol.* **1**:321.

Horner, W. D. (1942) Dinitrophenol and its relation to formation of cataract. *Arch. Ophthalmol.* **27**:1097.

Howland, J. W., and S. M. Michaelson (1959) Studies on the biological effects of microwave irradiation of the dog and rabbit. In: *Proceedings of the Third Annual Tri-Service Conference on Biological Effects of Microwave Radiating Equipments*, C. Süsskind (ed.). University of California, Berkeley, p. 191.

Kalant, H. (1959) Physiologic hazards of microwave radiation, survey of published literature. *Can. Med. Assoc. J.* **81**:575.

Keatinge, G. F., J. Pearson, J. P. Simons, and E. E. White (1955) Radiation cataract in industry: Review of the literature, discussion of the pathogenesis, and description of environmental conditions in an iron rolling mill. *Arch. Ind. Health* **11**:305, **12**:538.

Kenshalo, D. R. (1960) Comparison of thermal sensitivity of the forehead, lip, conjunctiva and cornea. *J. Appl. Physiol.* **15**:987.

Kikkawa, Y., and T. Sato (1963) Elastic properties of the lens. *Exp. Eye Res.* **2**:210.

Kinoshita, J. H., L. O. Merola, and E. Dikmak (1962) Osmotic changes in experimental galactose cataracts. *Exp. Eye Res.* **1**:405.

Kinoshita, J. H., L. O. Merola, E. D. Dikmak, and R. L. Carpenter (1966) Biochemical changes in microwave cataracts. *Doc. Ophthalmol.* **20**:91.

Koch, H., O. Hockwin, and E. Weigelin (1972) New aspects of cataractogenesis. *Isr. J. Med. Sci.* **8**:1562.

Kramar, P., A. F. Emery, A. W. Guy and J. C. Lin (1973) Theoretical and experimental studies of microwave induced cataracts in rabbits. In: *1973 IEEE G-MTT International Microwave Symposium—Digest of Technical Papers.* IEEE, New York, p. 265.

Kramar, P., A. Emery, A. W. Guy, and J. C. Lin (1975) The ocular effects of microwaves on hypothermic rabbits: A study of microwave cataractogenic mechanisms. *Ann. N.Y. Acad. Sci.* **247**:155.

Kramar, P. O., C. Harris, A. W. Guy, and A. F. Emery (1976) Mechanism of microwave cataractogenesis in rabbits. In: *Biological Effects of Electromagnetic Waves*, Vol. I, C. C. Johnson and M. L. Shore (eds.). HEW Publ. (FDA) 77-8010, pp. 49–60.

Langley, R. K., C. B. Mortimer, and C. McCulloch (1960) The experimental production of cataracts by exposure to heat and light. *Arch. Ophthalmol.* **63**:473.

Leeson, T. S. (1971) Lens of the rat eye: An electron microscope and freeze-etch study. *Exp. Eye Res.* **11**:78.

Lele, P. P., and W. Weddell (1956) The relationship between neurohistology and corneal sensibility. *Brain* **79**:119.

Lerman, S. (1962) Radiation cataractogenesis. *N.Y. State J. Med.* **62**:3075.

Liesmaa, M. (1972) Congenital cataract and Ectopia lentis. *Acta Ophthalmol. Suppl.* **112**:3.

Lubin, M., G. W. Curtis, H. R. Dudley, L. E. Bird, P. F. Daley, D. G. Cogan, and S. J. Fricker (1960) Effects of ultrahigh frequency radiation on animals. *Arch. Ind. Health* **21**:555.

Mantel, N., and W. R. Bryan (1961) "Safety" testing of carcinogenic agents. *J. Nat. Cancer Inst.* **27**:455.

McAfee, A. D., A. Longacre, Jr., R. R. Bishop, S. T. Elder, J. G. May, and M. G. Holland (1979) Absence of ocular pathology after repeated exposure of unanesthetized monkeys to 9.3 GHz microwaves. *J. Microwave Power* **14**:41.

McGuiness, R. (1967) Association of diabetes and cataract. *Br. Med. J.* **2**:416.

Matelsky, I. (1968) Non-ionizing radiation. In: *Industrial Hygiene Highlights*, Vol. 1, L. V. Cralley and G. D. Clayton (eds.). Industrial Hygiene Foundation of America, Pittsburgh, pp. 147–178.

Mellerio, J. (1971) Light absorption and scatter in the human lens. *Vision Res.* **11**:129.

Merola, L. O., and J. H. Kinoshita (1961) Changes in the ascorbic acid content in lenses of rabbit eyes exposed to microwave radiation. In: *Biological Effects of Microwave Radiation*, Vol. 1. M. F. Peyton (ed.). Plenum Press, New York, p. 285.

Michaelson, S. M. (1972) Human exposure to non-ionizing radiant energy—Potential hazards and safety standards. *Proc. IEEE* **60**:389.

Michaelson, S. M. (1978) Relevance of experimental studies of microwave-induced cataracts to man. In: *Current Concepts in Ergophthalmology*, B. Tengroth and D. Epstein (eds.). Soc. Ergophthalmologica Internationalis, pp. 105–124.

Michaelson, S. M., R. A. E. Thomson, and J. W. Howland (1961) Physiologic aspects of microwave irradiation of mammals. *Am. J. Physiol.* **201**:351.

Michaelson, S. M., R. A. E. Thomson, and J. W. Howland (1967) Biologic Effects of Microwave Exposure. Tech. Rep. RADC-TR-67-461, Griffiss AFB, Rome Air Development Center, Rome, N.Y.

Michaelson, S. M., J. W. Howland, and W. B. Deichmann (1971) Response of the dog to 24,000 and 1285 MHz microwave exposure. *Ind. Med. Surg.* **40**:18.

Muller, H. K., O. Kleifeld, O. Hockwin, and U. Dardenne (1956) Der Einfluss von Pilocarpin und Mintacol auf der Stoffwechsel der Linse. *Ber. Dtsch. Ophthalmol. Ges.* **60**:115.

Neidlinger, R. W. (1971) Microwave cataract. *IEEE Trans. Microwave Theory Tech.* **MTT-19**:250.

Newell, F. N., and J. T. Ernest (1974) *Ophthalmology: Principles and Concepts*, 3rd edition. Mosby, St. Louis, pp. 75, 317.

Ogino, S., and K. Yasukara (1957) Biochemical studies on cataract. VI. Production of cataracts in guinea pigs with dinitrophenol. *Am. J. Ophthalmol.* **43**:936.

Pirie, A. (1968) Color and solubility of the proteins of human cataracts. *Invest. Ophthalmol.* **7**:634.

Pirie, A. (1972) Cataract: An introduction. *Isr. J. Med. Sci.* **8**:1550.

Pirie, A., and R. van Heyningen (1964) The effect of diabetes on the content of sorbitol, glucose, fructose and inositol in the human lens. *Exp. Eye Res.* **3**:124.

Richardson, A. W., T. D. Duane, and H. M. Hines (1948) Experimental lenticular opacities produced by microwave irradiation. *Arch. Phys. Med.* **29**:765.

Richardson, A. W., T. D. Duane, and H. M. Hines (1951) Experimental cataracts produced by 3-centimeter pulsed microwave irradiation. *Arch. Ophthalmol.* **45**:382.

Rosenthal, S. W., L. Birenbaum, I. T. Kaplan, W. Metlay, W. Z. Snyder, and M. M. Zaret (1976) Effects of 35 and 107 GHz CW microwaves on the rabbit eye. In: *Biological Effects of Electromagnetic Waves*, Vol. I, C. C. Johnson and M. L. Shore (eds.). HEW Publ. (FDA) 77-8010, pp. 110–128.

Salit, P. W. (1936) Phospholipid content of cataractous and sclerosed human lenses; biochemical studies of lenticular changes. *Arch. Ophthalmol.* **16**:271.

Satoh, K. (1972) Age-related changes in the structural proteins of human lens. *Exp. Eye Res.* **14**:53.

Seth, H. S., and S. M. Michaelson (1965) Microwave cataractogenesis. *J. Occup. Med.* **7**:439.

Shilyayev, V. G. (1970) Effects of microwave radiation on the visual organ. In: *Influence of Microwave Radiation on the Organism of Man and Animals*, I. R. Petrov (ed.). Meditsina Press, Leningrad (NASA TT F-708), pp. 142–146.

Sliney, D. H., and B. C. Freasier (1973) Evaluation of optical radiation hazards. *Appl. Opt.* **12**:1.

Sorsby, A. (1962) Cataract: Some statistical and genetic aspects. *Exp. Eye Res.* **1**:296.

Sorsby, A. (1972) *Modern Ophthalmology*, 2nd edition, Vol. 1. Lippincott, Philadelphia, p. 649.

Stokinger, H. E. (1972) Concepts of threshold in standards setting: An analysis of the concept and its application to industrial air limits (TLV's). *Arch. Environ. Health* **25:**153.

Tarkkanen, A., and K. Karjakainen (1966) Kataraktbildung während einer Mioticabehandlung des chronischen Glaukoms mit offenem Winkel. *Acta Ophthalmol.* **44:**932.

van Heyningen, R. (1959) Formation of polyols by the lens of the rat with 'sugar' cataract. *Nature (London)* **184:**194.

van Heyningen, R. (1962) The sorbitol pathway in the lens. *Exp. Eye Res.* **1:**396.

van Heyningen, R. (1972) The human lens. III. Some observations on the post-mortem lens. *Exp. Eye Res.* **13:**155.

van Pelt, W. F., W. R. Payne, and R. W. Peterson (1973) A Review of Selected Bioeffects Thresholds for Various Spectral Ranges of Light. HEW Publ. (FDA) 74-8010.

van Ummersen, C. A., and F. G. Cogan (1965) Age as a factor in induction of cataract in the rabbit. *Arch. Environ. Health* **11:**177.

Vogt, A. (1932) Fundamental investigation of the biology of infrared. *Klin. Monatsbl. Augenheilkd.* **89:**256.

von Frey, M. (1895) Beitrage zur Sinnesphysiologie der Haut. *Ver. Sachs. Ges. Wiss. Math. Phys. Kl.* **47:**166.

Vos, J. J. (1966) Some Considerations on Eye Hazards with Lasers. TDCK-46027, National Defense Research Council, T.N.O., Medical Biological Lab., Rijswijk, Netherlands.

Waley, S. G. (1969) The lens: Function and macromolecular composition. In: *The Eye,* Vol. 1, H. Davson (ed.). Academic Press, New York, p. 299.

Wanko, T., and M. A. Gavin (1961) Cell surfaces in the crystalline lens. In: *The Structure of the Eye,* G. K. Smelser (ed.). Academic Press, New York, p. 221.

Weiter, J. J., E. D. Finch, W. Schultz, and V. Frattali (1975) Ascorbic acid changes in cultured rabbit lenses after microwave irradiation. *Ann. N.Y. Acad. Sci.* **247:**175.

WHO (1966) *WHO Epidemiol. Vital Stat. Rep.* **19:**433.

Williams, D. B., J. P. Monahan, W. J. Nicholson, and J. J. Aldrich (1955) Biological effects studies on microwave radiation time and power threshold for the production of lens opacities by 12.3 cm microwaves. *Arch. Ophthalmol.* **54:**863.

Zaret, M. M. (1959) Comments on papers delivered at Third Tri-Service Conference on Biological Effects of Microwave Radiation. In: *Proceedings of the Third Annual Tri-Service Conference on Biological Effects of Microwave Radiating Equipments,* C. Süsskind (ed.). University of California, Berkeley, p. 334.

Zaret, M. (1964) An experimental study of the cataractogenic effects of microwave radiation. Tech. Doc. Rep. RADC-TDR-64-273, Griffiss AFB, Rome Air Development Center, Rome, N.Y.

Zeller, E. A., K. G. Wakim, J. F. Herrick, W. L. Benedict, and L. Daily, Jr. (1951) Influence of microwaves on certain enzyme systems in the lens of the eye. *Am. J. Ophthalmol.* **34:**1301.

19

Epidemiological and Other Investigations in the Human

A number of retrospective studies have been done on human populations exposed or believed to have been exposed to RF/MW energies. There have been a few epidemiological studies of MW/RF exposure but these have generally been limited in scope (Silverman, 1979, 1980). Persons exposed while assigned to the military services or occupationally exposed in industrial settings have been the principal groups studied. A few other populations living or working near generating sources or exposed to medical diathermy have been or are being investigated (Silverman, 1979, 1980; Bureau of Radiological Health, 1980; Ruggera, 1980). Information about health status has come from medical records, questionnaires, physical and laboratory examination, and vital statistics. Sources of exposure data include personnel records, questionnaires, environmental measurements, equipment emission measurements, and (assumed adherence to) established exposure limits. Although there have been advances in measurement, microwave dosimetry still presents formidable problems for meaningful assessment in most epidemiological studies (Roberts and Michaelson, 1985; Silverman, 1979, 1980).

An early study on U.S. Navy personnel during World War II did not reveal any conditions that could be ascribed to radar exposure (Daily, 1943). Ten years later, a 4-year surveillance of a relatively large group of radar workers in the United States did not show any significant clinical or pathophysiological differences between exposed and control groups (Barron and Baraff, 1958; Barron et al., 1955). On the other hand, surveys of East European workers revealed functional changes in the nervous and cardiovascular systems (Gordon, 1960, 1966, 1970; Sadchikova, 1974).

Barron et al. (1955) reported results of a study conducted to evaluate changes in various physical and functional characteristics of radar personnel employed by an airframe manufacturer. The radars included S-band (2800 MHz) and X-band (9375 MHz). Exposure times and power densities for individuals were not given, but zones at various distances from the antenna were specified and used to define three ranges of power densities. The minimal average power density in Zone A was $13.1\,mW/cm^2$. Zone B ranged from 3.9 to $13.1\,mW/cm^2$. Zone C was $<3.9\,mW/cm^2$. The authors stated that because of the relatively low field power densities, personnel working in Zone C were eliminated from the study.

A total of 226 exposed subjects that had experience in Zone A were studied. The radar workers were characterized by their duration of exposure. Controls (88) were stated to have had no industrial radar exposure. Methods of selection of cases or controls were not specified. The age distribution of all subjects ranged from 20 to more than 50 years, with the majority under 40 years of age.

A decrease in polymorphonuclear cells was reported in 25% of the radar workers and 12% of the controls. An increase in monocytes and eosinophils was also observed for the exposed group, but in a later report (Barron and Baraff, 1958) these effects were attributed to a variation in interpretation. Platelet counts and urinalyses were similar between the two groups. Ophthalmological examinations revealed ocular anomalies of several diverse types in 12 exposed persons and 1 control.

The problems with this study that diminish its utility include the lack of statistical testing of the observed frequencies, the disproportionate number of exposed versus control subjects, questionable comparability of exposed and control subjects because of age, and lack of descriptive or adjustment techniques to handle potential lack of comparability, lack of information on attempts to control potential examiner or observer bias in examination, and lack of documentation of diagnostic criteria. In spite of these problems, since this is one of the earlier attempts at evaluation of human exposure, this report has considerable value.

In an extensive 12-year survey, 841 men, aged 20 to 40 years, occupationally exposed to microwaves for various periods, were examined for the incidence of functional disturbances and disorders considered as contraindications for occupational exposure to microwaves according to the criteria employed in Poland (Czerski and Piotrowski, 1972; Czerski and Siekierzynski, 1975; Czerski *et al.*, 1974; Siekierzynski *et al.*, 1974). The population worked under identical conditions except for the exposure levels, of which there were two subgroups. Workers in the first subgroup (507 individuals) were exposed to varying power densities between 0.2 and $6\,mW/cm^2$; in the second subgroup, power densities were below $0.2\,mW/cm^2$. No dependence of incidence of disorders, such as organic lesions of the nervous system, changes in translucency of the ocular lens, primary disorders of the blood system, neoplastic diseases, or endocrine disorders on exposure level, duration, or work history could be shown. The incidence of functional disturbances ("neurasthenic syndrome," gastrointestinal tract disturbances, cardiovascular disturbances with abnormal ECG) was found not to be related to the level or duration of occupational exposure. There were no instances of irreversible damage or disturbances caused by exposure to microwaves. (Czerski and Piotrowski, 1972).

Pazderova-Vejlupkova (1981) evaluated 95 employees (men and women) of radio-transmitting stations (0.3 to 30 MHz; 19-year mean exposure; mean intensity of electromagnetic field 80 V/m) and 58 employees of TV-transmitting stations (30 to 300 MHz; 7.2-year mean exposure; mean intensity of field, 2.9 V/m). No signs of morbidity were found. There were no reliable differences between these subjects and a nonexposed reference group.

Djordjevic et al. (1979) reported the medical evaluation of radar workers, aged 25 to 40 years, with a work history of 5 to 10 years. Specific frequencies of exposure were not cited but were stated to be within the whole range used in radar operations. Evaluation of the working environment was undertaken, including power density measurements. While the environmental analyses are not given, it was concluded that the workers were exposed to pulsed microwaves within a wide range of intensities but generally less than $5\,mW/cm^2$. The lower limit of this exposure may have been $1\,mW/cm^2$, but it is not clear from the discussion whether this estimate refers to the workers included in this study or to radar station personnel in general. The control group consisted of 220 persons reported to be similar in age, working environment, and socioeconomic status. The controls did not have work experience with microwave sources. Selection criteria or further descriptive information was not given for either the cases or controls.

Ten major endpoints or diagnoses were covered in the clinical evaluation, including ophthalmological examinations. The two groups were found not to differ with respect to the ten factors. The type of procedure was not reported. The groups also did not differ in terms of statistical electrocardiogram results or on multiple biochemical and hematological indicators. Radar workers did demonstrate more subjective complaints, including headache, fatigue, irritability, sleep disturbance, inhibition of sexual activity, and impairment of memory. Based on their survey of working conditions, the authors attribute the latter result to specific problems such as lighting or poor ventilation in the environment of radar workers.

The Medical Follow-up Agency of the National Academy of Sciences of the United States studied mortality and morbidity among 40,000 personnel of the United States Navy potentially exposed to radar. Graduates of technical schools for training in the use of radar and maintenance of equipment were compared with graduates of technical schools not involved with microwave energy. There was no indication that exposure to microwaves adversely affected mortality from all causes or from specific causes (Robinette and Silverman, 1977; Robinette et al., 1980). In this study the records of 40,000 U.S. Navy personnel who enlisted during the period 1950 to 1954 were examined. Approximately 20,000 had job classifications with maximum potential for exposure to radar, i.e., electronics technicians, fire control technicians, and aviation electronics technicians. A similar number of radio and radar equipment operators believed to have a minimal potential for exposure were used as a comparison group. No specific data on exposure or frequencies were provided; however, the authors state that the low-exposure group of radio and radar operators was exposed to levels well below $1\,\text{mW/cm}^2$, whereas the high-exposure occupations on the average may perhaps have involved levels below $1\,\text{mW/cm}^2$ for duty hours, but infrequently included exposures $>10\,\text{mW/cm}^2$, perhaps as high as $100\,\text{mW/cm}^2$. The authors found no apparent difference in the long-term mortality patterns between the two exposure groups more than 20 years postexposure.

This study was preceded by a survey to investigate physiological and physical effects among U.S. Navy crewmen who could have been exposed to $0.1-1\,\text{mW/cm}^2$ aboard on aircraft carrier (U.S. Senate, 1977). No significant differences were found with respect to task performance, psychological tests, or biological effects. Blood study findings were within the normal range.

A study was performed on 4388 employees and 8283 dependents of the U.S. Foreign Service with more than 1800 employees and 3000 dependents at the Moscow Embassy and 2500 employees with 5000 dependents at comparison posts (controls) (Lilienfeld et al., 1978; U.S. Senate, 1979). Exhaustive comparative analyses were made of all symptoms, conditions, diseases, and causes of death among the employees and dependent groups of adults and children assigned to the Moscow Embassy during the period from 1953 to 1976, when the Soviets beamed microwaves at the U.S. Embassy. Comparisons were made with employees at other U.S. embassies in Budapest, Leningrad, Prague, Warsaw, Belgrade, Sophia, and Zagreb. The comparison group was chosen to be as similar as possible to the 1800 employees in the Moscow group for selection (posting) criteria and environmental influences except that the posts were not subject to microwave exposure (Lilienfeld et al., 1978). Exposures that ranged between 2.56 and 4.1 GHz at a maximum power density of $5\,\mu\text{W/cm}^2$ were documented from August 1963 to May 1975; the frequency range was expanded to 0.6 to 9.6 GHz in May 1975, and maximum power density was increased to $18\,\mu\text{W/cm}^2$ from August 1975 to February 1976. Exposures ranged from a low of 0.5 hr/day to 20 hr/day (U.S. Senate, 1979). No evidence was found that the Moscow group had experienced any higher mortality or any differences in specific causes of death.

Extensive effort was exerted to identify and trace the populations. Information on illnesses, conditions, or symptoms was sought from two major sources: (1) employment medical records were fairly extensive, which reflected examination requirements for foreign duty, and (2) a self-administered health history questionnaire. Questionnaire responses were validated for a stratified sample by review of hospital, physician, and clinic records. Death certificates were also sought, although other sources also were used to ascertain mortality status.

Standardized mortality ratios for various subgroups were developed for each cause of death, standardized for age and calendar period, and specific for sex. Similar procedures were applied to develop summary morbidity indices.

Hundreds of comparisons between the Moscow and control posts were made from information in the medical records. Various health problems were generally similar with two exceptions. Moscow employees had a threefold greater risk of acquiring protozoal infections than comparison post employees. In general, both sexes in the Moscow group had somewhat higher frequencies of most of the common kinds of health conditions reported. The authors noted that these most common conditions represented a very heterogeneous collection and it is difficult to conclude that they could have been related to exposure to microwave radiation since no consistent pattern of increased frequency of morbidity in the exposed group could be found.

Some excesses were reported by Moscow employees in the health history questionnaire. Both sexes reported more eye problems due to correctable refractive errors. More psoriasis was reported by men and anemia by women. The Moscow employees, especially males, reported more symptoms such as irritability, depression, concentration difficulties, and memory loss. It is possible, however, that a bias due to awareness of potential adverse effects is operating, since the strongest differences were present in the subgroup with the least exposure.

For both male and female employees, the observed mortality was less than expected based on U.S. mortality rates, with males having a more favorable experience than female employees. In both sexes, cancer was the predominant cause of death. The Moscow and comparison groups did not differ appreciably in overall and specific mortality. The authors noted, however, that the population was relatively young, and it may be too early to detect long-term mortality effects.

The authors concluded that no convincing evidence was discovered to implicate microwaves in the development of adverse health effects at the time of the analysis. But they also carefully discussed the limitations inherent in the study. No differences in health status by any measure could be attributed to microwave exposure (Silverman, 1980, 1985).

The overall mortality experience of the Moscow group involving all causes of death was more favorable than the comparison group. However, the female death rate from malignant neoplasms was slightly, but not significantly, higher than expected in the Moscow group, and the incidence of malignant neoplasms other than skin was significantly higher in the Moscow female group. In both cases, the numbers were very small. In the former case, there were seven different cancer sites involved in eight cases, which—according to the authors—virtually eliminates a single causal factor. In the latter case, there were ten cases involving seven different sites, and when exposure to microwaves was considered, it was found that the rate was highest for those who had minimum exposure to microwaves.

This study was preceded by a cytogenetic evaluation for possible mutagenesis performed on 250 samples from 71 State Department employees and family members before, during, and after assignment at the U.S. Embassy in Moscow (U.S. Senate, 1979). No genetic or other adverse biological effect among employees and dependents attributable to microwave exposure could be established.

A study was also conducted to determine the blood lymphocyte counts of adult employees and dependents of the American Embassy in Moscow (U.S. Senate, 1979). About 350 adults who were Embassy employees during the study period were examined; approximately 1000 foreign service personnel in the United States served as a comparison group. The higher average lymphocyte count found in the Moscow population did not correlate with microwave irradiation in the Embassy and was believed to be of microbial or protozoal origin.

Considerable publicity has been given to a death alleged to be due to microwave exposure.* This case was a workmen's compensation award and not subjected to litigation. The individual apparently was suffering from Alzheimer's disease, which is not uncommon in the general population. Alzheimer's disease has been recognized since 1903 and is not related to MW/RF exposure. At necropsy the diagnosis was bilateral lower-lobe bronchial pneumonia; the brain was not examined. The subject was never exposed to significant levels of microwaves. His activities required him to work at the back of a television transmitting system. He was never required to work in front of the "antenna dish," although even in front of the antenna dish, the power density would not have been greater than $1\,mW/cm^2$.

Finland has had one of the highest rates of cardiovascular disease (CVD) mortality in the world with the eastern provinces having higher

---

* *The New York Times* March 3, 1981; April 21, 1981; *The Philadelphia Inquirer* March 4, 1981.

rates of CVD than those in the west. North Karelia, an eastern province bordering on the Soviet Union, had been identified in the 1950s as having a particularly high incidence of CVD. Zaret (1976) suggested that RF radiation from Soviet communications or radar might be contributing to the incidence of CVD. He also stated without supportive data or references that "a new finding, an increased incidence of cancer, also appears to be emerging in North Karelia." The major thrust of the article was directed to the possibility of exploiting the North Karelia Project to investigate the role of RF energy in the evolution of CVD and carcinogenesis. The abnormal cancer incidence has never been verified, although the CVD frequency had been reported previously. Contrary to Zaret's (1976) implication, the high incidence of coronary heart disease in the Kupio and North Karelia areas of eastern Finland noted as long as 20 years ago is *not* related to the presence of Soviet radars. This high incidence of acute myocardial infarction in North Karelia had been surveyed in the 1950s by an international team under the leadership of Professor Ancel Keys of the University of Minnesota. One of the reasons for selecting Finland for the survey is that this country has a well-organized medical system with reliable census data. These surveys were included in a series of publications entitled "Coronary Disease in Seven Countries," which appeared as *American Heart Association Monograph* **29**, 1970. In this series of articles, it is noted that there is a high incidence of coronary heart disease in eastern Finland as well as other parts of the world. There are many factors extant in eastern Finland such as elevated blood pressure, hypercholesterolemia, and heavy cigarette smoking, all three of which are established risk factors involved in coronary heart disease. Also related is a distinct rugged, northern-latitude-lumberman life style. In 1971, the Finnish government, in conjunction with the World Health Organization, began a program known as the "North Karelia Project" (Puska *et al.* 1978). Its objectives were to decrease CVD morbidity and mortality by identifying the causative factors, devising means for primary prevention, and strengthening treatment and secondary prevention. Cigarette smoking, elevated blood pressure, and serum cholesterol levels were identified as the three major risk factors. The Finnish Project program, which extended from 1972 to 1977, was responsible for significant changes in diet and life style, which correlated with significant reductions in mortality from CVD.

19.1. NERVOUS SYSTEM AND CARDIOVASCULAR EFFECTS

Nervous and cardiovascular system alterations and behavioral effects of exposure of humans to microwave energy have been reported mostly in the Eastern European literature (Marha et al., 1968; Petrov, 1970; Presman, 1968; Gordon, 1960) and have been reviewed by Michaelson (1972, 1974, 1975), Michaelson and Dodge (1971), Dodge and Glaser (1977), Silverman (1973, 1980), and Albrecht and Landau (1979). Soviet and other Eastern European publications describe subjective complaints consisting of fatigability, headache, sleepiness, irritability, loss of appetite, and memory difficulties (Marha et al., 1968; Petrov, 1970; Presman, 1968; Gordon, 1960). Psychic changes that include unstable mood, hypochondriasis, and anxiety have also been reported. Most of the subjective symptoms are reversible, and pathological damage to neural structures is insignificant (Orlova, 1971). Functional disturbances of the CNS have been described as "radiowave sickness"—the neurasthenic or asthenic syndrome. The symptoms and signs include headache, fatigability, irritability, loss of appetite, sleepiness, sweating, thyroid gland enlargement, difficulties in concentration or memory, depression, and emotional instability. The clinical syndrome is generally reversible if exposure is discontinued (Silverman, 1979, 1980, 1985; Roberts and Michaelson, 1985).

Another frequently described manifestation is a set of labile functional cardiovascular changes including bradycardia (or occasional tachycardia) arterial hypertension (or hypotension), and changes in cardiac conduction. This form of neurocirculatory asthenia is also attributed to nervous system influence. Effects indicated by hypotonus, bradycardia, delayed auricular and ventricular conduction, decreased blood pressure, ECG alterations in workers in RF/MW fields have been reported (Gordon, 1966; Sadchikova, 1974; Sadchikova and Orlova, 1958). The identification and assessment of these poorly defined, nonspecific complaints, and symptom-complexes is extremely difficult (Silverman, 1973). These changes, however, do not diminish the capacity to work and are reversible (Osipov, 1965). No serious cardiovascular disturbances have been noted in humans or animals as a result of microwave exposure (Edelwejn et al., 1974).

Several reviewers (Silverman, 1979, 1980; Michaelson, 1975; Michaelson and Dodge, 1971; Dodge and Glaser, 1977; Albrecht and Landau, 1979; Guskova and Kochanova, 1975) have noted the difficulties in establishing the presence of and quantifying the frequency and severity of "subjective" complaints. Individuals suffering from a variety of chronic diseases may exhibit the same dysfunctions of the central nervous and cardiovascular systems as those reported to be a result of exposure to microwaves (Guskova and Kochanova, 1975); thus, it is extremely difficult, if not impossible, to rule out other factors in attempting to relate microwave exposure to clinical conditions. Most of the subjective symptoms are reversible, and pathological damage to neural structures is insignificant (Orlova, 1971). The difficulties in establishing the presence of and quantifying the frequency and severity of "subjective" complaints cannot be stated too strongly (Roberts and Michaelson, 1985).

19.2. OCULAR EFFECTS

Numerous surveys of ocular effects of MW/RF energies in man have been made, especially in the United States (Silverman, 1979, 1980). Most investigations have involved military personnel and civilian workers at military bases and in industrial settings. The principal factors of interest have been the significance of minor lens changes in the cataractogenic process and cataracts (opacities impairing vision). Several cases of cataract attributed to microwave exposure have been reported, but substantiation has not been established. There is no clinical or experimental evidence that ocular lens damage allegedly due to microwave exposure is morphologically different from lens abnormalities from other causes, including aging. That cataract can be produced in rabbits by exposure to microwaves is well established. Extrapolating results from animal studies to the human is difficult, because the conditions, durations, and intensities of exposure on the lens can be explained on the basis of thermal injury (Michaelson, 1978).

Several cases of alleged cataract formation in persons exposed to microwaves have been reported, but the precise details of exposure are generally impossible to determine. It is also difficult to relate cause and effect, because lens imperfections do occur in otherwise healthy individuals, especially with increasing age. Numerous drugs, industrial chemicals, and certain metabolic diseases are associated with cataracts.

Barron et al. (1955), Barron and Baraff (1958), and Daily (1943) did not find changes in the eyes of people working with radar. A case has been reported where a technician exposed his eyes to 4000–5000 MHz for 1 year with resultant cataract production (Hirsch, 1970; Hirsch and Parker, 1952). He received frequent and lengthy exposures at close range directly in the field to estimated power densities in excess of 100 mW/cm^2. Bilateral posterior subcapsular opacities, as well as nuclear opacification, developed. He was also noted to have, in the left eye, cells in the aqueous and vitreous humors, vitreous opacities, and choroiditis. Hirsch (1970) believes that the significant exposure occurred in the 3 days prior to onset of symptoms. This seems to be an unconvincingly short latent period for production of moderately advanced cataracts. Also significant is the possibility that the patient had a recurrent uveitis and chorioretinitis associated with vitreous opacities and secondary cataracts. The case, therefore, would not appear to be conclusive of a cataractogenic effect of long-term, high-level microwave exposure (Milroy and Michaelson, 1972).

Zaret and Eisenbud (1961) selected 67 age-matched pairs as a subgroup for statistical analysis. They used a semiquantitative scoring method (rated 0–3) to describe findings and used a chi-square test of the differences between the number of microwave workers with the same, lower, or higher scores. These findings were significant at $p < 0.01$ for both opacities and posterior polar defects. No statistically significant relationship was found between the opacity score and a numerical exposure index.

Zaret et al. (1963) conducted a study on the frequency of occurrence of lenticular imperfections in the eyes of microwave workers. The number of defects showed a linear increase with age. Although an apparent statistical difference in the score of lens changes between exposed and control groups existed, the difference was considered not significant from a clinical standpoint. According to Zaret et al. (1963), the extent of minor lenticular imperfections does not serve as a useful clinical indicator of cumulative exposure.

Utilizing Veterans Administration hospital records and military personnel records, Cleary et al. (1965) conducted a case-control of cataract formation among Army and Air Force veterans. This is the only case-control study focused on clinically diagnosed cataracts. The frequency of microwave exposure as denoted by radar work history was similar between cases and control.

Cleary et al. (1965; Cleary and Pasternack, 1966) found that although repeated subthreshold exposures may produce minimal types of lens changes, it did not appear to increase the incidence of cataracts in military personnel following operational exposure. According to Cleary and Pasternack (1966), occupational exposure to microwaves may be implicated as a stress that increases the rate of lens aging.

More complete follow-up of the Zaret and Eisenbud (1961) study was reported by Cleary and Pasternack (1966). Multiple regression techniques were used. They studied 736 microwave workers and 559 controls. Their initial evaluation using linear regression analysis for controls and microwave workers suggested earlier appearance of minute lens findings in the worker group. Chi-square analysis, however, of the two groups revealed that there were statistically significant differences in the age composition in spite of a close match in mean ages. Subsequent multiple regression analysis including age, duration of microwave work, and exposure estimates, resulted in age regression coefficients that were not significantly different from controls. Statistically significant differences between lenticular findings and various exposure variables (e.g., duration of work, average power output of equipment, reported overexposures) were noted; however, they were not always positive correlations. The authors went to considerable length to explain away their negative data and emphasize their positive correlations. Given the possibility of statistical artifacts, and variability of their reported results, one might easily interpret their study in the opposite manner suggesting that no relationship between lenticular defects and microwave exposure was noted. Estimates of actual exposure in terms of power densities were not made.

Majewska (1968) studied the eyes of 200 Polish workers employed from 6 months to 12 years at installations using microwave generating equipment operated over a range from 600 MHz to 10.7 GHz (2.8 to 50 cm). Although cited as high intensity by the author, intensity levels were not specified. Two hundred comparably aged unexposed controls were also examined. No methods of subject selection nor the sex of the participants were reported. After dilation of the subjects' pupils, lenses were examined with an ophthalmoscope and a slit lamp. It was not stated whether "double-blind" procedures were applied to mask the group assignment of the subjects for the examiners. Lens changes were noted in 168 of the subjects and 148 of the controls. This difference was calculated as statistically significant. The result was presented as a summary measure over all ages; age-specific differences were not presented.

In the same study, the effects of longer-term exposure were evaluated by comparing 100 controls to 102 employees, drawn from the original group, who had worked with high-frequency electromagnetic wave generators for over 4 years. Subjects were graded on a five-point scale for degree of lens opacity. The mean grade of opacities in the exposed group was greater than in controls in each 5-year age group ranging from 20 to 50 years of age. Among microwave workers, the mean grade of lens changes, uncontrolled for age, also showed an increase with length of employment. Although this part of the study was stated to be focused on employees with 4 or more years of work experience, the data on lens scores and duration of employment list results for persons with under 4 years of employment. This evaluation also suffers from the lack of quantitative measures of exposure. However, no authentic cases of microwave-induced cataracts have been described in the Polish literature, nor was this lesion found in an extensive occupational survey among microwave workers (Czerski et al., 1974).

According to Zaret et al. (1970), preclinical signs of microwave injury consist of roughening, thickening, and minute areas of opacification in the posterior capsule. It should be noted, however, that thickening of the posterior capsule of the lens is not a reliable criterion of microwave exposure since such changes exist in a variable manner in the population at large; they occur in many individuals with no exposure to microwaves; and they could be due to numerous other factors, e.g., metabolic diseases, trauma, drugs, and so on.

All of the cases of microwave cataracts reported by Zaret et al.

(1970) occurred in individuals working in the immediate vicinity of microwave generating or propagating equipment. Most were engaged in research, development, testing, or maintenance of high-power radar systems, and according to the authors had multiple exposures to power densities far exceeding $10\,\text{mW/cm}^2$. Many of these people had repeated exposures at several different wavelengths.

In case reports of microwave-induced cataracts (Shimkovich and Shilyayev, 1959; Zaret et al., 1970), cause–effect relationships have not been established. The development or detection of cataract has only been coincidental with the exposure to microwaves and most likely due to other causes such as uveitis, congenital cataracts, or to metabolic diseases such as diabetes that could cause similar types of cataracts (Shilyayev, 1970). On the basis of our present knowledge of the conditions under which experimental "microwave cataract" arises and of its diagnosis, it must be acknowledged that none of the cases described in the literature is fully verified since the exposure of the individual was not accompanied by painful sensation or even mild sensation in the surrounding area of the eye (Michaelson, 1972; Shilyayev, 1970). It is highly unlikely that an individual can be exposed to high-intensity microwaves for a sufficient length of time that can prove harmful, since he would probably feel the heat due to energy absorption, which would serve as a warning (Michaelson, 1972, 1974).

In November 1970 the United States Air Force Radiological Health Laboratory was directed to survey several EC121 aircraft ("Radar Planes") for X-ray, RF, and UV radiation. Only in the navigator's dome very near the glass was the RF power density above $10\,\text{mW/cm}^2$ and with the sextant in place it was impossible to get one's head in the dome. On March 11, 1974, a group of scientists including seven certified ophthalmologists visited Letterman General Hospital at the Presidio in San Francisco at which time 8 of a group of 65 former EC121 servicemen were examined by the ophthalmologists. Although each subjected had lenticular lesions ranging from cataracts to lesser opacities to minor abnormalities, the consensus of the examining opthalmologists was that these lesions were not different from what any practicing ophthalmologist might find in patients of the same age group, i.e., 34–56 years of age, regardless of history. None of the opthalmologists observed changes that could be used to justify the assignment of an etiology to microwave exposure. Of the 65 EC121 personnel, there were 3 cases of cataract. Only one of these had a stated history of having served on a U.S. Air Force EC121 plane.

Odland (1972) reported results of a survey of ocular anomalies in personnel from eight military installations. The population consisted of 377 exposed individuals and 320 controls. Exposure conditions were not specified. Exposed personnel were defined as individuals whose primary duties involved the operation or maintenance of radar equipment. Selection criterion for controls was duty that did not permit actual or potential exposure to radar. The actual work assignments of control persons were not stated. Medical histories were taken, and opthalmological examinations were performed in a double-blind manner. The occurrence of lens anomalies was similar in the two groups; however, the frequency of anomalies between control and exposed groups was different for individuals who had a family history of diabetes, non-traumatic cataract, glaucoma, or defective vision. Lens changes were noted in 29% of the exposed individuals with such a history versus 17% in the controls with a family history of eye problems. No statistical tests were applied to any of the reported frequency distributions. He did note, however, that the incidence of cataract had remained stable over a 10-year period, and that minor variations were well within statistical limits of random variation. The results did not indicate significant trends in incidence of cataracts within age groupings, except the rise with age, which is consistent with the natural history of this abnormality. Joly and Servantie (1970) also reported that there was no evidence of radar-induced cataract in the French Air Force over an 8-year observation period.

In a study by Appleton and McCrossen (1972), 226 individuals, occupationally associated with microwaves to varying degrees, some of whom had been included in the series reported by Zaret *et al.* (1970), were subjected to ophthalmological examination and were compared to a population not associated to as great an extent with microwaves. Microwave-exposed workers were defined as those who worked with Signal Corps electronic communication, detection, guidance, and weather equipment. Controls did not report such a work history. Likely intensities or frequencies were not specified. There were 135 control and 91 exposed personnel. Examination was conducted in most cases semiannually over a 30-month period. Some of the workers examined were involved in this type of work for 25 years. The examination results were similar between the two groups over all age groupings, although no statistical tests were applied. Appleton and McCrossen (1972) concluded that the available clinical evidence does not support the assumption that cataracts that develop in personnel performing duties in the vicinity of microwave generating equipment are a result of microwave exposure, unless a specific instance or instances of severe exposure can be documented and correlated with subsequent cataract development.

The survey was later extended to six other installations (Appleton, 1973). The exposure of military personnel was classified as "likely" versus "unlikely." The latter group served as controls. Blind procedures were utilized for the examining ophthalmologists, i.e., they were not aware of the exposure classification of subjects. The same team of examiners performed all tests, except at one location, in an attempt to minimize observer variation. The same three endpoints used in the 1972 study were also examined here. Older age groups demonstrated a trend toward opacities among exposed personnel, but, since the numbers in some age groups were small, this result is questionable.

Aurell and Tengroth (1973) and Tengroth and Aurell (1974) reported that in a factory where microwave equipment was tested there was an increased incidence of lens opacities among the workers. The exposure levels were sometimes ten times above the safety level, and discomfort of heat sensation was reported (Tengroth, 1983). None of the lens lesions, however, resulted in a loss of vision and therefore do not fit the definition of a cataract. The authors also reported retinal lesions in the paramacular and macular regions, which were more frequent in the exposed than in the control subjects. Such retinal lesions had not been reliably reported previously or since this isolated report. It was also noted that changes in the retina resembling chorioretinal scars were present in a significant number of individuals. Regrettably, the authors gave no exposure data to permit proper assessment of this material. Tengroth (1983) has suggested that "temperature changes in the delicate neuronal tissues of the retina" must be considered in these cases. Appleton and McCrossen (1972) and Zydecki (1974) have noted that no particular morphological features distinguish lens opacities in microwave workers from those seen in a control population.

Zydecki (1974) proposed the establishment of criteria for the evaluation of lens translucency. To this end he examined three groups: 1000 subjects exposed to different levels of microwaves, about $0.1 \text{ mW}/\text{cm}^2$ or more and $0.01 \text{ mW}/\text{cm}^2$ or less; 1000 unexposed controls matched by age; and 1000 minors aged 5–17 years. Lens defects were more common in the higher exposure group. This study has several defects such as: there was no discussion of sample selection criteria, age distributions were not presented, and statistical testing for significant associations was mentioned but not discussed.

Siekierzynski et al. (1974) reported on a survey in which the incidence of lenticular opacities was examined in 841 microwave workers with various periods of occupational exposure at 2 to $60 \text{ W}/\text{m}^2$ (507 individuals) or at below $2 \text{ W}/\text{m}^2$ (334 individuals). The incidence of lenticular opacities was compared between these groups, as well as analyzed within each group, subdivided according to age or duration of occupational exposure. No dependence of the incidence of lenticular opacities on the exposure level or duration was found. A statistically significant correlation with age was found.

In a report by Czerski and Siekierzynski (1975), no authentic cases of "microwave cataracts" have been described in the Polish literature, nor was this lesion found in an extensive occupational survey among microwave workers. The authors suggest that in those reports where a higher incidence of lenticular opacities is noted (Zydecki, 1974; Majewska, 1968), these may possibly be related to poorly controlled exposure conditions.

Shacklett *et al.* (1975) reported eye examinations of 817 military and civilian personnel. There were 477 persons with a history of microwave exposure and 340 controls without exposure drawn from eight Air Force bases between November 1971 and December 1974. The authors stated detailed work histories were taken (including time with and type of equipment), but information on typical exposure settings is not given. Local unit commanders selected the subjects using criteria established by the examining team. Standard diagnostic criteria were established. The same ophthalmologists performed all examinations and were not aware of whether a subject was considered as exposed or a control. No differences were noted between the two groups in the frequency of opacities, vacuoles, and posterior subcapsular iridescence. The results were stated not to be statistically significant; the type of test was not stated. An age-dependent increase in lens changes was noted for both groups.

As noted by Hathaway *et al.* (1977), the U.S. Army began an organized and concerted effort to perform medical surveillance on microwave workers in 1968. Ocular examinations were performed on 705 microwave workers. The age range of workers was 20–65 years. The number of years of work with microwave equipment varied from less than 1 year to 35 years. A summary of the first 5 years of experience was reported by Appleton *et al.* (1975). They could not demonstrate any difference between potentially exposed workers and the control group. Completion of 6 years of examination did not reveal any evidence of lenticular or retinal defects that could be attributed to microwave exposure.

A study of 2946 patients born after 1910, who had been treated for cataracts in Veterans Administration Hospitals in the United States in the period 1950 to 1962, compared their exposure to radar with that of 2164 controls (men with adjacent hospital register numbers). No association between exposure to radar and risk of cataracts was found (Robinette *et al.*, 1980).

Daily and Daily (1965) have reviewed the application of microwave diathermy in the treatment of diseases of the eye. In addition, clinical application of 2450-MHz microwaves has been reported by Clark (1952), Burmeister (1956), and Raue (1963). Such information can no doubt be used to establish the criteria for alleged cataractogenesis in man from microwave exposure.

Clark (1952) generally used 90 to 240 mW/cm^2 (2450 MHz) and treated the open eyes daily for 15 min, sometimes as long as 9 months. Eye examination was performed at regular intervals during the course of treatment and for several months after treatment had been terminated. The author noted that although many of his patients received very large numbers of treatments, he never observed any damage to the crystalline lens.

Burmeister (1956) directed 150–180 mW/cm^2 (2450 MHz), from an 8-cm circular reflector at a distance of 5 cm from the eyes, 10 min daily for from 6 to 20 days, and in stubborn cases for 6 weeks. Careful examination of the eyes before and after exposures showed no pathological changes—neither dilatation of retinal vessels nor alteration of intraocular pressure. Davies (1952) and Clark (1952) noted that in 100 and 95 cases, respectively, in which microwave diathermy (ca. 175 mW/cm^2) was used to treat a variety of eye diseases, there was no evidence of lens damage from the treatment.

If one carefully reviews the human data that are available, information derived from human case reports and studies actually adds little to our knowledge of microwave cataractogenesis. The human data do not even provide very conclusive evidence that microwave exposure causes cataracts in man. None of the case reports of cataracts can be conclusively attributed to microwave exposure although in some cases there may possibly be an association. Retrospective studies of microwave workers have provided only a finding of clinically insignificant opacities, possibly representing an aging effect. Dosimetry generally has not been very good if available at all. In most cases, very rough estimates of intensity are given in terms of "exposure scores." No data are available on the frequencies to which workers have been exposed, and, in most cases, exposures have been in a wide range of frequencies. The scoring methods used for both degree of exposure and lenticular defects have not been particularly sound, and their validity has been questioned (Milroy and Michaelson, 1972).

Lens opacities have also been noted to appear at the locations of existing microscopic congenital changes and, on reaching a certain magnitude, progress no further even when there is no change in the occupational setting (Shilyayev, 1970). Such studies are only qualitative and do not give any relation between the actual power level and pathology. Thus, little can be concluded from the available human data case reports and surveys. Nothing at all can be said about cumulative effects, or nonthermal effects on the basis of these reports. Many of the microwave-exposed personnel may also have been exposed to X rays emitted from high-voltage tubes used in microwave generators. The extent and significance of these exposures are not adequately known. As ionizing radiation can also produce posterior subcapsular cataracts, it is possible that this could be an etiological factor in cataracts among microwave workers (Milroy and Michaelson, 1972). Similar types of posterior subcapsular cataracts have also developed in man after therapeutic administration of corticosteroids (Crews, 1963; Tarkkanen et al., 1966) as well as other drugs or exposure to various chemical agents (Gehring, 1971).

Neidlinger (1971) notes that there is no reason to believe that current guidelines are inadequate for the protection of personnel from cataract formation. Confusion has been created by reports that have alleged microwave injury without substantial proof. Great care should be taken to minimize confusion by avoiding exaggeration. At the same time, it is essential not to overlook any possibilities. Clarification as to the occurrence of cataract in a microwave worker population can be achieved in part by animal experimentation, by careful records of occupational exposure, as well as by visual and ophthalmological epidemiologic studies of microwave worker populations (Hathaway, 1978).

To date there is no known case in which microwave energy has been the proven cause of a human cataract. The fact that an individual develops posterior subcapsular cataracts and that at some previous time in his life had been, or may have been, exposed to microwaves does not automatically establish a cause–effect relationship. Even so, a number of retrospective studies have been done on human populations exposed to MW/RF energies. Cases of presumed microwave cataract have been reported in the literature (Hirsch and Parker, 1952; Hirsch, 1970; Shimkovich and Shilyayev, 1959; Zaret et al., 1970), but in no instance has convincing evidence been offered that microwaves are actually the causative agent. Most of the experimental evidence is based largely on studies with rabbits, dogs, and nonhuman primates. In these animal models, it appears that the level of microwaves that produces cataracts is so high that (except for the head) the animal's body must be shielded; otherwise, superficial burns and death due to hyperthermia would occur. It appears that microwave exposure at cataractogenic levels cannot be tolerated by experimental animals unless they have been previously anesthetized. The cataractogenic level in rabbits is many times higher than the maximum exposure allowed by our most permissive safety standards, and there is no experimental evidence to support the hypothesis that subthreshold exposures have late cumulative effects.

As noted by Appleton (1974a,b), there is no clinical or experimental evidence that lens damage due to microwave energy is morphologically different from lens abnormalities from other causes, including the aging process. The idea that there is a microwave radiation signature on the lens, i.e., that signs of microwave lens damage are pathognomonic, or even characteristic, has little support from the evidence at hand. Based on the available evidence, both clinical and experimental, the following conclusions appear reasonable:

1. Lens damage probably has not occurred in humans from repeated exposure to low levels of microwave energy.
2. Lens damage probably could not occur in a human from acute exposure to microwave energy without associated severe facial burns (Appleton, 1974b).

In the assessment of microwave radiation as a hazard to the human eye, it must be expected that any attempt to establish, ex post facto, a clear cause–effect relationship in suspected or alleged human cases will encounter difficulty. Nevertheless, the scientific scrutiny accorded these cases must be no less demanding than that applied to conclusions based on animal experimentation. Sensationalism and overspeculation must also be avoided. It does appear that microwave ovens, microwave diathermy, and military radar are safe to humans if existing standards of safety are observed, and there is an extremely wide margin of safety already built into these standards.

In 1972, Working Group 35 of the National Research Council on Ocular Effects of Microwave Radiation concluded that the effects of microwave exposure on the human eye appeared to be thermal in nature; at least nonthermal effects have not been specifically isolated. The time–temperature history of the lens probably determines the development of opacities in the lens. There is no current evidence that cataract production depends on the pulse modulation frequency of the absorbed radiation. Thus, average power measurements should be the most meaningful in practical situations.

Based on a review of all the information available, the Working Group stated that it could see no reason to deviate from the safety standard of $10\,\text{mW/cm}^2$ with regard to any potential ocular effect. No member of the Working Group knew of evidence that would justify stating that $10\,\text{mW/cm}^2$ is unsafe as far as the eye is concerned.

On the basis of what is known today, it is doubtful that there is such an entity as a clinical microwave cataract. It appears that the ophthalmologist must make a presumptive assignment of the etiology based on the possibility of previous exposure to what is often an unknown amount of radiation. The preponderance of evidence indicates that a minimum critical temperature must be exceeded to form a cataract. There is no known rate of progression for growth and development of a cataract. One is unable to conclude in any given instance that the cataract has or has not been accelerated in its rate of progression by reason of any insult.

According to Zaret, the first sign of a microwave cataract is a thickening and roughening of the posterior capsule of the lens. He considers the thickness of the capsule to be about 1 µm. According to most authorities, in the human the thickest portion of the capsule is at the posterior pole of the lens where it is 4 µm thick. It varies over the posterior capsule and at about 1 mm from the equator it may be 23 µm thick. The powers supplied by the slit lamp will not reveal this difference (Carpenter, 1975).

Although Zaret (Zaret *et al.*, 1970) mentions a latency of 10 or 20 years, there is no evidence in the literature that supports a long latency period for microwave cataractogenesis. Zaret has stated that "careful slit-lamp examination discloses that the microwave injured capsule becomes opaque, thickened and rough." According to Appleton (1975), Zaret's contention of capsulopathy is not supported by evidence in the literature nor by observations by those investigators performing microwave research. The thickness of the posterior capsule is such that it is almost unidentifiable under the biomicroscope or slit lamp. Therefore, to claim roughening and thickening is inappropriate (Appleton, 1975). Carpenter (1975) concurs in this statement. Donaldson (1975) has stated that to his knowledge, no ophthalmologist has ever seen the changes Zaret describes in the posterior capsule, and he has never seen a cataract that could unequivocally be attributed to microwave radiation. One should note, however, the report by Bouchat and Marsol (1967), which notes capsular thickening as a result of microwave exposure. Zaret has noted that "if seen for the first time it is impossible for the ophthalmologist to determine the etiology of the cataract except by presumptive history of exposure."

There is no clinical or experimental evidence that lens damage due to microwave energy is morphologically different from lens abnormalities due to other causes including the aging process. No particular morphological features distinguish lens opacities in microwave workers from those seen in a control population (Appleton, 1974a,b; Appleton and McCrossen, 1972; Zaret *et al.*, 1970; Zydecki, 1974). Based on the available evidence, both clinical and experimental, it can thus be concluded that lens damage probably has not occurred in humans from repeated exposure to low levels of microwave energy (Appleton, 1973, 1974a,b).

Lenticular defects too minor to affect visual acuity have been studied as possible early markers of microwave exposure or precursors of cataracts. The studies have been mainly prevalence surveys, although the time periods are often variable or not specified; reexamination data rarely permit estimates of incidence. Some generalizations, however, can be made about observations of lens changes in microwave workers and comparison groups:

1. Lens imperfections occur normally and increase considerably with age among employed males studied. There is evidence that lens changes increase with age even during childhood (Zydecki, 1974). By about age 50, lens defects have been reported in most comparison subjects, based on data from various studies.
2. Although a few suggestive differences have been reported (Zydecki, 1974; Cleary and Pasternack, 1966; Majewska, 1968), there is no clear indication that minor lens defects are a marker for microwave exposure in terms of type or frequency of changes, exposure factors, or occupation (Silverman, 1979, 1980). The reported earlier appearance of lens defects in microwave workers than in comparison groups is not convincing because there is considerable variation in the type, number, and size of defects recorded, in the scoring methods used by different observers, and in the number examined.
3. Clinically significant lens changes, which would permit selection of individuals to be followed up, have not been identified (Zaret et al., 1963).
4. There is no evidence from ophthalmological surveys to date that minor lens opacities are precursors of clinical cataracts (Silverman, 1979, 1980); a case control study of World War II and Korean War veterans was negative for cataract (Cleary et al., 1965).

Neither definition nor methods of detection of cataract are standardized (Silverman, 1979, 1980). The common meaning of cataract, a lens opacity that interferes with visual acuity, is open to many interpretations as to degree and nature of the opacity and loss of visual acuity. Specific disorders, physical agents, and injuries are known to cause cataracts but many cataracts are loosely called "senile" when they occur after middle age. Alleged "microwave cataracts" are not distinguishable from other cataracts, in the opinion of most opthalmologists (Shacklett et al., 1975; Hathaway et al., 1977; Hathaway, 1978; Appleton, 1973).

The most prominent characteristic of cataracts is their age distribution. Although estimates of frequency are not comparable because of differences in the population groups surveyed, as well as nonuniform methods of detection and definition, all point to low frequencies until about the fifth decade of life, when sharp increases occur. Although not comparable with general population figures, recorded mean annual incidence rates are of the order of 2 per 100,000 (Silverman, 1979, 1980).

In a preliminary national estimate by age of the total prevalence of cataracts in the civilian noninstitutionalized population aged from 1 to 74 in the United States, one or more cataracts was found in 9% of the population (U.S. DHEW, 1979). For the various age groups under 45, the frequency of the condition increased gradually from 0.4% in those aged 1–5 years to 4% in those aged 35–44. The pronounced increase that occurs after age 45 reaches a maximum in the oldest group examined: of those aged 65–74, over half had cataracts. Cataract data for personnel on active duty in the armed services (who are mainly healthy, relatively young men) are available as incidence rates that show similar age dependence up to about age 55 (Odland, 1972). Parenthetically, in the United States as of August 1981, no legal proceeding with regard to alleged microwave-induced cataract in man has been ruled in favor of the plaintiff. As noted by a Working Group of the U.S. National Research Council (NRC, 1981), retrospective studies of workers have not revealed any evidence of cataract attributable to microwave exposure.

19.3. FERTILITY AND STERILITY

Although studies indicate that high-power-density exposure can affect the testes and ovaries, these responses can be related to the heating of the organs; the sensitivity of the testes to heat is well known (van Demark and Free, 1973). The power densities associated with testicular damage are generally high; Baranski and Czerski's (1976) review of more than 20 experimental reports provides numbers that range from 10 to 400 mW/cm^2.

Reports of human sterility or infertility from exposure to microwaves are questionable. Barron *et al.* (1955; Barron and Baraff, 1958) found no evidence of changes in fertility among men occupationally exposed to microwaves. Their study, however, was not designed to assess adverse effects on the testes. There is one case report of altered fertility in a man from unusually large exposures to microwaves (Rosenthal and Beering, 1968). In this report, radar was implicated as being responsible for oligospermia and infertility in a young man previously demonstrated to be fecund. The difficulty in evaluating this report is that there was no preexposure examination of this individual, so any causal relationship is very tenuous. The authors did not designate an exposure level, but did note that the patient frequently performed maintenance on the radar antenna while the equipment was in operation; he did not wear protective clothing, and he was exposed repeatedly to microwave power densities more than 3000 times the protection guide number (10 mW/cm^2) of the U.S. Air Force at that time.

Lancranjan et al. (1975) studied a population of 31 adult males (mean age 33 years) with a mean exposure of 8 years (range 1 to 17 years) to 3.6- to 10-GHz electromagnetic fields that "frequently were in the range of tens to hundreds of $\mu W/cm^2$." A group of 30 men of similar mean age and no known exposure to microwaves served as a control for the semen and hormone analysis. Statistical analysis of the results showed no differences in urinary content of 17-ketosteroids or total gonadotropin between exposed and control groups. Statistically significant decreases were reported for exposed personnel in the number of sperm per milliliter of semen, percent of motile sperm in the ejaculate, and the percent of normal sperm.

Marha (1970) and Marha et al. (1968) have cited decreased spermatogenesis, altered birth sex ratios, changes in menstrual patterns, retarded fetal development, congenital defects in neonates, and decreased lactation in nursing mothers working in RF fields. According to these authors, such effects occur at microwave exposure intensities greater than $10\,mW/cm^2$. The influence of intervening or cofactors such as noise or general working conditions was not mentioned in these reports.

19.4. GROWTH AND DEVELOPMENT

Five cases of inborn defects in offspring of women exposed during the early stages of pregnancy to shortwave diathermy have been reported (Cocorra et al., 1960; Rubin and Erdman, 1959; Minecki, 1967). Assessment of these reports requires considerable circumspection. Neither conception nor pregnancy was disturbed by therapeutic microwave diathermy (Rubin and Erdman, 1959). Such therapeutic interventions by their very nature employ very high intensities. Also, the medical reason for treatment is not always clear.

A few human data are available from studies in which RF heating of the pelvic region was used to treat gonorrhea, pelvic inflammatory disease, endometriosis, carcinoma of the uterus, or pelvic peritonitis. In one report (Gellhorn, 1928), the pelvic temperature in women was raised to 115°F (46°C). Although the author was concerned about possible harmful effects, he did not allude to specific complications. In another report, four women were treated with microwave diathermy (2450 MHz, 100-W output) for chronic pelvic inflammatory disease before or during pregnancy (Rubin and Erdman, 1959). Three women delivered normal infants; the fourth, who received eight treatments during the first 59 days of pregnancy, aborted on day 67 but delivered a normal baby after a subsequent pregnancy during which she again received microwave treatment. The authors concluded that microwaves did not interfere with ovulation, conception, or pregnancy.

Microwave heating has been used to relieve the pain of uterine contractions during labor (Daels, 1973, 1976). The analgesic effect was found helpful in 2000 selected patients without obstetric pathology, and the babies were born healthy with good circulation. No evidence of injury was manifested in a 1-year follow-up of the children; there was no evidence of mental retardation. Four cases of chromosome anomalies in controls and two cases in the irradiated group were noted. It is important to note that the human fetus at parturition is almost fully developed, and thus gross structural defects at this late stage of development would not be expected.

There are reported case studies of increases in congenital abnormalities in women working in RF fields in Eastern Europe (Marha et al., 1968), but there are no unequivocal reports of microwave-induced human teratologies.

A case-control study of Down's syndrome in relation to exposure to ionizing radiation yielded an unexpected finding regarding paternal exposure to radar (Sigler et al., 1965). Apparently, fathers of children with Down's Syndrome gave more frequent histories of occupational exposure to radar during military service than did fathers of unaffected children, a difference that was of borderline statistical significance. Exposure during military service occurred before the birth of the affected child. An excess of military service was seen for fathers of the children with Down's syndrome. This increase in military experience was not statistically significant. An increased history of paternal radar exposure as either radar technicians or operators was, however, significant for case fathers. After publication of the first report in 1965, expansion of the study group, follow-up of all fathers to obtain more detailed information about radar exposure, and a search of available military personnel records were undertaken. Cohen et al. (1977) enlarged the study, attempted to validate parental exposure/work histories, and examined karyotypes for evidence of chromosomal effects. The suggestive excess of radar exposure to fathers of babies with Down's syndrome was not confirmed in this later study (Cohen et al., 1977).

A report of congenital anomalies at a U.S. Army base (Peacock et al., 1971) suggested that during the 3-year period 1968–1971 the communities surrounding the base had reported a number of cases of clubfoot among white babies that greatly exceeded the expected number (based on birth certificate notifications for the State). This base was a training facility for fixed-wing and helicopter aircraft, situated within 35 miles (56 km) of dozens of radar stations. A more detailed investigation showed that in the six-county area surrounding the base, there was, during the same time period, a considerably higher rate of anomalies (diagnosed within 24 hr after birth) among births to military personnel than in the State as a whole. Analysis showed that apparently there were errors in the malformation data on the birth certificates and a probable overreporting from the Army base. Thus, convincing evidence was lacking that radar exposure was related to congenital malformations (Burdeshaw and Schaffer, 1973). The higher malformation rate across a group of counties of the State was presumably environmentally induced but no specific agent was suggested (Silverman, 1979, 1980, 1985).

19.5. CANCER

Microwave-induced cancer has not been reported or suspected in medical surveillance examinations of microwave workers or service personnel (Silverman, 1979, 1980). Two cohort epidemiological studies (Robinette and Silverman, 1977; Robinette et al., 1980; Lilienfeld et al., 1978) that looked into the question systematically did not show an excess of any form of cancer that could be interpreted as microwave related (Silverman, 1979, 1980, 1985).

19.6. CRITIQUE OF EPIDEMIOLOGICAL STUDIES

There is considerable difficulty in establishing the presence of and quantifying the frequency and severity of "subjective" complaints. Individuals suffering from a variety of chronic diseases may exhibit the same dysfunctions of the central nervous and cardiovascular systems as those reported to be a result of exposure to microwaves; thus, it is extremely difficult, if not impossible, to rule out other factors in attempting to relate microwave exposure to clinical conditions.

Although cataract has been incriminated for many years as one of the chief hazards of exposure to microwaves, it is not possible to accept the reports as proven. There is no clinical or experimental evidence that lens damage allegedly due to microwave energy is morphologically different from lens abnormalities from other causes, including the aging process.

If the available human data are carefully reviewed, information derived from human case reports and studies actually add little to our knowledge of microwave cataractogenesis. None of the case reports of cataracts can be conclusively attributed to microwave exposure. The scoring methods used, both for degree of exposure and for lenticular defects, have not been particularly sound, and their validity has been questioned.

Reports of effects in man must be put in perspective. Most epidemiological and incidence studies suffer from inadequate design and examination as well as lack of substantiation of actual power levels and duration of microwave exposure. It is essential that the multiple environmental factors be evaluated that may interact among themselves and with personal characteristics of the individual. There is always the danger that real factors may be overlooked, leading to a false association with factors of initial interest (Roberts and Michaelson, 1985).

An important concept of disease causation is that, in general, disease is not caused by a single factor or agent, but rather is influenced by multiple, interactive factors such as the subject and his environment. Health effects or manifestations of disease have a spectrum of intensity ranging all the way from the barely discernible and rapidly reversible symptomatic disorders, through an increasing gradient of severity to the point of irreversibility, to disease states of such gravity as to ultimately cause death. For electromagnetic fields, in common with most other agents, biological or physical, the trivial end of this severity scale includes detectable physiological effects, which are well within the range of physiological adaptation and do not constitute disease in any meaningful sense. The validity of application of the epidemiological method to the study of the health impact of an agent is largely determined by the ascertainability and definition of an effect.

There are numerous problems in designing epidemiological or incidence studies. Even if these problems could be overcome, it might involve an inordinate, even astronomic, cost. One problem is to select paired populations that are not systematically loaded with some other bias. The control or comparison group should be comparable with the case or exposed group in all relevant characteristics, except for the exposure itself. The report of the study should provide the data needed to assess whether the study has met these requirements, and should note potential biases in selection of subjects, in measurements, and in follow-up that may affect the inferences being derived regarding the effects of the fields. The sample must also be large enough to make it possible to detect an increased risk.

An outstanding problem of epidemiological studies of MW/RF exposure is related to exposure assessment. Typical of the situations existing in the literature are studies that provide no documentation of the basic elements of exposures such as frequency, modulation, and power density. Often only broad categorizations such as "exposed" or "nonexposed" are provided. Most of the reports on humans demonstrate a lack of adherence to rigorous study design, analyses, and discussion. Control groups are frequently lacking. Population selection criteria and methods are usually not described. Control of confounding variables, such as age, is often not considered. Applied statistical methods may not be described or largely because of study design do not measure the strength of association via relative risk or odds ratios. The majority of the studies are descriptive or cross-sectional in nature. It is thus often necessary to study a population of many thousands to get significant results. Perhaps the main limitation of epidemiological studies of RF/MW exposure is the lack of recognized pathophysiological manifestations at realistic levels of exposure as indicators for measuring the effects of the fields on man.

If reasonably controlled, occupational comparisons can be made for sufficiently long periods of time with groups that are comparable in important demographic, social, and health characteristics, possible health effects associated with electromagnetic fields can be evaluated. For example, if it can be demonstrated that highly exposed workers do indeed have more ill-defined complaints and illnesses, higher rates of absenteeism due to illness, poorer performance records, greater hospital clinic or physician attendance rates, increased liability to accidents, and the like, such leads are a valuable source for further investigations of specific electromagnetic effects. Psychosocial factors are important in assessing the effects of environmental or occupational insults. Weintraub (1975) found a significant overall relationship between job dissatisfaction and psychosomatic complaints.

Reports of occupational surveys of workers exposed to electromagnetic fields in the USSR and other Eastern European countries have engendered concern regarding "safe levels" of exposure to these fields. In general, the epidemiological or incidence studies from these countries may be criticized as being inadequate in scope and detail, lacking in statistical power, and not subject to review or criticism by peer scientists. Moreover, they often appear oriented to emphasize particular preconceived ideas. For example, functional disturbances of the CNS are repeatedly cited to explain a host of ill-defined symptoms and signs. In general, one can have little confidence in these studies and the environmental standards that have emerged from them. The philosophical approaches both to science and to safety standards differ so much from those accepted in the West that it is difficult to make comparisons.

Soviet and other Eastern European investigators describe such symptoms as listlessness, excitability, headache, drowsiness, and fatigue in persons occupationally exposed to electromagnetic fields. These symptoms are also caused by many other occupational factors, so it is not possible to define a cause–effect relationship. Many other factors in the industrial setting or home environment as well as psychosocial interactions can cause similar symptoms. The Soviets consider the CNS to be especially sensitive to all sorts of environmental insults. Their conceptual basis for the above viewpoint is largely centered about Pavlovian "nervism". Very briefly, this theory can be interpreted to mean that the

CNS exerts a controlling influence over all types of reactions in the organism, including various local tissue reactions. Other reactions are considered to be of only secondary importance. Thus, Soviet physiologists have persistently attributed environmental effects to a CNS mechanism that might be responsible for each environmentally induced phenomenon.

As with other areas of scientific research, Soviet publications typically lack descriptions of study methods and the selection and characteristics of controls in the detail that is standard for the West. They often fail to provide results that can be scientifically evaluated by the reader, and employ an idiosyncratic vocabulary that mixes empirical observations with hypothetical processes. Thus, any review of the Soviet literature must be read with appropriate caution.

The symptoms and signs commonly described in the Soviet and other Eastern European studies are regarded as functional disturbances of the CNS and are called the neurasthenic or asthenic syndrome. The term "neurasthenia" originated a century ago, but has been almost obsolete in the medical literature of North America for some decades. Another frequently described manifestation of exposure to electromagnetic fields is a set of labile functional cardiovascular changes. This form of neurocirculatory asthenia or vagotonic reaction, known as the vegetative dystonia or autonomic dystonia syndrome, is attributed to neural influence mainly from the parasympathetic division of the autonomic nervous system. A third group of findings, more serious but less frequent than the others, that includes hallucinations, insomnia, syncope, and inhibition of visceral functions is associated with electromagnetic radiation exposure and is called the diencephalic syndrome. In the clinical appraisal, routine neurological examination appears to add little to the history and general physical findings beyond descriptions of hand tremors, dermographism, and rare ataxia. Correlations between EEG changes and other clinical observations and subjective complaints have been made but do not appear consistent.

Studies of exposed working groups that report finding a neurological or behavioral character present serious difficulties. The difficulties stem from the many kinds of publications in which pertinent material is not presented, and the variability of the data presented. Most investigators do not describe how they selected controls for the exposed subjects; how one selects controls can affect the results markedly. In looking for emotional instability, psychological difficulties, and cardiovascular change, it is essential that proper instruments, techniques, and interpretations be used. These factors, added to the lack of objective criteria for assessing many of the observed clinical phenomena, the problems of subject variation and observer variability, and the inadequacies and uncertainties of field measurement and exposure data, make it impossible to determine from existing clinical studies whether electromagnetic fields can or cannot induce neural or behavioral changes in man.

In this context, Guskova and Kochanova (1975) dispute earlier Soviet reports of the relationship of cardiovascular diseases to electromagnetic radiation. According to these authors, it is very difficult to make etiological diagnoses of pathology of the circulatory system in groups of workers who deal with sources of superhigh-frequency radiations. This work involves tuning radio equipment or operating of radar stations, which requires a high degree of nervous and emotional tension and involves other deleterious factors. The incidence of hypertension with chronic exposure to SHF fields is comparable to the findings of a Moscow population survey according to WHO criteria. In addition to smoking and obesity, genetic factors and emotional stress, psychological personality factors that determine an individual's reactivity to environmental conditions are proven risk factors in the development of cardiac ischemia.

Guskova and Kochanova (1975) suggest, when diagnosing cardiovascular pathology in individuals exposed to UHF, in addition to assessing working conditions, it is also imperative to take into consideration frequently encountered causes of cardiopathy. When investigating working conditions, this should not be limited to demonstrating a high level of UHF fields; one must also pay attention to the extent of nervous and emotional stress, related to the occupation and the environment as well as to night shifts. They state: "as for the effects of microwave radiation on onset of cardiovascular pathology, in our opinion it may take a certain place among other deleterious factors. However, for the time being there is no reason to relate development of disease to it alone."

To draw causal inferences from results of prevalence studies is inherently difficult. This is so because the match between the empirical and the ideal population is unnecessarily poor. The investigator can exert no experimental control, since he cannot ascertain the time order of the changes in his independent and dependent variables. He is not able to refine his measures of exposure to the required degree.

A very cogent analysis of the problem in surveys of human exposure has been made by Czerski and Siekierzynski (1975), who noted that analysis of occupational exposure to microwave radiation is fraught with many difficulties. Of utmost importance is assessment of the relationship between microwave exposure levels and the health status of the examined groups of workers. The possible role of other environmental factors and of socioeconomic conditions must be taken into account. As often happens in such studies, it is difficult to demonstrate a causal relationship between a disease and the influence of environmental factors, at least in individual cases.

The problem of adequate control groups is controversial and hinges mostly on what one considers "adequate." Quantitation of occupational exposure is extremely difficult. This is particularly true when personnel move around in the course of their duties and are exposed to nonstationary fields, i.e., moving beams or antennas, as well as to near and far fields at random.

An important concept of disease causation is that, in general, disease is not caused by a single factor or agent, but rather is influenced by multiple, interactive components including the subject and his environment. Health effects or manifestations of disease have a spectrum of intensity ranging from the barely discernible and rapidly reversible symptomatic disorders, through an increasing gradient of severity to the point of irreversibility, and finally, to disease states of such gravity as ultimately to cause death. For electromagnetic fields, in common with most other agents, biological or physical, the trivial end of this severity scale includes detectable physiological effects, which are well within the range of physiological adaptation and do not constitute disease in any meaningful sense.

REFERENCES

Albrecht, R. M., and E. Landau (1979) Microwave radiation: An epidemiologic assessment. *Rev. Environ. Health* **3**:44.

Appleton, B. (1973) Results of Clinical Surveys for Microwave Ocular Effects. HEW Publ. (FDA) 73-8031.BRH/DBE 73-3.

Appleton, B. (1974a) Experimental microwave ocular effects. In: *Biological Effects and Health Hazards of Microwave Radiation*, P. Czerski, K. Ostrowski, M. L. Shore, C. Silverman, M. J. Suess, and B. Waldeskog (eds.), Polish Medical Publishers, Warsaw, pp. 186–188.

Appleton, B. (1974b) Microwave cataracts. *J. Am. Med. Assoc.* **229**:407.

Appleton, B. (1975) Comment. *Ann. N.Y. Acad. Sci.* **247**:133.

Appleton, B., and G. C. McCrossen (1972) Microwave lens effects in humans. *Arch. Ophthalmol.* **88**:259.

Appleton, B., S. Hirsch, R. O. Kinion, M. Soles, G. C. McCrossen, and R. M. Neidlinger (1975) Microwave lens effects in humans. *Arch. Ophthalmol.* **93**:257.

Aurell, E., and B. Tengroth (1973) Lenticular and retinal changes secondary to microwave exposure. *Acta Ophthalmol.* **51**:764.

Baranski, S., and P. Czerski (1976) *Biological Effects of Microwaves*. Dowden, Hutchinson & Ross, Stroudsburg, Pa.

Barron, C. I., and A. A. Baraff (1958) Medical consideration of exposure to microwaves (radar). *J. Am. Med. Assoc.* **168**:1194.

Barron, C. I., A. A. Love, and A. A. Baraff (1955) Physical evaluation of personnel exposed to microwave emanations. *J. Aviat. Med.* **26**:442.

Bouchat, J., and C. Marsol (1967) Bilateral capsular cataracts from radar. *Arch. Ophtalmol.* **27**:593.

Bureau of Radiological Health (1980) Annual Report of the Division of Biological Effects. Fiscal Year 1979, HHS Publ. (FDA) 81-8152, p. 34.

Burdeshaw, J. A., and S. Schaffer (1973) Factors Associated with the Incidence of Congenital Anomalies: A Localized Investigation. Environmental Protection Agency, Final Report, Contract No. 68-02-0791.

Burmeister, H. (1956) Results of irradiating the eyes with microwaves. *Klin. Monatsbl. Augenheilkd.* **129:**336.

Carpenter, R.L. (1975) Comment. *Ann. N.Y. Acad. Sci.* **247:**154.

Clark, W. (1952) Microwave diathermy in ophthalmology: Clinical evaluation. *Trans. Am. Acad. Ophthalmol. Otolaryngol.* **56:**600.

Cleary, S. F., and B. S. Pasternack (1966) Lenticular changes in microwave workers, a statistical study. *Arch. Environ. Health* **12:**23.

Cleary, S. F., B. S. Pasternack, and G. W. Beebe (1965) Cataract incidence in radar workers. *Arch. Environ. Health* **11:**179.

Cocorra, G., A. Blasio, and B. Nunziata (1960) Remarks on embryopathies induced by shortwaves. *Pediatria—Riv. Igiene, Med. Chir Infanzia* **68:**7.

Cohen, B., A. M. Lilienfeld, S. Kramer, and L. C. Hyman (1977) Parental factors in Down's syndrome: Results of the second Baltimore case-control study. In: *Population Cytogenetics: Studies in Humans,* E. B. Hook and I. H. Porter (eds.). Academic Press, New York, p. 301.

Crews, S. J. (1963) Posterior subcapsular lens opacities in patients on long term corticosteroid therapy. *Br. Med. J.* **1:**1644.

Czerski, P., and M. Piotrowski (1972) Proposals for specification of allowable levels of microwave radiation. *Med. Lotn.* **39:**127.

Czerski, P., and M. Siekierzynski (1975) Analysis of occupational exposure to microwave radiation. In: *Fundamental and Applied Aspects of Nonionizing Radiation,* S. M. Michaelson, M. W. Miller, R. Magin, and E. L. Cartensen (eds). Plenum Press, New York, pp. 367–377.

Czerski, P., M. Siekierzynski, and A. Gidynski (1974) Health surveillance of personnel occupationally exposed to microwaves. I. Theoretical considerations and practical aspects. *Aerosp. Med.* **45:**1137.

Daels, J. (1973) Microwave heating of the uterine wall during parturition. *Obstet. Gynecol.* **42:**76.

Daels, J. (1976) Microwave heating of the uterine wall during parturition. *J. Microwave Power* **11:**166.

Daily, L. (1943) A clinical study of the results of exposure of laboratory personnel to radar and high frequency radio. *U.S. Nav. Med. Bull.* **41:**1052.

Daily, L., and R. K. Daily (1965) Heat in diseases of the eye. In: *Therapeutic Heat and Cold,* 2nd edition, S. Licht (ed.). E. Licht, New Haven, Conn., p. 491.

Davies, R. H. (1952) Comment in Clark, W. (1952) Microwave diathermy in ophthalmology: Clinical evaluation. *Trans. Am. Acad. Ophthalmol. Otolaryngol.* **56:**600.

Djordjevic, A., A. Kolak, M. Stojkovic, N. Rankovic, and P. Ristic (1979) A study of the health status of radar workers. *Aviat. Space Environ. Med.* **50:**396.

Dodge, C. H., and Z. R. Glaser (1977) Trends in nonionizing bioeffects research and related occupational health aspects. *J. Microwave Power* **12:**319.

Donaldson, D. D. (1975) Comment. *Ann. N.Y. Acad. Sci.* **247:**134.

Edelwejn, Z., R. L. Elder, E. Klimkova-Deutschova, and B. Tengroth (1974) Occupational exposure and public health aspects of microwave radiation. In: *Biological Effects and Health Hazards of Microwave Radiation,* P. Czerski, K. Ostrowski, M. L. Shore, C. Silverman, M. J. Suess, and B. Waldeskog (eds.). Polish Medical Publishers, Warsaw, pp. 330–331.

Gehring, P. J. (1971) The cataractogenic activity of chemical agents. *CRC Crit. Rev. Toxicol.* **1:**93.

Gellhorn, S. (1928) Diathermy in gynecology. *J. Am. Med. Assoc.* **90**:1005.

Gordon, Z. V. (1960) The problem of the biological action of UHF. *Tr. Gig. Tr. Prof. AMN SSR* **1**:5.

Gordon, Z. V. (1966) Biological Effect of Microwaves in Occupational Hygiene. Izd. Med., Leningrad (TT 70-50087, NASA TT F-633, 1970).

Gordon, Z. V. (1970) Occupational health aspects of radio-frequency electromagnetic radiation. In: *Ergonomics and Physical Environmental Factors*. Occupational Safety and Health Series, No. 21, International Labour Office, Geneva, pp. 159–172.

Guskova, A. K., and Y. H. Kochanova (1975) Some aspects of etiological diagnostics of occupational diseases as related to the effects of microwave radiation. *Gig. Tr. Prof. Zabol.* **3**:14 (JPRS L/6135, 1976).

Hathaway, J. A. (1978) The needs for medical surveillance of laser and microwave workers. In: *Current Concepts in Ergopthalmology*, B. Tengroth and D. Epstein (eds.). Societas Ergophthalmologica Internationalis, Stockholm, pp. 139–160.

Hathaway, J. A., H. Stern, E. M. Sales, and E. Leighton (1977) Evaluation of ocular medical surveillance of microwave and laser workers. *J. Occup. Med.* **19**:683.

Hirsch, F. G. (1970) Microwave cataracts. In: *Electronic Products and the Health Physicist*. BRH, DEP Rep. 70-26, pp. 111–40.

Hirsch, F. G., and J. T. Parker (1952) Bilateral lenticular opacities occurring in a technician operating a microwave generator. *Arch. Ind. Hyg.* **6**:512.

Joly, R., and B. Servantie (1970) Biological effects of ultra-high frequency electromagnetic radiation (radar). Advisory Group for Aerospace Research and Development (AGARD), NATO, Conference Preprint No. 95, p. C9-1.

Lancranjan, I., M. Maicanescu, E. Rafaila, I. Klepsch, and H. I. Popescu (1975) Gonadic function in workmen with long-term exposure to microwaves. *Health Phys.* **29**:381.

Lilienfeld, A. M., J. Tonascia, S. Tonascia, C. H. Libauer, G. M. Canthen, J. A. Markowitz, and S. Weida (1978) Foreign Service Health Status Study: Evaluation of Health Status of Foreign Service and Other Employees from Selected Eastern European Posts. Final Report. July 31, 1978. Contract No. 6025-619073, Department of Epidemiology, Johns Hopkins University, Baltimore, NTIS PB-288, p. 1963.

Majewska, J. (1968) Study of effects of microwaves on visual organs. *Klin. Oczna* **38**:323.

Marha, K. (1970) Maximum admissible values of HF and UHF electromagnetic radiation at work places in Czechoslovakia. In: *Biological Effects and Health Implications of Microwave Radiation*, S. F. Cleary (ed.). HEW, PHS, BRH/DBE 70-2, p. 188.

Marha, K., J. Musil, and H. Tuha (1968) *Electromagnetic Fields and the Living Environment*. State Health Publishing House, Prague (Transl. SBN 911302-13-7, San Francisco Press, 1971).

Michaelson, S. M. (1972) Human exposure to non-ionizing radiant energy—Potential hazards and safety standards. *Proc. IEEE* **60**:389.

Michaelson, S. M. (1974) Effects of exposure to microwaves: Problems and perspectives. *Environ. Health Perspect.* **8**:133.

Michaelson, S. M. (1975) Radiofrequency and microwave energies, magnetic and electric fields. In: *The Foundations of Space Biology and Medicine*, Vol. II, Book 2, M. Calvin and O. G. Gazenko (eds.). NASA, Washington, D.C., pp. 409–452.

Michaelson, S. M. (1978) Relevancy of experimental studies of microwave-induced cataracts to man. In: *Current Concepts in Ergophthalmology*, B. Tengroth and D. Epstein (eds.). Societas Ergophthalmologica Internat., pp. 105–124.

Michaelson, S. M., and C. H. Dodge (1971) Soviet views on the biologic effects of microwaves: An analysis. *Health Phys.* **21**:108.

Milroy, W. C., and S. M. Michaelson (1972) Microwave cataractogenesis: A critical review of the literature. *Aerosp. Med.* **43**:67.

Minecki, L. (1967) *High Frequency Electromagnetic Radiation*: *Biological Effect and Health Protection*. Wydawnictwo Zwiazkowe CRZZ Press, Warsaw.

National Research Council (1981) Effects of Microwave Radiation on the Lens of the Eye. Working Group 35 Committee on Vision. Assembly of Behavioral and Social Sciences, National Academy Press, Washington, D.C.

Neidlinger, R. W. (1971) Microwave cataract. *IEEE Trans. Microwave Theory Tech.* **MTT-19**:250.

Odland, L. T. (1972) Observations on microwave hazards to USAF personnel. *J. Occup. Med.* **14**:544.

Orlova, T. N. (1971) Clinical aspects of mental disorders following protracted human exposure to super-high frequency electromagnetic waves. In: *Cerebral Mechanisms of Mental Illnesses*, Kazan, pp. 16–18.

Osipov, Y. A. (1965) *Occupational Hygiene and the Effects of Radio-Frequency Electromagnetic Fields on Workers*. Izvestiya Meditisina Press, Leningrad, pp. 78–103.

Pazderova-Vejlupkova, J. (1981) Update on epidemiology: Europe. In: *XXth Assembly of URSI*, Washington, D.C.

Peacock, P. B., J. W. Simpson, C. A. Alford, and F. Saunders (1971) Congenital anomalies in Alabama. *J. Med. Assoc. State Ala.* **41**:42.

Petrov, I. R. (ed.) (1970) *Influence of Microwave Radiation on the Organism of Man and Animals*. Meditsina Press, Leningrad (NASA TT F-708).

Presman, A. S. (1968) *Electromagnetic Fields and Life*. Izd-vo Nauka, Moscow (Transl. Plenum Press, 1970).

Puska, P., J. Tuomilehto, J. Salonen, A. Nissinen, J. Virtamo, S. Bjorkqvist, K. Doskela, L. Noittaanmaki, T. Takalo, T. Kottke, J. Maki, P. Siplia, and P. Varvikko (1978) The North Karelia Project: Evaluation of a comprehensive community programme for control of cardiovascular diseases in 1972–1977 in North Karelia, Finland. Research Institute for Community Health, University of Kupio, Finland.

Raue, N. (1963) The use of microwaves in ocular therapeutics. *Klin. Monatsbl. Augenheilkd.* **142**:533.

Roberts, M. J., Jr., and S. M. Michaelson (1985) Epidemiological studies of human exposures to radiofrequency radiation. *Int. Arch. Environ. Health* **56**:169.

Robinette, C. D., and C. Silverman (1977) Cause of death following occupational exposure to microwave radiation (radar) 1950–1974. In: *Biological Effects and Measurement of Radiofrequency/Microwaves*, D. G. Hazzard (ed.). HEW Publ. (FDA) 77-8026, pp. 337–344.

Robinette, C. D., C. Silverman, and S. Jablon (1980) Effects upon health of occupational exposure to microwave radiation (radar) 1950–1974. *Am. J. Epidemiol.* **112**:39.

Rosenthal, D. S., and S. C. Beering (1968) Hypogonadism after microwave radiation. *J. Am. Med. Assoc.* **205**:245.

Rubin, A., and W. J. Erdman (1959) Microwave exposure of the human female pelvis during early pregnancy and prior to conception. *Am. J. Phys. Med.* **38**:219.

Ruggera, P. S. (1980) Measurements of Emission Levels During Microwave and Shortwave Diathermy Treatments. BRH, HHS Publ. (FDA) 80-8119.

Sadchikova, M. N. (1974) Clinical manifestations of reactions to microwave irradiation in various occupational groups. In: *Biological Effects and Health Hazards of Microwave Radiation*, P. Czerski, K. Ostrowski, M. L. Shore, C. Silverman, M. J. Suess, and B. Waldeskog (eds.). Polish Medical Publishers, Warsaw, pp. 261–267.

Sadchikova, M. N., and A. A. Orlova (1958) Clinical picture of the chronic effects of electromagnetic microwaves. *Gig. Tr. Prof. Zabol.* **2**:16.

Shacklett, D. E., T. J. Tredici, and D. L. Epstein (1975) Evaluation of possible microwave-induced lens changes in the United States Air Force. *Aviat. Space Environ. Med.* **46**:1403.

Shilyayev, V. G. (1970) Effects of microwave radiation on the visual organ. In: *Influence of Microwave Radiation on the Organism of Man and Animals,* I. R. Petrov (ed.). Meditsina Press, Leningrad (NASA TT F-708), pp. 142–146.

Shimkovich, I. S., and V. G. Shilyayev (1959) Cataract of both eyes which developed as a result of repeated short exposures to an electromagnetic field of high density. *Vestn. Oftalmol.* **72:**12.

Siekierzynski, M., P. Czerski, H. Milczarek, A. Gidynski, C. Czarnecki, E. Dziuk, and W. Jedrzescak (1974) Health surveillance of personnel occupationally exposed to microwaves. II. Functional disturbances. *Aerosp. Med.* **45:**1143.

Sigler, A. T., A. M. Lilienfeld, B. H. Cohen, and J. E. Westlake (1965) Radiation exposure in parents of children with mongolism. *Bull. Johns Hopkins Hosp.* **117:**374.

Silverman, C. (1973) Nervous and behavioral effects of microwave radiation in humans. *Am. J. Epidemiol.* **97:**219.

Silverman, C. (1979) Epidemiologic approach to the study of microwave effects. *Bull. N.Y. Acad. Med.* **55:**1166.

Silverman, C. (1980) Epidemiologic studies of microwave effects. *Proc. IEEE* **68:**78.

Silverman, C. (1985) Epidemiology of microwave radiation effects in humans. In: *Epidemiology and Quantitation of Environmental Risk in Humans from Radiation and Other Agents.* A. Castellani (ed.). Plenum Press, New York, pp. 433–458.

Tarkkanen, A., R. Esila, and M. Liesmaa (1966) Experimental cataracts following long-term administration of corticosteroids. *Acta Ophthalmol.* **45:**665.

Tengroth, B. M. (1983) Caractogenesis induced by RF and MW energy. In: *Biological Effects and Dosimetry of Nonionizing Radiation Radiofrequency and Microwave Energies.* M. Grandolfo, S. M. Michaelson, and A. Rindi (eds.). Plenum Press, New York, pp. 485–500.

Tengroth, B., and E. Aurell (1974) Retinal changes in microwave workers. In: *Biological Effects and Health Hazards of Microwave Radiation,* P. Czerski, K. Ostrowski, M. L. Shore, C. Silverman, M. J. Suess, and B. Waldeskog (eds.), Polish Medical Publishers, Warsaw, pp. 302–305.

U.S. Department of Health, Education and Welfare (1979) Health Examination Statistics. HEW, National Center for Health Statistics, Medical Statistics Branch, March 2, 1979.

U.S. Senate (1977) Radiation Health and Safety. Hearings before the Committee on Commerce, Science, and Transportation. 95th Congress, First Session on Oversight of Radiation Health and Safety, June 16, 17, 27, 28, and 29, 1977, Serial No. 95–49, pp. 284, 1195, 1196.

U.S. Senate (1979) Committee on Commerce, Science, and Transportation. Committee Print. Microwave Irradiation of the U.S. Embassy in Moscow. April (43-949), U.S. Government Printing Office, Washington, D.C.

van Demark, W. R., and J. R. Free (1973) Temperature effects. In: *The Testis,* Vol. III, A. D. Johnson, W. R. Gomes, and M. L. van Demark (eds.). Academic Press, New York, pp. 233–312.

Weintraub, J. R. (1975) The relationship between job satisfaction and psychosomatic disorders. Presented at the Western Psychological Association Convention, Sacramento, April.

Zaret, M. M. (1976) Electronic smog as a potentiating factor in cardiovascular disease: A hypothesis of microwaves as an etiology for sudden death from heart attack in North Karelia. *Med. Res. Eng.* **12:**13.

Zaret, M. M., and M. Eisenbud (1961) Preliminary results of studies of lenticular effects of microwaves among exposed personnel. In: *Proceedings of the Fourth Annual Tri-Service Conference on Biological Effects of Microwave Radiation,* M. F. Peyton (ed.), Vol. I, Plenum Press, New York, pp. 293–308.

Zaret, M. M., S. Cleary, B. Pasternack, M. Eisenbud, and H. Schmidt (1963) A Study of Lenticular Imperfections in the Eyes of a Sample of Microwave Workers and a Control Population. Final Rep. RADC-TDR-63-125, New York University, New York, 142 pp.

Zaret, M. M., I. T. Kaplan, and A. M. Kay (1970) Clinical microwave cataracts. In: *Biological Effects and Health Implications of Microwave Radiation*, S. Cleary (ed.). HEW, PHS, BRH/DBE 70-2, p. 82.

Zydecki, S. (1974) Assessment of lens translucency in juveniles, microwave workers and age-matched groups. In: *Biological Effects and Health Hazards of Microwave Radiation*, P. Czerski, K. Ostrowski, M. L. Shore, C. Silverman, M. J. Suess, and B. Waldeskog (eds.). Polish Medical Publishers, Warsaw, pp. 306–308.

20

Personnel Protection, Protection Guides, and Standards

20.1. PROTECTIVE CLOTHING AND EYE SHIELDS

Although protective clothing and eye shields have been developed and demonstrated as providing effective shielding in some circumstances (Glaser and Heimer, 1971; Christianson and Rutkowski, 1967; Wadey, 1956), their use is not recommended. Reflections can increase the hazard to other people, and faults, such as open circuits, can act as secondary sources to actually increase the hazard to the wearer. In high-radiation fields, arcing problems may arise (Klascius, 1971).

20.2. PERSONAL MONITORS

Several attempts have been made to develop devices to record individual cumulative exposures to microwaves, or to give warning when predetermined exposure levels are exceeded. These are not in common use and are probably best suited to establishing whether people are being exposed to possibly significant amounts of MW/RF radiation so that their working practices should be investigated. Because of inadequate calibration and other technical difficulties, these have not been accepted as reliable recordings of exposure.

20.3. ANCILLARY HAZARDS ASSOCIATED WITH ELECTROMAGNETIC INTERFERENCE

Aside from the primary biological hazard of direct irradiation by RF/MW energy, there is a more subtle influence that can affect users of electronic prosthetic devices such as cardiac pacemakers and diagnostic medical equipment, e.g., electroencephalographs, electrocardiographs, electromyographs, and so on (Ruggera and Elder, 1971). This effect is termed electromagnetic interference (EMI), which may cause a variety of malfunctions. EMI occurs when signals generated by one or more electronic or electromechanical devices adversely affect the operation of other electronic devices. The offending signals can be products of intended radiation, such as radio, television, and radar transmission, or unintended signals generated by internal combustion engine ignition systems, electric razors, electromechanical relays, and so on. The characteristic of electronic equipment that permits undesirable responses when subjected to EMI is called susceptibility and the technology that has evolved to solve the problems of EMI is called electromagnetic compatibility (EMC). Of greatest concern has been the possibility of interference with the function of implanted electronic cardiac pacemakers (see Chapter 13). Improvements in pacemaker design have largely eliminated their susceptibility problems (Smyth, 1974). Pacemakers are typically tested for EMI at least at a frequency of 450 MHz (where susceptibility is generally considered to be the greatest).

20.4. EXPOSURE STANDARDS

There is a need to set limits on the amount of exposure to radiant energies individuals can accept with safety. The objective of protection is to prevent injury to people. Protection standards should be based on scientific evidence, but are quite often the result of empirical approaches to various problems reflecting current qualitative and quantitative knowledge. A numerical value for a standard implies a knowledge of the effect produced at a given level of stress, and that both effect and stress are measurable. One problem is the definition of what an "effect" is and whether it can ultimately be shown to modify man's "way of life" or that of his offspring (Taylor, 1971).

If there were a clear-cut relationship between exposure level and pathophysiological effect, the problem of setting standards would be greatly simplified. not only are there numerous variables to be considered, but it is often difficult or impossible to obtain the necessary data to draw valid conclusions concerning effects of exposure to noxious agents.

In most biological processes, there is a certain range between those levels that produce no effects and those that produce detectable effects. A detectable effect is not necessarily one that is irreparable or even a sign that the threshold for damage has been reached. Ultimately, a clear differentiation has to be made between biological effects *per se* that do not result in short-term or latent functional impairment against which the body cannot maintain homeostasis and effectiveness, and injury that may impair normal body activity either temporarily or permanently.

To ensure uniform and effective control of potential health hazards from microwave exposure, it is necessary to establish uniform effect or threshold values. Ideally, effect or threshold values should be predicated on firm human data. If such data are not available, however, extrapolation from well-designed, adequately performed, and properly analyzed animal investigations is required.

In considering standards, it is necessary to keep in mind the essential differences between a "personnel exposure" standard and a "performance" or "emission" standard for a piece of equipment. An exposure standard refers to the maximum level of power density and exposure time for the whole body or for any of its parts and incorporates a safety factor. An emission standard (or performance standard) refers not to people but to equipment, and specifies the maximum emission (or leakage) from a device at a specified distance. Emission standards are such that human exposure will be at levels considerably below personnel exposure limits.

Microwave exposure standards are generally based, with some variation, on those developed in the United States, Russia, Poland, and Czechoslovakia. The U.S. Protection Guide of 10 mW/cm^2 was suggested about 20 years ago by Schwan and his associates, which was based on the "thermal load" that a standard (healthy) adult could tolerate and dissipate under usual environmental conditions without a rise in body temperature. Intensive investigation was subsequently carried out by the U.S. Department of Defense into the biological effects of microwave radiation (Michaelson, 1971). None of these investigations produced any evidence of a hazard at the proposed limit of 10 mW/cm^2. Indeed, no conclusive evidence was established for any effect below the level of 100 mW/cm^2 that could be considered hazardous for man.

Very few countries have promulgated MW/RF standards, and in those cases where standards exist, very few have legal backing. Most standards issued have been of a voluntary or consensus nature and thus provide only guidelines for exposure, e.g., the U.S. ANSI standard (ANSI, 1966, 1982).

The first standards for controlling exposure to MW/RF radiation were introduced in the 1950s in the USA and USSR. The maximum permissible exposure levels that were proposed then have remained substantially unchanged, i.e., for continuous exposure these are respectively 10 mW/cm^2 and $10 \mu\text{W/cm}^2$. Most countries that have developed national standards based them on either the USA (ANSI, 1966) or the Soviet (USSR, 1958) values. Subsequently, some countries have proposed standards that are intermediate between these.

The basis for the USA (ANSI, 1966, 1982) and U.K. standards is the thermal consequences of exposure. Exposure to 10 mW/cm^2 (>100 MHz) is considered to result in an additional heat load comparable to the metabolic rate (Durney *et al.*, 1978). This thermal load should be readily accommodated under normal circumstances. The $10 \, \text{mW/cm}^2$ level was felt to be about a factor of 10 or more lower than the exposure considered as a risk factor. ANSI (1982) modified the standard on the basis of SAR.

The USSR standard derives from experiments on small laboratory animals and surveys of people occupationally exposed. Functional changes were reported in animals after exposure to energies in the frequency range 1 to 10 GHz at about $1 \, \text{mW/cm}^2$ over a period greater than 1 hr. One-tenth of this value was recommended as the safe level for exposure throughout the working day, and applying a safety factor of 10 to allow for individual variation in sensitivity, and taking into account the human studies, yielded an occupational exposure standard of $10 \, \mu\text{W/cm}^2$ for the working day (Baranski and Czerski, 1976; Petrov, 1970; Minin, 1974). The USSR standard allows incremental increases in exposure, each by a factor of 10, for exposure durations shorter than 2 hr, and for 20 min, respectively (Table 20-1).

Most of the biological investigations relevant to the development of exposure standards have been carried out over the approximate frequency range 1 to 10 GHz. There is, however, a considerable divergence in the frequency range over which the standards of individual countries apply. Reference should generally be made to the standards themselves for detailed information, but the tables below provide summaries of some existing standards. Table 20-1 summarizes the occupational and general public exposure standards existing in the USSR, Poland, and Czechoslovakia. Table 20-2 summarizes the standards existing in the USA (ANSI), Canada, Sweden, and United Kingdom. Information on the type (general public or occupational) of standard, applicable frequency range, exposure limit, exposure duration, and MW/RF source characteristics is provided for comparison purposes.

20.4.1. Occupational Standard (USA)

The OSHA standard, adopted in 1972, applies to employees in the private sector. An addendum, adopted in 1975, applies to work conditions particularly in the telecommunications industry. OSHA standards are mandatory for federal employees including the military. Maximum permissible exposure limit was $10 \, \text{mW/cm}^2$, for durations greater than 6 min, over the frequency range 10 MHz–100 GHz. The OSHA standard, however has been challenged as being unenforceable.

20.4.2. Product Emission Standard

The "Radiation Control for Health and Safety Act of 1968" (PL 90-602), administered by HEW/FDA (BRH), provides authority for

PROTECTION GUIDES

TABLE 20-1
USSR, Polish, and Czechoslovakian Exposure Standards

Standard	Type	Frequency	Exposure limit	Exposure duration	CW/pulsed	Antenna stationary/rotating	Remarks
USSR Government 1976	Occupational	10–30 MHz	20 V/m	Working day	Both	Both	Military units and establishments of Ministry of Defense excluded
		30–50 MHz	10 V/m	Working day	Both	Both	
			0.3 A/m	Working day	Both	Both	
		50–300 MHz	5 V/m	Working day	Both	Both	
		0.3–300 GHz	10 μW/cm^2	Working day	Both	Stationary	
			100 μW/cm^2	Working day	Both	Rotating	
			100 μW/cm^2	2 hr	Both	Stationary	
			1 mW/cm^2	2 hr	Both	Rotating	
			1 mW/cm^2	20 min	Both	Stationary	
	General public	0.3–300 GHz	1 μW/cm^2	24 hr	Both	Both	
Czechoslovakian government 1970	Occupational	10–30 MHz	50 V/m	Working day	Both	Both	Max. peak 1 kW/cm^2
		30–300 MHz	10 V/m	Working day	Both	Both	
		0.3–300 GHz	25 μW/cm^2	Working day	CW	Both	
			10 μW/cm^2	Working day	Pulsed	Both	
			1.6 mW/cm^2	1 hr	CW	Both	
			0.64 mW/cm^2	1 hr	Pulsed	Both	
	General public	30–300 MHz	1 V/m	24 hr	Both	Both	
		0.3–300 GHz	2.5 μW/cm^2	24 hr	CW	Both	
			1 μW/cm^2	24 hr	Pulsed	Both	
		30–300 MHz	1 V/m	24 hr	Both	Both	
		10–30 MHz	2.5 V/m	24 hr	Both	Both	
Polish government 1972	Occupational	0.3–300 GHz	0.2 mW/cm^2	10 hr	Both	Stationary	P-power density in W/m^2
			0.2–10 mW/cm^2	32/P^2 (hr)	Both	Stationary	
			1 mW/cm^2	10 hr	Both	Rotating	
			1–10 mW/cm^2	800/P^2 (hr)	Both	Rotating	
	General public	0.3–300 GHz	10 μW/cm^2	24 hr	Both	Stationary	
			0.1 mW/cm^2	24 hr	Both	Rotating	
Polish government 1977	Occupational	10–300 MHz	20 V/m	Working day	Both	Both	E-electric field intensity in V/m
	General public	10–300 MHz	20–300 V/m	3200/E^2 (min)	Both	Both	
			7 V/m	24 hr	Both	Both	

TABLE 20-2
United States, Canadian, Swedish, and U.K. Exposure Standards

Standard	Type	Frequency	Exposure limit	Exposure duration	CW/pulsed
USA—ANSI 1982	Occupational and general public	0.3–3 MHz 3–30 MHz 30–300 MHz 300–1500 MHz 1500–100,000 MHz	100 mW/cm^2 900/f 1.0 mW/cm^2 f/300 5 mW/cm^2	>6 min	Both
Canada—Health and Welfare 1978	Occupational	10 MHz–1 GHz 1–300 GHz 10 MHz–300 GHz	1 mW/cm^2 5 mW/cm^2 25 mW/cm^2 (max.)	No limit No limit 2.4 min	Both Both Both
	General public	10 MHz–300 GHz	1 mW/cm^2	No limit	Both
Sweden—Worker Protection Authority 1976	Occupational	0.3–300 GHz 10–300 MHz 10 MHz–300 GHz	1 mW/cm^2 5 mW/cm^2 1–25 mW/cm^2 25 mW/cm^2 (max.)	8 hr 8 hr $60/X$ (min)^a	Both Both Both CW, pulsed average over 1 sec
U.K.—MRC 1971	General public	30 MHz–30 GHz	10 mW/cm^2 1 mW hr/cm^2	No limit 0.1 hr	Both Both

^{a} X = power density in mW/cm^2.

controlling radiation from electronic devices. The BRH microwave oven standard, effective October 1971 (U.S. Department of Health, Education and Welfare, 1974) states that microwave ovens may not emit (leak) more than 1 mW/cm^2 at time of manufacture and 5 mW/cm^2 subsequently, for the life of the product—measured at a distance of 5 cm and under conditions specified in the standard. The Canadian standard (Repacholi, 1978; Canadian Department of National Health and Welfare 1974) restricts the maximum leakage to 1 mW/cm^2 at 5 cm from the oven (consumer, commercial, and industrial). These standards have been adopted in Japan and most of Western Europe (IEC, 1976). The exposure levels from these standards are consistent with standards for the general population in the USSR and Poland (Baranski and Czerski, 1976).

20.4.3. American National Standards Institute (ANSI)

There are nongovernment organizations that have developed recommended standards and safety criteria. For example, ANSI is a voluntary body with members from government, industry, various associations, and the academic community that develops consensus standards (guides) in various areas. ANSI issued a safety standard in 1966 with maximum permissible exposure of 10 mW/cm² averaged over any 6-min period for frequencies from 10 MHz to 100 GHz, which was essentially adopted by OSHA. This standard was reviewed and reissued with minor modifications in 1975. ANSI must review and withdraw, revise, or reissue ANSI standards every 5 years. New recommendations (ANSI, 1982) are based on frequency dependence and specific absorption rates (SARs). For human exposure to electromagnetic energy of radiofrequencies from 300 kHz to 100 GHz, the RF protection guides, in terms of equivalent plane wave free space power density and in terms of the mean squared electric (E^2) and magnetic (H^2) field strengths as a function of frequency, are given in Table 20-3.

For near-field exposure, the only applicable RF protection guides are the mean squared electric and magnetic field strengths given in columns 3 and 4. For convenience, these guides may be expressed in equivalent plane wave power density (column 2).

For both pulsed and nonpulsed fields, the power density and the mean squares of the field strengths, as applicable, are averaged over any 0.1-hr period and should not exceed the values given in Table 20-3. For situations involving exposure of the whole body, the RF protection guide is believed to result in energy deposition averaged over the entire body mass for any 0.1-hr period of about 144 J/kg or less. This is equivalent to an SAR of about 0.40 W/kg spatially and temporally averaged over the entire body mass.

The National Institute for Occupational Safety and Health (NIOSH) is developing a criteria document with recommended standards for occupational MW/RF exposures, which is, except for certain modifications, comparable to that recommended by ANSI. The ANSI standard applies to the total population, occupational as well as nonoccupational but not to the purposeful exposure of patients by or under direction of practitioners of the healing arts.

TABLE 20 3
USA Exposure Standards

Frequency, f (MHz)	Power density (mW/cm²)	E^2 (V²/m²)	H^2 (A²/m²)
0.3–3	100	400,000	2.5
3–30	900/f²	4,000 (900/f²)	0.025 (900/f²)
30–300	1.0	4,000	0.025
300–1500	f/300	4,000 (f/300)	0.025 (f/300)
1500–100,000	5	20,000	0.125

20.4.4. Standards in Various Countries

The Radiation Protection Bureau of Health and Welfare, Canada is considering "Emission and Exposure Standards for Microwave Radiation." The maximum permissible levels (MPLs) are 1 mW-hr/cm^2 average energy flux for whole-body exposure over 1 hr, and a maximum exposure during any 1 min of 25 mW/cm^2 in occupational settings. The MPLs would apply over the frequency range 10 MHz–300 GHz (Table 20-4). No distinction is made between CW and pulsed waveforms (Health and Welfare, Canada, 1978, 1979; Repacholi, 1978).

The State Committee on Standards of the Council of Ministers of the USSR has promulgated "Occupational Safety Standards for Electromagnetic Fields of Radiofrequency" (GOST 12.1.006-76), effective January 1, 1977. It specifies the maximum permissible magnitudes of voltage and current density of an electromagnetic field in the workplace (Table 20-5). It does not, however, apply to personnel of the Ministry of Defense. Maximum permissible RF fields in the workplace must not, during the course of the workday, exceed the limits given in Table 20-5.

The USSR Ministry of Protection (1984) has endorsed guidelines for maximum exposure limits for the general population, which stipulate the maximum allowable levels of electromagnetic energy in human habitation, as given in Table 20-6.

The Polish Ministries of Work, Wages and Social Affairs and of Health and Social Assistance (1972, 1977) promulgated a change in the Polish occupational exposure standard. For the general population, the

TABLE 20-4
Canadian Standards

	Frequency	Limits			Comments
		Power density (mW/cm^2)	rms E strength (V/m)	rms H strength (A/m)	Safety code 6 (1979)[a]
Occupational	10 MHz–1 GHz	1	60	0.16	Average over 1 hr
		25	300	0.8	Average over 1 m
	1–300 GHz	5	140	0.36	Average over 1 hr
		25	300	0.8	Average over 1 m
General public	10 MHz–300 GHz	1	60	0.16	Average over 1 m

[a] Additional provisions for exposure shorter than 1 hr and exposure of extremities.

TABLE 20-5
Soviet Standards[a]

Frequency range	P (mW/cm²)	E (V/m)	H (A/m)
60 kHz–1.5 MHz			5
0.06–3.0 MHz		50	
3.0–30 MHz		20	
30–50 MHz		10	0.3
50–300 MHz		5	
300 MHz–300 GHz	0.01	(Entire workday)	
	0.10	(2-hr period during workday)	
	1.00	(20-min period during workday)	

[a] GOST 12.1.006-76; USSR, 1984.
Note 1: Also applies in environments with ambient temperatures above 28°C, in the presence of X-radiation, except that, under these conditions, the maximum during a 20-min period is restricted to 0.1 mW/cm².
Note 2: The workday level was raised from $10\,\mu\text{W/cm}^2$ to $25\,\mu\text{W/cm}^2$ in January 1982 (USSR Committee on Science and Technology).

values of 10 and 100 $\mu\text{W/cm}^2$ were adopted for continuous and intermittent exposures, respectively. These values were taken as the upper limits of a safe zone, in which occupation is unrestricted. Three other zones are also defined, based on power density. For stationary (continuous) fields, these are defined as follows:

1. *Safe zone*—the mean power density cannot exceed 10 $\mu\text{W/cm}^2$; human exposure is unrestricted.
2. *Intermediate zone*—minimal value 10 $\mu\text{W/cm}^2$, upper limit 200 $\mu\text{W/cm}^2$; occupational exposure is allowed during a whole workday (normally 8 hr, but in principle can be extended to 10 hr).
3. *Hazardous zone*—minimal value 200 $\mu\text{W/cm}^2$, upper limit 10 mW/cm²; occupational exposure time per 24 hr is determined by the formula:

$$t = 32p^2$$

TABLE 20-6
Soviet Population Exposure Standards[a]

Frequency range	P (μW/cm²)	E (V/m)
30–300 kHz		25
300 kHz–3.0 MHz		15
3.0–30 MHz		10
30–300 MHz		3
300 MHz–300 GHz	1	

[a] USSR (1984).

where t is the exposure time in hours and p is the mean power density in W/cm^2.
4. *Dangerous zone*—mean power density in excess of 100 W/cm^2 (10 mW/cm^2); human exposure is forbidden.

For exposures to nonstationary fields, i.e., intermittent exposure, the following values were adopted:

1. *Safe zone*—mean power density does not exceed 1 W/cm^2 (100 μW/cm^2).
2. *Intermediate zone*—minimal value 1 W/cm^2 (100 μW/cm^2), upper limit 10 W/m^2 (1 mW/cm^2).
3. *Hazardous zone*—minimal value 10 W/m^2 (1 mW/cm^2), upper limit 100 W/m^2 (10 mW/cm^2); occupational exposure time per 24 hr is determined by the formula:

$$t = 800/p^2$$

where t and p are as given above.
4. *Dangerous zone*—mean power density in excess of 100 W/m^2 (10 mW/cm^2); human exposure is forbidden. In 1977, the Polish Standard for occupational exposure (WHO, 1981) extended the frequency range down from 300 to 0.1 MHz (Table 20-7).

In 1976, the Swedish National Board for Industrial Safety promulgated a nonionizing RF standard (Worker Protection Authority Instruction No. 111) effective January 1, 1977. This regulation applies to all work that may involve exposure to RF energy between 10 MHz and 300 GHz. The instruction specifically excludes applications involving the treatment of patients. Maximum permissible exposures (as averaged over a 6-min period) are given in Table 20-8.

TABLE 20-7
Polish Standards [a]

Frequency range	Hazardous zone			Intermediate zone		Safe zone	
		T_p		T_p		T_p	
0.1–10 MHz(max)	250 A/m	40/H	10 A/m	Entire workday		2 A/m	No limit[b]
	1000 V/m	560/E	20 V/m			20 V/m	
10–300 MHz(max)	300 V/m	3200/E^2	20 V/m			7 V/m	

[a] T_p, permissible time of exposure per workday (min); E, electric field (V/m); H, magnetic field (A/m).
[b] General public.

TABLE 20-8
Swedish Standards[a]

Frequency range	Power density (mW/cm^2)
10–300 GHz	5
300 MHz–300 GHz	1

[a] The maximum permissible momentary exposure is 25 mW/cm^2 Royal Swedish Academy of Engineering Sciences (1976).

According to the World Health Organization and the International Radiation Protection Association (WHO, 1981), the exposure range of 0.1 to 1 mW/cm^2 for workers has a high enough safety factor to permit continuous exposure over the whole frequency range (100 kHz–300 MHz), whole- or partial-body exposure to continuous or pulsed energies. Higher exposures may be permissible over part of the frequency range and for intermittent or occasional exposures. Environmental exposure should be based on the ALARA principle—as low as reasonably achievable—with social and economic benefits considered.

20.4.5. Criteria for Setting Tolerance Levels and Exposure Standards

When developing standards or regulations to control exposure levels to the general public and/or persons exposed occupationally, a number of points should be considered (Repacholi, 1978):

1. Does there or could there exist a problem where MW/RF exposure levels could rise uncontrolled to unsafe levels? If so:
2. Who is being exposed and under what conditions?
3. What are the potentially dangerous sources of MW/RF energy, how rapidly are these sources proliferating, and how are they being controlled?
4. Would the existence and implementation of standards alleviate problems?

In order for a promulgated standard to be understood with respect to technical detail and measurement for compliance, careful consideration should be paid to the following points:

1. There should be a clear distinction between emission and exposure standards.
2. Dependent on the frequency range addressed by the standard, there should be clear definitions of electric and magnetic field strengths and power density. If possible, there should be ref-

erences on how these values are measured. If this cannot be incorporated into the standard, there should be literature references where this information can be obtained.
3. The meaning of the permitted exposure duration should be described, e.g., the allowed times and levels for exposure to continuous or pulsed fields. Clear explanations should be made on accepted levels for intermittent exposures and whether higher levels are allowed for short durations.
4. In general, present exposure standards refer to whole-body exposure. Partial-body exposures should be addressed.
5. Frequency dependence should be considered. It is generally felt that existing standards oversimplify the frequency dependence of the biological effects, health hazards, and thus safety limits. Sufficient information is available today to expect the introduction of greater frequency dependence into future revisions of standards.

According to Gordon (1970) and Gordon *et al.* (1974), the criteria for setting occupational personnel exposure standards in the USSR represent complex investigations consisting of three major components:

1. Hygienic evaluation of the working conditions of persons working with sources of RF electromagnetic waves, i.e., determination of the actual intensities of radiation.
2. Dynamic clinical observations on the state of health of people working with sources of RF radiation over a period of several years (five or more).
3. Experimental studies on the nature of the biological effects of microwaves to determine threshold values for lethal effects and potentially hazardous reactions.

Unfortunately, the concept of "threshold reaction" in the context of medical evaluation of a biological effect, and especially in the setting of standards, remains indefinite. There are as yet no clear-cut and widely applicable pathophysiological criteria for distinguishing between protective adaptive reactions and compensatory reactions, between regulatory reactions in an emergency situation, and pathological reactions at various system levels, including the CNS. This results in significant difficulties in the analysis of homeostasis, in the analysis of the differentiated threshold characteristics of biological reactions that are determined by the general level of excitability and reactivity, and in the analysis of pathological reactions, which are determined by adaptational and compensatory capabilities existing in a biological system (Gordon, 1970).

Experimental investigations, dealing at least in part with protection standards, are largely directed toward establishing threshold intensities for microwaves which elicit either known adverse biological effects, or a reaction that cannot with complete certainty be regarded as reflecting a disturbance in the homeostatic mechanisms. It is in this sense that one must appreciate experimental data on biological effects of low-intensity microwaves, which deal with threshold effects that are considered when protection standards are being set (Gordom, 1970).

These concepts have enabled Soviet authorities to recommend MW/RF standards for workers, and even in recent years, to update some of them. They have also proposed a protection standard for the general population of 1 $\mu W/cm^2$ for occupational groups (Gordon, 1973).

A search of Soviet publications fails to reveal any basis for limiting exposure time to 2 hr or 20 min in a 24-hr period to levels of 100 and 1000 $\mu W/cm^2$, respectively, although Petrov and Subbota (1970) suggest the Soviet standard is based on reports noting that some disturbances occur in experimental animals at exposure levels in the vicinity of 1 mW/cm^2. Taking this value as a limiting value and considering a full workday as rounded off to 10 hr, a permissible exposure level of 0.1 mW/cm^2 seemed reasonable. Introducing an additional safety factor of 10, a level of 0.01 mW/cm^2 (10 $\mu W/cm^2$) was derived. In general, it would appear that the values obtained in this manner from experimental studies indicate a large safety factor and can be applied to the general population; but it seems that the values are too conservative for personnel subjected to periodic medical examination such as in the industrial setting (Czerski and Piotrowski, 1972).

It appears to a large degree that the apparent differences between USA and Eastern European standards are based not on actual factual information but on differences in basic philosophy. These differences appear in the areas of industrial hygiene.

The basic industrial hygiene philosophy of the USSR can be summarized as follows (Magnuson *et al.*, 1964):

1. The maximum exposure is defined as that level such that daily work in the environment will not result in *any deviation in the normal state* as well as not result in disease. Temporary changes in conditional responses are considered deviations from normal.
2. Standards are based entirely on presence or absence of biological effects without regard to the feasibility of reaching such levels in practice.
3. The values are maximum exposures rather than time-weighted averages.
4. Regardless of the value set, the optimum value and goal is zero.

5. Deviations above maximum permissible exposures "within reasonable limits" are permitted.
6. Maximum permissible exposure levels represent desirable values or ideals for which to strive.

In order to properly extrapolate the laboratory results, it is necessary to convert electromagnetic field exposure level information used for laboratory experiments into the rate of energy absorption in the bodies of the exposed test animals. In addition, it is also necessary to relate human exposure under various levels and conditions to the rate of energy absorption or specific absorption rate (SAR) in the tissues. The SAR rather than the exposure field is the quantity most directly related to the biological effect in the tissues of exposed subjects. Engineering work over the past several years allows easy calculation and prediction of the average SAR in man and animals exposed under various conditions and, in many cases, the actual SAR distribution over the entire body may be quantifiable (Durney *et al.*, 1978).

The SAR is the mass-normalized rate at which the potential energy of an electromagnetic field is coupled to an absorbing body. The ultimate fate of absorbed RF energy is an increase in kinetic energy. The SAR is predicated on the axiom that it is absorbed energy and not incident energy that is responsible for biological reactions.

MW/RF safety standards in general do not take into account this extrapolation process and, as a result, many are too conservative over some portions of the frequency spectrum and not conservative enough over other portions.

In its 1979/80 recommendation, the ANSI C95.1 committee used engineering advances made over the previous decade to more accurately extrapolate laboratory data from test animals for recommending maximum incident power density or electromagnetic field strength for human exposure. The ANSI C95.1 committee analyzed pertinent publications for thresholds of effects. There was general agreement among many of the papers reporting effects at 0.5 W/kg of average SAR and above. On the other hand, the reported thresholds for effects below 0.5 W/kg varied over a wide range with no general agreement among publications or internal consistency of results. Decrement in working ability by test animals began to occur when rats were subjected to average SAR levels of 4 to 10 W/kg. It was felt that the average SAR allowed for human exposure should be at least an order of magnitude below the threshold level of the most replicated and least controversial of the effects in animals. This corresponds to a whole-body average SAR of approximately 0.36 W/kg, which was later rounded off to one significant figure, 0.4 W/kg. The committee then set allowable exposure levels to values that would prevent the average SAR in an exposed human from exceeding 0.4 W/kg. This resulted in the proposed standard of 1 mW/cm^2 over the frequency range 30–300 MHz. At frequencies below 30 MHz, the exposure level is allowed to rise as a function of 900 divided by the square of the frequency or up to 100 mW/cm^2 at a frequency of 300 MHz. From this frequency to 300 kHz, it was proposed to limit the exposure level to 100 mW/cm^2. At frequencies above 300 MHz, the exposure standard is allowed to rise with frequency according to the formula: frequency divided by 300—until it reaches a level of 5 mW/cm^2 at 1500 MHz. At frequencies above 1500 MHz, the allowed exposure level is held constant at 5 mW/cm^2 to a frequency of 300 GHz. This was approved in 1982 (American National Standards Institute, 1982).

A major problem that requires resolution is that of partial-body exposure. The criteria discussed up to this point are based on whole-body exposure to a plane-wave field. Thus, in terms of a stated maximum power density, the standard should be relaxed for partial-body exposures to account for the large decrease in energy absorbed by the body tissues under such exposure conditions. This could be accounted for by allowing the peak or maximum SAR (hot spots) to increase in magnitude for decreasing average SAR. It would be inconsistent to have a partial-body standard that serves as the whole-body standard, since it would be more conservative than the whole-body exposure standard and unnecessarily restrict the use of many sources, the total output power of which is far less than that which the body would absorb under plane-wave exposure conditions. The local electric and magnetic field strength and "apparent" power densities could greatly exceed those specified in standards based on whole-body exposure conditions.

It should be pointed out that all biological effects are not necessarily hazardous. Many substances or conditions produce biological changes in the human that are not considered hazardous. Philosophically, we could also say that all conditions including life itself have profound effects upon biological systems that eventually lead to the organism's death. Therefore, we should be practical and define a hazard as an apparent unfavorable effect that leads to injury, disease, illness, or premature death (Tyler, 1976).

In many countries, initial and periodic medical examinations of workers are a legal requirement. In the USSR, Poland, and Czechoslovakia, for example, special requirements are mandatory for workers occupationally exposed to MW/RF energy either in periodicity of examinations or in the type of medical examination. When overexposure occurs, depending on the circumstances, a medical examination may be required. In this case, a special examination can be conducted.

In countries where initial and periodic medical examinations of workers are required by regulations, the type of examination to be performed is generally defined. Such exams include physical evaluation, hematology and urinalysis, and sometimes a chest X-ray examination. Some countries, e.g., Poland, require more specific examinations for people working with MW/RF energy, which can include electrocardiography, neurological examination with electroencephalography, and ophthalmological examination using a slit lamp.

Tyler (1976) suggests a medical surveillance program should be designed to elicit early signs and symptoms of biological effects before any serious health damage has occurred. As noted before, this requires a detailed knowledge of how the substance or condition affects the biological organism. Unfortunately, in the case of electromagnetic radiation, this knowledge is far from complete, and thus any present system of health surveillance must be viewed as preliminary in nature.

From a purely medical viewpoint, there may be limited rationale for the proposal and establishment of a medical surveillance program for microwave workers at the present time. On the other hand, in light of the present controversy concerning biological effects, it may be wise from a legal standpoint to institute a surveillance program for the future protection of both the employer and workers. With the institution of a microwave health surveillance program in a large worker population, adequate medical data would become available that could be evaluated for trends. This trend analysis would then provide a basis for conducting specific research programs. The major drawback to this approach is the requirement for compatible data from many different sources and the need to collect data over a period of years (Tyler, 1976). Data obtained through health monitoring could, however, provide insight into potential problem areas that should be subjected to careful epidemiological study.

The establishment of a tolerable level of exposure to a potentially hazardous physical or chemical agent, below which man is capable of dealing with the imposed stress without significant health risk, is a fundamental need in the design and operation of practical control programs against environment health hazards. This has led to doubts as to the long-term safety of any level of exposure that gives rise to a demonstrated biological response of whatever kind or degree. The possibility is emphasized that an agent, quite apart from its specific effect, may contribute over a long period of exposure to the development and progression of one or another of the chronic diseases that commonly accompany aging. This may occur even though the exposure level was below the established tolerance limit.

Standards must be based on scientific facts, realistically derived, and not on political feasibility, expedience, emotion of the moment, or unsupported information. If necessary data are not available, studies should be made to supply them. Meanwhile, provisional, tentative, or best judgment standards clearly marked and recognized as such, should be proposed, but only upon definite need (Stokinger, 1971).

While a numerical value is ultimately decided upon, the nonabsolute nature of the data upon which it is based should suggest that such value must not be taken to represent an *absolute* boundary between the positively safe and the positively unsafe. Thus, for example, if the "safe" value is 50, this cannot be taken to mean that 49 is always safe or that 51 represents an unsafe area. At best, such values represent guides for protective action (Dinman, 1973).

It is difficult to conceive of an existence free of any displacement from the steady state, for even the process of digestion implies a "new" cellular amino acid, hexose, or fatty acid environment. Yet without such process, there is no life. Therefore, the living organism must—and does—possess the ability to permit limited displacements from homeostasis. Do such costs involved in reestablishing the steady state necessarily impose an indelible decrement on a fixed lifetime quantum of energy generation? This assumption implies that biological systems operate within exceedingly narrow if nonexistent rate limits. Even minimally, that there is such a concept as "rate limits" strongly suggests the hazard of ignoring quantitative parameters when dealing with any life process. The finding that DNA repair can occur after ultraviolet irradiation, or that bacterial cells can utilize an "abnormal" carbon source by, for example, enzyme induction, belies the concept that biological systems have exceedingly narrow ranges of response to environmental challenge (Dinman, 1972).

"Effect" is a neutral word, implying neither benefit nor harm. Confusion has arisen because of the frequent implication that an "effect" is *per se* deleterious. Confusion that equates the presence of a biological effect with a deleterious implication ignores several concepts. To believe that a single molecule's presence in a cell implies a definite potential for deleterious effect disregards stochastic considerations. To believe that such molecules cause an undesirable effect disregards the presence of multiplicity of interfering substances (Dinman, 1972).

There are profound differences of opinion as to what constitutes a no-effect level of an environmental agent for man. The preponderant opinion in the United States holds that slight deviations within homeostatic limits of biological change are not deleterious (Hatch, 1972). All necessary life processes required by living organisms are associated with perturbations of a steady state. For all bodily functions, there are constant deviations from a steady state. Such deviations represent necessary accommodative change to environmental alterations in its broadest sense (Dinman, 1973). There has been a rather uncritical tendency by some to interpret demonstrated biological response, of whatever kind and intensity, as evidence of impending loss of health and, in the extreme, to regard the response itself as a direct expression of injury (Hatch, 1973).

To avoid confusion, there is need for deeper understanding of the actual "threat-to-health" implications associated with changes, which are detected far below the region of real illness. One must start with a full assessment of the strengths and limitations of the various protective mechanisms that operate in the homeostatic and compensatory zones to offset such insults. For it is the successful operation of these mechanisms within permissible limits that makes it possible to deal with exposure levels above zero without a threat to health. In the United States, we have accepted a certain degree of dependence upon these mechanisms, which, it is believed, can be drawn upon safely and repeatedly, as normal physiological functions, provided they are not overloaded (Hatch, 1973).

Regulatory officials in the USSR, in contrast, have set a dividing line between health and potential ill health at the point of earliest change from the normal physiological behavior exhibited by healthy animals prior to exposure, as revealed by the most sensitive means available to detect any kind of response to the agent. This point is selected so as to make no demands upon either the compensatory mechanisms or the processes of adaptation in the homeostatic zone. These, they feel, should be kept in reserve, so far as possible, to meet the emergency needs of unexpected encounters with environmental stresses (Hatch, 1973).

In the USSR, the major scientific basis utilized for setting standards derives from reactions of the higher nervous system and physiological alteration. Feasibility does not seem to be considered in the standard setting process, although there is some question as to whether such standards represent goals or working realities (Dinman, 1973). Because such minimal functional changes are considered as designating the borderline between harm and safety, and since a safety margin is then applied, Soviet standards in general tend to be lower than those found in the United States.

While such generalizations are useful, the problem becomes more difficult when one attempts to define the actual limits beyond which change becomes deleterious. Though practically any change is considered as being potentially detrimental by the regulatory officials of the USSR, it becomes difficult to reconcile this position with the concept of a normal range associated with homeostasis. In the strictest sense, a no-effect level does not exist; however, for operational purposes, the range of biological response that exceeds homeostatic limits must be ascertained. The problems of defining the effect such stresses (within homeostatic limits) may have over a long period, should be appreciated (Dinman, 1973).

The no-effect level is a puristic concept, because there is some biological response when the organism encounters some exogenous material (Dinman, 1972; Hatch, 1972). Whereas in the United States it is clearly understood that such responses are not deleterious *per se,* in the USSR this is not explicitly recognized. Nevertheless, in the United States a no-effect level is implied to be one that does not produce any deleterious or undesirable effect upon human health and well-being or overload the normal protective mechanism of the body (Hatch, 1972).

In this context, some comments by Ryazanov (1962, 1965), a leading Soviet toxicologist, are noteworthy: "It is well known that between toxic and harmless concentrations there lies a broad range of concentrations that do not provoke pathological, but adaptational and protective reactions. Although, at these concentrations, no pathological manifestations are shown and morbidity is not increased in the population, they must, nevertheless, also be regarded as inadmissible. The appearance of protective reactions bears witness to the fact that the condition of the external environment has deviated from the physiological optimum" (Ryazanov, 1965).

"It is not always possible to reach very rapidly the levels suggested by the use of very low standards. For that reason, the goal for a certain period of time is to bring about the use of these standards. These standards are for the purpose of use in the future, not today. They cannot be reached today. The standards must serve as the goal" (Ryazanov, 1962).

Because of problems inherent in interpretation of toxicological data, the approach that is used in the United States is that it is desirable to have a margin of safety between the lowest effective dose and the proposed threshold limit value. This is the concept that is used in occupational exposures. Expressed mathematically, threshold limit value (TLV) = the lowest effective dose divided by a safety factor. The safety factor depends upon the nature of the response produced by the lowest effective doses of the insult. What constitutes evidence of a response varies. In the United States, biochemical, physiological, or even reversible changes in organ morphology may constitute the minimal response. In the USSR, on the other hand, more credence is placed upon subtle neurophysiological change as evidence of a deleterious alteration (Dinman, 1973).

Principles of standard setting include:

1. Protection standards must be established by a process of balancing biological risk and the derived benefits.
2. A standard must relate to man's health and well-being: it must speak to the prevention or control of a health hazard.

3. The standard must be attainable; it must be a reasonable standard both in terms of the state of the art and economic factors involved.
4. The standard should be matched to the degree of the actual hazard that may exist.
5. A standard should not contain overly restrictive, arbitrary, and capricious rules and regulations.
6. A standard should have a *reasonable* margin of safety, i.e., a standard of protection against *excessive* potential health hazards, while still enjoying the benefits of modern technology.
7. Standards should be responsive to the latest and best and most reliable medical and scientific data.
8. A standard should be reasonable and, in light of the state of the art, technically feasible.
9. Environmental control may be looked upon as a balancing of the risks to human health and well-being against benefits derived from technological achievements.

Guidelines for development of standards include:

1. Standards should express the best scientific knowledge available at the time regarding the known cause-and-effect relationship between specific conditions in the environment and man's health. Hence, standards are always subject to revision in light of new knowledge.
2. Consideration should also be given to any effects on human health and safety that arise from the action of environmental factors on living systems.
3. Conditions such as duration of exposure of a given intensity, the well-being of the receptor prior to exposure, and other circumstances having a bearing on dose–effect relationship should be considered.
4. The standard should be truly relevant to the health or general welfare of people, and should be addressed to the prevention or control of a hazard.
5. The standard must be realistic and attainable. The standard should contain the best available methods of measurement and control that are economically feasible and that do not constitute unacceptable risks to human health.

REFERENCES

American National Standards Institute (1966) Safety Level of Electromagnetic Radiation with Respect to Personnel. C95.1–1966, C95.1–1974, ANSI, New York.

American National Standards Institute (1982) American National Standard Safety Levels with Respect to Human Exposure to Radiofrequency Electro-magnetic Fields, 300 kHz to 100 GHz. C95.1-1982, ANSI, New York.

Baranski, S., and P. Czerski (1976) *Biological Effects of Microwaves*. Dowden, Hutchinson & Ross, Stroudsburg, Pa.

Canadian Department of National Health and Welfare (1974) Radiation emitting devices regulations. SRD/74-061 23. October 1974, Part III, Microwave Ovens, Canada Gazette, Part V, 1974: **108**:2822-2825.

Christianson, C., and A. Rutkowski (1967) Electromagnetic Radiation Hazards in the Navy. Nav. Appl. Sci. Lab. Tech. Memo No. 3 AD 645-696.

Czerski, P., and M. Piotrowski (1972) Proposals for specification of allowable levels of microwave radiation. *Med. Lotn.* **39**:127.

Dinman, B. D. (1972) The "non-concept" of "no threshold": Chemicals in the environment. *Science* **175**:495.

Dinman, B. D. (1973) Principles and use of standards of quality for the work environment. In: *The Industrial Environment—Its Evaluation and Control*. NIOSH, HEW, PHS, Washington, D.C., p. 75.

Durney, C. H., C. C. Jacobson, P. W. Barber, H. Massoudi, M. F. Iskander, J. L. Lords, D. K. Ryser, S. J. Allen, and J. C. Mitchell (1978) Radiofrequency Radiation Dosimetry Handbook, 2nd edition. Tech. Rep. SAM-TR-78-22, Brooks AFB, Texas.

Glaser, Z. R., and G. M. Heimer (1971) Determination and elimination of hazardous microwave fields aboard naval ships. *IEEE Trans. Microwave Theory Tech.* **MTT-19**:232.

Gordon, Z. V. (1970) New data and tasks in work hygienic and experimental study of the effects of radiofrequency electromagnetic fields. In: *Biological Effects of Radiofrequency Electromagnetic Fields. Gig. Tr. Provzaholevaniya* **14**:32.

Gordon, Z. V., A. V. Roscin, and M. S. Byckov (1974) Main directions and results of research in the USSR on the biologic effects of microwaves. In: *Biological Effects and Health Hazards of Microwave Radiation*, P. Czerski, K. Ostrowski, M. L. Shore, C. Silverman, M. J. Suess, and B. Waldeskog (eds.). Polish Medical Publishers, Warsaw, pp. 22-35.

Hatch, T. F. (1972) Permissible levels of exposure to hazardous agents in industry. *J. Occup. Med.* **14**:134.

Hatch, T. F. (1973) Criteria for hazardous exposure limits. *Arch. Environ. Health* **27**:231.

Health and Welfare, Canada (1978) Health aspects of radiofrequency and microwave radiation exposure. Part II. Ottawa, HEW (DOC 78-EHD-22).

Health and Welfare, Canada (1979) Recommended safety procedures for the installation and use of radiofrequency and microwave radiation devices in the frequency range 10 MHz-300 GHz. Ottawa, HEW (Safety Code Publ. 79-EHD-30).

International Electrotechnical Commission (1976) Particular Requirements for Microwave Cooking Appliances. IEC 335-25, part 2.

Klascius, A. F. (1971) Microwave radiation protective suit. *Am. Ind. Hyg. Assoc. J.* **32**:771.

Magnuson, H. J., D. W. Fassett, H. W. Gararde, V. K. Rowe, H. F. Smyth, and H. E. Stokinger (1964) Industrial toxicology in the Soviet Union—Theoretical and applied. *Am. Ind. Hyg. Assoc. J.* **25**:185.

Michaelson, S. M. (1971) The tri-service program—A tribute to George M. Kanuf, USAF (MC). *IEEE Trans. Microwave Theory Tech.* **MTT-19**:131.

Minin, B. A. (1974) Microwaves and Human Safety—Parts I and II. JPRS 65506-1 and 2, 1975.

Petrov, I. R. (ed.) (1970) *Influence of Microwave Radiation on the Organism of Man and Animals*. Meditsina Press, Leningrad (NASA TT F-708).

Petrov, I. R., and A. G. Subbota (1970) Conclusion. In: *Influence of Microwave Radiation on the Organism of Man and Animals,* I. R. Petrov (ed.). Meditsina Press, Leningrad (NASA TT F-708).

Polish Council of Ministers (1972) Order dated 25 May 1972 concerning safety and hygiene of work while using equipment generating electromagnetic fields in the microwave range. (*In Polish*). Dziennik Ustaw PRL No. 21, pp. 193–195.

Polish Ministers of Labor, Wages, and Social Affairs and of Health, and Social Assistance (1977) Order dated 19 February 1977 concerning safety and hygiene of work while using equipment generating electromagnetic fields in the range of 0.1 MHz to 300 MHz. Dziennik Ustaw PRL No. 8, 73–75.

Repacholi, H. H. (1978) Proposed exposure limits for microwave and radiofrequency radiations in Canada. *J. Microwave Power* **13**:199.

Royal Swedish Academy of Engineering Sciences (1976) Biological Effects of Electromagnetic Fields. Stockholm, RSAES **160** (ISBN91.7082.123.2).

Ruggera, P. S., and R. L. Elder (1971) Electromagnetic Radiation Interference with Cardiac Pacemakers. HEW Publ. (BRH/DEP) 71-5.

Ryazanov, V. A. (1962) Sensory physiology as a basis for air quality standards. *Arch. Environ. Health* **5**:480.

Ryazanov, V. A. (1965) Criteria and methods for establishing maximum permissible concentrations of air pollution. *Bull. WHO* **32**:389.

Smyth, H. (1974) The pacemaker patient and the electromagnetic environment. *J. Am. Med. Assoc.* **227**:1412.

Stokinger, H. E. (1971) Sanity in research and evaluation of environmental health. *Science* **174**:662.

Taylor, L. S. (1971) Radiation protection trends in the United States. *Health Phys.* **20**:499.

Tyler, P. E. (1976) Microwave radiation—Medical surveillance. Presented at the 1976 International Microwave Symposium, Cherry Hill, N.J.

U.S. Department of Health, Education and Welfare (1974) *Regulations for Administration and Enforcement of the Radiation Control of Health and Safety Act of 1968.* Paragraph 1030.10, Microwave Ovens, HEW Publ. (FDA) 75-8003, pp. 36–37.

USSR (1958) *Temporary Sanitary Rules for Working with Centimeter Waves.* Ministry of Health Protection of the USSR.

Wadey, W. G. (1956) Magnetic shielding with multiple cylindrical shells. *Rev. Sci. Instrum.* **27**:910.

World Health Organization/International Non-Ionizing Radiation Committee of the International Radiation Protection Association (1981) Environment Health Criteria 16 Radiofrequency and Microwaves. WHO/INIRC IRPA, Geneva.

21
Problems and Recommendations

Elucidation of the biological effects of microwave exposure requires a careful review and critical analysis of the literature. This requires differentiating established effects and mechanisms from speculative and unsubstantiated reports. Most of the experimental data support the concept that the effects of microwave exposure are primarily, if not wholly, a response to hyperthermia or altered thermal gradients in the body. There are, nevertheless, large areas of confusion, uncertainty, and actual misinformation.

Although there is considerable agreement among scientists concerning the biological effects and potential hazards of microwaves, there are areas of disagreement. There also is a philosophical question about the definition of hazard. One objective definition of injury is an irreversible change in biological function as observed at the organ or system level. With this definition, it is possible to define a hazard as a probability of injury on a statistical basis. It is important to differentiate between the hazard levels at which injury may be sustained and effect or perception. All effects are not necessarily hazards. In fact, some effects may have beneficial applications under appropriately controlled conditions. Microwave-induced changes must be understood sufficiently so that their clinical significance can be determined, their hazard potential assessed, and the appropriate benefit/risk analyses applied. It is important to determine whether an observed effect is irreparable, transient, or reversible, disappearing when the electromagnetic field is removed or after some interval of time. Of course, even reversible effects are unacceptable if they transiently impair the ability of the individual to function properly or to perform a required task.

A critical review of studies on the biological effects of microwaves shows that many of the investigations suffer from inadequacies of either technical facilities and energy measurement skills, or insufficient control of the biological specimens and the criteria for biological change. More sophisticated conceptual approaches and more rigorous experimental design must be developed. There is a great need for systematic and quantitative comparative investigation of the biological effects, using well-controlled experiments. This should be done by using sound biomedical and biophysical approaches at the various organizational levels, from the whole animal to the subcellular level on an integrated basis, with full recognition of the multiple associated and interdependent variables.

More sophisticated assessment of the predictive value of animal testing for human responses is needed. This should be specifically directed toward comparing responses in several species to determine whether there is anything unique about a particular test animal. A systematic examination of several species is needed so that answers may be provided as to whether the use of several species is better than one in predicting human response.

It is important that research be conducted so that all aspects of the study are quantified: the type and degree of the effect, whether the effect is harmful, harmless, or merely an artifact, and how it relates to the results obtained by other investigators. For microwave bioeffects, body size of the experimental animal must be taken into account. Since body-absorption cross sections and internal heating patterns can differ widely, an investigator may think he is observing a low-level or a "nonthermal" effect in one animal because the incident power is low, while in actuality the animal may be exposed to as much absorbed power in a specific region of the body as another larger animal is with much higher incident power. In performing experimental studies on animals for extrapolation to man, interspecies scaling factors must be considered.

The question of whether reported CNS changes in man (if they are validated) would be important enough to affect human performance should be resolved. Better understanding of local, regional, and whole-body thermoregulation is required. More precise and better controlled long-term, low-level laboratory studies have been suggested. But these have to be rigidly controlled to obviate circadian rhythm and biological drift over time, which will influence responses.

Particular attention should be paid to instrumentation problems, such as developing more adequate probes for making measurements in the presence of electromagnetic fields. Essential are field strength, electrophysiological, and thermal probes that will give artifact-free readings, that will not distort the field in any way, and that will not give rise to inadvertent stimulation of the tissue due to induced currents.

Well-designed and appropriately controlled epidemiological and clinical investigations of groups of workers and others exposed to microwaves should be encouraged. Studies of workers and individuals exposed to MW/RF energies, along with appropriate control groups, should include a thorough analysis of the exposure environment, including cofactors as well as electromagnetic fields. Epidemiological study is applicable not only to disorders in which there may be a major, definable, etiological agent, but is also useful in evaluating disorders in which multiple environmental factors may interact. There is always the danger that real factors may be overlooked, leading to false associations with factors included in the study. Such interacting factors could be heat, cold, toxic agents, hypoxia, noise, other radiant energy such as X rays, chronic disease state, and/or medication (Roberts and Michaelson, 1985).

Because of the difficulties in extrapolating from animal experiments to man, epidemiological studies, including appropriate clinical and laboratory examinations, are essential to improve our understanding of possible health hazards from exposure to MW/RF energies. As noted by Silverman (1979, 1980, 1985), it is difficult to identify exposed populations, select suitable controls, and obtain exposure data. Some study groups already characterized can be improved by the acquisition of additional exposure data, some groups should be followed for longer periods, and some should be investigated for additional endpoints.

The reports from Eastern Europe of a wide variety of functional changes and possible nervous system effects have yet to be confirmed. In appropriate epidemiological studies, medical reports should be augmented to include an assessment of emotional and psychological status.

A careful search should be made for exposed groups not yet investigated or considered for study. In epidemiological studies, as in experimental or clinical work, there is rarely a single study, positive or negative, that can be accepted as definitive. Replication and validation are needed at all exposure levels (Roberts and Michaelson, 1985).

Above all, there is a need for scientific competence and integrity. It is important to maintain a proper perspective and assess realistically the biomedical effects of microwave exposure, so that the worker or the general public will not be unduly exposed, nor will research, development, and beneficial utilization of this energy be hampered or unnecessarily restricted.

REFERENCES

Roberts, N. J., Jr., and S. M. Michaelson (1985) Epidemiologic studies of human exposures to radiofrequency radiation. *Int. Arch. Environ. Health* **56**:169–178.
Silverman, C. (1979) Epidemiologic approach to the study of microwave effects. *Bull. N.Y. Acad. Med.* **55**:1166.
Silverman, C. (1980) Epidemiologic studies of microwave effects. *Proc. Inst. Electr. Electron. Eng.* **68**:78.
Silverman, C. (1985) Epidemiology of microwave radiation effects in humans. In: *Epidemiology and Quantitation of Environmental Risk in Humans from Radiation and Other Agents*. A. Castellani (ed.). Plenum Press, New York, pp. 433–458.

Index

Abortions, spontaneous, association of microwave exposure with, 294
Adaptation, as sign of physiological adjustment to thermal effects of microwave exposure, 339
Adenosarcoma
  pulmonary papillary
    dielectric data for tumor tissues in, 134
  renal tubular
    dielectric data for tumor tissues in, 134
Adrenocortical hormones, neuroendocrine effects on production and suppression of, 430–434
Adrenocorticotropic hormone (ACTH), association of stress with increased production of, 319
Age, as factor in development of cataracts in humans, 566–568, 569, 623
Agrobacterium tumefaciens, 253
Albumin, effects of microwave exposure on serum levels of, 530, 532, 533
Algesireceptors, and pain perception by skin, 546
American National Standards Institute (ANSI), 642–643, 650
Ames's Test, for detection of chemical mutagens, 250
Ampere's law, 12, 13
Anechoic chambers, design and applications for whole-body irradiation, 63–65, 66
Angle of incidence, as factor determining fate of plane waves at tissue interfaces, 138
Animal experimentation, criteria for evaluation of, 223–225
Antenna modeling theorem, 115
Antennas
  as means of distribution of electromagnetic energy, 36–45
  receiving characteristics, 43–45
Aplysia, in vitro neurological studies of, 370–371, 372

Aspergillus nidulans, 255, 256
Aspergillus niger, 248
Atherosclerosis, rabbit studies of effects of MW/RF energies on, 459

Bacillus subtilis, 247, 249
Bacteria, studies of effects of MW/RF exposure on, 245–247, 249, 250, 251, 252, 254
Basal metabolic rate (BMR)
  ratio to human specific absorption rates, 237
  and thermoregulation, 343, 353
Beeswax, electric properties at 25°C, 99
Behavior, effects of MW/RF exposure on, 413–420
Biochemical changes, association of MW/RF exposure with
  enzyme activities, 524–527
  histamine release, 530–531
  metabolism, 527–530
  serum chemistry, 531–534
Biological effects, contrasting of hazards with, 227–228
Biological literature, criteria for evaluation of
  analysis of scientific reports, 225
  animal experiments, 223–225
  evaluation of causal nature of observed associations, 228–230
  extrapolation of animal data for human applications, 230–238
Birth defects, association of microwave exposure with, 294, 625–626
Blood
  depth of electromagnetic wave penetration, in, 141
  dielectric properties of, 120–121
    temperature dependence of, 130, 131
  effects on hematopoiesis and hematology
    animal experiments, 492–505
    in vitro studies, 489–492
    observed effects in humans, 505–508

663

Blood (cont.)
    reflection coefficient at 37°C at tissue interfaces, 139
    studies of diathermic effects on histamine content of, 530–531
    studies of effects of MW/RF exposure on clinical chemistry of, 530–534
Blood–brain barrier, effects of microwave exposure on permeability of, 389–395
Blood pressure
    association of atherogenesis with elevated, 459
    association of microwave exposure with changes in, 451, 452, 453, 457, 460–461, 462, 463, 464, 466, 470, 471
Blood urea nitrogen, microwave effects on values of, 530, 531, 532, 533
Blood uric acid, effects of microwave exposure on values of, 531
Body mass, proportional relationship of mammalian metabolic activities to, 233–234
Bone growth, studies of effects of diathermy on, 306
Bone marrow, aplasia of, as consequence of microwave exposure, 501
Boundary conditions, as contributing factor in wave propagation, 14–16
Brain, role in physiologic thermal regulation, 317
Brain tissue
    dielectric properties, 122, 124, 128–129
    temperature dependence of, 130, 131
Brewster angle, 27, 141
Bryson, V., and formulation of principles of biological impedance, 4
BUN: see Blood urea nitrogen
Burns: see Skin pathology

Calcium, and neural excitation, 374
Caloreceptors, and thermal perception by skin, 542
Calorimetry, in measurement of whole body absorption, 75–76, see also Twin-well Calorimetry
Canada, microwave exposure standards in, 642, 644
Cancer, association of microwave exposure with development of, 626
Carbon dioxide, effects of microwave exposure on serum levels of, 532

Cardiovascular system
    disorders of, and heat tolerance, 341–342
    and neuroendocrine activity, 439
    studies of microwave effects on
        animal experiments, 451–460
        electronic cardiac pacemaker interference, 472–484
        observed effects on humans, 460–472
Cataracts
    among children, 573–574
    association of aging with development of, 566–568, 623
    association of diabetes with development of, 571–573
    association of radiation with development of, 571, 572–579
    classification and diagnosis, 565–566
    definitions, 563–565
    epidemiology, 568–570
    etiology, 570–574
    frequency specificities for development of, 586–587
    opacification mechanisms in development of, 568
    thermal aspects of development of, 569–592
    threshold and cumulative effects in development of, 592–595
Cats, neurological studies of, 373, 378, 382, 384
Cavities
    coupling of waveguides with, 35–36
    excitation of waves within, 35
    properties and functions, 32–35
Cell membranes, changes in permeability of, association of exposure to RF energy with, 268
    studies of the effects of MW/RF exposure on, 244
Cells, studies of hyperthermic effects of RF energy on, 269–272
Cellular differentiation, embryonic association of MW/RF exposure with inhibition of, 295
Chest pains, association with MW/RF exposure in humans, 462, 465, 466, 471
Children, development of cataracts in, 573–574
Chlorides, effects of microwave exposure on serum levels of, 532
Cholesterol, effects of RF exposure on serum levels of, 529

INDEX

Chromosome aberrations, sources of error in estimating frequency of, 263
Circular polarization of plane waves, 18
Circulation
  influence of drugs on, 249
  and thermoregulation in humans, 335, 336, 337, 343–344, 348
  and thermoregulation in mammals, 333, 339, 419
Cole, K. S., and formulation of principles of biological impedance, 4
Colony-forming ability of *Escherichia coli*, effects of RF energy on, 264
Conducting media: *see* Lossy media
Conduction, as passive thermoregulatory mechanism, 326
Conductivity, as factor influencing propagation of electromagnetic waves in tissue, 137
Convection, as passive thermoregulatory mechanism, 326
Cooling, evaporative, as passive thermoregulatory mechanism, 326
Core temperature, measurement of, 331
Corticosteroids, association of development of cataracts with, 571
Coturnix coturnix japonica: *see* Quail
Coupling of cavities to waveguides, 35–36
Crayfish, *in vitro* neurological studies of, 371
Critical angle, 28
Curtis, H. J., and formulation of principles of biological impedance, 4
Czechoslovakia, microwave exposure standards in, 641, 651

D'Arsonval, M. A., research on physiological effects of high-frequency currents, 3
Debye equations, 118, 123
Deoxyribonucleic acid: *see* DNA
Developmental stages, association of variables of tolerances to thermal energy in insects with, 275, 276
Dextran, studies of brain uptake of, 391, 392, 394
Diabetes
  as causative factor in development of cataracts, 571, 573
  and effects of RF exposure on carbohydrate metabolism, 529
Diathermy, therapeutic applications, 349–352
Dielectric constants, as factor influencing propagation of electromagnetic waves in tissue, 137

Dielectric properties
  methods of measuring
    microwave techniques, 111–117
    radiofrequency techniques, 104–111
  temperature dependence of, 102–103, 118–119
  of tissue, 120–132
  of tumors, 132–134
  of water, 117–120
Direct-contact applicators, for partial-body irradiation, 48–52
Dispersion,
  α, 93
  β, 93–94
  σ, 94
  γ, 94
  in tissue, 93–95
DNA
  studies of radiation effects on metabolism of, 241–242
  synthesis in rabbit lens epithelium following MW/RF exposure, 269
Dogs
  cardiovascular studies in, 451, 457–458, 459–460, 477
  comparative specific absorption rates, 238
  GH stress response in, 320
  hematopoietic and hematological studies of, 495–496, 501–504
  neurological studies of, 378
  pathological studies of skin of, 550–555
  studies of diathermic effects on bone growth in, 306
  studies of diathermic effects on histamine release in, 530–531
  studies of lethality of MW/RF exposure in, 346, 347
  studies of microwave effects on metabolism in, 528, 529
  studies of microwave effects on ocular lens and cataractogenesis in, 581, 590
  studies of microwave effects on reproduction, development, and growth in, 291–292, 306–307
  studies of microwave effects on serum chemistry in, 532–533
  studies of MW/RF effects on hypothalamic–hypophysial–adrenal response in, 430, 431
  studies of MW/RF effects on hypothalamic–hypophysial–thyroidal in, 436

Dogs (cont.)
  studies of neonatal subcellular changes in retinas of, 306–307
  studies of response to local MW/RF exposure in, 348
  studies of thermoregulation in, 341
Dominant lethal test, for study of mutagenic potential of microwave energy in mammals, 265
Doses and dose rates, as exposure factors used in microwave diathermy, 351
Drugs
  association of development of cataracts with, 571–572
  and circulatory function, 459

E polarizations, 26
Egg production, microwave exposure and, 287, 295
Electrode polarization, in conductivity measurements, 107
Electrolytes, microwave effects on metabolism of, 532–533
Electromagnetic energy, radiation of
  near fields, 39–43
  short dipole, 37–39
Electromagnetic interference (EMI), in electronic cardiac pacemakers, 472–484
Electro-thermia Monitor, 81
Elliptical polarization, of plane waves, 18–19
Embryonic development, animal studies of effects of MW/RF exposure on
  dogs, 306–307
  domestic fowl, 294–295
  Guinea pigs, 309
  insects, 294
  mice, 297–300
  monkeys, 307
  quails, 295–296, 297
  rabbits, 306
  rats, 301–306, 309
Endocrine system
  interrelationship with immunity, 319
  interrelationship with nervous system, 425–430
  and maintenance of homeostasis, 318, 320, 321, 425
  and thermoregulation in mammals, 334
Energy absorption
  methods of measuring, 74–83
  relationship to basal metabolic rate, 236–237
  and thermoregulation in humans, 342

Energy flux, as exposure factor utilized in microwave diathermy, 350, 351
Energy storage, and wave propagation, 16–17
Enzyme activity, association of MW/RF exposure with changes in, 524–527
Epinepherine, association of microwave exposure with increased serum levels of, 527
Epithelium, lens, studies of microwave effects on maturation of, 269
Erythrocytes, *in vitro* studies of effects of microwave irradiation on, 489–492
Escherichia coli
  genetic studies of effects of MW/RF exposure on, 246, 247, 249, 250, 251, 252, 254, 264
  studies of effects of RF energy on colony forming ability and molecular structures of B cells of, 264
  studies of inhibitory and stimulatory effects on expression of genetically regulated enzyme synthesis, 263
Estrous cycle, and radiosensitivity to microwaves, 287, 289, 297
Exencephaly, as consequence of microwave exposure, 297
Extrapolation of data from animal to human, as criterion for assessing reliability of laboratory studies, 229, 230–238
  in hazard assessment, 234
  physical variables to be considered in, 232–234
  in toxicology, 233
Eyes
  anatomy and physiology, 559–574
  spectral transmission of ocular media in, 574–575

Faraday's law, 12, 13
Fat
  depth of electromagnetic wave penetration at tissue interfaces, 240
  dielectric properties, 123, 124
  temperature dependence of, 130, 131
  reflection coefficient at 37°C in interface with bone, 139
  and thermoregulation, 343
Fertility, temperature effects on, 293–294
Fetal death, as consequence of microwave exposure, 297

INDEX

Fever
  association of fetal malformation and abortion with, 308
  as form of heat integration, 318
  role in immune response, 519
Fibroleiomyoma, vaginal, dielectric data for tumor tissues in, 134
Field strengths, as means of measuring field specific biological interactions, 48
Fluoroptic thermometers, 83–84
Fourier analysis, application to propagation of plane waves, 18
Fowl, domestic
  in vitro studies of microwave effects on brains of, 373–374, 375
  studies of effects of microwave exposure on embryonic heart rate of, 451–452
  studies of effects of microwave exposure on reproduction and development in, 291, 294–295
Free space, propagation of plane waves in, 17–20
Frequency, as factor determining fate of plane waves at tissue interfaces, 138
Frequency dependence
  as characteristic of electrical properties of biological materials, 95
  of energy absorption, 149
Frequency scaling, as method for extrapolation of animal data, 235–236
Fricke, H., and formulation of principles of biological impedance, 4
Frigidoreceptors, and thermal perception by skin, 542
Frogs
  cardiovascular studies, 452
  in vitro neurological studies of, 572
  in vivo neurological studies of, 578
  studies of skin biochemistry in, 549
Fruit fly
  studies of genetic effects resulting from microwave exposure in, 273–275
  studies of reproductive efficiency in, 287
Fungi
  effect of MW/RF exposure on, 248–249, 254
Fusarium solani, 248

Gastric mucosa, blanching of, as response to superficial heat application to gastrointestinal tract, 337

Gauss's electric law, 12, 13
Gauss's magnetic law, 12, 13
General adaptation syndrome, 428
Glass–soda borosilicate, dielectric properties at 25°C, 99
Globulins, effects of microwave exposure on serum levels of, 530, 532, 533
Glucocorticoids, association with immune response, 319
Glucose, association of microwave exposure with changes in production of, 527–529, 531, 532
Growth hormone
  impact of stress on production of, 319, 320, 428, 437–438
  neuroendocrine effects on production and suppression of, 437–438
Growth-hormone-inhibiting factor (GIF) in feedback mechanism resulting in production of ACTH and glucocorticoids, 319, 428
Growth inhibition, embryonic, and MW/RF exposure
  in domestic fowl, 295
  in mice, 297
Guinea pigs
  hematopoietic and hematological studies of, 500, 504–505
  immunological studies of, 514, 517
  neurological studies of, 381
  studies of microwave effects on enzyme activity in, 524
  studies of microwave effects on ocular lens and cataractogenesis in, 579
  studies of microwave effects on reproduction and development of, 292, 309
  studies of skin biochemistry in, 549

H polarizations, 26, 27
Hamsters
  hematological and hematopoietic studies of, 498
  neurological studies of, 385, 386
  studies of hematopoietic effects of microwaves in, 496
  studies of hyperthermic cell damage in, 270–271
  studies of microwave effects on lung cells of, 268–269
  studies of microwave effects on protein metabolism in, 529–530

Hamsters (cont.)
  studies of occurrence of chromosome aberrations in, 262
Hazard assessment, effects research and, 234
Hazards, contrasting of biological effects with, 227–228
Heart rate
  as function of internal temperature, 460
  physiological regulation of, 472–473
  studies of effects of MW/RF exposure on
    chick embryos, 451–452
    dogs, 457–458, 460
    frogs, 452
    humans, 461, 463, 464, 466, 470, 471
    Japanese quail embryos, 452
    rabbits, 454–455, 456–457, 459
    rats, 454, 459–60
Heat stroke, definition, 340
Heat tolerance, relationship to degree of development of nervous system, 275
Helic pomatia, in vitro neurological studies of, 371–372
Hemangiopericytoma, dielectric data for tumor tissue in, 134
Hematoma, splenic, dielectric data for tumor tissues in, 134
Hemorrhages, occurrence in mouse embryos exposed to microwaves, 297
Histamine release, studies of diathermic effects on, 530–531
Hober, R., contributions to research on electrical properties of tissues, 4
Hodgkin, A. L., and formulation of principles of biological impedance, 4
Hodgkin–Huxley equations, derivation from principles of biological impedance, 4
Holaday model H1 1500 survey meter, design and applications for measuring microwave radiation, 73–74
Humans
  comparative specific absorption rates, 238
  epidemiological studies, 603–631
  guides and standards for MW/RF protection of, 637–656
  hematological and hematopoietic studies of, 491, 492, 505–508
  neurological studies of, 395–399, 610–611
  problems associated with studies of cataractogenesis in, 595–597, 623
  ratio of specific absorption rate to basal metabolic rate: *see* Basal metabolic rate

Humans (cont.)
  studies of cardiovascular effects of MW/RF exposure in, 460–472, 611
  studies of cutaneous pain perception in, 547–548
  studies of cutaneous thermal perception in, 544–545
  studies of electromagnetic cardiac pacemaker interference in, 472–484
  studies of lymphoblastoid transformations in, 514
  studies of microwave effects on metabolism in, 529
  studies of microwave effects on reproduction and development in, 293–294, 623–626
  studies of neurological effects of microwave exposure in, 395–399, 610–611
  studies of ocular effects of microwave exposure in, 611–623
  studies of response to local exposure to MW/RF energies, 348, 349
  thermoregulation in, 334–338
Huxley, A. F., and formulation of principles of biological impedance, 4
Hyperthermia
  association with microwave exposure, 269–270
  in cancer therapy, 270, 352
  comparative studies of microwaves and infrared effects on development of, 349
  and inhibition of tumor growth, 517
Hypophysis: *see* Pituitary gland
Hypothalamic temperature, as stimulus for thermoregulatory behavior, 324
Hypothalamic–hypophysial–adrenal response (HHA), 425, 430–434
Hypothalamic–hypophysial–somatic response (HHS), 425, 437–438
Hypothalamic–hypophysial–thyroidal response (HHT), 425, 434–437
Hypothalamus
  and neuroendocrine maintenance of homeostasis, 318
  and production of pituitary hormones, 427, 430–438
  role in thermoregulation, 322, 419

Immune system, studies of relationship between microwave exposure and altered responses in, 513–520

INDEX 669

Insects
  studies of genetic effects of microwave exposure on, 272–277
  studies of microwave effects on reproduction and development in, 287, 294
Insulin, studies of brain uptake of, 31, 392, 394
Interfaces, reflection and transmission at, 23–26
Invertebrates
  effects of RF energy on, 272–277
Irradiation, partial-body, methods and procedures, 48–52
Isotropic instruments for measurement of power densities, 66–72

Kidney tissue, temperature coefficients of dielectric constant and conductivity, 130, 131
Kramers–Koenig relationship, 101

Lactation, association of MW/RF exposure with decreased, 294, 625–626
Larvae
  studies of effects of microwave exposure on, 273, 274, 276
  tolerance to thermal energy in, 275–276
Leiomyosarcoma, dielectric data for tumor tissues in, 134
Lens, ocular
  opacification of, in development of cataracts, 568, 571
  studies of microwave effects on
    animal experiments, 579–588
    biochemical changes, 585
    far-field exposure effects, 587–588
    maturation, 269
Lethality, of thermal stress from MW/RF exposure in
  dogs, 346, 347
  mice, 344–345
  rabbits, 346
  rats, 345, 346, 347
Lethal heat stress and enzyme inactivation, 331
Liebesny, P., and research on therapeutic applications of radiofrequency energy, 4

Linear polarization, of plane waves, 18
Lipids, effects of RF exposure on serum levels of, 529
Literature, scientific, criteria for evaluation of, 225–228
Liver tissue, dielectric properties, 124
  temperature dependence of, 130, 131
Lizards, behavioral studies of thermoregulation in, 323, 420
Lossy media, propagation of plane waves in, 20–23
Lungs
  depth of electromagnetic wave penetration in tissues of, 140
  reflection coefficient at 37°C in tissue interfaces of, 139
Lymphoblastoid transformation, association of microwave exposure with, 513–514
Lymphocytes, studies of response to microwave exposure in, 268, 497, 479, 499, 500, 501, 505, 506, 507, 515, 517–518
Lymphocytopenia, association of microwave exposure with
  in dogs, 502
  in humans, 506
Lymphopenia, association of microwave exposure with, 519
Lymphopoiesis, association of microwave exposure with increased, 517
Lysozyme levels, association of microwave exposure with decreases in, 516

Macromolecular structure, studies of effects of MW/RF exposure on, 241–244
Mammals
  studies of fetal resorption in, 303, 308, 309
  temperature regulation in, 333–334, *see also* Cats, Dogs, Guinea pigs, Humans, Mice, Monkeys, Rabbits, Rats, Sheep
Mannitol, studies of brain uptake of, 391, 392, 394
Mating behavior, and microwave exposure in mice and rats, 289
Maxwell's equations
  applications to boundary conditions between different media, 14–15
  applications to calculations involving Lossy dielectrics of low frequencies, 100
  applications to wave behavior within cavities, 32
  applications to wave propagation, 11–15

Maxwell's equations (*cont.*)
  integral forms of, 12
Meloidogyne javanica, 249
Menstrual disorders, association of microwave exposure with, 294, 624
Metabolism
  association of MW/RF exposure with changes
    in carbohydrates and lipids, 527–529
    in proteins, 529–530
  effects of thyroid hormones on, 320, 435
  and thermoregulation in animals, 438–439
  and thermoregulation in humans, 337
Metamorphosis, of insects, studies of microwave exposure effects in relation to stages of, 275–277
Mice
  comparative specific absorption rates of, 238
  immunological studies of, 514, 516, 517, 518–519
  neurological studies of, 378
  studies of chromosome translocations and mutagenesis in sperm cells of, 265–266, 267
  studies of diathermic effects on histamine release in, 530
  studies of hematological and hematopoietic effects of microwaves in, 492–495, 496–497
  studies of increased [^{35}S]methionine incorporation in spleens, thymus glands, and livers of, 263
  studies of lethality of MW/RF exposure in, 344–345
  studies of metabolic adjustment to MW/RF exposure in, 439
  studies of microwave effects on metabolism in, 529
  studies of microwave effects on ocular lens and cataractogenesis in, 588
  studies of microwave effects on reproduction, growth, and development in, 287, 288, 292, 297–300
  studies of microwave effects on serum chemistry in, 533
  studies of microwave stimulation of B lymphocytes in spleens, 265
  studies of occurrence of stimulated splenic lymphopoiesis in, 263
  studies of radiation-based changes in thermal denaturation profiles and base composition of testicular DNA in, 266–267

Microorganisms, studies of effects of MW/RF exposure on
  bacteria, viruses and fungi, 245–250
  mechanisms of microbial action, 250–256
Microstrip exposure systems, design and applications, 55–56
Microwave energy
  behavioral effects, 413–420
  biochemical effects, 523–534
  cardiovascular effects, 451–484
  cytological effects, 241–245, 269–272
  and development of hyperthermia, 349
  dosimetry, 47–88
  effects on immune system, 513–520
  effects on invertebrates, 272–277
  effects on macromolecular cell structure, 241–244
  effects on microorganisms, 245–256
  effects on reproduction, development, and growth, 287–310
  effects on skin, 539–555
  effects on unicellular organisms, 256–258
  epidemiological studies of effects of, 605–631
  factors contributing to temperature increases during exposure to, 324–327
  genetic effects, 258–269
  hematological and hematopoietic effects, 489–508
  history of research on, 1–6
  neural effects, 361–402
  neuroendocrine effects, 425–445
  ocular effects, 559–597, 611–623
  physical properties of, 11–45
  propagation and absorption in tissue media
    in complex tissue models, 171–195
    in laboratory animal models, 204–218
    in models of the human body, 177–195
    in multiple layers of tissue, 141–195
    in planar tissue structures, 138–145
    in prolate spheroidal tissue models, 160–171
    in scaled dielectric bodies, 195–204
    in spherical tissue structures, 146–160
  recommendations for future research on, 659–661
  standards for controlling exposure to, 637–656
  thermal effects of absorption of, 270–271
Miniature swine, heat tolerance experiments involving, 340
Mitochondria, studies of effects of MW/RF exposure on, 244–245

INDEX

Mitotics, association of development of cataracts with, 571, 572
Monkeys
  Rhesus
    behavioral studies of, 416
    comparative specific absorption rates of, 238
    hematological and hematopoietic studies of, 504–505
    neurological studies of, 377
    studies of microwave effects on enzyme activity in, 525–526
    studies of microwaves effects on serum chemistry of, 533
  Squirrel
    behavioral studies of, 416, 420
    studies of neonatal deaths in, 307
    studies of microwave effects on ocular lens and cataractogenesis in, 579
MRP (midbrain raphe) neurons, and thermoregulation, 338
Multimode cavities, design and application for whole-body irradiation, 62–63
Muscle tissue
  depth of electronic wave penetration in, 140
  dielectric properties, 122, 124
    comparison with dielectric properties of sarcoma tissue, 133, 134
    temperature dependence of, 130, 131
  reflection coefficient at 37°C in interfaces with skin, 139
Mutations, genetic, association of microwave exposure with increased occurrences of, 274–275, 290–291

Naphthalene, as cataractogenic agent, 572
National Institute for Occupational Safety and Health (NIOSH), 643
Nervous system
  anatomy and physiology, 361–401
  interaction of electromagnetic energy with tissues of, 366–371
  interrelationship with endocrine system, 425–430
  in vitro studies of microwave effects on, 370–376, 379
  in vivo studies of microwave effects on
    biochemical changes, 379–384
    changes in effects of drugs, 387–388
    electroencephalographic changes, 377–379
    histopathological damage, 384–387

Nervous system (*cont.*)
  and maintenance of homeostasis, 318, 320–321, 362–363, 425
  and thermoregulation in mammals, 334, 419
  and tolerance to heat resulting from microwave exposure, 275
Network analyzers, applications in permittivity measurement, 133
Neurospora, 249
Neurotransmitters, and central nervous system functions, 317
Neutrophilia, association of microwave exposure with, 519
Norepinephrine, role in development of fever, 318

Ohm's law, 367
Oldendorf technique, 392, 393, 395
Oncley, J. L., contributions to study of effect of electrical fields on biopolymers, 4
Opalina ranarum, 257
Organogenesis, and teratogenic susceptibility, 298
OSHA standard, 640
Osswald, K., and research on tissue properties, 4
Ovaries, studies of uptake of tritiated thymidine in tissues of, 264

Passive ion transport, in rabbit erythrocytes exposed to microwaves, 491
Pätzold, J., and research on therapeutic applications of radiofrequency energy, 4
Pavlov, I., and research on reflexes, integrative action of nervous system, 363, 364, 400–401
Permittivity: *see* Dielectric properties
Personnel Exposure Standards, 637–640
Phagocytic activity, association of microwave exposure with changes in, 516
Phenylthiazines, association of development of cataracts with, 571
Phosphorus, effects of microwave exposure on serum levels of, 532
Photobacterium fischeri, 252
Physarum polycephalum, studies of genetic and metabolic changes following microwave exposure of, 264
Phytohemagglutinin (PHA), 262, 515
Piersol, G. M., and research on tissue properties, 4

Pituitary gland
  and central nervous system functions, 317
  embryonic development, 427
  studies of effect of microwave exposure on gonadotropin secretion by, 289
Plane waves: *see* Waves, plane
Poland, microwave exposure standards in, 641, 644–645, 651
Polarization, as factor determining fate of plane waves at tissue interfaces, 138
  see also specific polarizations (e.g., *E, H*)
Polystyrene, foamed, electric properties at 25°C, 99
Potassium, alterations in metabolism of, association of microwave exposure with, 489–490, 532
Power density
  definition, 47
  methods and instruments for measurement of, 66–68
  of plane waves propagating through conducting media, 22
Power flow, and wave propagation, 17
Power series equations, 123
Poynting vector, 47
Prawn, *in vitro* neurological studies of, 371
Primates, GH stress response in, 320, *see also* Humans, Monkeys
Probes, for measuring permittivity, 105–106, 108, 109, 111
Product Emission Standard, 640–642
Propagation factor, for plane waves in Lossy media, 21–22
Prostaglandin E, role in development of fever, 318
Proteins, effects of microwave exposure on metabolism of, 529–530, 533–534
Pseudomonas aeruginosa, 252
Pupae, studies of effects of microwave exposure on, 266–277

Quail
  hematological studies, 499
  studies of MW/RF effects on embryonic development of, 295–297
  studies of MW/RF effects on heart rate in, 452
Quartz, fused, electrical properties at 25°C, 99

Rabbits
  behavioral studies of, 417

Rabbits (*cont.*)
  cardiovascular studies of, 451, 454–457, 459–460
  comparative specific absorption rates of, 238
  hematological and hematopoietic studies of, 490, 491, 492, 501
  immunological studies of, 514, 516
  neurological studies of, 376, 377, 378, 379, 380, 387, 388
  pathological studies of, skin of, 550
  studies of diathermic effects on histamine release in, 531
  studies of diathermic effects on offspring of, 306
  studies of effects of RF energy on enzyme activity in, 524–525, 527
  studies of erythrocytes and peritoneal granulocytes for irradiation effects in, 268
  studies of lethality of MW/RF exposure in, 346
  studies of microwave effects on maturation of lens epithelium in, 269
  studies of microwave effects on metabolism in, 527–528, 529, 530
  studies of microwave effects on ocular lens and cataractogenesis in, 579, 581–590, 591–592, 593, 595
  studies of microwave effects on reproduction and development in, 289, 306
  studies of microwave effects on serum chemistry in, 531, 532, 533
  studies of MW/RF effects on hypothalamic–hypophysial–adrenal response in, 431, 432
  studies of MW/RF effects on hypothalamic–hypophysial–throidal response in, 435
  studies of response to local exposure to MW/RF energies, 348
Radiation
  heat, as passive thermoregulatory mechanism, 326
  radiofrequency
    history of research on biological effects of, 1–6
    therapeutic use of, 3–4
Radiometry, microwave, in detection of subcutaneous tumors, 132
Rajewsky, B.
  and research on therapeutic applications of radiofrequency energy, 4
  and research on tissue properties, 4

Raman spectroscopy, in studies of effects of MW/RF exposure on cell membranes, 244

Rats
  behavioral responses contributing to thermal regulation in, 323
  behavioral studies of microwave effects in, 413–415, 416
  cardiovascular studies of, 451, 452–454, 460
  comparative specific absorption rates of, 238
  cytokinetic studies of thymidine uptake during pregnancy and effects on fetuses of, 264
  hematological and hematopoietic studies of, 497–500
  immunological studies of, 514–515, 517
  in vitro neurological studies of, 373, 375–376
  in vivo neurological studies of, 376, 377, 378, 380, 383–384, 385, 387–388, 390, 391–393
  pathological studies of skin of, 550
  studies of effects of MW/RF exposure on mitochondria in, 244
  studies of effects of MW/RF exposure on nucleic acid metabolism in, 241, 242, 243
  studies of effects of MW/RF on hypothalamic–hypophysial–adrenal response in, 431, 432, 434
  studies of effects of 2450 MHz microwaves on cellular elements in peritoneal fluid and peripheral blood of, 265
  studies of effects of uptake of tritiated thymidine in ovarian and intestinal tissues of, 264
  studies of germ cell mutagenesis and reproduction efficiency in, 267
  studies of growth hormone inhibition in, 438
  studies of lethality of MW/RF exposure in, 345, 346, 347
  studies of microwave effects on enzyme activity in, 526–527
  studies of microwave effects on hepatic tumors in, 270
  studies of microwave effects on metabolism in, 529, 530
  studies of microwave effects on reproduction and development in, 288, 289, 290, 291, 293, 294
  studies of microwave effects on serum chemistry in, 531–532
  studies of MW/RF effects on hypothalamic–hypophysial–thyroidal response in, 435, 436

Relaxation mechanism
  and frequency dependence of electrical properties of physical materials, 95
  in Lossy dielectric materials at low frequencies, 96–102
  in low-loss dielectric materials, 97–98
  in tissues, 102

Reproduction and development
  studies of effects of MW/RF exposure on, 287–310
    dogs, 291–292
    domestic fowl, 287
    Drosophila, 287
    guinea pigs, 292
    humans, 293–294, 623–626
    mice, 287, 288, 289, 292
    rabbits, 289
    rats, 288, 289, 290, 291, 293, 294

Resorptions of embryos exposed in microwaves, 297, 303, 304, 308–309

Respiration, as active thermoregulatory mechanism, 327, 419

Rhizocetonia soloni, 249

Ribonucleic acid: *see* RNA

RNA, studies of effects of radiation on metabolism of, 241, 530

Rodents: *see* Hamsters, Mice, Rats

Saccharomyces cerevisiae, 249, 251, 252, 253, 254

Salmonella typhimurium, 250

Sarcoma, dielectric properties of tissues in rats at 28° C, 133

Scaling: *see* Extrapolation

Schaefer, H.
  and research on therapeutic applications of radiofrequency energy, 4
  and research on tissue properties, 4

Schereschewsky, J. W., and introduction of ultrashortwave therapy, 3

Schliephake, E., and research applications of radiofrequency energy, 3

Schwan, H.
  and formation of principles of biological impedance, 4
  and research on therapeutic applications of radiofrequency energy, 4
  and research on tissue properties, 4

Sensors, in measurement of internal energy absorption, 79–84

Serratia marcescens, 247

Sex ratios, association of microwave exposure with alterations in, 294, 624
Sheep
  studies of microwave effects on ocular lens and cataractogenesis in, 579
  studies of relationship of diathermy irradiation to cardiac pacemaker interference in, 477
  studies of thermoregulation in, 341
Shell temperature measurement of, 331–332
Skin
  anatomy and physiology, 539–541
  biochemistry, 549
  pain perception in, 546–548
  pathology, 550–555
  and temperature regulation, 539–540
  thermal perception in, 542–546
Skin temperature, as stimulus for thermoregulatory behavior, 324
Skin tissue, dielectric properties of, 122, 123
Skull, neuroendocrine effects of localized MW/RF exposure to, 439–441
Sodium, effects of microwave exposure on serum levels of, 532
Somatostatin, and production of growth hormone, 320
Specific absorption rate (SAR)
  comparative studies of animals and humans with respect to, 238
  definition, 47–48, 238
  in establishment of MW/RF exposure standards, 650
  as exposure factor in microwave diathermy, 350–351
  factors influencing biological response to, 231
  as function of frequency for species of different sizes, 236
  and performance of direct-contact applicators for partial-body irradiation, 50, 52
  ratio to human basal metabolic rate: see Basal metabolic rate in spherical tissue models, 147–148
Sperm, association of MW/RF exposure with increased chromosome translocation in, 267
Spermatogenesis, studies of effects of microwave exposure on, 289–293, 294, 310
Staphylococcus aureus, 247
Sterility, association of microwave exposure with, 290, 293, 623–624
Stillbirths, studies of association of microwave exposure with, 308

Stray capacitance, in conductivity measurements, 108, 109
Streptococcus faecalis, 249, 250
Stress, involvement of endocrine system in response to, 319, 425, 428, 429
Sweating, as active thermoregulatory mechanism, 327, 335, 337, 419
Sweden, microwave exposure standards in, 642, 646–647

Takashima, and research on effects of electrical fields on biopolymers, 4
Teflon (polytetrafluoroethylene), dielectric properties at 25° C, 99
Temperature dependence, of dielectric properties, 102–103, 129–132
Temperature humidity index (THI), association of decreases in average lethal doses of radiation with, 297
Tenebrio molitor
  studies of effects of microwave exposure on larvae of, 276
  studies of effects of microwave exposure on pupae of, 276–277
Testes, studies of effects of microwave exposure on, 266–267, 289–293, 294
Thermal equilibrium
  behavioral responses contributing to, 322–323
  physiologic responses contributing to, 322
Thermal stress, studies of responses of homeothermic animals to, 339–344
Thermocouples, in studies of distribution of absorbed energy, 79
Thermography, applications in evaluation of SAR distribution over a surface, 84–88
Thermoreceptors, in skin, 542
Thermoregulation
  active mechanisms for, 327
  behavioral, 321, 417–420
  in birds, 327
  definitions, 321
  in humans, 328
  in mammals, 327
  and metabolic rates, 329–330
  passive mechanisms for, 326
  physiologic advantages and disadvantages of, 327–328
  physiology of, 317–321
Thymidine uptake
  studies of effects in rat ovarian and intestinal tissues, 264

INDEX

Thymidine uptake (*cont.*)
  studies of effects on rat fetuses, 264–265
Thyroid hormones
  and basal and resting metabolic rates, 320
  neuroendocrine effects on production and suppression of, 434–437
Thyrotropin-releasing hormone (TRH)
  in feedback mechanism resulting in thyroid hormone production, 319, 428, 435
  functions, 435
Time dependence, association of relaxation processes in biological materials with, 95
Tissues
  dielectric properties of, 102
  electromagnetic properties of, 93–134
  irradiation methods
    anechoic chambers, 63–65
    applicators for partial-body irradiation, 48–52
    microstrip exposure system, 55–56
    multimode cavities, 62–63
    TEM (transverse electromagnetic) chambers, 52–55
    waveguide chambers, 56–62
  studies of hyperthermic effects of RF exposure on, 269–272
  wave propagation and energy absorption in, 137–218
Toxicology, applications of extrapolation of data in, 233
Transverse electromagnetic (TEM) chambers, design and application in whole-body irradiation, 51–55
Trauma, association of development of cataracts with, 571, 574
Triglycerides, effects of microwave exposure on serum levels of, 529
Tumor tissue, dielectric properties of, 132–134
Twin-well calorimetry, applications in specific absorption, 76–79

Unicellular organisms, effects of MW/RF exposure on, 256–258
United States, microwave exposure standards in, 640, 642–643, 654, 655
U.S. Office of Naval Research, and initiation of research on effects of microwaves, 5
USSR
  approach to biology and medicine in, 399–401
  microwave exposure standards in, 640, 641, 644, 645, 649, 651, 654, 655

Vector analysis, in applications of Maxwell's equations, 13
Viruses, effects of MW/RF exposure on, 248

Water, permittivity of, 117–120
Water content, relationship to dielectric properties of tissues, 124, 125, 126, 130–131, 134
Wave equations, applications to wave propagation, 16
Waveguide chambers, design and applications in whole-body irradiation, 56–62
Waveguides
  coupling with cavities, 35–36
  field structure and operation, 28–32
Waves
  electromagnetic, refraction, 26–28
  plane
    polarization, 18–19
    propagation, 17–18, 19–28
    reflection and transmission in tissue media, 138–141
    transmission at interfaces between differing media, 24–26

Yeast, effect of MW/RF exposure on, 249, 251, 253, 254